$97.95

# EMERGENCY MEDICINE
## Self-Assessment and Review

D1733248

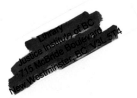

*Visit our website at* **www.mosby.com**

# EMERGENCY MEDICINE
## Self-Assessment and Review

### HAROLD THOMAS, JR., MD, FACEP
Associate Professor, Department of Emergency Medicine
Oregon Health Sciences University
Chief, Emergency Medical Services
Portland Veteran Affairs Medical Center

### ROBERT E. O'CONNOR, MD, MPH, FACEP
Program Director, Emergency Medicine Residency
Christiana Care Health System
Newark, Delaware
Clinical Associate Professor of Surgery (Emergency Medicine)
Jefferson Medical College, Thomas Jefferson University
Philadelphia, Pennsylvania

### GWEN L. HOFFMAN, MD, FACEP
Program Director, Emergency Medicine Residency
Spectrum Health–Downtown
Grand Rapids, Michigan
Associate Professor of Medicine, Michigan State University
College of Human Medicine
East Lansing, Michigan

### EARL SCHWARTZ, MD, FACEP
Chairman, Department of Emergency Medicine
Wake Forest University School of Medicine
Winston-Salem, North Carolina

**FOURTH EDITION**

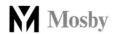 Mosby

A *Harcourt Health Sciences Company*
St. Louis   Philadelphia   London   Sydney   Toronto

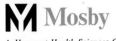

A *Harcourt Health Sciences Company*

Publisher: Laura DeYoung
Developmental Editor: Robin Sutter
Project Manager: Patricia Tannian
Project Specialist: Ann E. Rogers
Design Manager: Gail Morey Hudson
Manufacturing Manager: David Graybill

**FOURTH EDITION**

Mosby, Inc.
11830 Westline Industrial Drive
St. Louis, Missouri 63146

Library of Congress Cataloging-in-Publication Data
Emergency medicine: self-assessment and review / [edited by] Harold
    Thomas . . . [et al.]. —4th ed.
       p.    cm.
    ISBN 0-323-00538-1
    1. Emergency medicine—Examinations, questions, etc.
    [DNLM: 1. Emergencies examination questions.   2. Emergency
Medicine—methods examination questions.   WB 18.2 E533 1999]
    RC86.9.E45   1999
    616.02'5'076—dc21
    DNLM/DLC
    for Library of Congress               CIP

00   01   02   03  /  9  8  7  6  5  4  3

# CONTRIBUTORS

The authors wish to acknowledge the following emergency physicians for their contributions to this text.

Sharon C. Amaya, M.D.
M. Greg Amaya, M.D.
Shobhit Arora, M.D.
E. David Bailey, M.D.
Janice K. Balas, M.D.
Michael Baram, M.D.
Suzanne F. Beavers, M.D.
Martin A. Bennett, M.D.
Lars Blomberg, M.D.
James K. Bouzoukis, M.D.
Kevin Bristowe, M.D.
Michael D. Brown, M.D.
Patrick Brunett, M.D.
James Bryan, M.D.
Michael S. Buchsbaum, M.D.
Brian E. Burgess, M.D.
Leo W. Burns, M.D.
Scott A. Carlson, M.D.
Chih Chen, M.D.
Stephanie L. Ciccarelli, M.D.
Gregory P. Cuculino, M.D.
Sandra K. Dettmann, M.D.
Joseph B. Dore, M.D.
Denise L. Dunlap, M.D.
Eric Gallagher, M.D.
Dana A. Ger, M.D.
Angelo Grillo, M.D.
Robert D. Hagan, D.O.
Greg Harders, M.D.
Richard J. Harper, M.D.
Richard S. Hartoch, M.D.
Carol L. Henderson, M.D.
Anita H. Hodson, M.D.
Gwen L. Hoffman, M.D.
Jack Horowitz, M.D.
Brian Hoyt, M.D.
Leonardo Huertas, M.D.
David Hughes, M.D.
Neil B. Jasani, M.D.
Jeffrey S. Jones, M.D.
Norm Kalbfleisch, M.D.
Kenneth D. Katz, M.D.
Evelyn Kim, M.D.
Scott P. Krall, M.D.
Ryan M. Kramer, M.D.
Steven Kushner, M.D.
Andrew Langsam, M.D.

Warren F. Lanphear, M.D.
Craig Lauder, D.O.
Greg Ledbetter, M.D.
J. Leibovitz, M.D.
John R. Leisey, M.D.
Brian K. Lentz, M.D.
Brian J. Levine, M.D.
Bret M. Levy, M.D.
John F. Madden, M.D.
Robert T. Maroko, M.D.
Bonnie B. Matthaeus, M.D.
Dale E. McNinch, D.O.
Ross E. Megargel, D.O.
Christine Milosis, M.D.
David M. Morrison, M.D.
Usamah Mossallam, M.D.
Elizabeth A. Moy, M.D.
Christopher J. Murphy, M.D.
Sunanda Nabha, M.D.
Jason E. Nace, M.D.
Leonard A. Nitowski, M.D.
Hans Notenboom, M.D.
Bruce W. Nugent, M.D.
Robert E. O'Connor, M.D.
Brent Passarello, M.D.
Dale J. Ray, M.D.
Gordon D. Reed, M.D.
Daron P. Riley, M.D.
Robert A. Rosenbaum, M.D.
Howard Rubinstein, M.D.
Philip N. Salen, M.D.
Earl Schwartz, M.D.
Donnita M. Scott, M.D.
Michael D. Shertz, M.D.
R. Alan Shubert, M.D.
Paul R. Sierzenski, M.D.
Michael E. Silverman, M.D.
Matthew P. Sullivan, M.D.
Thomas A. Sweeney, M.D.
Harold Thomas, Jr., M.D.
James E. Thompson, M.D.
Jeffrey M. Tiongson, M.D.
Maria C. Vergara, M.D.
Tuananh Vu, M.D.
Henry E. Wang, M.D.
Barbara N. Wynn, M.D.
George R. Zlupko, M.D.

# Contents

# ANSWERS

# EMERGENCY MEDICINE
## Self-Assessment and Review

# QUESTIONS

**PART ONE   GENERAL CONCEPTS**

**SECTION 1   RESUSCITATION**

 **1  Airway Management**

*E. David Bailey and Brian E. Burgess*

Select the appropriate letter that correctly answers the question or completes the statement.

1. Which of the following is not indicative of a potentially difficult airway?
   A. Edentulousness
   B. Immobilized trauma patient
   C. Prominent upper incisors
   D. Receding mandible
   E. Short neck

2. Which of the following is *not* a requirement for rapid-sequence intubation?
   A. Emergent intubation is necessary
   B. If intubation fails, ventilation is predicted to be successful
   C. Intubation is predicted to be successful
   D. Resources are available for a rescue airway such as cricothyrotomy if both intubation and ventilation fail
   E. The patient has an empty stomach

3. Which of the following neuromuscular blocking agents has the shortest onset of action?
   A. Atracurium besylate
   B. Cisatracurium besylate
   C. Pancuronium bromide
   D. Succinylcholine
   E. Vecuronium bromide

4. Which of the following is true regarding hyperkalemia associated with succinylcholine administration?
   A. Can be severe and occurs shortly after administration in burn and trauma patients
   B. Increases in serum $K^+$ usually exceed 0.5 mEq/L
   C. Is contraindicated in renal failure patients
   D. Should be used with caution in patients with known hyperkalemia
   E. The hyperkalemia associated with succinylcholine occurs with all neuromuscular blocking agents

5. A 22-year-old male is brought to the emergency department following a motor vehicle collision. The patient has a Glasgow Coma Scale score of 6, his pulse is 120, and his blood pressure is 80/40; he has head, chest, and abdominal injuries. Which of the following is the most appropriate induction agent for rapid-sequence intubation?
   A. Etomidate
   B. Fentanyl
   C. Ketamine
   D. Midazolam
   E. Thiopental

6. Laryngoscopy is associated with a reflex sympathetic response to laryngoscopy (RSRL). Which of the following is true regarding RSRL?
   A. Decreases myocardial oxygen demand
   B. Fentanyl enhances the RSRL
   C. Is associated with a decrease in intracranial pressure
   D. Is usually not blunted by administration of beta blockers
   E. Is usually tolerated by healthy patients

7. Laryngoscopy is associated with an increase in intracranial pressure (ICP). Which of the following statements regarding the associated increase in ICP is true?
   A. Blind nasal tracheal intubation does not have the associated increase in ICP found with laryngoscopy
   B. Blind nasal tracheal intubation is easier and safer, and it carries a lower complication rate
   C. Giving a defasciculating dose of a competitive neuromuscular blocker can increase ICP
   D. Intravenous lidocaine can blunt the ICP response
   E. Succinylcholine and other neuromuscular blockers decrease ICP

8. Which of the following is *not* true of the pediatric airway?
   A. The airway is short, and care should be taken not to intubate the bronchi
   B. The epiglottis is high and firm
   C. The larynx is higher in the neck
   D. The narrowest portion of the airway is the cricoid ring
   E. The prominent occiput of the small child brings the mouth too far anterior of the larynx; visualization is aided by a slight lifting of the torso

9. Even under ideal conditions, some intubations are unsuccessful. Which of the following statements regarding the failed airway is false?
   A. Airways such as the laryngeal mask airway and esophageal obturator airway are available in the event of a failed airway
   B. Awake intubation may be accomplished by nasal tracheal intubation
   C. Care should be taken before intubation to access the airway for ease of ventilation as well as intubation
   D. Cricothyrotomy is the crucial rescue procedure when intubation and ventilation have failed
   E. In those cases when ventilation with bag mask is likely to fail, rapid-sequence intubation is the procedure of choice

10. Which of the following is *not* true regarding cricothy-rotomy?
    A. Can be done by emergency physicians trained in the procedure
    B. Is indicated when intubation and ventilation have failed
    C. Is quicker and more likely to succeed than tracheostomy
    D. Procedure in the pediatric patient is similar to that in adults
    E. Relative contraindications include coagulopathy, distorted anatomy, and infection

# 2 Mechanical Ventilation and Noninvasive Ventilatory Support

### Greg Ledbetter

Select the appropriate letter that correctly answers the question or completes the statement.

1. Which of the following is not a criterion of acute respiratory failure?
   A. Acute dyspnea
   B. $PaCO_2$ greater than 50 mm Hg
   C. Room air $PaO_2$ less than 50 mm Hg
   D. Significant respiratory alkalosis
2. The major advantage of synchronized intermittent ventilation (SIMV) is that it prevents:
   A. Decreased venous return to the heart and decreased cardiac output
   B. Nosocomial infections of the lungs and sinuses
   C. Respiratory alkalosis
   D. Stacking breaths, which can lead to barotrauma
3. Advantages of noninvasive ventilatory support versus more invasive measures include all of the following except which one?
   A. Ease of weaning
   B. Reduced risk of airway injury
   C. Reduced risk of nosocomial infection
   D. Reduced risk of pulmonary barotrauma
4. Adding positive end-expiratory pressure (PEEP) has all of the following advantages except:
   A. Decreasing intrapulmonary shunting
   B. Helping prevent atelectasis
   C. Improving respiratory acidosis
   D. Reducing oxygen requirements
5. An increase in peak inspiratory pressure (PIP) can be due to all of the following except:
   A. Airway occlusion by secretions or kinking of the endotracheal tube
   B. Air leak around an uncuffed tube in children
   C. Pneumothorax
   D. Pulmonary edema

6. In managing chronic obstructive pulmonary disease (COPD) exacerbations, which is true?
   A. Intrinsic positive end-expiratory pressure (PEEP) should be minimized by using extrinsic PEEP
   B. The I/E ratio should be 1:1 or 1:2 to maximize inspiratory time
   C. Tidal volume should be increased to maximize $CO_2$ exchange
   D. Respiratory acidosis should be corrected quickly to minimize the adverse effects on the body

# 3 Cardiopulmonary Arrest

### Kevin Bristowe and Brian Burgess

Select the appropriate letter that correctly answers the question or completes the statement.

1. Which of the following statements is true regarding the epidemiology of cardiac arrest in the United States?
   A. All patients surviving to discharge will have some degree of neurologic impairment
   B. Approximately 25% of cases are attributed to cardiovascular causes, with 75% attributed to non-cardiac causes
   C. Cardiac arrest accounts for 75% of all non-traumatic deaths
   D. Of all patients admitted to the hospital after pre-hospital cardiac arrest, less than 50% survive to discharge
   E. The pre-hospital system has no impact on survival in sudden cardiac death
2. A 59-year-old hypertensive man collapses after complaining of severe substernal chest pressure. Which of the following is the most likely etiology for his collapse?
   A. Asystole
   B. Bradysystolic cardiac arrest
   C. Pulseless electrical activity
   D. Respiratory arrest
   E. Ventricular fibrillation
3. When considering the causes of non-traumatic cardiac arrest, which of the following is most correct?
   A. Circulatory obstruction (i.e., tension pneumothorax or cardiac tamponade) initially presents as bradycardia and hypertension, which progresses to pulseless electrical activity (PEA), ventricular fibrillation (VF), or asystole
   B. Drowning is a form of asphyxia resulting in hypoxia and immediate ventricular fibrillation
   C. Hypomagnesemia is the most common metabolic cause of cardiac arrest and results in progressive widening of the QRS complex that can deteriorate into VT, VF, asystole, or PEA
   D. Hypothermia is not associated with any cardiac arrhythmias

E. Lighting injuries can produce massive direct current electrocution that can result in asystole and prolonged apnea

4. When considering the results of cardiopulmonary arrest, which of the following statements is most correct?
   A. All organ systems show evidence of damage within the first 5 minutes of cardiopulmonary arrest
   B. Beta-one and Beta-two receptors are primarily activated by endogenous catecholamines to preferentially shunt blood from nonessential vascular beds
   C. Cardiopulmonary resuscitation must produce approximately the same amount of blood flow as the pre-arrest state to provide successful resuscitation
   D. Cardiopulmonary resuscitation represents a period of globally reduced blood flow, with cardiac outputs generally less than 30% of normal
   E. The epicardium is much more sensitive than the endocardium to the ischemia of cardiac arrest

5. Ventricular fibrillation is the presenting rhythm in more than 50% of patients with pre-hospital cardiac arrest. Which of the following is the most important initial therapy in a patient with ventricular fibrillation?
   A. Cardiopulmonary resuscitation
   B. Cardioversion
   C. Defibrillation
   D. Establishment of a secure airway
   E. Intravenous access

6. When considering electrical therapy, which of the following is most correct?
   A. A precordial thump has a 10% to 25% success rate in converting pulseless ventricular tachycardia (VT) to a perfusion rhythm
   B. Precordial thump is the method of choice to convert patients with VT and a pulse to sinus rhythm
   C. The goal of cardioversion in cardiac arrest is to electrically terminate ventricular fibrillation (VF) or pulseless VT, with the hope that an organizing rhythm will result
   D. Too much current is never harmful to the heart muscle
   E. Transthoracic impedance is increased by pressing firmly on the paddles with approximately 25 pounds of force and using a coupling gel between the skin and paddles

7. When administering pharmacologic therapy, which one of the following statements is correct?
   A. Central venous access via the femoral vein is the safest and most effective form of access
   B. Drugs that can be administered via endotracheal routes are epinephrine, atropine, and lidocaine in the standard intravenous dose
   C. Intracardiac epinephrine injection is recommended and often preferred as an alternative to peripheral access
   D. Intraosseous (IO) drug infusion during CPR is effective, but IO access may be difficult in adults and is associated with delayed circulation

E. Peripheral access should be obtained only after administration of medicines via the endotracheal route

8. When considering pharmacotherapy in cardiopulmonary arrest, which of the following is correct?
   A. Atropine is effective in ventricular fibrillation (VF) because of its ability to decrease the VF threshold
   B. Bretylium is a class I antidysrhythmic neuronal blocking agent that elevates the VF threshold
   C. Lidocaine is effective in shortening action potential duration in nonischemic zones and can slow conduction and prolong refractoriness in ischemic zones
   D. Procaine in doses of 17 mg/min up to 30 mg/kg works to increase the VF threshold
   E. Sodium bicarbonate therapy is effective in countering the respiratory acidosis of cardiac arrest

9. A 79-year-old man arrives at the emergency department with the complaint of chest pain and shortness of breath. A wide complex tachycardia is noted on the monitor, and no pulse is obtainable. Which of the following is the most appropriate initial therapy for this patient?
   A. ABCs
   B. Cardioversion
   C. Defibrillation
   D. Epinephrine
   E. Lidocaine

10. When caring for the patient with cardiac arrest, which of the following is true?
    A. Establishment of an airway with appropriate end tidal $CO_2$ measurements during cardiac arrest and CPR have not been proven useful
    B. Historical information as to the nature and/or etiology of the cardiac arrest adds little information to alter treatment
    C. In evaluating and treating a patient in cardiac arrest, reestablishment of normal sinus rhythm always indicates a pulse
    D. Once cardiac arrest is established, it is not necessary to complete a thorough physical examination
    E. Restoration of normal brain function is the defining factor of successful resuscitation

# 4 ▼ Neonatal Resuscitation

*Dale J. Ray*

Select the appropriate letter that correctly answers the question or completes the statement.

1. Which of the following is the major indicator of inadequate ventilation?
   A. Color
   B. Heart rate
   C. Lethargy
   D. Respiratory rate
   E. Systolic blood pressure

2. An infant at 35 weeks' gestation has just been delivered in the emergency department. The child's temperature is 33° C. Because of this, what is most likely to develop?
   A. Apnea
   B. Decreased oxygen consumption
   C. Hyperglycemia
   D. Metabolic alkalosis
   E. Sepsis

3. A 4.5-kg boy whose mother is a diabetic is delivered in the emergency department. He is 38 weeks' gestational age and is lethargic with a blood sugar of 22. What is the most appropriate management?
   A. 4.5 ml of D10W
   B. 4.5 ml of D25W
   C. 9 ml of D25W
   D. 18 ml of D10W
   E. 45 ml of D10W

4. In the delivery room, meconium is noted in the amniotic fluid. What is the most appropriate initial treatment?
   A. Give two quick breaths, intubate, and suction
   B. Intubate as rapidly as possible and then ventilate
   C. Nasal oxygen, suction, then intubate
   D. Suction mouth and then nose as head is delivered
   E. Wipe off face then suction nose and mouth

5. Which of the following accurately describes management of neonatal resuscitation?
   A. Administer atropine for heart rate less than 50
   B. Bag and mask ventilate if heart rate is less than 100
   C. Begin chest compressions when heart rate is less than 90
   D. Give epinephrine for heart rate less than 80
   E. Hyperextend the head to intubate

6. Which of the following is appropriate in a neonate who is being adequately ventilated?
   A. Atropine for heart rate <50
   B. Dextrose 50% for Dextrostick <50
   C. Epinephrine 1:10,000 at 0.1 to 0.3 ml/kg for heart rate <80
   D. Sodium bicarbonate 8.4% at 2 mEq/kg
   E. Whole blood at 20 ml/kg

# 5 Pediatric Resuscitation

*Dale J. Ray*

Select the appropriate letter that correctly answers the question or completes the statement.

1. In the pediatric population, what is the approximate percent mortality following out-of-hospital cardiac arrest?
   A. 50 to 55
   B. 60 to 65
   C. 70 to 75
   D. 80 to 85
   E. 90 to 95

2. Advanced life support personnel bring in a 1-year-old boy in asystole. While in the field he was intubated, but attempts at peripheral venous access were unsuccessful. By what method should the emergency physician administer the resuscitation medications?
   A. Central venous line
   B. Endotracheal tube
   C. Femoral vein
   D. Intraosseous line
   E. Saphenous vein

3. In a 2-year-old girl in cardiac arrest, what is the preferred site of drug administration?
   A. Endotracheal
   B. Intracardiac
   C. Intravascular or intraosseous
   D. Oral
   E. Subcutaneous

4. Which of the following best describes the use of epinephrine in pediatric resuscitation?
   A. At large doses, the beta-adrenergic effects predominate.
   B. Data demonstrates that patients without organized cardiac activity after two rounds of epinephrine may leave the hospital alive; those without activity after four rounds do not.
   C. Drug of choice for treatment of bradycardia caused by hypoxia or ischemic insult to the heart.
   D. Not indicated in asystole.
   E. Recommended initial IV dose is 0.1 mg/kg of 1:1000 solution, one fourth of the endotracheal dose.

5. Which of the following may be exacerbated by administering glucose during resuscitation?
   A. Bradycardia
   B. Cerebral injury
   C. Hypertension
   D. Hypoxia
   E. Tachycardia

6. A 3-month-old, 4.5-kg girl, born 1 month premature, presents bradycardic. Despite pre-hospital intubation, what is the most appropriate mg dose of IV atropine?
   A. 0.04
   B. 0.08
   C. 0.12
   D. 0.40
   E. 1.00

7. Treatment with calcium is indicated for which of the following?
   A. Asystole
   B. Electromechanical dissociation
   C. Hyperkalemia
   D. Hypomagnesemia
   E. Ventricular fibrillation

8. Which of the following best describes the airway of a young child as compared with that of an adult?
   A. Inferior and posterior position of laryngeal opening.
   B. Less risk for occlusion secondary to smaller occiput.
   C. Narrowest portion of trachea is at cricoid ring.

D. Proportionately smaller head.

E. Proportionately smaller tongue.

9. What is the correct endotracheal tube size in mm for a 4-year-old?

   A. 3
   B. 3.5
   C. 4
   D. 4.5
   E. 5

10. A 4-year-old, 20-kg near-drowning victim is intubated and stabilized in the emergency department. A sudden drop in oxygen saturation is noted as well as bradycardia. Which of the following would be least appropriate?

    A. Atropine 0.2 mg IV
    B. Checking pressure from oxygen source
    C. Needle thoracostomy
    D. Reintubation
    E. Suctioning of endotracheal tube

11. In a 6-year-old girl, what is the lower limit of normal systolic blood pressure in mm Hg?

    A. 52
    B. 62
    C. 72
    D. 82
    E. 92

12. What is the most common pediatric arrest rhythm?

    A. Asystole
    B. Coarse ventricular fibrillation
    C. Electromechanical dissociation
    D. Fine ventricular fibrillation
    E. Pulseless ventricular tachycardia

13. A 5-month-old, 6-kg boy has been resuscitated successfully. He is intubated and oxygenating well, with a systolic blood pressure of 54 and pulse of 148. What is the most appropriate next step?

    A. Atropine 0.1 mg
    B. Dobutamine 5 mg/kg/minute
    C. Dopamine 5 mg/kg/minute
    D. Epinephrine 0.05 mg/kg/minute
    E. Normal saline 120 ml

14. A 10-kg child is hypotensive post-resuscitation. An epinephrine drip is desired. In order to set an epinephrine drip so that 1 ml/hr delivers 0.1 mg/kg/minute, how many milligrams of epinephrine would be added to normal saline to make a final volume of 100 ml?

    A. 0.1
    B. 0.6
    C. 1
    D. 1.6
    E. 6

# 6 Shock

*Chih Chen and Leo W. Burns*

Select the appropriate letter that correctly answers the question or completes the statement.

1. Which is the resuscitative fluid of choice for persistent hemorrhagic shock?

   A. 5% Albumin
   B. 6% Hydroxyethyl hetastarch
   C. Normal saline
   D. Packed red blood cells
   E. Ringer's lactate

2. Which of the following treatments of septic shock is appropriate?

   A. Giving colloid fluid for hypoperfusion unresponsive to crystalloid boluses
   B. Giving corticosteroids to decrease the cascade of cytokines from the systemic inflammatory response syndrome (SIRS)
   C. Providing initial volume replacement of 10-15 ml/kg of crystalloid
   D. Providing presumptive monotherapy treatment with an aminoglycoside antibiotic
   E. Supplementing the blood hematocrit to at least 50%-55% in order to increase oxygen-carrying capacity

3. Which of the following is the most effective immediate treatment of anaphylactic shock?

   A. Cimetidine 2 mg/kg IV
   B. Diphenhydramine 1 mg/kg IV
   C. Epinephrine (1:1000) 0.3 ml SQ
   D. Epinephrine (1:10,000) 1 mg IV
   E. Hydrocortisone 5 mg/kg IV

4. With regard to neurogenic shock, which of the following is true?

   A. Bradycardia is prominent in spinal cord lesion rostral to $T_1$ but is usually transient and self-limiting
   B. Bradycardia and hypotension should first be treated with oxygen and crystalloid infusion
   C. Central neurogenic hypotension results from spinal injury that stimulates vagal efferent fibers
   D. Spinal cord lesions below $T_4$ typically cause both hypotension and bradycardia
   E. Epinephrine is the preferred vasopressor agent

5. Which of the following measurements is the most sensitive indicator of hypovolemic shock?

   A. Decrease in orthostatic systolic blood pressure of 20 mm Hg
   B. Hypotension
   C. Hypoxemia
   D. Increase in orthostatic pulse rate of 20 beats/min
   E. Tachypnea

6. With regard to cardiogenic shock, which of the following is true?
   A. Amrinone is the initial inotrope of choice
   B. Intraaortic balloon pumps are contraindicated in the presence of mitral regurgitation
   C. For sedation and anxiety, benzodiazepine and morphine can be used in standard doses
   D. Tachycardia is an early signal of cardiogenic shock in an anterior MI
   E. Thrombolysis should be withheld if the patient could undergo percutaneous transluminal coronary angioplasty (PTCA) within 2 to 3 hours

7. With regard to hemorrhagic shock, which is true?
   A. An increased diastolic pressure is usually a late sign
   B. As hemorrhage worsens, the pulse pressure widens
   C. Hypotension is an early sign in children
   D. Once vascular decompensation occurs, the mortality rate approaches 50%
   E. Sympathetic nervous activation occurs early and increases heart rate, myocardial contraction, and ejection fraction

8. Tris(hydroxymethyl)-aminomethane (THAM) is a(n):
   A. Drug delivery modality using artificial lipid membrane
   B. Inotrope with combined adrenergic and dopaminergic activity
   C. Organic buffer that improves cardiac function during acidemia
   D. Potent calcium channel antagonist
   E. Potent free radical scavenger

9. Which of the following statements is true regarding magnesium administration?
   A. $Mg^{++}$ has a low volume of distribution
   B. $Mg^{++}$ potentiates the activity of $Ca^{++}$ channels
   C. $Mg^{++}$ should be used with caution in the patient with renal impairment and in cases of cyclic antidepressant overdose
   D. The empiric use of magnesium is contraindicated
   E. Total plasma concentrations of $Mg^{++}$ correlate well with the ionized concentration of $Mg^{++}$ and intracellular stores

10. During shock, which organ has the highest preserved blood flow?
    A. Brain
    B. Heart
    C. Kidneys
    D. Liver
    E. Lungs

11. A 25-year-old man is an unrestrained driver involved in a motor vehicle collision. He is unresponsive on arrival at the emergency department with the following vital signs; T, 37.1° C; HR, 110/min; RR, 10/min; BP, 80/60. Proper initial management would include which of the following?
    A. Intubation and mechanical ventilation with at least 5 cm $H_2O$ PEEP
    B. Inotropic agents given concurrently with the initial volume infusion

C. The use of 100% oxygen until the hypotension is corrected
D. Midazolam in a standard induction dosage to facilitate intubation
E. Volume infusion to a normal CVP level of 8 cm $H_2O$

12. Which of the following indicators represents effective resuscitation?
    A. Initially low end-tidal $CO_2$ that increases
    B. Lactate level that increases
    C. Mixed venous oxygen saturation that decreases
    D. Serum bicarbonate level that decreases
    E. Supplemental oxygen requirement that increases

13. Which of the following is an inappropriate reason for early intubation of a patient in shock?
    A. Decrease the work of breathing
    B. Prevent aspiration
    C. Protect the airway during transport
    D. Relieve bronchospasm of a patient in status asthmaticus
    E. Treat systemic acidosis

 7 Brain Resuscitation

*Carol L. Henderson and Leo W. Burns*

Select the appropriate letter that correctly answers the question or completes the statement.

1. The EEG initially becomes silent when the cerebral blood flow (CBF) falls below what percentage of normal?
   A. 20%
   B. 30%
   C. 40%
   D. 50%

2. A 58-year-old insulin-dependent-diabetic man is successfully resuscitated after a witnessed arrest with bystander CPR. Methods of optimizing his neurologic recovery include which of the following?
   A. Administering phenytoin to prevent anoxic seizures
   B. Allowing permissive hypercarbia as long as oxygenation is adequate
   C. Insulin administration to maintain euglycemia or even mild hypoglycemia
   D. Using vasopressors to keep his mean arterial pressure between 100 and 120 mm Hg

3. With respect to CPR and cerebral blood flow (CBF), which is true regarding neurologic recovery?
   A. CPR begun 5 minutes after circulatory arrest results in 0% CBF
   B. If CPR is started within 2 minutes of arrest, almost 50% of CBF can be achieved
   C. Standard CPR generates 40%-50% of normal cardiac output
   D. The success rate of resuscitation is proportional to the arrest duration

4. With total ischemia, the brain's concentration of ATP decreases by 90% within how many minutes?
   A. 1
   B. 2
   C. 5
   D. 10

5. When the $PaO_2$ is less than 25 mm Hg, patients usually present with which of the following conditions?
   A. Coma
   B. Difficulty with coordination
   C. Seizures
   D. Short-term memory loss

6. The effect of calcium on cerebral ischemia includes which of the following?
   A. Blocks free-radical formation by stabilizing cell membranes
   B. Increases red cell deformability and microcirculatory flow
   C. Optimizes production from oxidative phosphorylation
   D. Releases glutamate and is linked to the effects of other excitatory amino acids such as aspartate

7. A 68-year-old nursing home resident falls in the bathroom. She has an initial Glasgow Coma Scale score of 6. She is intubated in the field. A CT scan reveals a large subdural hematoma. During her work-up, her glucose is found to be 389. Optimal management includes which of the following?
   A. Aggressively hydrate the patient with normal saline solution to hasten blood sugar correction at the expense of hypervolemia
   B. Avoid lowering the blood sugar; hyperglycemia is permitted due to the stress the injury puts on the body. It will self-correct without being detrimental
   C. Hydrate the patient with normal saline and give an oral hypoglycemic agent through her nasogastric tube
   D. Put the patient on a sliding-scale insulin regimen or a continuous insulin drip if necessary to maintain euglycemia

8. Which is true about barbiturates?
   A. They act as potent free-radical scavengers to protect neuronal cell membranes from lipid peroxidation
   B. They decrease cerebral metabolism, edema formation, and intracranial pressure
   C. They block excitatory amino acid receptors thereby mitigating damage to ischemic neuronal cells
   D. They block the influx of calcium into ischemic neuronal cells to impede calcium's destructive cascade of effects

9. Which of the following treatment modalities consistently demonstrates protective cerebral effects in laboratory models following nontraumatic cardiac arrest?
   A. Corticosteroids to stabilize cell membranes as well as scavenger for free radicals generated by post-ischemic reperfusion
   B. Hypotension via vasoactive agents to decrease cerebral demand and prevent delivery of calcium to cells during reperfusion
   C. Moderate hypothermia, to 30° C, by suppressing cerebral metabolic activity thus improving the balance between oxygen supply and demand
   D. Using no PEEP during mechanical ventilation to aid cerebral venous drainage and decrease ICP

10. With regard to an ischemic insult, the ischemic penumbra is:
    A. The brain area where cells are dead
    B. The brain area where cells are functioning but will inevitably die
    C. The brain area where cells are unaffected
    D. The brain area where cells are viable but have lost function

11. A 34-year-old man is hit in the head and chest with a baseball bat. His airway is intact, and breath sounds are decreased, with wheezing on the right. His vital signs on arrival are HR, 125; BP, 90/77; RR, 44; GCS, 12; and pupils are 3 mm, reactive, and equal. During the secondary survey, his GCS deteriorates to 8 and his left pupil dilates to 6 mm and fixed. Immediate interventions include which of the following?
    A. Administer vasopressors if hydration alone cannot keep the mean arterial pressure between 90 and 100 mm Hg
    B. Give dexamethasone (Decadron) 10 mg IV prophylactically to protect neuronal cell membranes and reduce cerebral edema
    C. Hyperventilate the patient to maintain a $PaCO_2$ <25 to decrease ICP
    D. Intubate immediately, using ketamine as an induction agent to facilitate anesthesia

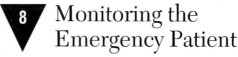

## 8 ▼ Monitoring the Emergency Patient

### David Hughes

Select the appropriate letter that correctly answers the question or completes the statement.

1. Which of the following demonstrates the most to least accurate method of measuring blood pressure, especially at the extremes?
   A. Auscultation, intraarterial catheter, oscillometric cuff
   B. Intraarterial catheter, auscultation, oscillometric cuff
   C. Intraarterial catheter, oscillometric cuff, auscultation
   D. Oscillometric cuff, intraarterial catheter, auscultation

2. If the true arterial saturation of hemoglobin is 70%, which of the following may be falsely elevated on pulse oximetry?
   A. Methemoglobinemia
   B. Carboxyhemoglobinemia
   C. Both A and B
   D. None of the above

3. End-tidal carbon dioxide detection may be affected by which of the following?
   A. Cheyne-Stokes respirations
   B. Fever
   C. Obstructive airway disease in a mechanically ventilated patient
   D. Shock
   E. All of the above

4. Which of the following does not warrant intraarterial blood pressure monitoring?
   A. Anatomic difficulties obtaining cuff pressures
   B. Frequent need for arterial blood gases
   C. Nitroprusside use
   D. Patient who is rapidly progressing to shock

# 9 ▼ Blood and Blood Component Therapy

*Jack Horowitz and Denise L. Dunlap*

Select the appropriate letter that correctly answers the question or completes the statement.

1. The majority of acute hemolytic transfusion reactions result from which of the following?
   A. A clerical error resulting in the transfusion of the wrong unit of blood to the patient
   B. Antibodies in the donor's type O serum against the recipient's A or B antigen
   C. Antigen-antibody reaction to the Rh factor
   D. Emergent use of type O blood with subsequent reaction to Kell, Kidd, and Duffy antigens
   E. Untyped transfusions of large amounts of fresh frozen plasma

2. If an intravascular hemolytic transfusion reaction is suspected, which of the following actions is appropriate?
   A. Eliminate or slow fluids at once to minimize the threat of disseminated intravascular coagulation
   B. Realize that liver failure may occur because of increased bilirubin from hemolysis
   C. Maintain urine output of at least 3 ml/kg/hr
   D. Stop the transfusion and give 80-100 mg furosemide with fluids
   E. Stop the transfusion and give mannitol to eliminate haptoglobin

3. The essential difference between a "type and crossmatch" and a "type and screen" is what?
   A. The "crossmatch" includes both ABO and Rh identification, whereas the "screen" only includes ABO grouping
   B. The "crossmatch" involves mixing donor cells with recipient serum and serves as a check on ABO group compatibility
   C. The "screen" alone is indicated in urgent blood transfusions since it can be done in less time
   D. The "screen" identifies other hemolytic antibodies that the "crossmatch" may miss
   E. The "screen" is more costly and therefore should be ordered only if transfusion is a certainty

4. A 12-year-boy with classic hemophilia arrives at the emergency department with a bleeding laceration to his leg after a fall from his bicycle. He is in no distress and has normal vital signs. The preferred treatment for this patient would be:
   A. Cryoprecipitate
   B. Factor VIII concentrate
   C. Factor IX concentrate
   D. Fresh frozen plasma
   E. Whole blood

5. Which is true of one unit of cryoprecipitate?
   A. Carries no risk of disease transmission
   B. Contains 80 units of factor VIII and 200 to 300 mg of fibrinogen
   C. Contains high proportions of all coagulation factors
   D. Is indicated in all patients who have received 5 units of packed RBCs
   E. Is of no use in hemophilia A, Von Willebrand disease, or acute disseminated intravascular coagulation

6. Which of the following cases is most suitable for autotransfusion?
   A. A 12-year-old boy with a hemothorax and a diaphragmatic rupture following a MVC
   B. A 5-year-old girl with abdominal trauma and a positive diagnostic peritoneal lavage
   C. A 78-year-old man receiving daily aspirin therapy who has a traumatic hemothorax
   D. A patient with COPD and pneumonia who has a hemothorax following a bleb rupture
   E. A spontaneous hemothorax in a patient with metastatic lung cancer

7. Using standard storage techniques, the storage life of whole blood is about how long?
   A. 2-6 days
   B. 8-15 days
   C. 20-40 days
   D. 60-80 days
   E. 80-120 days

8. Which of the following is a true statement?
   A. Blood banks routinely screen blood for CMV and EBV
   B. Cryoprecipitate is an acceptable treatment for a hemorrhaging patient with hemophilia A when factor VIII is not available
   C. Spontaneous bleeding is common in patients with platelet counts of 40,000-80,000
   D. The most common posttransfusion infection is hepatitis B

9. Which of the following statements regarding immune globulin is true?
   A. It can provide passive immunization against diseases such as rabies, tetanus, and hepatitis B
   B. It is a form of active immunization that promotes life-long immunity from a particular disease
   C. It should be given to all Rh-positive women after miscarriage, abortion, or severe antepartum hemorrhage
   D. Patients who are bitten by a potentially rabid animal require the rabies human diploid cell vaccine alone since the immune globulin will not help acutely
   E. Tetanus hyperimmune globulin is indicated in very dirty, contaminated wounds regardless of prior immunizations

10. Which of the following is a potential complication of multiple unit red blood cell transfusions?
    A. A reactive thrombocytosis secondary to coagulation activation
    B. Hypercalcemia secondary to citrate toxicity
    C. Hypermagnesemia causing dysrhythmias
    D. Hypothermia
    E. Shortening of the QT segment on an ECG

## SECTION 2  PRACTICE OF EMERGENCY MEDICINE

### 10 Approach to the Patient in the Emergency Department

*No questions*

### 11 Clinical Decision Making and "Best Practice" Systems

*No questions*

### 12 Geriatrics: Unique Concerns

*Norm Kalbfleisch*

Select the appropriate letter that correctly answers the question or completes the statement.

1. Which of the following statements regarding the elderly is false?
   A. Emergency providers order more than 45% more ancillary tests for their elderly patients than for their younger patients given an identical presenting complaint
   B. The elderly make up 13% of the population yet account for more than 45% of intensive care admissions
   C. The percentage of elderly in the population will nearly double in the next 30 years
   D. The elderly make up 13% of the population yet account for more than 25% of ED visits
   E. The elderly make up 13% of the population yet account for more than 35% of ambulance transports

2. Physiologic changes and laboratory values attributable to the normal effects of aging include which of the following?
   A. Mild to moderate normocytic anemia
   B. Mild renal insufficiency
   C. Q waves, particularly in an inferior distribution on an ECG
   D. All of the above
   E. None of the above

3. Regarding myocardial infarction or unstable angina in the elderly, which of the following statements is true?
   A. Atypical presentations of AMI occur more frequently in elderly men than women of the same age
   B. Confusion without chest pain or shortness of breath may be the initial presenting sign of elderly patients with acute myocardial infarction
   C. The majority (>50%) of patients age 85 or older have chest pain as part of their initial presentation of acute myocardial infarction
   D. All of the above
   E. None of the above

4. Which of the following statements is true regarding the elderly with trauma?
   A. Falls experienced by the elderly result in less mortality and morbidity when compared to falls experienced by middle-aged patients
   B. Elderly patients should typically be admitted to an intensive care unit if they have a significant mechanism of injury, except when their vital signs remain within normal limits in the ED
   C. Head trauma without focal neurologic findings is associated with intracranial hemorrhage less commonly in the elderly as compared with middle-aged patients
   D. The elderly can tolerate brief periods of hypovolemic shock if promptly and aggressively resuscitated
   E. The elderly patient with multiple rib fractures should be considered for admission

**13** ## Approach to the Immunocompromised Patient in the Emergency Department

*Lars Blomberg*

Select the appropriate letter that correctly answers the question or completes the statement.

1. Which of the following statements concerning humoral immunity is incorrect?
    A. IgG and IgM, when in contact with an antigen, activate the alternative complement pathway
    B. Inappropriate B cell antibodies are thought to be responsible for autoimmune processes
    C. Opsonization is important in defense against infection with *S. pneumoniae* and *H. influenzae*
    D. Secretory IgA is the predominant Ig present in GI fluids
2. A 50-year-old man who has undergone autologous bone marrow transplantation following treatment for non-Hodgkin's lymphoma presents with increasing shortness of breath and a chest x-ray consistent with interstitial pneumonitis. The most likely etiologic pathogen is:
    A. Aspergilloses
    B. Cytomegalovirus
    C. *P. carinii*
    D. *S. pneumoniae*
3. Disseminated toxoplasmosis is a significant risk in which of the following transplant patients?
    A. Bone marrow
    B. Heart
    C. Kidney
    D. Liver
4. All of the following commonly prescribed drugs raise cyclosporin levels except which one?
    A. Diltiazem
    B. Erythromycin
    C. Ketoconazole
    D. Rifampin
5. Which of the following antibiotics is not recommended for empiric treatment of the neutropenic cancer patient?
    A. Ceftazidime
    B. Ciprofloxacin
    C. Imipenem
    D. Ticarcillin/clavulanate
6. A 53-year-old female with end-stage renal disease on hemodialysis presents to the ED with general malaise and a temperature of 102° F. What is the most likely bacterial pathogen?
    A. *E. coli*
    B. *H. influenzae*
    C. *S. aureus*
    D. *S. pneumoniae*
7. A 32-year-old male with sickle cell disease and functional asplenia presents in septic shock, with disseminated intravascular coagulation, purpura, and multiple organ dysfunction. All of the following are likely pathologic organisms except which one?
    A. *H. influenzae*
    B. *N. meningitidis*
    C. *S. aureus*
    D. *S. pneumoniae*

 **14** ## Emergency Ultrasound

*Patrick Brunett*

Select the appropriate letter that correctly answers the question or completes the statement.

1. Which of the following characterizes acoustically dense structures such as gallstones?
    A. Bright or dark depending on calcium content
    B. High impedance, appear dark
    C. High reflectivity, appear bright
    D. Low reflectivity, appear bright
    E. Low impedance, appear dark
2. The 3.5 MHz probe is best suited for which application?
    A. Abdominal aorta
    B. Foreign bodies
    C. Testicles
    D. Uterus
    E. Vasculature of the neck
3. Diagnostic prenatal ultrasound has been associated with which of the following adverse effects in humans?
    A. Diminished school performance
    B. Increased childhood cancers
    C. Microcavitation if pulsed sound waves are used
    D. Speech delay
    E. There are no adverse effects associated with prenatal ultrasound
4. A hyperdynamic myocardium in the setting of pulseless electrical activity (PEA) signifies which of the following?
    A. Hyperkalemia
    B. Hypothermia
    C. Hypovolemia
    D. Massive myocardial infarction
    E. Pulmonary embolism
5. Which of the following is the most reliable bedside ultrasound finding in traumatic pericardial tamponade?
    A. Diastolic collapse of the right atrium
    B. Diastolic collapse of the right ventricle
    C. Failure of inferior vena cava collapse with inspiration
    D. Fluid in the pericardial sac
    E. Myocardial rupture

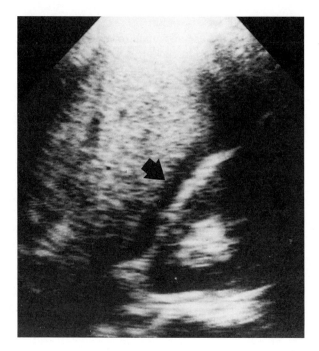

FIG. 14-1

6. A 46-year-old male is the unrestrained driver in a motor vehicle collision. An emergency abdominal ultrasound of the right upper quadrant is performed, with the accompanying image obtained. Which of the following statements is true?
   A. The patient needs immediate laparotomy
   B. There is at least 2000 cc of fluid in the abdomen
   C. This is a more specific test than CT scan
   D. This is a more sensitive test than diagnostic peritoneal lavage
   E. The patient may have preexisting ascites

7. A 42-year-old female patient reports right upper quadrant pain and vomiting after a fatty meal. An emergency physician performs ultrasound examination of the right upper quadrant to detect which of the following?
   A. Cholelithiasis
   B. Dilated common bile duct
   C. Pericolic fluid
   D. Sludge
   E. Thickened gall bladder wall

8. Which of the following may cause a false negative ultrasound study for hydroureter?
   A. Bowel gas
   B. Dehydration
   C. Obesity
   D. Staghorn calculi
   E. All of the above

9. A 63-year-old male presents with left flank pain radiating to the left groin. Urinalysis is positive for blood. A plain abdominal film is negative for ureteral stones. What is the next step in management of this patient?

   A. Contrast computed tomography
   B. Emergency ultrasound for detection of ureteral stone
   C. Emergency ultrasound for detection of hydroureter
   D. Intravenous pyelogram
   E. Urologic consultation

10. What is/are the indication(s) for immediate surgical intervention in a 70-year-old male patient with an abdominal aortic aneurysm (AAA) detected on ultrasound?
    A. Abdominal pain
    B. AAA greater than 3.0 cm and abdominal pain
    C. AAA size greater than 3.0 cm in caliber
    D. Hemodynamic instability and abdominal pain
    E. The presence of Murphy's sign on ultrasound examination

11. What level of β-human chorionic gonadotropin (β-hCG) is required to detect an intrauterine pregnancy using transabdominal ultrasound?
    A. 600
    B. 1000
    C. 1800
    D. 3000
    E. 6500

12. What advantage does transvaginal ultrasound have over transabdominal ultrasound for obstetric examination?
    A. Provides a wider and deeper view
    B. Uses the commonly available 3.5 MHz probe
    C. Provides easier spatial orientation with minimal training
    D. Detects intrauterine pregnancy at earlier gestation ages
    E. Not as reliable in detecting cornual pregnancy

13. What is the goal of bedside ultrasound performed by emergency physicians?
    A. Decrease patient exposure to ionizing radiation
    B. Expedite definitive treatment
    C. Provide definitive diagnosis
    D. Reduce adverse reactions to intravenous contrast dye
    E. Replace formal ultrasound studies

 **15** Life and Death

*No questions*

 **16** Bioethics

*No questions*

# 17 Approach to Administration in the Emergency Department

*No questions*

# 18 Legal Issues in Emergency Medicine

*No questions*

# 19 Clinical Forensic Medicine

*No questions*

# 20 The Medical Literature: A Reader's Guide

*No questions*

**SECTION 3   ANESTHESIA AND PAIN MANAGEMENT**

# 21 Pain Management

*Ryan M. Kramer and Denise L. Dunlap*

Select the appropriate letter that correctly answers the question or completes the statement.

1. Meperidine (Demerol) and morphine, both opioid agonists, provide similar degrees of pain relief when administered in equianalgesic doses. What is the advantage of using morphine?
    A. Less CNS toxicity as evidenced by a lower incidence of seizures, hallucinations, and psychosis
    B. Less potential for abuse
    C. Less respiratory depression
    D. Requires lower doses of naloxone to reverse hypotension caused by decreased peripheral vascular resistance
2. A 35-year-old male currently being treated with an albuterol inhaler and prednisone for asthma presents with an anterior shoulder dislocation. Why is fentanyl (Sublimaze) the preferred opioid analgesic?

    A. It can be given by mouth
    B. It does not cause histamine release
    C. It does not produce chest wall muscle rigidity that may interfere with ventilation
    D. Its short duration of action minimizes the risk of respiratory depression
3. Pentazocine (Talwin) is a potent opioid agonist-antagonist analgesic. What characteristic of this drug has limited its clinical usefulness?
    A. It can precipitate biliary tract spasm
    B. It has increased risk of abuse
    C. It presents a risk of respiratory depression equal to that of opioid agonists
    D. It produces visual or auditory hallucinations, disorientation, dysphoria, and feelings of depersonalization in a small percentage of patients
4. Inhaled nitrous oxide is safe and effective in the emergency department. Which of the following statements regarding nitrous oxide is true?
    A. It can be administered to patients with altered level of consciousness or head injury
    B. It may be self-administered, so the patient controls the level of analgesia
    C. Scavenging devices are not necessary, because nitrous oxide levels in the patient are at low levels
    D. The nitrous oxide/oxygen ratio does not have to be adjusted for altitude; hence it may have aeromedical applications
5. A patient arrives with a facial laceration requiring suture repair, but he reports an allergy to lidocaine. Which local anesthetic can be used?
    A. Bupivacaine
    B. Etidocaine
    C. Mepivacaine
    D. Procaine
6. A 10-year-old (30 kilogram) boy presents with multiple facial lacerations after a motor vehicle crash. What is the maximum safe dose of 1% lidocaine with epinephrine that can be used as a local anesthetic for repair of his wounds?
    A. 2.1 mL
    B. 21 mL
    C. 210 mL
    D. 2100 mL

# 22 Sedation and Analgesia for Procedures

*Brian J. Levine and Angelo Grillo*

Select the appropriate letter that correctly answers the question or completes the statement.

1. What is believed to be most responsible for muscular and glottic rigidity associated with fentanyl (Sublimaze) use?

A. Concurrent benzodiazepine administration
B. Excessive dosing (50-100 μg/kg)
C. Histamine release
D. Intramuscular injection

2. A patient received fentanyl and midazolam intravenously before incision and drainage of a perianal abscess. Why should observation and pulse oximetry be continued after completion of the procedure?
   A. Midazolam is lipophilic, and a late release of drug from fat stores may occur
   B. Respiratory depression may increase in the absence of painful stimuli
   C. The effective half-life of fentanyl is prolonged when co-administered with midazolam
   D. There is a risk of a delayed hypersensitivity reaction

3. What is the major advantage of nitrous oxide use in the emergency department?
   A. Can be used at high altitudes without dose adjustment
   B. Hypoxia is not a concern at concentrations of 70%-80%
   C. It is a very effective analgesic while having minimal sedating and anxiolytic effects
   D. It may be self-administered, so the patient controls the level of analgesia

4. A 27-year-old male has just undergone a closed shoulder reduction for a glenohumeral dislocation. Multiple doses of meperidine (Demerol) were used for conscious sedation. It has been 10 minutes since reduction, and the patient's oxygen saturation falls to 86% despite oxygen via nasal cannula. What should the next step be?
   A. Apply a 100% non-rebreather mask and observe
   B. Intubate with neuromuscular blockade
   C. Prepare for positive pressure ventilation, administer small (0.1 mg) doses of naloxone until the patient responds and observe
   D. Prepare for positive pressure ventilation, administer small (0.2 mg) doses of flumazenil until the patient responds and observe

5. Ketamine is a dissociative anesthetic characterized by deep analgesia and amnesia. Clinical usefulness is limited, however, by which of the following side effects?
   A. Cardiovascular instability, including hypotension and paradoxical bradycardia
   B. Dreams and hallucinations on awakening from anesthesia
   C. Increased incidence of bronchospasm
   D. Loss of airway reflexes

6. Which of the following regarding flumazenil is true?
   A. Can be used in a patient with polypharmacy overdose to reverse respiratory depression
   B. Its effectiveness decreases the need for monitoring for respiratory depression
   C. May precipitate withdrawal in patients who have received repeated doses of benzodiazepines
   D. Since it competitively binds GABA-benzodiazepine receptors in the CNS, resedation is rare

7. Patients can be safely discharged after conscious sedation when they meet which of the following criteria?
   A. The patient can understand and follow directions, speak clearly, and walk without assistance
   B. The patient has been completely reversed with naloxone and is immediately awake and alert and follows commands
   C. The patient states he or she feels in safe condition to leave
   D. The patient will have someone at home to watch him or her

8. What is the most important consideration regarding conscious sedation in children?
   A. Benzodiazepines should not be used since they usually cause paradoxical hyperactivity
   B. Fentanyl should be combined with a benzodiazepine since respiratory depression is decreased
   C. The agents have different pharmacokinetics in children, and age-dependent responses may vary
   D. With a variety in the routes of administration (IV, IM, nasal, oral, rectal), fentanyl is ideal

---

**SECTION 4 | EMS**

---

## 23 ▼ EMS: Overview and Ground Transport

*Daron P. Riley and Angelo Grillo*

Select the appropriate letter that correctly answers the question or completes the statement.

1. Which of the following is true regarding EMS communications?
   A. 911 Service was introduced in 1973 and has been adopted nationwide
   B. About 35% of all EMS calls are considered to be potentially life threatening or critical
   C. New studies have shown that emergency medical dispatchers are unable to identify patients as being pulseless and apneic when speaking to callers
   D. A priority-based dispatch system has been proven to be more financially efficient at allocating resources than a criteria-based dispatch service
   E. Systems status management has been shown to be beneficial when used in all EMS systems regardless of population served or resources available

2. Which of the following is true regarding indirect or off-line medical control?

A. Deviations from a specified protocol usually indicate a problem with the individual EMT

B. Ensuring access to critical incidence stress debriefing following emotionally traumatic events is an important responsibility of the off-line medical director

C. Off-line medical control includes reference to retrospective patient care review between a receiving physician and EMT once the patient has reached the ED

D. The use of standing orders for trauma patients has dramatically reduced scene times

3. Which of the following medicolegal situations best illustrates competency with on-line medical command?

A. A 20-year-old male was involved in a motor vehicle crash head on with a brick wall. He appears intoxicated, and his girlfriend states that they had an argument earlier in the day and he stated he was going to kill himself. He denies any suicidal ideation now and states he ran off the road. He is alert and oriented and is refusing care. On-line medical direction allows release to the local police station for outstanding traffic violations and DUI offense.

B. A 30-year-old male is thrown from his car and is noted to be comatose and hypotensive. A pediatric intensive care physician is on scene requesting to insert a subclavian line. The on-line physician instructs medics to intubate, hyperventilate, and allow him to proceed with the procedure.

C. A 40-year-old diabetic woman on oral hypoglycemic agents was found unresponsive by family members. On medic arrival, fingerstick glucose was 20 and intravenous glucose revived the patient, but she is still mildly confused. The patient's family is refusing transport to the hospital. The on-line physician states that the family can observe and feed the patient and may not transport.

D. A 50-year-old male is being transported with chest pain. A 12-lead ECG performed by medics reveals ST elevation in the anterior leads. The closest hospital with catheterization facilities is on divert to critical patients, but the patient is receiving Coumadin for recent DVT and had a CVA 3 months ago. The on-line physician commands medics to proceed to the diverting hospital regardless.

E. A 90-year-old male with h/o prostate cancer is found in a neighbor's yard pulseless and apneic. The neighbors are performing CPR when medics arrive. The patient's son states he is a DNR but no papers are available and the wife is not at home. The on-line physician requests to abort resuscitative efforts.

4. Which of the following is correct about the levels of EMS provider recognized by the United States Department of Transportation/National Highway Traffic Safety Administration (DOT-NHTSA)?

A. A first responder (FR), usually a police officer or firefighter, is a non-transport provider who is skilled in basic life support and possibly automatic external defibrillation (AED) operation who receives didactic instructions and serves a clinical rotation for certification

B. Emergency medical technician–basic (EMT–B) has increased survival in out-of-hospital cardiac arrest through the adoption of endotracheal intubation

C. Emergency medical technician–intermediate (EMT–I) is especially suited for inner-city communities by providing advanced skills and procedures (e.g., Combitube) with less educational time expenditure

D. Emergency medical technician–paramedic (EMT–P) scope of practice includes defibrillation, endotracheal intubation, and administration of many scientifically proven acute life support medications

E. Emergency medical technician–paramedic (EMT–P) training requires between 700 and 1100 hours of didactic and clinical field training in order to incorporate procedures such as transthoracic pacing, needle cricothyrotomy, and needle decompression of tension pneumothorax

5. Which statement about EMS system design is most correct?

A. Basic life support crews should be skilled in spinal immobilization, fracture splinting, assisting childbirth, performing CPR, establishing intravenous, access, and hemorrhage control

B. Hospital-based EMS systems are the most prevalent, with EMTs participating in ED patient care when not responding to calls

C. Most public EMS systems are incorporated as subdivisions of the municipal fire service

D. Multi-tiered systems are most appropriate for rural and suburban areas

E. The EMS governing council is responsible for licensing and certifying EMS providers, establishing standards of practice, and investigating all patient care or systems complaints

6. A 22-year-old female who is pregnant presents to the ED complaining of labor pains and states that her "water broke." There are no obstetric capabilities at this hospital, and the patient needs to be transferred. Which of the following meets COBRA regulations?

A. A hospital-based ambulance crew is instructed to "scoop and run" with this patient to the nearest hospital with obstetric capabilities

B. After the accepting hospital is notified, the patient is transported with a nurse and obstetric supplies

C. The emergency physician examines the patient and gives strict instructions to the patient's husband to proceed directly to the accepting hospital

D. The patient is interviewed by a nurse who agrees that the patient is in labor and arrangements are made for transfer

E. The patient is found to be fully dilated, and the accepting hospital is 30 minutes away. The transfer arrangements are completed

**24** Disaster Preparedness
and Response

*Philip N. Salen and Anita H. Hodson*

Select the appropriate letter that correctly answers the question or completes the statement.

1. Which one of the following clinical scenarios best typifies a medical disaster?
   A. A bomb blast in a building resulting in more than 1000 casualties in a large city
   B. A fire at a suburban office building resulting in dozens of casualties
   C. A multiple vehicle accident several miles from a small rural community results in 6 critical patients and 12 minor patients
   D. A plane crash occurs on the outskirts of a mid-sized city resulting in close to 100 casualties
   E. All of the above

2. In multiple-casualty triage, rescue personnel often use a simple triage and rapid-treatment technique for initial patient triage that depends on a quick assessment of what?
   A. Patients' ability to survive current injuries
   B. Age and current injuries of patients
   C. Age and medical history of patients
   D. Patients' airway status and Glasgow coma scale
   E. Patients' respirations, perfusion, and mental status

3. What is the only patient care intervention provided during the process of triage of mass casualty situations?
   A. C-spine immobilization of patients with possible neck injuries
   B. Cardiopulmonary resuscitation of witnessed deaths
   C. Opening of obstructed airways and direct pressure on obvious external hemorrhage
   D. Pain control that can be done as part of the triage process
   E. Rapid procedures, such as splinting of fractures, that can be done quickly in the field

4. The following patients in a multi-patient disaster scenario should be triaged into which order of treatment (choices are below)?
   (1) 40-year-old confused male with third-degree burn wounds to 60% of BSA
   (2) 25-year-old paramedic with a fractured right arm and second-degree burn wounds to 5% of BSA
   (3) 8-year-old girl with no spontaneous respirations, no pulse, and third-degree burn wounds to 20% of her body
   (4) 20-year-old male with third-degree burn wounds to 30% of BSA
   (5) 70-year-old female with first- and second-degree burn wounds to 10% of BSA and chest pain
   A. 1, 3, 5, 4, 2
   B. 1, 5, 3, 2, 4
   C. 1, 5, 4, 2, 3
   D. 3, 1, 5, 4, 2
   E. 3, 5, 1, 4, 2

5. Which statement best characterizes the incident commander at a disaster scene?
   A. Has overall management responsibility for the incident
   B. Has responsibility for non-medical aspects of disaster scenes
   C. Is expected to handle public information, safety, and inter-agency issues
   D. Is expected to make final decisions on key triage issues
   E. Should be the most experienced physician on hand

6. Which one of the following statements best characterizes an internal disaster?
   A. An event occurring in the community in an indoor setting that results in a sudden influx of patients requiring emergency care
   B. Any event occurring in the community that results in a sudden influx of patients requiring emergency care
   C. An event that disrupts daily routine community functions
   D. An event that disrupts daily routine hospital functions and occurs within the confines of the hospital
   E. An event that disrupts daily routine hospital functions

7. Basic components of a hospital disaster plan must include which of the following?
   A. A roster of all critical positions and personnel and a reliable method for their mobilization
   B. An interdepartmental planning group that is responsible for disaster assessment and planning
   C. Contingency plans to compensate for lost resources
   D. Redundant communication systems
   E. All of the above

8. Disasters involving toxic substances pose special challenges for caregivers. Which of the following statements regarding toxic disasters are most accurate (choices are below)?
   (1) Effective decontamination of victims and the need for effective safety measures on the part of rescue personnel are important in preventing secondary contamination
   (2) Critically ill contaminated patients who need immediate lifesaving procedures should bypass immediate decontamination and go straight to regular patient areas
   (3) Contaminated patients should be brought to a predesignated decontamination site containing a warm-water shower with a container to hold drainage water
   (4) Air intake vents in rooms in which there are contaminated patients should be opened so that caregivers are not put at risk by toxic fumes
   A. 1, 2, and 3
   B. 2, 3, and 4
   C. 1 and 3
   D. 1 only
   E. 2 and 4

9. What is the goal of critical incident stress debriefing (CISD) for emergency caregivers after providing care in a disaster situation?
   A. CISD allows all the participants involved in the disaster to review any negative outcomes in a private setting
   B. CISD allows the incident commander and his or her liaisons to review quality control issues in order to improve planning and hospital response
   C. CISD is a forum for review of the disaster situation in order to determine how to provide more effective care
   D. The purpose of CISD is to assist the caregiver in regaining emotional control by facilitating ventilation of feelings and reactions through listening and support
   E. All of the above

10. Which of the following statements best characterizes the Federal Emergency Management Agency (FEMA)?
    A. FEMA's primary goal is to provide the medical response element that will bring organized aid to disaster-affected areas, set up an evacuation system, and put into effect a network of precommitted hospital beds throughout the United States
    B. FEMA has no specific funding for particular emergencies and disasters and must petition the federal government for funding when crises arise
    C. FEMA intervenes with state and local organizations' preparation for and response to emergencies when petitioned by state and local government
    D. FEMA is the federal government's focus for emergency preparedness and response in the United States and has a responsibility that encompasses the entire spectrum of disasters and emergencies
    E. All of the above

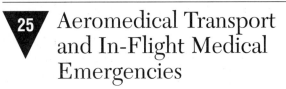

# ▼ 25 Aeromedical Transport and In-Flight Medical Emergencies

### *Matthew P. Sullivan and Anita H. Hodson*

Select the appropriate letter that correctly answers the question or completes the statement.

1. Transportation of a trauma patient stabilized in an outlying emergency department to a higher level facility constitutes which level of aeromedical response?
   A. Primary
   B. Quaternary
   C. Secondary
   D. Tertiary

2. Boyle's law, as it applies to altitudes, states what?
   A. As altitude decreases and atmospheric pressure increases, air expands and volume increases
   B. As altitude increases and atmospheric pressure decreases, air contracts and volume decreases
   C. As altitude increases and atmospheric pressure decreases, air expands and volume increases
   D. As altitude increases and atmospheric pressure decreases, air remains constant in volume

3. At altitude, the molecules that compose air are farther apart and there are fewer oxygen molecules per unit area. The normal physiologic response is best characterized by which one of the following?
   A. Increased cardiac stroke volume and increased tidal volume
   B. Increased cardiac stroke volume and tachypnea
   C. Tachycardia and increased tidal volume
   D. Tachycardia and tachypnea

4. What is the relationship between altitude and temperature as predicted by Charles' law and increasing altitude?
   A. Decreases temperature
   B. Does not affect temperature
   C. Has a variable effect on temperature
   D. Increases the temperature

5. During ascent to flight altitude, which of the following consequences may be predicted by Boyle's law?
   A. Air leak around cuffed endotracheal tubes
   B. Artificial compartment syndrome related to air splints
   C. Artificial decrease in the rate of intravenous infusion
   D. Inadequate pressure support provided by the pneumatic antishock garment

6. Aeromedical transport is contraindicated in all of the following patients except which one?
   A. Patients at risk of childbirth in flight
   B. Patients in full cardiac arrest before transport
   C. Patients prone to psychotic or violent behavior
   D. Patients suffering from decompression sickness

7. In a commercial aircraft, cabin pressure at cruising altitude will approximate pressures at what altitude?
   A. 1000 to 4000 feet
   B. 5000 to 8000 feet
   C. 9000 to 12,000 feet
   D. Sea level

8. The Federal Aviation Administration (FAA) establishes standards for medical equipment aboard U.S. commercial aircraft. Which of the following is required by law?
   A. Defibrillator
   B. Dextrose injection
   C. Laryngoscope
   D. Lidocaine injection

9. All of the following are contraindications to commercial flight except which one?
   A. Anemia (hemoglobin <8.5mg/dL)
   B. Contagious disease
   C. Immobility
   D. Pregnancy <36 weeks' gestation

# 26 ▼ Multiple Trauma

*Jeffrey M. Tiongson and Neil B. Jasani*

Select the appropriate letter that correctly answers the question or completes the statement.

1. A 70-kg male has sustained a large scalp laceration. Witnesses reported massive blood loss. His pulse is 114 beats/min, respiratory rate is 22, BP is 124/93, and capillary refill is 1-2 seconds. What is the most accurate assessment of his degree of hemorrhage?
   A. Class I, up to 15% of blood volume
   B. Class II, 15%-30% of blood volume
   C. Class III, 30%-40% of blood volume
   D. Class IV, >40% of blood volume

2. A 6-year-old girl is treated for injuries sustained after falling off her bicycle. The handlebars struck her across the abdomen, and she is now complaining of diffuse abdominal pain. Vitals are HR, 110; RR, 24; BP, 110/73; pulse oximetry, 99%; and she has good capillary refill. Which of the following injuries is most likely?
   A. Duodenal hematoma
   B. Lumbar vertebral compression fracture
   C. Pericardial tamponade
   D. Splenic rupture

3. The creation of trauma centers and trauma designations has had a significant impact on the practice of emergency medicine. Which is most true regarding the impact of trauma centers?
   A. All 50 states now have level I trauma centers
   B. Pre-hospital care has been dramatically decreased, thus reducing arrival times to receive definitive care
   C. The care of a trauma patient begins on arrival at the trauma center
   D. Trauma centers dramatically reduce the incidence of preventable death from trauma

4. A 41-year-old man ingested LSD and then jumped off of a four-story building. He landed on his feet. After initial management of the ABCs, what subsequent radiographic evaluation is most appropriate?
   A. C-spine, chest
   B. C-spine, chest, pelvis
   C. C-spine, chest, pelvis, thoracolumbar spine
   D. C-spine, chest, thoracolumbar spine, pelvis

5. A 25-year-old man is injured in a motor vehicle collision. Which of the following signs would mandate transport to a trauma center?
   A. Ejection from the vehicle
   B. Femur fracture
   C. Intrusion of passenger compartment by 6 inches

   D. Isolated rib fracture
   E. Systolic BP 98 mm Hg

6. Trauma resuscitation can be chaotic and complicated. The trauma team is ultimately in charge of the resuscitation of patients. Which of the following actions should be performed by the trauma captain?
   A. Auscultation of breath sounds
   B. Delegation of the components of the resuscitation
   C. Digital rectal examination
   D. Placement of endotracheal tube
   E. Placement of peripheral IV catheters

7. A 34-year-old male is brought to the hospital after being thrown and then trampled by a horse. He is confused and combative, mumbling incoherently. His BP is 75 mm Hg by palpation, RR is 30, HR is 140 beats/min, and pulse oximetry is 88% on a non-rebreather mask. His breath sounds are equal bilaterally. His jaw is swollen and deformed. Which of the following interventions takes highest priority?
   A. C-spine immobilization
   B. Examination of lumbosacral spine
   C. High-dose methylprednisolone
   D. Large-bore IV access and saline bolus
   E. Rapid-sequence intubation

8. A 24-year-old 70-kg man is brought to the hospital 1 hour after jumping off a local bridge. Witnesses report he fell approximately 100 feet before striking the water. He is awake, asking that he be allowed to die. Primary survey is intact and secondary survey reveals priapism, stool incontinence, and no movement of lower extremities. What is the most appropriate next intervention?
   A. Cross-table lateral x-ray of lumbosacral spine
   B. Methylprednisolone 125 mg IV
   C. Methylprednisolone 2.1 g IV
   D. MRI of the spine
   E. Immediate consultation with psychiatrist

9. A 45-year-old woman complains of abdominal pain immediately after a motor vehicle collision. She was restrained in the back seat with a lap belt. After she has received 3 liters of saline IV, her vitals are BP, 80 systolic; HR, 133; RR, 23; pulse oximetry, 99% on a non-rebreather mask. The radiologist on call for CT scan is en route to the hospital and is approximately 20 minutes away. What is the most appropriate next step?
   A. Give repeated saline boluses and reassess in 20 minutes
   B. Start transfusion with type-specific PRBCs and perform diagnostic peritoneal lavage
   C. Start transfusion with type-specific PRBCs, place Foley catheter and nasogastric tube, and perform diagnostic peritoneal lavage
   D. Start transfusion with type-specific PRBCs and wait for abdominal CT scan

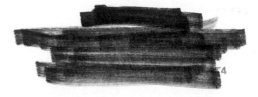

10. Which of the following patients is least likely to benefit from emergent thoracotomy?
    A. Man with blunt chest trauma with Hamann's crunch
    B. Teen with gunshot wound to the upper back
    C. Pedestrian struck by an auto with no signs of life before arrival at hospital
    D. Woman with a stab wound to the left chest with faint carotid pulses

11. Care of the elderly trauma victim can be challenging. Regarding head trauma in the elderly, which of the following is most correct?
    A. Altered mental status in elderly trauma victims can be safely attributed to senility
    B. Atrophy is protective against cerebral edema
    C. Bridging subdural veins may be ruptured secondary to minor trauma
    D. Use of head CT scan should be based on the same indications for younger patients

12. A 5-year-old boy is brought to the hospital after diving head first into shallow water. He is crying and unable to cooperate with the examination. His father states he complained of shooting pains in his arms immediately after the accident. His primary survey is intact and he is moving all extremities. Which of the following statements is most accurate?
    A. A small towel should be place under his head to properly align his cervical spine
    B. He can be released from C-spine immobilization after an adequate cross-table lateral cervical spine x-ray
    C. Lower cervical injuries are more common than upper cervical injuries in children
    D. Spinal cord injury without radiographic abnormality should be ruled out before removal of spinal immobilization

## 27 ▼ Trauma in Pregnancy

*Stephanie L. Ciccarelli and Neil B. Jasani*

Select the appropriate letter that correctly answers the question or completes the statement.

1. A primigravida in her fourteenth week of pregnancy is the front seat passenger involved in a motor vehicle collision and sustains moderate blunt abdominal trauma. She is having severe abdominal pain and is known to be Rh negative.
    A. At 14 weeks, the fetal blood volume is insufficient to cause fetal-maternal hemorrhage beyond the protection of a single 300 μg dose of RhoGAM
    B. It takes at least 5 cc of fetal blood exposure for 50% of mothers to become Rh sensitive
    C. RhoGAM must be administered within 4 hours of the transfusion to prevent sensitization, so quick laboratory turnaround time is essential

D. The Kleihauer-Betke test cannot be used in circumstances in which there is persistence of fetal hemoglobin in the maternal circulation
    E. This patient should have the Kleihauer-Betke test to calculate the dosage of RhoGAM needed to prevent sensitization

2. Which of the following is true in obstetric traumas?
    A. If the maternal saturation is 100%, supplemental oxygen need not be given
    B. Maternal pulse and blood pressure are not reliable predictors of fetal well-being
    C. Risk of aspiration is equal to that in a non-pregnant patient
    D. When mechanical ventilation is instituted, the same parameters/settings should be used as those in a non-pregnant patient

3. In blunt abdominal trauma during pregnancy, which is true?
    A. Diagnostic peritoneal lavage (DPL) by open technique can be done safely only in the first two trimesters
    B. Fetal blood flow is reduced by 10% to 20% before maternal blood pressure is affected
    C. The most common cause of fetal death is premature delivery
    D. The mother can lose 40% of her blood volume before showing signs of shock

4. What is the most common result of obstetric trauma?
    A. Maternal hemorrhage
    B. Abruptio placentae
    C. Uterine contractions
    D. Uterine rupture

5. A 27-year-old pregnant woman who recently immigrated from India presents with a dirty wound. She is unaware of ever having received a tetanus immunization.
    A. Both the tetanus toxoid and the immunoglobulin are safe in pregnancy and should be administered
    B. Neither the tetanus toxoid nor the immunoglobulin should be administered
    C. Tetanus toxoid should be given, but the immunoglobulin should not because the antibody crosses the placenta
    D. There are insufficient data to dictate a standard of care regarding tetanus toxoid or immunoglobulin in obstetric patients

6. How does maternal cardioversion affect the fetus?
    A. Because the amount of energy reaching the fetal heart is significant, fetal monitoring is recommended
    B. Cardioversion can be safely performed during the first and second trimesters but not in the third
    C. It should not be performed unless the situation is imminently life threatening
    D. Studies have shown no need for fetal monitoring during maternal cardioversion

7. A 32-year-old woman in her twenty-fifth week of gestation fell down 6 steps, with the impact isolated to her back. She has no abdominal complaints. Vital signs are

HR, 96; BP, 100/62; RR, 16. Exam is remarkable only for mild to moderate tenderness over T10 to L2 and a gravid uterus. The urine is negative for blood. Which of the following is true?

A. Absence of direct abdominal trauma and no clinical evidence of abdominal injury preclude fetal injury, and the patient may be discharged from the emergency department with acetaminophen and close follow-up

B. Fetal monitoring may be helpful in monitoring maternal well-being because fetal hemodynamics are more sensitive to fluid status and oxygenation than maternal parameters

C. Patient and fetus should be monitored for 2 hours and if normal, may be discharged with acetaminophen and close follow-up

D. There is no indication to monitor because the fetus is not viable at 25 weeks' gestation and management would not change even if fetal distress were detected

8. Which of the following is true about maternal/fetal fatalities after trauma?

A. Because the time since maternal circulation ceases is the critical factor in fetal outcome, emergency physicians should be capable of performing perimortem C-sections

B. Even if maternal death occurs or is imminent, consent must be obtained before a C-section can be performed

C. Fetal death is an indication for C-section

D. Maternal death rate is greater than fetal death rate

9. Which of the following statements is true for maternal carbon monoxide exposure?

A. Fetal carboxyhemoglobin concentrations plateau 12 hours after exposure

B. Fetal carboxyhemoglobin elimination half-life is approximately equal to maternal elimination half-life

C. Hyperbaric oxygen is contraindicated in pregnancy

D. The mother is at greater risk than the fetus

E. Treatment with 100% oxygen is recommended for five times as long as is needed to reach acceptable maternal levels

# 28 ▼ Principles of Wound Management

*Michael E. Silverman and Scott P. Krall*

Select the appropriate letter that correctly answers the question or completes the statement.

1. Which one of the following statements is true regarding the physiology of wound healing?

A. In a surgically repaired laceration, epithelialization bridges the defect by 12 hours

B. Lacerations perpendicular to skin folds, lines of expression, and joints do not impair functions or cause unappealing scars

C. Sharp debridement, converting a jagged wound to a linear laceration, should be done to improve the potential scar

D. Static forces of skin are demonstrated clinically by the gaping of wounds following incision

E. Static forces of skin tension of a given area of skin are variable based on an individual's body position and movements

2. Which of the following statements is true concerning risk factors for wound infection?

A. Because of their high velocity and thermic reaction, missile injuries usually sterilize the wound on skin entry

B. Because soil fractions cause an immune response, foreign matter left in a wound doesn't change the risk of infection

C. Crush mechanism, high-velocity missiles, and deep penetrating wounds all are increased risk factors for wound infection

D. It takes at least 6 hours for bacterial proliferation to reach a level that may result in infection after acute trauma

E. Laceration produced by fine cutting forces increases risk of infection compared with crush injuries

3. Glass greater than what thickness is visible on x-ray when appropriate views are done?

A. 0.5 mm

B. 1.0 mm

C. 2.0 cm

D. 2.0 mm

E. Glass cannot be seen on x-ray

4. In regards to anesthesia in wound management, which is the correct statement?

A. Digital artery vasospasm that was accidentally induced by local infiltration of epinephrine can successfully be reversed with a local injection of phenylephrine

B. Laceration of the hands, fingers, feet, and toes are poor candidates for regional anesthesia because of poor blood supply

C. Lidocaine with epinephrine should be avoided in wounds with higher risks of infection because some studies show a lower resistance to infection when epinephrine is used

D. The onset of action of lidocaine with direct infiltration is seconds and lasts 3-5 minutes

E. When Lidocaine is administered as a regional nerve block, onset occurs in 15-20 minutes and lasts approximately 75 minutes

5. Which of the following statements is true regarding local anesthesia?
   A. Lidocaine-bicarbonate mixture should last for 6 months if kept refrigerated
   B. TAC (tetracaine, adrenaline, cocaine) may be effective for anesthesia of face and scalp lacerations
   C. TAC needs to be applied for 2-3 minutes before suturing to allow for adequate anesthesia
   D. Larger gauge needles (e.g., 18 gauge) allow for quick administration and less pain
   E. When buffering lidocaine with bicarbonate, a ratio of 1:100 is appropriate

6. A man comes to the ED with a 7-cm laceration to his left forearm from a box cutter. Examination of his left upper extremity reveals normal motor and sensory function, with a capillary refill of 1 second. He had a tetanus booster 3 years ago but says he developed anaphylactic shock after receiving lidocaine for local anesthetic. Which local anesthetic is best to use?
   A. Bupivacaine
   B. Hydroxyzine
   C. Lidocaine
   D. Normal saline
   E. Tetracaine

7. A woman was struck in the head with a softball, resulting in a 5-cm laceration involving the superior right eyelid, eyebrow, and forehead. History and physical examination reveal no loss of consciousness and a normal exam except for the laceration. Preparation for primary wound closure should include all of the following except what?
   A. Cleaning the wound with high-pressure irrigation
   B. Cleansing the surrounding skin
   C. Debridement of devitalized tissue
   D. Removing hair to clean and examine the wound adequately
   E. Using local anesthetic

8. Which of the following suture materials is considered absorbable?
   A. Nylon
   B. Prolene
   C. Silk
   D. Stainless steel wire
   E. Vicryl

9. Stapling wounds is an alternative to suturing. Which of the following statements is true about staples?
   A. Because of the strength of the steel, staples perform better on skin subject to large amounts of tension
   B. Stapled wounds take longer to gain tensile strength and thus must be left in 1-3 days longer than sutures
   C. Staples are more comfortable while in situ compared with sutures
   D. Monofilament stainless steel staples may increase the risk of infection
   E. The time necessary for closure is significantly less compared with sutures

10. Tetanus can be a serious complication of wounds. Which of the following statements is true?

A. Immunization must be given within 24 hours of injury
B. Tetanus immune globulin must be give 24 hours before tetanus toxoid to avoid binding and neutralization
C. Tetanus toxoid should never be given during pregnancy
D. The majority of patients that get tetanus are unimmunized as children before entering school
E. Up to 40% of all cases of tetanus occur in individuals who have either minor wounds or no recollection of any injury

# 29 Injury Control

### *Christine Milosis and Scott P. Krall*

Select the appropriate letter that correctly answers the question or completes the statement.

1. Regarding injury and the injury triangle (host, agent, and environment), which of the following is true?
   A. Most injuries are random events, and no consistently useful relationship exists among the three elements of the triangle
   B. Most injuries are the result of human error; therefore, only changes in the host through education can be expected to decrease the number of injuries yearly
   C. Most injuries are the result of human negligence and, as a result, no meaningful changes can be expected until society as a whole cares about the issue of injury
   D. Most injuries may be viewed within the disease paradigm; therefore, all three elements of the triangle are interrelated and modifiable

*Match the following using a phase factor matrix model of injury analysis (using the example of a toddler's interaction with a poisonous substance).*
   A. Event agent
   B. Event environment
   C. Event host
   D. Post-event agent
   E. Post-event environment
   F. Post-event host
   G. Pre-event agent
   H. Pre-event environment
   I. Pre-event host

2. Ability to reach object     _____
3. Adult supervision     _____
4. Age     _____
5. Cognitive function     _____
6. Height of storage     _____
7. Overdose instructions on bottle     _____
8. Poison control availability     _____
9. Safety cap     _____
10. Tendency for toxicity     _____

11. Which of the following is true regarding motor vehicle-related trauma?
    A. In the United States, approximately 10,000 deaths involving motor vehicle crashes occur annually
    B. In the United States, firearms are associated with the largest source of injury fatalities and motor vehicle crashes are the second largest source of injury fatalities
    C. In the United States, motor vehicle crashes are the leading cause of death and disability for teenagers of driving age
    D. Persons age 70 and older make up the lowest risk driving group due to conservative driving characteristics

12. In studying the biomechanics of motor vehicle crashes, it has been shown that maximizing the stopping distance is the most important means to minimize energy transfer to the body. Which of the following contributes to maximizing stopping distance?
    A. Air bag deployment
    B. Cars constructed of deformable metals
    C. Collapsible steering wheel columns
    D. Seat belt use
    E. All of the above

13. Regarding firearms, which of the following is false?
    A. All guns are firearms
    B. Despondent elderly persons in a home with guns constitute a high-risk environment
    C. Firearm-related suicides account for 78% of suicide fatalities
    D. In the 15- to 24-year-old age-group, 25% of all deaths are related to firearms
    E. The most common cause of death for African-American men in the United States is a firearm-related event

14. What is the leading cause of accidental death for those ages 1 to 44 years of age in the United States?
    A. Falling
    B. Motor vehicle collision
    C. Penetrating trauma
    D. Poisoning
    E. Recreational injury

15. An injury event can best be characterized in terms of which of the following?
    A. ED management
    B. Influence of alcohol or other drugs
    C. Methods for prevention in the future
    D. Responsible societal factors
    E. Three phases: pre-injury, injury, post-injury

16. An injury event can be most usefully and completely analyzed in terms of which of the following?
    A. Attributing fault
    B. Environmental contribution (such as roadway conditions)
    C. Host factors, agent-related factors, and environment factors
    D. Prevention of recurrences
    E. Time of day and season of year

17. Which of the following statements is true regarding seat belts?
    A. Abdominal injuries occur only with misuse
    B. Clavicle and rib fractures with concurrent cardiac contusions occur only with misuse
    C. Lap and shoulder belts are 75% effective in reducing fatalities
    D. Child safety seats are required in 34 states
    E. Wearing seat belts under the arm, too loose, or too high may cause unique injuries

18. Which of the following statements is true of homicide?
    A. It is due to firearms in 25% of all cases
    B. It is perpetrated by strangers more commonly than by acquaintances
    C. It is the leading cause of death for African-American males age 15-24 years
    D. It occurs at the same rate throughout all metropolitan areas
    E. Gang-related activity is most likely involved when women are murdered

 **30** ## Youth and Gang Violence

*No questions*

**SECTION 2   HEAD AND SPINAL TRAUMA**

 **31** ## Head Trauma

*Usamah Mossallam and Andrew Langsam*

Select the appropriate letter that correctly answers the question or completes the statement.

*The following paragraph applies to Questions 1 through 3:*
    A 59-year-old alcoholic male was found by police on the sidewalk of a downtown street. Witnesses report the patient fell from a standing position. They report that he appeared intoxicated. Upon paramedic arrival the patient was unresponsive. His eyes opened only to pain, he was moaning and pulled away from painful stimuli.

1. What is this patient's Glasgow Coma Scale score?
    A. 5
    B. 6
    C. 7
    D. 8
    E. 10

2. The patient is likely to have suffered which type of CNS bleed?
   A. Epidural hematoma
   B. Intracerebral hematoma
   C. Subdural hematoma
   D. Traumatic subarachnoid hemorrhage

3. What are the chances of survival for the patient?
   A. 10%-20%
   B. 35%-50%
   C. 55%-70%
   D. 70%-85%
   E. 85%-100%

4. A significant finding on physical examination of a patient suspected of having a basilar skull fracture might include all of the following except which one?
   A. Battle's sign (postauricular blood)
   B. CSF rhinorrhea
   C. Hemotympanum
   D. Nasal fracture
   E. Raccoon's eyes (periorbital ecchymoses)

5. Which of the following statements is true regarding closed head injury?
   A. Anticonvulsant administration is indicated for patients who are iatrogenically paralyzed and intubated
   B. Barbiturates should be administered early to patients with severe head injury, especially in the setting of multiple trauma
   C. Hypotension resulting from a severe head injury is a common finding in trauma patients
   D. Mannitol is neuroprotective and should be given early
   E. Steroids have been shown to improve survival in patients with elevations in intracranial pressure associated with closed head injury

6. For which of the following minor head injury patients is a CT scan recommended?
   A. A 4 year old
   B. Initial GCS of 14
   C. Loss of consciousness less than 2 minutes
   D. Normal pupils
   E. Skull fracture

7. A 30-year-old man comes to the ED with a history of falling off a ladder and hitting his head. He was unconscious briefly but soon awoke and returned to his normal mental state. Over the course of the next hour he became confused and then lapsed into unconsciousness again. Which of the following injury patterns does this patient probably have?
   A. Epidural hematoma
   B. Intracerebral hemorrhage
   C. Normal
   D. Subarachnoid hemorrhage
   E. Subdural hematoma

8. The Cushing's reflex, a late finding of intracranial pressure elevation, is best described by which of the following findings?

A. Extension posturing and tachycardia
B. Flexion posturing and bradycardia
C. Hypertension and bradycardia
D. Hypotension and bradycardia
E. Hypotension and tachycardia

9. All of the following are early interventions in the unconscious victim of head trauma with a hemotympanum except which one?
   A. Insertion of a Foley catheter to measure urine output
   B. Insertion of a nasogastric tube to prevent aspiration
   C. Intubation to prevent airway compromise and consequent elevation in $Pco_2$
   D. Neurosurgical consultation
   E. Stabilization of the C-spine

10. What is the fastest therapeutic intervention available for decreasing intra-cranial pressure?
    A. Dexamethasone 10 mg IV
    B. Hyperventilation of the lungs
    C. Intravenous barbiturates
    D. Lasix 40 mg IV
    E. Mannitol 1 mg/kg IV

11. Which of the following is the diagnostic study of choice in acute head trauma?
    A. CT scan
    B. Lumbar puncture
    C. MRI
    D. Skull radiograph
    E. Ultrasound

12. What is the most common CT scan abnormality found after severe closed head injury?
    A. Epidural hematoma
    B. Intracerebral hemorrhage
    C. Subdural hematoma
    D. Traumatic subarachnoid hemorrhage

---

 **32 Facial Trauma**

*Joseph B. Dore and Andrew Langsam*

Select the appropriate letter that correctly answers the question or completes the statement.

1. What is the most common cause of facial trauma?
   A. Altercations
   B. Animal bites
   C. Child abuse
   D. Motor vehicle collisions
   E. Work-related injuries

2. Which of the following studies is the best for the initial evaluation of the maxilla, maxillary sinuses, floors, and inferior rims of the orbits, and the zygomatic arches?
   A. Axial CT scan of the head
   B. Coronal CT scan of the head
   C. Lateral view of the facial bones
   D. Posteroanterior view of the facial bones
   E. Waters' projection

3. A 32-year-old man was involved in a barroom altercation. He arrived at the emergency department complaining of double vision and right-sided facial numbness after sustaining numerous blows to the head and face. Physical examination reveals right-sided enophthalmos and an inability to gaze upward with the right eye. What would be appropriate emergency department management of this patient's condition?
   A. Careful follow-up with the ophthalmologist for an orbital blowout fracture
   B. Immediate neurosurgical consultation for traumatic intracranial hemorrhage
   C. Nonsteroidal antiinflammatory agents and reassurance that his vision will improve once the swelling resolves
   D. Blood alcohol level since these symptoms are most likely secondary to ethanol intoxication
   E. Serum Lyme titers and an infectious disease consult

4. A 17-year-old intoxicated unrestrained front seat passenger was thrown from a convertible when it struck a tree. Respirations are agonal, blood pressure is 60 and palpable, Glasgow Coma Scale score is 7, blood is present from the right ear canal, the maxilla and nasal bones are freely mobile on both sides, and rhinorrhea is present. Which of the following would be a treatment priority?
   A. Immediate orotracheal intubation or surgical cricothyrotomy
   B. Nasotracheal intubation with direct laryngoscopy and Magill forceps
   C. Opening the airway with the head-tilt/chin-lift method
   D. Immediate portable cross-table lateral radiograph of the cervical spine
   E. Surgical consultation for tracheostomy in the operating room

5. Which of the following principles regarding the management of facial wounds is true?
   A. Beveled lacerations should be debrided parallel to the lacerated edges to preserve orientation with the opposite side and allow for improved closure
   B. Debris embedded in a traumatic abrasion should be removed by a consulting plastic surgeon 3 to 4 days after the accident to allow easier removal and facilitate a better cosmetic outcome
   C. Dog bite puncture wounds to the face should be copiously irrigated, explored for deep tissue injury, and closed primarily
   D. Relatively clean facial wounds may be repaired up to 24 hours after injury
   E. Quality of the final result is compromised in facial fractures not treated within 48 hours of the accident

6. Which of the following facial injuries should be referred to an appropriate specialist?
   A. Laceration near the medial canthus not involving the lacrimal system
   B. Laceration of the outer ear, including cartilage
   C. Laceration of the cheek with blood at the opening of Stinson's duct
   D. Through-and-through laceration of the lip crossing the vermilion border
   E. Through-and-through laceration of the nose with associated fractured cartilage

7. All of the following management principles are true for soft tissue injury except which one?
   A. Debridement of facial wounds should be avoided because this may extend wound margins and aggravate bleeding
   B. Facial wounds should be carefully explored before closing
   C. Tetanus prophylaxis is an initial concern
   D. The width of the wound edges before skin sutures are placed is an approximate gauge of the width of the resultant scar
   E. Wounds up to 24 hours old may be closed on the face

8. Which of the following is true regarding the management of facial wounds?
   A. Deep layers are best closed with running locked stitches for added strength
   B. Monofilament synthetic nonabsorbable sutures are the preferred choice for skin closure on the face
   C. Nonabsorbable sutures of 4-0 or 5-0 size should be used to approximate deep layers
   D. The skin does not regain adequate tensile strength for 2-3 weeks after repair

9. A 32-year-old woman playing tennis sustains a blow to her left eye. She complains of pain in her left eye but denies flashes of light, floaters, diplopia, or decrease in vision. Initial examination reveals 20/20 vision in both eyes, functioning extraocular muscles, and an intact globe. Orbital emphysema is noted surrounding her left eye however, and the patient begins to complain of decreased visual acuity in that eye. What step should be taken next?
   A. Ballottement of the globe started immediately in an attempt to dislodge the clot causing the central retinal artery occlusion
   B. Intraorbital needle aspiration or lateral canthotomy with cantholysis to release pressure under the orbit
   C. Ophthalmologic consult for traumatic retinal tear with vitreous hemorrhage
   D. Topical cycloplegics (5% homatropine) to the affected eye for treatment of traumatic iridocyclitis with an ophthalmologic follow-up

10. A 27-year-old woman was the unrestrained driver of a car that was rear ended just before arrival at the emergency department. She complains of a sore nose. Examination reveals mild tenderness but no crepitance nor deformity of the external nose. Internal examination reveals a large grape-like swelling over the left side of the nasal septum. What is the most appropriate action?
    A. Checking prothrombin time and partial thromboplastin time for possible coagulopathy
    B. Closed reduction of the nasal septum with follow-up by an otorhinolaryngologist
    C. Incision and drainage of a septal hematoma with anterior packing
    D. Referral to an otorhinolaryngologist advising the patient to be seen within 1 week
    E. Referral to an otorhinolaryngologist for treatment of her nasal polyps

 **33** Spinal Injuries

*Robert T. Maroko and John F. Madden*

Select the appropriate letter that correctly answers the question or completes the statement.

1. Which of the following statements is true regarding spinal injuries?
    A. A normal neurologic examination excludes the possibility of cord injury
    B. A spinal injury should be suspected in a trauma victim with a femur fracture
    C. A vertebral bony injury must be present in order for a spinal cord injury to exist
    D. Central cord syndrome is most commonly seen in children

2. Which of the following spinal injuries is considered unstable?
    A. Bilateral facet dislocation
    B. Burst fracture of vertebral body
    C. Clay shoveler's fracture
    D. Isolated fracture of vertebral body
    E. Wedge fracture

3. The patient shown in this x-ray (Figure 33-1) was thrown into extreme hyperextension as a result of abrupt deceleration. What is his injury commonly referred to as?
    A. Clay shoveler's fracture
    B. Hangman's fracture
    C. Jefferson fracture
    D. Odontoid fracture
    E. Tear drop fracture

4. A Jefferson fracture is caused by what forces?
    A. Extension
    B. Flexion
    C. Rotation
    D. Vertical compression

5. The patient in Figure 33-2 has a fracture of which portion of the vertebrae?
    A. Anterior arch of C1
    B. Body of C2
    C. C1 spinous process
    D. Odontoid process of C2
    E. Posterior arch of C1

6. The maximum neurologic deficit following spinal cord injury is seen at what time?
    A. At time of initial injury
    B. During the following hours
    C. During the following days
    D. During the following weeks
    E. During the following months

7. A construction worker arrives at the emergency department after a fall from a roof. Which of the following injuries is most likely to be associated with a compression fracture of the lumbar spine?

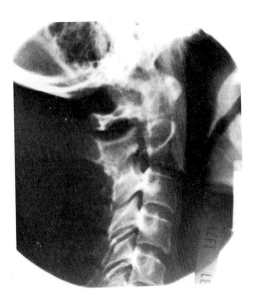

**FIG. 33-1**

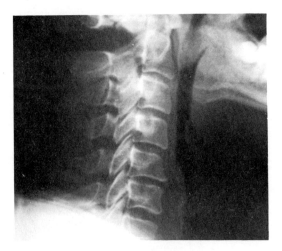

**FIG. 33-2**

A. Bilateral ankle and foot fractures
B. Bilateral radial fractures
C. Facial and mandibular fractures
D. Scapular fracture and humeral fracture

8. A patient presents to the emergency room after a motor vehicle collision. He is awake and complaining of shortness of breath. On physical examination he has abdominal breathing in the absence of thoracic breathing. Which level of spinal cord injury would explain these findings?
A. Brain stem
B. C2
C. C6
D. L4
E. S1

9. A young football player presents to the emergency department after a tackle that left him briefly unconscious. Which of the following complaints is most likely be attributed to injury of the spine at the C6 and C7 level?
A. Blurred vision
B. Occipital pain
C. Hand tingling
D. Nausea
E. Perioral tingling

10. In patients with complete spinal cord lesions that persist longer than 24 hours after the injury, approximately what is the likelihood of having functional recovery?
A. 0%-10%
B. 30%-40%
C. 50%-60%
D. 90%-100%

11. An elderly woman presents to the emergency department after a fall from standing in which she struck her forehead against a desk on her way down. She is almost quadriplegic but has worse deficit on upper extremity testing compared to lower extremity testing and has sacral sparing. Which co-morbid disease is this patient likely to have associated with this syndrome?
A. Arthritis
B. Coronary artery disease
C. Hypertension
D. Hyperthyroidism

12. A patient presents to the emergency department after a gunshot injury to his back. Which set of symptoms would be most consistent with Brown-Séquard syndrome?
A. Bilateral motor and sensory deficit
B. Bilateral motor deficit only
C. Bilateral sensory deficit only
D. Ipsilateral motor and sensory deficit
E. Ipsilateral motor deficit and contralateral sensory deficit

13. Which of the following is the preferred method of airway management for patients with traumatic cardiopulmonary arrest even with evidence of spinal injury?
A. Nasotracheal intubation
B. Obturator airway
C. Orotracheal intubation
D. Tracheostomy

14. Which of the following patients has the least risk for cord injury?
A. Isolated spinal process fracture of C5 without neurologic deficit
B. Isolated spinal process fracture of C6 and tingling of his left arm
C. Posterior atlantoaxial dislocation without a fracture
D. Tear drop fracture of C4

---

 ## 34 ▼ Neck Trauma

*M. Greg Amaya and John F. Madden*

Select the appropriate letter that correctly answers the question or completes the statement.

1. Injury to which zone of the neck leads to the highest mortality rate?
A. Zone I
B. Zone II
C. Zone III
D. Zone IV

2. A young male comes to the ED with a stab wound to the neck, resulting in a large hematoma that is distorting normal airway anatomy. Vital signs are recorded as follows: heart rate, 95; respiratory rate, 28; and blood pressure, 140/95. There is no evidence of stridor. What would be the proper technique for controlling the airway in this patient?
A. Awake oral intubation with local anesthesia
B. Blind nasotracheal intubation
C. Immediate cricothyrotomy
D. Rapid-sequence induction with endotracheal intubation
E. Immediate consult of a trauma surgeon for placement of a tracheostomy

3. A previously stable patient with a gunshot wound to the neck suddenly develops tachypnea, tachycardia, hypotension, and a machinery-like heart murmur. What should the physician do immediately?
A. Perform a needle aspiration of the right ventricle of the heart
B. Place bilateral chest tubes
C. Place the patient in a seated upright position
D. Place the patient in the left lateral decubitus position in Trendelenburg
E. Administer a fluid challenge of 20 cc/kg

4. Paramedics radio in about a 25-year-old female with a stabbing injury to the right side of her neck just under her chin. The patient is awake and is tachypneic to 28 but is maintaining her airway. Her pulse is 115 and blood pressure 93/50. Paramedics report she is bleeding briskly, and they have an 8-minute transport. What should orders include?
   A. Assessment of wound depth and tissue involvement in order to evaluate the extent and nature of hemorrhage
   B. Direct transfer to the operating room on arrival, with early notification of the OR staff and trauma surgeon
   C. Immediate intubation because the patient is tachypneic and in danger of losing her airway
   D. Placement of two intravenous catheters for volume resuscitation, with frequent assessment of vital signs and placement of MAST trousers should bleeding continue
   E. Placement of two intravenous catheters for volume resuscitation and direct application of external pressure to the site of bleeding

5. A tachycardic, hypotensive patient with penetrating neck trauma and bleeding into the oropharynx presents to a low-volume, single-coverage emergency department. The nearest appropriate trauma center is 15 minutes away and is ready to accept the patient. Before transfer, what should the physician do?
   A. Rapidly prepare the patient for transport without further delay and send the patient with a transport nurse certified in ACLS.
   B. Secure an airway, pack the oropharynx with heavy gauze, and establish intravenous access with fluid and blood product resuscitation
   C. Secure an airway, place an orogastric tube to decompress the stomach of both air and swallowed blood, and establish intravenous access with fluid and blood product resuscitation
   D. Transfer the patient only after completing full primary and secondary surveys, including C-spine, chest, and pelvis radiographs
   E. Transfer the patient only if the platysma has been penetrated

6. A patient who was struck in the side of the head and face with a crowbar is experiencing decreasing levels of consciousness, with unilateral limb paresis and Horner's syndrome. What is the most likely diagnosis?
   A. Air embolus
   B. Brachial plexus injury
   C. Carotid artery thrombosis
   D. Cervical spine fracture
   E. Thrombosis of the cavernous sinus

7. What do fractures of the thyroid cartilage caused by blunt injury result in?
   A. Aphonia because the anterior vocal cord attachment is invariably disrupted

   B. Exacerbation of the normal anatomic landmarks of the neck
   C. Mandatory tracheostomy for airway stabilization
   D. The need for aggressive diagnostic imaging consisting of computed tomography and rigid bronchoscopy
   E. The need for voice rest, humidified air, and prophylactic antibiotics with delayed surgical repair acceptable assuming a secured airway

8. In managing strangulation injuries, which of these is true?
   A. Calcium boluses have been shown to improve the postanoxic cerebral circulation, helping to decrease long-term ischemic sequelae
   B. Because of the high frequency of respiratory complications, prophylactic antibiotics should be routinely given
   C. Intubation is an important adjunct even in the absence of unstable airways
   D. Phenobarbital is the drug of choice for postanoxic seizures
   E. Steroids have been shown to be effective treatment for both cerebral edema and central neurogenic ARDS

---

**SECTION 3   CHEST TRAUMA**

---

 **35   Thoracic Trauma**

*Sharon C. Amaya and Bonnie B. Matthaeus*

Select the appropriate letter that correctly answers the question or completes the statement.

1. Isolated fracture of the first rib:
   A. Is associated with a higher rate of pneumothorax compared with fractures of other ribs
   B. Is often easier to visualize on the AP cervical spine radiograph than on chest radiograph
   C. Requires angiographic evaluation of the aorta
   D. Requires surgical intervention
   E. Results in a tenfold increase in morbidity and mortality compared with fractures of other ribs

2. Patients sustaining sternal fractures:
   A. Are commonly diagnosed by AP chest radiograph
   B. Can usually be discharged if ECG and initial CPK-MB enzymes are otherwise normal
   C. Have an associated mortality of 5% to 7%
   D. Should be admitted and evaluated for cardiac contusion
   E. Should be electively intubated

3. Which of the following is the major cause of respiratory insufficiency in a patient with a flail chest?
   A. Associated pulmonary contusion
   B. Decreased cardiac output
   C. Mediastinal shift

D. Paradoxical chest wall movement

E. Pendelluft effect

4. A 52-year-old woman presents after sustaining a fall onto her right side. She is complaining of right sided chest pain. Her oxygen saturation is 99% on a non-rebreather mask and her vital signs are stable. She is found to have six consecutive rib fractures with paradoxical motion of the right chest. What does treatment for this injury include?

A. Immediate intubation

B. Immediate referral to orthopedics for external fixation of the ribs

C. Placement of a chest tube in the midclavicular third intercostal space

D. Restriction of intravenous pain medication to prevent hypercarbia

E. Trial of continuous positive airway pressure (CPAP)

5. A young man presents to the ED after having his upper chest under the full weight of a steel beam for several minutes. The skin of his head and neck is a deep violet color, and he has significant facial edema. What is the most clinically significant worry in this patient?

A. Intracranial hemorrhage from increased intracranial pressure

B. Pulmonary injury from high intrathoracic pressure

C. Retinal edema causing permanent vision loss

D. Tympanic membrane rupture potentially causing permanent hearing loss

E. Venous thrombosis of the great neck veins from stagnation of blood flow

6. Which of the following is a characteristic of a pneumomediastinum?

A. Commonly progresses to tension pneumomediastinum

B. Is associated with Beck's triad

C. May result from an esophageal tear

D. Requires immediate pericardiocentesis with aspiration of air

E. Typically causes subcutaneous emphysema over the anterior chest wall

7. Which of the following is a characteristic of pulmonary contusion?

A. Always associated with rib fractures

B. Associated with hemoptysis in approximately 90% of patients

C. Tends to last less than 24 hours

D. Usually evident on initial chest radiograph

E. Very uncommon in children

8. What is the earliest and most accurate means of assessing the status and progress of a patient with a pulmonary contusion?

A. CT scan of the chest

B. Pulmonary artery pressure measurements

C. Serial chest radiographs

D. Serial measurement of the alveolar-arterial oxygen gradient

E. Serial pulmonary function tests

9. Which of the following is a treatment for pulmonary contusion and $PaO_2 < 60\%$ on room air?

A. Aggressive fluid resuscitation to increase venous return

B. Chest tube thoracostomy

C. Intubation and ventilation

D. Lasix intravenously every 6 hours to decrease pulmonary edema

E. Vigorous tracheobronchial suctioning, pain relief measures, and steroids

10. Indications for chest tube thoracostomy include all of the following except which one?

A. Bilateral small pneumothorax

B. Hemothorax associated with a small pneumothorax

C. Increase in the size of a small pneumothorax despite therapy with oxygen

D. Multiple consecutive rib fractures

E. Tachypnea or desaturations with a small pneumothorax

11. A patient who has sustained blunt chest trauma has a chest radiograph that reveals two rib fractures but no other obvious injury. He suddenly complains of dyspnea and desaturates to 86% on a non-rebreather mask. His pulse is 120 and blood pressure is 110/62. What should the physician do?

A. Immediately perform needle decompression

B. Immediately repeat a chest radiograph with an expiratory view

C. Intubate

D. Order a CT scan of the chest

E. Prepare for a chest tube thoracostomy

12. The condition of an intubated patient who was involved in a motor vehicle crash suddenly deteriorates. What is the earliest sign of a potential tension pneumothorax in this patient?

A. Cyanosis

B. Distended neck veins

C. Hypotension

D. Increased resistance to ventilation

E. Tracheal deviation

13. A chest tube is placed for a hemothorax in a trauma patient. What are the indications to proceed to a thoracotomy?

A. Initial chest tube drainage >10 ml/kg of blood

B. No decrease in the size of the hemothorax on repeat chest radiograph

C. Patient had initially required 4 units of red cells for resuscitation

D. Patient was hypotensive during chest tube placement, requiring multiple fluid boluses

E. Persistent bleeding at a rate >7 ml/kg/hr

14. A young man is evaluated in the ED following blunt chest trauma. Physical examination reveals hemoptysis, subcutaneous emphysema, and decreased breath sounds on the right. A chest tube is placed for a large pneumothorax, but the patient fails to improve. A chest radiograph following chest tube placement shows persistence of the pneumothorax. What is the most likely diagnosis?
    A. Communicating pneumothorax
    B. Diaphragmatic rupture
    C. Laryngeal fracture
    D. Pneumothorax associated with flail chest
    E. Tracheobronchial disruption

# 36 Cardiovascular Trauma

### *Shobhit Arora and Bonnie B. Matthaeus*

Select the appropriate letter that correctly answers the question or completes the statement.

*The following paragraph applies to Questions 1 through 3:*
   Paramedics bring a 38-year-old man to the emergency department after he has crashed his automobile head-on into a telephone pole. He was an unrestrained driver traveling at approximately 45 mph. Paramedics report considerable front-end damage to the car, as well as a bent steering wheel. The patient is complaining of chest pain and has a contusion overlying his sternum. The ECG shows sinus tachycardia at 110, with occasional ectopic beats and no significant ST-T wave changes. CPK-MB isoenzymes are elevated. The emergency physician suspects a possible myocardial contusion.

1. In this patient, which of the following is the most common sign of myocardial contusion on initial presentation?
    A. Chest contusion
    B. Chest tenderness
    C. Ectopy
    D. Elevated CPK-MB isoenzymes
    E. Sinus tachycardia

2. A definitive diagnosis of myocardial contusion can be made based on which of the following?
    A. CT scan
    B. ECG
    C. Echocardiography
    D. Serial CPK-MB isoenzymes
    E. None of the above

3. The patient is discharged from the ED after a period of observation with a diagnosis of myocardial contusion. Ten days later, he returns to the ED complaining of chest discomfort and dyspnea on exertion. What is the most likely complication of a myocardial contusion that could be causing these symptoms?
    A. Atrial rupture
    B. Pericardial effusion

C. Post-contusion myocardial infarction
D. Pulmonary embolus
E. Ventricular rupture

*The following paragraph applies to Questions 4 through 8:*
   A 23-year-old man is brought in by paramedics after being assaulted. The patient was kicked and punched several times, struck in the chest with a baseball bat, and stabbed in the epigastric and periumbilical regions. He complains of chest and abdominal pain as well as shortness of breath. His vital signs are HR, 120; RR, 30; BP, 80/60. A CVP line reveals a pressure of 18 cm $H_2O$. A pulsus paradoxus is measured as 14 mm Hg. Examination reveals no neck vein distention. During the noisy ED resuscitation, heart tones and breath sounds are present but very difficult to auscultate.

4. Which of the following should the emergency physician be concerned about as possible life-threatening injuries that this patient may have sustained?
    A. Acute pericardial tamponade
    B. Myocardial rupture
    C. Tension pneumothorax
    D. Traumatic aortic rupture
    E. All of the above

5. Which of the following injuries would put this patient at greatest risk for acute pericardial tamponade?
    A. Blunt chest trauma from a baseball bat
    B. Kick to the sternum
    C. Stab wound to the epigastrium
    D. Stab wound to the periumbilical area
    E. C and D

6. What are the most reliable signs of pericardial tamponade?
    A. Diminished heart sounds, distended neck veins, and hypotension
    B. Diminished heart sounds, tachycardia, and elevated pulsus paradoxus
    C. Elevated CVP, tachycardia, and elevated pulsus paradoxus
    D. Elevated CVP, tachycardia, and hypotension

7. During the resuscitation, an ECG and a chest x-ray are obtained. The ECG shows a sinus tachycardia without ectopy or ST-T wave changes. There is no electrical alternans. The chest x-ray reveals a normal cardiac silhouette and no pneumothorax. Which of the following statements is most accurate?
    A. A normal cardiac silhouette on chest x-ray effectively rules out acute pericardial tamponade
    B. Despite the ECG and chest x-ray findings, the patient likely has acute pericardial tamponade based on clinical findings
    C. The lack of electrical alternans on ECG indicates that this patient does not have acute pericardial tamponade
    D. The patient likely has a pneumothorax that is causing his symptoms but is not visualized on chest x-ray

8. During resuscitation, the patient becomes apneic and pulseless. What immediate action should the emergency physician take?

A. Bilateral needle decompression
B. Closed-chest cardiopulmonary resuscitation
C. Left lateral thoracotomy
D. Pericardiocentesis

9. If the chest x-ray in this patient had shown an enlarged cardiac silhouette, what concomitant process might this represent?
    A. Acute aortic rupture
    B. Acute myocardial rupture
    C. Preexisting cardiac or valvular disease
    D. A, B, and C
    E. B and C

*The following paragraph applies to Questions 10 through 12:*

A 60-year-old man is brought to the ED after falling off a ladder from a height of 20 feet. He fell onto his back and is now complaining of interscapular back pain and difficulty breathing. The emergency physician notes that the patient's voice is rather hoarse. Heart and lung sounds are normal on examination. The patient's vital signs are HR, 90; BP, 180/110; RR, 20.

10. In this patient, which of the following signs or symptoms would suggest the diagnosis of traumatic aortic rupture?
    A. Dyspnea
    B. Hoarse voice
    C. Hypertension
    D. Interscapular pain
    E. All of the above

11. A chest x-ray reveals mediastinal widening. The patient's vital signs have been stable since arrival to the ED. What is the appropriate next step in management?
    A. Aortography
    B. Chest CT with contrast
    C. Transfer to the operating room for definitive repair of aortic tear
    D. Transthoracic echocardiography

12. The patient is diagnosed with an aortic tear just distal to the take-off of the left subclavian artery. A surgeon has been consulted and will be available in 30 minutes. What further interventions must the emergency physician perform while awaiting the surgeon?
    A. No further action is required by the emergency physician
    B. Place the patient on 100% oxygen via non-rebreather mask
    C. Reduce the patient's heart rate with medication
    D. Treat hypertension
    E. Provide vigorous fluid resuscitation

 Esophageal and Diaphragmatic Trauma

*Suzanne F. Beavers and Ross E. Megargel*

Select the appropriate letter that correctly answers the question or completes the statement.

1. Which one of the following statements is true?
    A. Esophageal perforation due to a foreign body is equally likely at any point along the esophagus
    B. NG tubes have not been associated with esophageal perforation
    C. The liquefaction necrosis associated with acid burns is more damaging to the esophagus than the liquefaction necrosis caused by alkali burns
    D. The most common cause of esophageal perforation is trauma
    E. The most common cause of iatrogenic esophageal perforation is endoscopy

2. Which statement is true regarding Boerhaave's syndrome?
    A. Always associated with a history of profuse vomiting
    B. It is the esophageal injury associated with the worst prognosis because the force involved causes mediastinal soiling in association with the injury
    C. The diagnosis of Boerhaave's syndrome is readily made by history and physical
    D. The esophageal tear in Boerhaave's syndrome is usually horizontal and occurs at the GE junction
    E. The pressure caused by vomiting leading to Boerhaave's syndrome is generally 10-20 psi

3. Which of the following statements is true with regard to the use of contrast medium in the radiographic evaluation of esophageal perforation?
    A. Barium should be used before Gastrografin
    B. Endoscopy after a contrast study of the esophagus readily allows for identification of the esophageal tear
    C. Gastrografin causes less mediastinal soiling than barium
    D. Gastrografin shows better definition of mucosal detail
    E. Gastrografin will obscure visualization on subsequent endoscopy

4. Select the true statement regarding diaphragmatic injury:
   A. A common complication of diaphragmatic hernia is strangulated abdominal viscera
   B. Diaphragmatic tears are more common in women than men because their diaphragms are weaker
   C. Herniation of abdominal contents into the chest cavity almost always occurs within 6 months of the diaphragmatic injury
   D. Most defects caused by blunt injury are relatively small, whereas those caused by penetrating trauma are large
   E. The most common organ to herniate through a right-sided diaphragmatic tear is the colon

5. Which of the following statements about diaphragmatic trauma is correct?
   A. A liver-spleen scan is often helpful in the diagnosis of diaphragmatic trauma
   B. CT and ultrasound are both sensitive for diaphragmatic tears in the acute phase of injury
   C. Herniation of abdominal contents occurs intermittently, making diagnosis difficult
   D. In the acute phase of this injury, DPL is diagnostic if greater than 100,000 RBC/mm$^3$ are found
   E. Instilling contrast through a DPL catheter is an excellent way of evaluating for a diaphragmatic tear

6. Which of the following statements is true with regard to traumatic diaphragmatic hernia?
   A. A patient with a history of a penetrating wound to the lower chest or flank who is more than 3 to 6 years old is at low risk for developing a diaphragmatic hernia
   B. Blunt trauma occurs with greater incidence than penetrating trauma

   C. Defects caused by penetrating trauma that are less than 2 cm in size heal spontaneously
   D. Diaphragmatic trauma caused by penetrating trauma is usually due to gunshot wounds
   E. Left-sided injuries predominate in blunt trauma
   *Fig. 37-1 applies to Questions 7 and 8:*

7. Which of the following is true?
   A. A NG tube can be helpful in therapy of this injury but is not useful for diagnosis
   B. CT would likely be better than chest x-ray for evaluation of this injury
   C. Giving this patient contrast material might lead to aspiration and would not be helpful in diagnosis
   D. If the initial chest x-ray in someone suspected of having a diaphragmatic tear is normal, there is no need to repeat it
   E. This entity can lead to tension viscerothorax, which acts similarly to a tension pneumothorax

8. In the diagnosis and management of this injury:
   A. An NG tube seen in the chest is for diagnostic purposes
   B. If this injury leads to tension viscerothorax, placement of a chest tube is necessary for treatment
   C. Surgical repair of this injury is required
   D. Trocars should not be used to place a chest tube if a tension viscerothorax is present because of the risk of visceral perforation
   E. All of the above

# 38 Abdominal Trauma

*Gregory P. Cuculino and Ross E. Megargel*

Select the appropriate letter that correctly answers the question or completes the statement.

1. A 52-year-old restrained driver involved in an motor vehicle accident complains of abdominal pain radiating to both testicles. What injury must be suspected?
   A. Duodenal injury
   B. Hepatic injury
   C. Renal colic
   D. Splenic injury
   E. Testicular torsion

2. During the evaluation of a trauma patient, an upright chest x-ray reveals the gastric bubble shifted to the right. No free air is present. What is the main concern?
   A. Bowel obstruction
   B. Duodenal hematoma
   C. Gastric injury
   D. Retroperitoneal hematoma
   E. Splenic injury

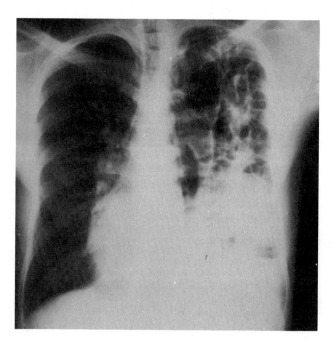

FIG. 37-1

3. A 36-year-old female comes to the emergency department complaining of a subjective fever, runny nose, muscle aches, and a cough. Past medical history is significant for a closed head injury suffered in a motor vehicle accident 3 days earlier. Chest x-ray is negative, but CBC demonstrates a WBC of 18,000 and 6 bands. What is the first action?
   A. CT scan of the abdomen looking for an abscess
   B. Discharge with the diagnosis of a viral illness
   C. Empirically treat with antibiotics
   D. Reevaluate for signs of infection
   E. Repeat the complete blood cell count

4. A 30-year-old male unrestrained driver presents for evaluation after a motor vehicle accident. Vital signs are temperature 37.8° C; pulse, 105; respiratory rate, 16; blood pressure, 120/70; pulse oximetry, 98% on room air. The patient is intoxicated, and the physical examination rendered no significant findings. Laboratory values follow. Which value causes the most concern?

| WBC | 15,000 |
| Amylase | 200 (elevated) |
| Hemoglobin | 11 |
| Hematocrit | 37 |
| Platelets | 236,000 |
| Blood alcohol | 0.280 |
| Sodium | 145 |
| Potassium | 4.2 |
| ABG: pH/Pco$_2$/Po$_2$ | 7.47/18/100 |
| Chloride | 106 |
| Bicarbonate | 12 |
| BUN | 11 |
| Creatinine | 0.8 |
| Glucose | 142 |

   A. Amylase
   B. Base deficit
   C. Blood alcohol
   D. Hemoglobin
   E. White blood cell count

5. A patient enters the emergency department with a stab wound to the anterior abdomen. A 3-centimeter laceration to the anterior abdominal wall has a small piece of omentum protruding through. Vital signs are heart rate, 98; blood pressure, 140/80; respirations, 18. What is the preferred next step?
   A. Celiotomy
   B. CT scan
   C. DPL
   D. Ultrasound
   E. Wound exploration

6. Which of the following will not cause a falsely positive DPL?
   A. Abdominal wall hematoma
   B. Inadequate hemostasis
   C. Pelvis fracture
   D. Retroperitoneal injury

7. A 17-year-old male is assaulted with a baseball bat. When he arrives at the emergency department, his vital signs are pulse, 153; respiratory rate, 24; blood pressure, 80/40. The abdomen is firm and diffusely tender. During evaluation the blood pressure becomes unobtainable. Which of the following is not a goal of ED thoracotomy and cross-clamping of the aorta?
   A. Atrial access for rapid fluid administration
   B. Proximal bleeding control
   C. Shunting of blood flow to coronary and cerebral vessels
   D. Stabilization of the patient to allow for a CT scan

8. A 25-year-old male presents with a stab wound to the upper abdomen. Vital signs are stable. The abdomen is soft, nondistended, and nontender; bowel sounds are present. Upright chest x-ray does not demonstrate a pneumothorax or free air under the diaphragm. What should the next step be?
   A. Evaluation of peritoneal entry by local wound exploration
   B. Performing a DPL
   C. Proceeding directly to laparotomy
   D. Suturing the wound and discharging the patient with clear discharge instructions

9. Which of the following most strongly points against a diaphragmatic injury?
   A. Chest x-ray
   B. Clinical examination
   C. DPL with lavage fluid RBC of 300
   D. Ultrasound

10. A patient suffers a glancing high-velocity gunshot wound to the abdomen. When can this patient be discharged from the emergency department?
   A. After a negative DPL
   B. After local wound exploration demonstrates no evidence of peritoneal injury
   C. After serial examinations demonstrate no peritoneal signs
   D. After ultrasound demonstrates no hemoperitoneum

11. What is the next step in the evaluation of the patient pictured in Figure 38-1?
   A. Celiotomy
   B. DPL
   C. Serial abdominal exams
   D. Serial ultrasounds

12. Which of the following is *not* an advantage of using ultrasound in the evaluation of a trauma patient?
   A. Can be done quickly
   B. Has no radiation hazard
   C. Instrument is portable and can be used at the bedside
   D. Is very sensitive for detecting intraperitoneal fluid
   E. Is very sensitive in detecting bowel and solid viscera damage

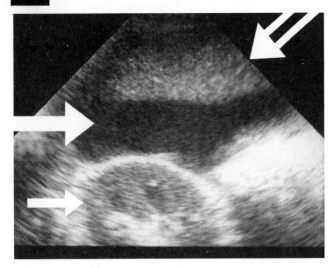

**FIG. 38-1**

13. A patient comes into the emergency department following blunt abdominal trauma. A DPL is performed. Which of the following red blood cell counts is the lowest that would be specific for an intraabdominal injury?
    A. $1000/mm^3$
    B. $5000/mm^3$
    C. $25,000/mm^3$
    D. $50,000/mm^3$
    E. $120,000/mm^3$
14. All of the following are clinical indicators for urgent laparotomy for patients presenting with abdominal stab wounds except which one?
    A. Bowel protrusion or evisceration
    B. Evidence of diaphragmatic injury
    C. Indeterminate local wound exploration
    D. Peritoneal irritation on physical examination
    E. Significant gastrointestinal bleeding
15. With regard to exploring local abdominal stab wounds in hemodynamically stable patients, which of the following statements is true?
    A. Blind probing with digits or instruments is an accurate method of determining the depth of penetration
    B. Cotton-tipped applicators are safe to use when exploring wounds
    C. If the peritoneum is violated, other diagnostic tests are indicated
    D. The stab wound should never be extended
    E. The wound should be explored without anesthesia

---

**39** Genitourinary Trauma

*Eric Gallagher and Christopher J. Murphy*

Select the appropriate letter that correctly answers the question or completes the statement.

1. The next step in management of a trauma patient with an identified partial urethral tear should be:
    A. Abdominal CT to look for associated injuries
    B. Attempt to carefully pass a 12 or 14 French catheter coudé
    C. Placement of a suprapubic catheter
    D. Proceed to operating room for repair
    E. Urologic consult if the urine does not clear within 6 hours
2. A 25-year-old male presents with a gunshot wound to the left flank. Vital signs are stable. A urine dipstick is negative for blood. Which of the following statements is correct regarding analysis of the urine in this case?
    A. More than 5 RBC/HPF is considered significant if the patent was hypotensive at any time
    B. Only gross hematuria is of significance
    C. The presence or absence of hematuria is more important than anatomic location of the injury in guiding further evaluation
    D. The presence or absence of hematuria is not a helpful screen for injury
3. Which of the following is correct regarding urologic injury in children?
    A. A child with <5 RBC/HPF on urine microscopy and no history of hypotension is safe to discharge with close follow-up
    B. Any degree of hematuria in a child mandates a full urologic evaluation
    C. Children generally require much greater force than adults to cause significant urologic injury
    D. CT using IV contrast is the diagnostic tool of choice in the evaluation of suspected urologic injury in a child
4. A 35-year-old male arrives at the emergency department after having been ejected from his auto. He has an obvious pelvic fracture, gross hematuria, and an expanding retroperitoneal hematoma. He also has a large abdominal wound with small bowel protruding. Vital signs are blood pressure, 90/40; pulse, 130; respirations, 30; temperature, 37° C. Which of the following is correct regarding evaluation of the urinary system in this patient?
    A. A bladder rupture should be assumed, and a suprapubic catheter should be placed to monitor urine output
    B. A retrograde urethrogram should be performed before taking the patient to the operating room; a single-shot IVP done in the trauma bay is adequate to demonstrate the vascular integrity of the kidneys
    C. Intraoperative bolus IVP should be performed to evaluate the integrity of the kidneys if the patient is stable enough to tolerate the procedure
    D. CT using IV contrast should be performed to asses the full extent of abdominal injury before operative management
5. Which of the following is correct concerning bladder rupture?
    A. In patients with a pelvic fracture, the absence of gross hematuria virtually eliminates the possibility of bladder rupture
    B. Mortality associated with bladder rupture is as high as 75%
    C. Most extraperitoneal bladder ruptures are associated with femur fractures

D. The classification of bladder rupture as intraperitoneal or extraperitoneal is academic because the management options are the same

E. The evaluation of bladder rupture should be done in an antegrade fashion, using a clamped Foley catheter and IV contrast CT

6. Which of the following is correct regarding external genital trauma?
   A. Any patient with a complaint of testicular trauma must have a color Doppler ultrasound to demonstrate blood flow
   B. Bleeding from the proximal stump in traumatic penile amputation is usually not controllable by direct pressure
   C. In cases of testicular dislocation, the testicle is most often found in the anterior thigh
   D. Most penile fractures respond to conservative, nonoperative management
   E. Testicular dislocation is usually the result of a direct blow, and associated injuries are uncommon

7. Which of the following is correct?
   A. In a patient with a suspected urethral tear, retrograde urethrography must be completed before taking the patient to the operating room
   B. Proper oblique views are critical to interpretation of retrograde urethrography
   C. Retrograde urethrography is not useful in evaluation of the female urethra
   D. Retrograde urethrography usually consists of two x-rays—one after instillation of contrast and one after voiding

8. Which of the following physical examination findings mandates retrograde urethrography?
   A. A high-riding prostate
   B. A seat-belt bruise across the lower abdomen
   C. Flank bruising
   D. Gross blood on rectal examination
   E. Pelvic fracture

# 40 Orthopedic Injuries: Management Principles

### *Leonardo Huertas and Christopher J. Murphy*

Select the appropriate letter that correctly answers the question or completes the statement.

1. A 42-year-old man who was seen 3 hours earlier in the emergency department for a left forearm contusion presents again complaining of severe increasing pain described as burning. On examination, he is found to have a significant contusion to the forearm and pain with passive stretching of the muscles. The initial x-rays were read as negative. Which of the following is most correct?
   A. Doppler ultrasound showing excellent flow would rule out a significant compartment syndrome
   B. Immediate fasciotomy should be considered
   C. Pain relief, splinting, and follow-up with orthopedics the following day should be arranged
   D. Repeat x-ray of the arm with special views would rule out an occult fracture

2. A 16-year-old male injured his left elbow while snowboarding. He arrives at the emergency department with an obvious left elbow dislocation. Which of the following nerves or arteries are most often associated with an elbow dislocation?
   A. Axillary nerve injury
   B. Distal radial head fracture
   C. Median and ulnar nerve injury
   D. Musculocutaneous nerve injury

3. Which describes the fracture shown in Figure 40-1?
   A. Radius fracture with dorsal angulation
   B. Radius fracture with volar angulation
   C. Ulnar fracture with dorsal angulation
   D. Ulnar fracture with volar angulation

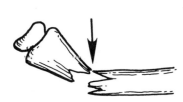

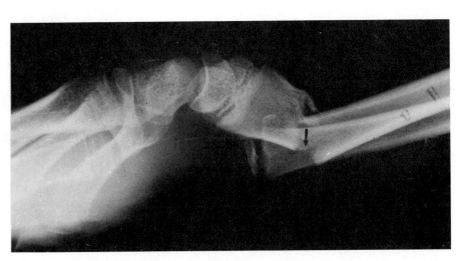

**FIG. 40-1**

4. A 28-year-old healthy female involved in a motor vehicle accident presents with a left tibial and fibular fracture. She is seen by an orthopedist in the emergency department and a cast is applied. She returned 2 days after the accident complaining of fever and shortness of breath. The pulse oxymetry reads 100%, the chest x-ray is read as normal, and the lower extremity Doppler ultrasounds are negative for any signs of DVT. Which of the following would be the correct course of action?

A. Admit patient for possible fat embolism syndrome

B. Give heparin to prevent any further pulmonary embolus

C. Reassure her that all test results are normal and that her fever and shortness of breath are most likely due to a viral infection

D. Treat with antibiotics and have her follow up with her primary care physician the following day

# 41 The Hand

*Bret M. Levy and Sunanda Nabha*

Select the appropriate letter that correctly answers the question or completes the statement.

1. Which of the following statements is true regarding anatomy of the hand?

A. Injury to the median nerve occurs most frequently at the wrist

B. Some of the bones of the hand cannot be directly examined by palpation

C. The flexor digitorum profundus flexes the DIP joint

D. The radial nerve and the tendons of the extrinsic flexors pass through the carpal tunnel

E. The radial nerve can be tested by opposition of the thumb and index finger

2. A 26-year-old bicyclist sustains a fall and has a 3-4 cm laceration on the medial aspect of her wrist. What is the easiest way to assess ulnar nerve integrity?

A. Assess her ability to pronate her hand

B. Check sensation over the anatomic snuff box

C. Have her extend her wrist and point her index finger

D. Have her pinch a piece of paper between her thumb and index finger and apply traction to the paper

E. Radially deviate the wrist when in neutral position

3. A mechanic presents with a complaint of finger pain after smashing his finger with a wrench. Examination reveals a 25% subungual hematoma with an intact nail bed. X-ray examination reveals a transverse fracture of the distal nail tuft. What should treatment include?

A. Antibiotics with therapy aimed at covering gram-negative organisms

B. Immobilizing the DIP joint for 6-8 weeks

C. Kirschner wire placement

D. Removal of nail and subsequent nail bed repair

E. Trephination of the hematoma for symptomatic relief

4. At a concert, a 21-year-old male bends over to tie his shoe. His hand is stepped on by an obese concert goer. On presentation, he is triaged to radiology. Examination reveals tenderness over the middle phalanx of his index finger. The x-ray reveals an oblique fracture through the middle phalanx. The skin is intact. Which of the following statements is true regarding the fracture?

A. Proper immobilization should not require a short arm cast with an attached outrigger

B. The flexed finger normally points to the lunate

C. These fractures are usually unstable after reduction

D. Up to 30 degrees of malrotation is well tolerated

5. A 19-year-old male complains of hand pain. His mother reports a fist-size hole in his bedroom wall, but the patient refuses to provide additional history. Which of the following statements is true concerning the radiograph shown in Figure 41-1?

A. Analgesia may be achieved via radial nerve block

B. Angulation of up to 40 degrees is generally well tolerated

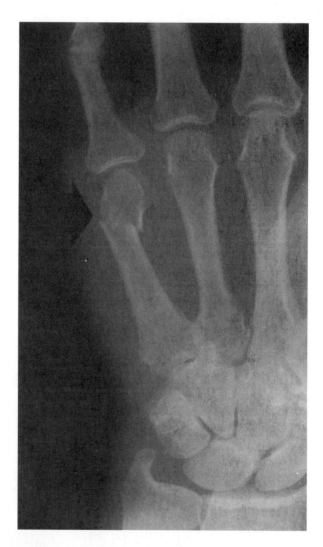

FIG. 41-1 From Harris JH Jr, Harris Wm, Norelline RA: *The radiology of emergency medicine,* Baltimore, 1995, Williams & Wilkins.

C. Fracture is likely due to a direct blow to the back of the hand

D. Metacarpal neck fractures are treated in a similar manner regardless of which metacarpal is involved

E. Treatment of this fracture consists of analgesics, ulnar gutter splint, and orthopedic follow-up

6. A 17-year-old female presents with a complaint of "jammed" index finger. There is marked swelling over the PIP joint. Which of the following statements is true?

A. Partial volar plate avulsion is rarely associated with lateral PIP dislocation

B. DIP joint dislocations are more common than PIP joint dislocations

C. Partial tears of the PIP are treated by open repair

D. The joint should be stressed in three planes to assess ligamentous stability

E. The joint should not be x-rayed since associated fracture is rare

7. A 50-year-old male sustains a fall while skiing. On presentation, his chief complaint is thumb pain. X-ray findings are normal. PE reveals tenderness over the ulnar aspect of the MCP joint. Which of the following statements is true concerning this injury?

A. A tear of the ulnar collateral ligament should be suspected

B. Avulsion fracture of the volar base frequently accompanies this injury

C. Complete rupture of the ulnar collateral ligament is treated with thumb spica for 2-3 weeks

D. This injury is easily diagnosed on x-ray

E. This may have been the result of forced ulnar deviation (adduction)

8. A 36-year-old carpenter is working on a new home and is temporarily distracted. He misses a nail with his hammer and hits his distal phalanx, which was hanging over the end of a board. Examination reveals erythema and swelling of the DIP joint. The skin and nail are intact. Which of the following is true (Figure 41-2)?

A. Antibiotics are indicated

B. If not properly treated, this may result in boutonniere deformity

C. Optimal management is K-wire fixation

D. There is likely involvement of the flexor tendon

E. This represents a zone III injury

9. Concerning injuries to the hand, choose the correct treatment method:

A. Closed distal tuft fracture requiring symptomatic treatment

B. Closed mallet finger deformity without intraarticular involvement of fracture; requires splint in mild hyperflexion

C. Flexor tendon laceration; treatment is antibiotics, superficial skin closure, referral

D. Injection of solvent via high-pressure gun requiring immediate operative debridement

E. Roofing nail driven through the thumb causing intraarticular PIP joint fracture; removal of foreign

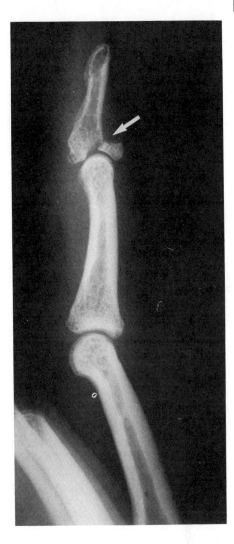

**FIG. 41-2** From Rosen P: *Diagnostic radiology in emergency medicine,* St Louis, 1992, Mosby.

body, first-generation cephalosporin, and follow-up with specialist within 72 hours will be required

10. A 14-year-old girl presents to the ED after having her finger caught in a printing press. Her x-ray reveals an intact distal tuft. She is quite upset and is bleeding from the injured site. Examination reveals avulsion of the distal one third of the nail and fingertip. Which of the following is true concerning treatment?

A. If exposed bone is present, primary closure is the treatment of choice

B. Injuries 1 cm proximal to the eponychium may be re-implanted

C. Lidocaine 1% with epinephrine injected at the base of the digit should be used to achieve good hemostasis within the wound site

D. This is the third most common injury to the upper extremity

E. Reimplantation of avulsed segments distal to the nail is generally indicated, but only in adults

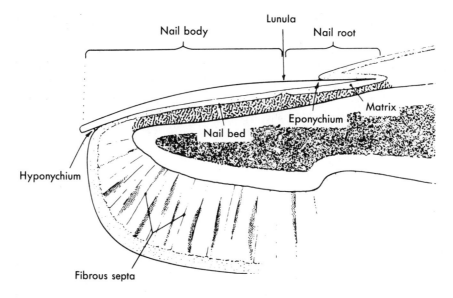

Nail body    Lunula    Nail root

Matrix

Eponychium

Nail bed

Hyponychium

Fibrous septa

**FIG. 41-3**    From Siegel DB, Gelberman RH: *Orthop Clin North Am* 19(4): 779, 1988.

11. Regarding Figure 41-3, choose the correct matching pair:
    A. Eponychium: where nail substance is made
    B. Matrix: if avulsed should be allowed to heal by secondary intention
    C. Nail bed: requires loose approximation since nail deformity is rare
    D. Nail body: provides support for volar fingertip during "pinching"
    E. Zone I line: injury at this zone must be closed primarily

12. Concerning infections involving the hand, which is the correct statement?
    A. A paronychia is usually due to blunt trauma
    B. An early paronychia may be treated with warm soaks, Cephalexin, and immobilization
    C. An eponychia may be treated with warm soaks and antibiotics
    D. Diabetic patients should be treated with an aminoglycoside alone because of the high incidence of gram-negative infections
    E. In human bite wounds, infection with *Staphylococcus aureus* should be suspected, but antibiotics are usually not indicated

13. A 58-year-old male with a history of hypertension complains of pain, swelling, and redness of his right index finger. Examination reveals a tense, erythematous distal phalanx with abscess involving the lateral nail space with extension into the pulp of the fingertip. Concerning treatment of this infection, which of the following statements is true?
    A. Osteomyelitis is a common complication
    B. The wound should be thoroughly irrigated and the skin edges approximated with non-absorbent sutures
    C. Treatment includes first-generation cephalosporin, incision and drainage along the ulnar aspect of the wound, and splinting
    D. Treatment includes penicillinase-resistant oral penicillin, incision and drainage along the radial aspect, and splinting
    E. Treatment mandates incision and drainage of the abscess, IV antibiotics, and immediate consultation with a hand surgeon

## 42 ▼ Forearm and Wrist

*R. Alan Shubert and Sunanda Nabha*

Select the appropriate letter that correctly answers the question or completes the statement.

1. Which of the following is the most commonly fractured carpal bone?
   A. Hamate
   B. Lunate
   C. Scaphoid
   D. Trapezium

2. Approximately what percentage of scaphoid fractures are not detected on plain radiography?
   A. 5%
   B. 10%
   C. 15%
   D. 20%

3. Which test should be performed, at 2 weeks after injury, to rule out a scaphoid fracture after repeat plain x-rays are negative?
   A. MRI
   B. Nothing
   C. Plain tomogram
   D. Technetium bone scan
   E. Ultrasound

4. According to the Mayfield and Yeager four-stage classification of carpal dislocations, lunate dislocations are associated with which stage?
   A. Stage I
   B. Stage II
   C. Stage III
   D. Stage IV
5. Colles' fracture, the most common wrist fracture, involves which of the following bones?
   A. Distal radius
   B. Hamate
   C. Proximal ulna
   D. Radial head
6. What is the most sensitive test for diagnosing carpal tunnel syndrome on physical examination?
   A. Forced extension maneuver
   B. Phalen's test
   C. Reilly manipulation
   D. Tinel's test
7. What is a fracture involving the junction of the proximal and middle thirds of the ulna with associated anterior dislocation of the radial head called?
   A. Bado's fracture
   B. Galeazzi fracture
   C. Monteggia's fracture
   D. Nightstick fracture
8. A 45-year-old female presents to the emergency department complaining of pain in her wrists. She says she has had worsening discomfort over the past 2 months and also has some tingling sensations in her index finger. She doesn't understand why, but the pain is worse at night. She is an executive secretary and reports no other serious medical problems. On physical examination, the patient is found to have mild thenar wasting of the right hand, and when asked to flex the wrists she complains of increasing numbness in the index and middle finger. What is the most likely diagnosis?
   A. Carpal tunnel syndrome
   B. Flexor tenosynovitis
   C. Osteoarthritis
   D. Raynaud's phenomenon
9. A 27-year-old man has fallen on his out-stretched right arm. His only complaint is wrist pain. He is exquisitely tender over the anatomic snuffbox but has full range of motion and an intact neurologic and circulatory examination of the affected extremity. A radiograph of his wrist fails to reveal a fracture or a dislocation. Which of the following treatments is most appropriate?
   A. Ace wrap and sling
   B. Long arm cast
   C. Short arm cast
   D. Short arm thumb spica cast
   E. Sugar-tong splint and repeat x-ray in 10 days
10. All of the following are true of a perilunate dislocation except which one?
   A. A triangular "piece of pie appearance" of the lunate on the PA film is pathognomonic

B. Clinical findings may be subtle and overlooked
C. It is a midcarpal dislocation resulting from a violent hyperextension injury
D. All of the above

# 43 ▼ Humerus and Elbow

*Paul R. Sierzenski and Leonard A. Nitowski*

Select the appropriate letter that correctly answers the question or completes the statement.
1. The posterior compartment of the upper arm (humerus), contains which of the following structures?
   A. Biceps brachei
   B. Brachial artery
   C. Median nerve
   D. Radial nerve
   E. Ulnar nerve
2. An 8-year-old boy presents with complaints of left arm pain after a football injury. Physical examination reveals a "carrying angle" of 30 degrees, which is 15 degrees greater than his right arm. This finding is most consistent with:
   A. Anterior elbow dislocation
   B. Axillary nerve injury
   C. Early compartment syndrome
   D. Supracondylar fracture
   E. None of the above
3. What is the most reliable early sign of compartment syndrome?
   A. Pain in the involved extremity
   B. Pallor of the extremity
   C. Paralysis of the extremity
   D. Paresthesias of the extremity
   E. Pulselessness on examination
4. A 37-year-old woman falls forward, landing on her outstretched arm. She presents with pain on active flexion, extension, pronation, and supination. The x-ray finding most specific for an occult radial head fracture is:
   A. Anterior fat pad sign
   B. Carrying angle of 12 degrees
   C. Periosteal elevation of the radius
   D. Posterior fat pad sign
   E. Superficial soft tissue swelling
5. Bowman's angle, as assessed on anteroposterior (AP) x-rays, is the intersection of a line drawn through the midshaft of the humerus and the growthplate of the capitulum. Bowman's angle should measure approximately how many degrees?
   A. 25
   B. 45
   C. 75
   D. 90
   E. 180

6. Midshaft humerus fractures often result in which of the following neurovascular complications?
   A. Brachial artery injury
   B. Compartment syndrome
   C. Median nerve injury
   D. Radial nerve injury
   E. Ulnar nerve injury
7. What is the most common mechanism of injury for supracondylar fractures in children?
   A. Avulsion injury: longitudinal pull on the arm in pronation
   B. Extension injury: fall on an outstretched hand
   C. Flexion injury: direct blow to the olecranon
   D. Spiral injury: twisting of the arm
   E. None of the above
8. Motor weakness of the interossei, or loss of sensation over the palmar aspect of the fifth digit and hypothenar eminence suggests which of the following?
   A. Carpal tunnel syndrome
   B. Median nerve injury
   C. Musculocutaneous nerve injury
   D. Radial nerve injury
   E. Ulnar nerve injury
9. What do the x-rays pictured in Figure 43-1 reveal?
   A. Anterior dislocation of the elbow
   B. Medial epicondyle fracture
   C. Olecranon fracture
   D. Posterior dislocation of the elbow
   E. Radial head dislocation (Nursemaid's elbow)
10. A serious complication of the injury pictured in Figure 43-1 is:
    A. Brachial artery injury
    B. Compartment syndrome
    C. Radial nerve injury
    D. Ulnar artery injury
    E. Ulnar nerve injury
11. A 12-year-old boy presents with elbow pain after pitching nine innings of baseball. His examination reveals tenderness over the medial aspect of the affected elbow. His injury is most likely:
    A. Avulsion of the medial epicondyle
    B. Fracture of the capitulum
    C. Olecranon bursitis
    D. Ulnar dislocation
    E. None of the above
12. What is the best treatment of radial head subluxation (nursemaid's elbow)?
    A. Immediate referral to an orthopedist
    B. Longitudinal traction and forearm pronation only
    C. Pressure over the radial head only
    D. Pressure over the radial head with forearm supination and elbow flexion
    E. Pressure over the radial head with longitudinal traction and forearm pronation

# 44 Shoulder

*Greg Ledbetter*

Select the appropriate letter that correctly answers the question or completes the statement.

1. All of the following statements regarding the radiologic examination of the shoulder are correct except which one?
   A. Proper radiologic examination requires a minimum of two views at right angles to one another

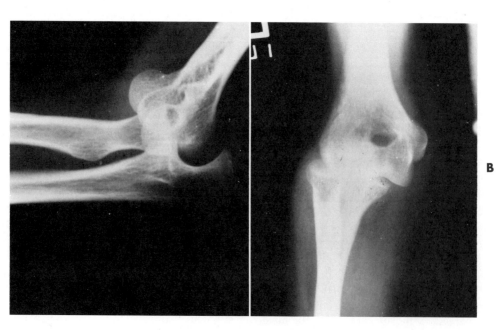

**FIG. 43-1**

B. Standard AP projections in internal and external rotation are inadequate because they project the humerus in a single (frontal) plane

C. The axillary lateral view projects the glenohumeral joint in the cephalocaudal plane

D. The transthoracic lateral view is the preferred and most useful orthogonal projection

E. The true AP view projects the glenohumeral joint without any overlap

2. All of the following statements regarding scapular fractures are correct except which one?

A. Severely comminuted and displaced fractures will usually require operative repair

B. Scapular fractures account for 1% of all fractures and less than 5% of all shoulder girdle injuries

C. The presence of a scapular fracture mandates a thorough search for associated injuries of the ipsilateral lung, chest wall, and shoulder girdle complex

D. The incidence of associated pneumothorax is 12% to 62%; pneumothorax may become evident 2 to 3 days after the initial injury

3. All of the following statements are true concerning proximal humerus fractures except which one?

A. More than 80% can be handled with close orthopedic follow up

B. Salter Harris I or II fractures through the proximal humerus in children are common fractures that require only routine orthopedic follow up

C. The classic mechanism producing proximal humerus fractures is falling on an outstretched, abducted arm

D. The most common complication is adhesive capsulitis

4. Which of the following statements regarding proximal humeral epiphyseal fractures is incorrect?

A. The fracture occurs through the hypertrophic zone of the epiphyseal growth plate

B. The injury is most common in young males between 4 and 10 years of age

C. The strength of the joint capsule is two to five times greater than that of the epiphyseal growth plate

D. The usual etiologic factors are contact sports or falls from heights

5. All of the following statements regarding injuries of the sternoclavicular joint are correct except which one?

A. A grade II injury (subluxation) is characterized by rupture of the sternoclavicular and costoclavicular ligaments

B. Anterior dislocations are far more common (9:1 ratio)

C. Posterior dislocations are associated with severe pain, and the neck is frequently flexed toward the injured side

D. Posterior dislocations may be associated with life-threatening injuries within the superior mediastinum

6. A 24-year-old male with a history of epilepsy complains of left shoulder pain. The shoulder has a flat, squared-off appearance, and the arm is fixed in adduction and internal rotation. Abduction is limited, and external rotation is completely blocked. What is the most likely diagnosis?

A. Inferior dislocation (luxatio erecta)

B. Subacromial posterior dislocation

C. Subcoracoid anterior dislocation

D. Subglenoid anterior dislocation

7. All of the following statements regarding the Hill-Sachs deformity are correct except which one?

A. The deformity is best visualized on an internal rotation view of the glenohumeral joint

B. The deformity is reported to be present in 11%-50% of all anterior dislocations

C. The deformity represents a compression fracture of the anteromedial aspect of the humeral head

D. Recurrent anterior dislocations have a higher incidence of Hill-Sachs deformity

8. After reduction of a subcoracoid anterior glenohumeral dislocation, a patient complains of numbness over the lateral aspect of the shoulder and inability to abduct the shoulder. Which is the most likely diagnosis?

A. Adhesive capsulitis

B. Axillary nerve injury

C. Brachial plexus injury

D. Rotator cuff tear

9. Radiologic findings with a posterior dislocation can include all of the following except which one?

A. Abnormal overlap of the humeral head with the glenoid fossa on a true AP (45-degree) film

B. An increased distance between the anterior glenoid rim and the articular surface of the humeral head on a standard AP film (rim sign)

C. Compression fracture of the posterolateral aspect of the humeral head (Hill-Sachs deformity)

D. Internal rotation and a "light bulb" appearance of the humeral head on the standard AP film

10. What is the most common muscle injured in a rotator cuff tear?

A. Infraspinatus

B. Subscapularis

C. Supraspinatus

D. Teres minor

11. The following are all true about rotator cuff tears except:

A. Decrease in flexion and abduction are early signs of a rotator cuff tear.

B. Drop arm test is positive in significant tears.

C. Hallmark of a complete tear on AP shoulder x-ray is superior displacement of the humeral head.

D. Most rotator cuff tears are associated with an acute traumatic event.

12. Following a recent fracture of the right wrist, a 45-year-old woman complains of pain and stiffness in the right shoulder. The pain localizes over the deltoid area and is most severe at night. There is uniform limitation of all active glenohumeral motion and a sense of mechanical restriction of joint motion on passive testing. What is the most likely diagnosis?

A. Adhesive capsulitis

B. Bicipital tendinitis

C. Calcific tendinitis

D. Rotator cuff tear

# 45 Pelvis and Hip

*Greg Ledbetter*

Select the appropriate letter that correctly answers the question or completes the statement.

1. Which is true concerning radiographic views of the pelvis?
   A. Anteroposterior (AP) view is used to demonstrate the extent of fractures and the degree of bony displacement
   B. On the AP view, the symphysis is normally less than 10 mm wide and the sacroiliac joint less than 5 mm wide
   C. The CT scan has not been shown to be superior to standard x-rays of the pelvis
   D. The inlet and outlet views help visualize hard to see sacral fractures and SI joint disruption
2. A pelvic fracture is often associated with all of the following except:
   A. Blood at the urethral meatus
   B. Maisonneuve's fracture
   C. Rotation of the iliac crest or leg length discrepancy
   D. Turner's sign
3. A 49-year-old female has pain in her hip after a fall. The AP pelvis and lateral hip x-rays are normal. To detect an occult acetabular fracture, what should the doctor order next?
   A. CT scan of the pelvis
   B. Inlet/outlet views of the pelvis
   C. Judet views of the hip
   D. Reorder the AP view of the pelvis
4. Avascular necrosis of the femoral head occurs most commonly after which of the following conditions?
   A. Acetabular fractures
   B. Congenital dislocation of the hip
   C. Intracapsular femoral neck fractures
   D. Septic arthritis of the hip joint

*Match each of the following terms with the appropriate statement.*
   A. Avascular necrosis of the femoral head
   B. Septic arthritis of the hip joint
   C. Transient synovitis of the hip

5. A 25-year-old man with a history of a hip dislocation that occurred in an auto accident. The patient now has pain in the groin and restriction of internal rotation and abduction of the previously dislocated hip _____
6. This is often attributed to a mild traumatic episode or a low-grade febrile illness such as tonsillitis or otitis media _____
7. A 10-year-old boy with a normal temperature and the insidious onset of pain in his left hip that radiates down into the left thigh and knee _____
8. A 65-year-old female missed a step and fell down in her home. On examination, her right leg appeared short-

ened, flexed, adducted, and internally rotated. On questioning she complains of pain in her right buttock radiating down the back of her leg. What is the most likely diagnosis?
   A. Anterior dislocation of hip
   B. Posterior dislocation of hip
   C. Pubic rami fracture
   D. Sacral fracture
   E. Slipped capital femoral epiphysis

# 46 Injuries of the Proximal Femur

*Greg Ledbetter*

Select the appropriate letter that correctly answers the question or completes the statement.

1. An open femur fracture that occurred on a farm requires which antibiotic regimen?
   A. Gentamicin
   B. Kefzol
   C. Penicillin
   D. All of the above
2. Avascular necrosis of the femoral head is a relatively common complication (>10%) in all femur fractures except for which of these?
   A. Femoral head fracture with posterior dislocation
   B. Femoral neck fracture (Garden I)
   C. Femoral neck fracture (Garden IV)
   D. Intertrochanteric fracture
3. The treatment of muscle strains includes all of the following except:
   A. Analgesics and antiinflammatory agents
   B. Early mobilization to prevent traumatic myositis ossificans
   C. Orthopedic consultation or follow-up in suspected third-degree sprains
   D. X-rays to rule out an associated avulsion fracture
4. All of the following are true regarding femoral head fractures except which one?
   A. The mechanism of injury is most commonly a fall
   B. The patient is usually unable to bear weight
   C. They are usually associated with hip dislocations
   D. They occur most commonly in young patients
5. Which of the following is true regarding femoral neck fractures?
   A. The majority of fractures are the result of only minor trauma
   B. They occur most commonly in elderly patients
   C. They occur most frequently in women
   D. With Garden I and II fractures, the patient may be able to ambulate
   E. All of the above
6. Which is the most common fracture of the femur?
   A. Femoral head

B. Femoral neck

C. Intertrochanteric

D. Subtrochanteric

E. None of the above

7. All of the following are frequently associated with femoral shaft fractures except which one?

A. Hip dislocation

B. Large volume blood loss

C. Ligamentous knee injuries

D. Nerve injuries

E. Patellar fracture

8. A 14-year-old obese boy comes to the ED complaining of left hip pain. He relates a 3-week history of groin and left medial thigh pain that has gradually increased, becoming more severe after he tripped and fell while running. There is tenderness over the left hip and decreased range of motion. An AP radiograph of the hip reveals no obvious abnormalities. What is the most likely diagnosis?

A. Anterior hip dislocation

B. Femoral stress fracture

C. Legg-Calvé-Perthes disease

D. Posterior hip dislocation

E. Slipped capital (proximal) femoral epiphysis

9. Which of the following is a contraindication to application of a Hare traction splint in a patient with a femur fracture?

A. Evidence of sciatic nerve injury

B. Large thigh hematoma

C. Open fracture with exposed bone ends

D. Both A and B

E. Both A and C

10. All of the following may be initially treated on an outpatient basis except which one?

A. Femoral stress fractures

B. Isolated greater trochanteric fractures

C. Isolated lesser trochanteric fractures

D. Slipped capital femoral epiphysis

E. All of the above

11. Which of the following is not true regarding greater and lesser trochanter fractures?

A. Lesser trochanter fractures are usually treated with bed rest followed by early mobilization

B. Lesser trochanter fractures with more than 2 cm separation of the avulsed fragment are usually treated with open reduction and internal fixation

C. Greater trochanter fractures can usually be treated like soft tissue injuries, with several days of bed rest followed by partial weight bearing

D. Greater trochanter fractures with more than 1 cm separation of the avulsed fragment are usually treated with open reduction and internal fixation

E. All of the above

12. Which of the following regarding femoral stress fractures is true?

A. Diagnosis is important because stress fractures may progress to displaced fractures if treated inappropriately

B. Orthopedic consultation is not necessary

C. Some stress fractures may require internal fixation

D. Treatment initially involves narcotic analgesia and weight bearing as tolerated

E. Both A and C

F. Both B and D

*Match each of the following terms with the appropriate statement.*

A. Femoral arterial injury

B. Femoral venous injury

C. Both

D. Neither

13. The presence of distal pulses excludes this injury _____

14. The most appropriate initial treatment is ligation or clamping of the injured vessel _____

15. May cause hemorrhagic shock _____

---

 # 47 Knee and Lower Leg

*Greg Ledbetter*

Select the appropriate letter that correctly answers the question or completes the statement.

1. A college football player comes to the ED with his athletic trainer, who is worried about a hyperextension injury with possible posterior dislocation of the patient's knee. The patient's knee has a small joint effusion and good pulses distally. Which of the following is required in the work-up?

A. Arteriogram of the affected knee

B. Arthrocentesis of the affected knee

C. Arthroscopy of the affected knee

D. MRI of the affected knee

2. Any disruption of the quadriceps mechanism requires which of the following?

A. Immobilization for partial disruption

B. Immobilization only for complete disruption

C. Surgical repair for partial or complete disruption

D. Non-weight bearing only

3. A long-distance runner comes to the ED with the complaint of gradual onset of pain in his knee, which now affects his running. When the patient is questioned about the point of maximum tenderness, he points to an area over and above the lateral epicondyle of his femur. The remainder of his joint examination is normal. What is the diagnosis?

A. Anterior cruciate ligament tear

B. Baker's cyst

C. Iliotibial band tendinitis

D. Lateral meniscal tear

4. A 13-year-old boy with no history of trauma has an insidious onset of infrapatellar pain. Which of the following is the most likely diagnosis?
   A. Anserine bursitis
   B. Baker's cyst
   C. Osgood-Schlatter disease
   D. Popliteal artery aneurysm

5. A patient complains of painful swelling in his right knee. He states the swelling is sometimes very pronounced and painful. Other times he barely feels anything. A tense, fluid-filled sac is palpable in the popliteal fossa. What does this most likely represent?
   A. Anserine bursitis
   B. Gouty arthritis
   C. Inflammation of the semimembranous or medial gastrocnemius bursa
   D. Tibial artery aneurysm

6. The Segond fracture or (lateral capsular sign) is a small vertical avulsion injury of the lateral aspect of the proximal tibia just distal to the plateau. Which ligaments are most commonly injured in association with a Segond fracture?
   A. Lateral collateral and anterior cruciate ligaments
   B. Lateral collateral and posterior cruciate ligaments
   C. Medial collateral and anterior cruciate ligaments
   D. Medial collateral and posterior cruciate ligaments

7. A patient is diagnosed as having patellar bursitis following knee trauma. After several days of immobilization, local heat, and antiinflammatory drugs, the patient returns complaining of increased swelling and pain. What would the appropriate treatment be?
   A. Aspirate the fluid and send for appropriate studies
   B. Order radiographs to check for osteomyelitis and if results are negative, reassure the patient
   C. Reassure the patient that this is to be expected
   D. Do a work-up for deep venous thrombosis

8. A runner comes to the ED with the complaint of persistent dull ache over the anterior aspect of his lower extremities. Upon physical examination the patient is found to have point tenderness over the anterior tibia. Plain radiograph shows no signs of fracture. Findings and diagnosis are consistent with a stress fracture. With regard to stress fractures, all the following statements are true except which one?
   A. A high incidence of stress fractures is seen in premenopausal female athletes who are amenorrheic
   B. In the athlete the most common site of stress fractures is the metatarsals
   C. Most tibial stress fractures are along the middle third of the tibial shaft
   D. The most important clinical diagnostic sign is point tenderness over the bony structure

9. A young female high school athlete complains of bilateral, poorly localized knee pain. She states that she just began training after a period of inactivity and denies any trauma. The pain is worse when she climbs stairs. The patella compression test is positive. This is consistent with which condition?
   A. Anserine bursitis
   B. Baker's cyst
   C. Chondromalacia patella
   D. Osgood-Schlatter disease
   E. Stress fracture

10. What is the best test for determining the integrity of the anterior cruciate ligament?
    A. Anterior drawer test
    B. Knee x-ray
    C. Lachman's test
    D. Posterior drawer test

11. All of the following statements about tibial plateau fractures are true except:
    A. A fat-fluid level on lateral knee x-ray is highly suggestive of an occult fracture
    B. Ligament injuries occur in 20%-25% of tibial plateau fractures, usually involving the anterior cruciate ligament and the medial collateral ligament
    C. Peroneal nerve injuries should be considered in tibial plateau fractures
    D. Vascular injuries are rare in tibial plateau fractures because of the location of the popliteal artery in relation to the tibial plateau

12. What is the Q angle useful in?
    A. Anterior cruciate ligament injuries
    B. Calcaneus fractures
    C. Patella dislocations
    D. Tibial plateau fractures

13. A football player comes to the emergency department with knee pain after being tackled by a 200-pound linebacker. The patient has a positive Lachman's test and valgus laxity. The rest of the physical examination findings are normal. What has the patient most likely damaged?
    A. Anterior cruciate ligament, lateral collateral ligament, and the lateral meniscus
    B. Anterior cruciate ligament, lateral collateral ligament, and the medial meniscus
    C. Anterior cruciate ligament, medial collateral ligament, and the lateral meniscus
    D. Posterior cruciate ligament, medial collateral ligament, and the medial meniscus

# 48 Ankle and Foot

*Greg Ledbetter*

Select the appropriate letter that correctly answers the question or completes the statement.

1. A 19-year-old basketball player comes to the ED complaining of an acute ankle injury. He describes an eversion mechanism and has tenderness over the deltoid and anterior tibiofibular ligaments. Which of the following radiograph views should be included in the work-up in addition to routine ankle views?

A. Calcaneal views
B. Fibular views
C. Navicular views
D. Plantar and dorsiflexion

2. A patient with a grade II ankle sprain would have all of the following except which one?
   A. Initially no pain and then increasing pain
   B. Moderate flexion loss
   C. Partial ligamentous tear
   D. Swelling and localized hemorrhage

3. Peroneal tendon dislocations of the ankle usually result from forceful passive dorsiflexion with slight inversion, resulting in a violent reflex contraction of the peroneal tendons. The patient may complain of a snapping or popping sensation during activities such as jogging or walking on uneven ground. When the diagnosis of superior peroneal retinaculum injury is entertained, the patient should initially be splinted in which of the following positions?
   A. Dorsiflexion with eversion
   B. Full dorsiflexion
   C. Full plantar flexion
   D. Midplantar flexion

4. A patient complains of the insidious onset of burning pain on the plantar surface of the foot. The pain radiates superiorly along the medial side of the calf. Rest decreases the pain. What does this suggest?
   A. Cuboid ligament sprain
   B. Plantar fascitis
   C. Tarsal tunnel syndrome
   D. Tenosynovitis of the extensor digitorum longus

5. How should nondisplaced distal third phalangeal fractures of the foot should be treated?
   A. Cast to the ankle
   B. Dynamic splinting
   C. Internal fixation
   D. Open-toe orthopedic shoe

6. The Ottawa Ankle Rules state that ankle radiographs are indicated in all of the following situations except which one?
   A. Bone tenderness at the medial or lateral malleolus
   B. Bone tenderness at the posterior edge of the distal 6 cm of the ankle
   C. Inability to bear weight on the ankle now or at the time of the accident
   D. Soft tissue swelling over the medial or lateral malleolus

7. Which of the following ankle fractures could be handled on an outpatient basis with close orthopedic follow up?
   A. Displaced medial malleolar fracture
   B. Lateral malleolar fracture with point tenderness over the deltoid ligament
   C. Nondisplaced bimalleolar fracture
   D. Weber type A lateral malleolar fracture

8. The test for Achilles tendon rupture is the:
   A. Anterior drawer test
   B. McMurray test
   C. Talar tilt test
   D. Thompson test

9. All of the following are true statements about calcaneal fractures except which one?
   A. 10% of calcaneal fractures have associated vertebral compression fractures
   B. Boehler's angle is useful in diagnosing calcaneal compression fractures
   C. Most calcaneal fractures can be handled on an outpatient basis with close orthopedic follow-up
   D. The calcaneus is the most commonly fractured tarsal bone

## SECTION 6 SOFT-TISSUE TRAUMA

## 49 Foreign Bodies

*Greg Ledbetter*

Select the appropriate letter that correctly answers the question or completes the statement.

1. A 30-year-old man comes to the ED complaining of foreign-body sensation in the right eye. A brief examination confirms penetrating globe injury. What action would be appropriate for the emergency physician?
   A. Give next-day ophthalmologic referral
   B. Instill a cycloplegic solution
   C. Instill antimicrobial drops
   D. Patch the opposite eye
   E. Perform a thorough slit-lamp examination

2. Which of the following would best facilitate removal of a foreign body from the ear canal?
   A. Avoiding the use of forceps to grasp the object
   B. Directing irrigation at the periphery of the object
   C. Placing the patient in Trendelenburg's position
   D. Pulling the pinna anteriorly to straighten the canal
   E. Reassuring the patient of the canal's insensitivity

3. Which patient is least likely to have a nasal foreign body?
   A. 2-year-old girl whose father says, "I saw her put a raisin in her nose."
   B. 3-year-old boy whose mother says, "He is always picking at his nose."
   C. 4-year-old girl whose father says, "She has body odor worse than mine."
   D. 5-year-old boy whose grandmother says, "He has bad smelling mucus from his right nostril."
   E. 6-year-old girl referred by her dentist with suspected nasal foreign body on dental x-ray.

4. An upper esophageal foreign body is most often oriented in which plane?
   A. Anteroposterior
   B. Coronal
   C. Oblique
   D. Sagittal
   E. Transverse

5. Review the radiographs in Figure 49-1, which were obtained on a child with a history suggestive of an aspirated foreign body. A is an inspiratory chest film; B is a forced expiratory chest film. What diagnosis is most likely?
   A. Early complete obstruction of left mainstem bronchus
   B. Early complete obstruction of right mainstem bronchus
   C. Late complete obstruction of left mainstem bronchus
   D. Partial obstruction of left mainstem bronchus
   E. Partial obstruction of right mainstem bronchus

6. A 35-year-old woman is eating in the hospital snack bar when she suddenly chokes and is unable to breathe. Several trained bystanders correctly perform the Heimlich maneuver and oropharyngeal finger sweep without effect. The patient is rushed to the ED, where she is found to be unconscious and apneic. What is the next step for the emergency physician?
   A. Emergency cricothyrotomy
   B. Emergency tracheostomy
   C. Four chest thrusts
   D. Indirect laryngoscopy
   E. Repeat Heimlich maneuver

7. A 55-year-old woman comes to the ED and says, "I choked on a fish bone, and now it's stuck in my throat." She complains of pain in the throat but has no respiratory compromise. Palpation of the neck reveals subcutaneous emphysema. What procedure would not be appropriate?
   A. Barium radiographic contrast study
   B. Direct laryngoscopy
   C. Endoscopy by a qualified gastroenterologist
   D. Indirect laryngoscopy
   E. Soft tissue lateral cervical spine radiography

8. A 65-year-old man comes to the ED 10 hours after eating steak. He complains of severe chest pain on swallowing and is noted to be drooling. A Gastrografin study confirms complete esophageal obstruction. What treatment option is best?
   A. Enzymatic degradation with oral papain solution
   B. Extraction under direct endoscopic visualization
   C. Glucagon 0.5 to 2.0 mg by rapid IV infusion
   D. Passage of bolus by oral ingestion of gas-forming agents
   E. Removal by Foley catheter balloon technique

9. A 3-year-old boy is brought to the ED after swallowing a disk (button) battery containing mercury. Abdominal radiograph confirms an intact disk battery in the stomach. What should the emergency physician recommend next?
   A. Chelation therapy to prevent mercury poisoning
   B. Immediate endoscopic extraction of the battery
   C. Ipecac administration to induce emesis and battery removal

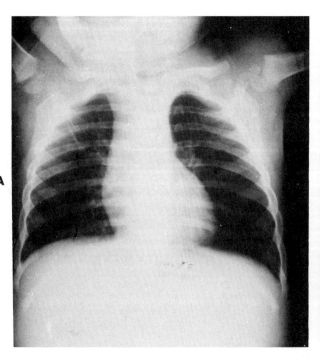
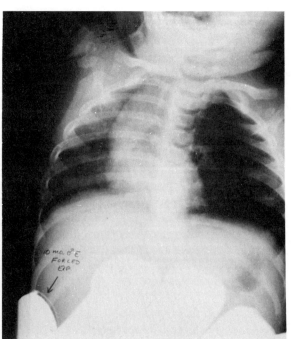

FIG. 49-1

D. Parents' observation of stools with no formal follow-up
E. Referral for a follow-up radiograph

10. A 24-year-old man comes to the ED complaining of abdominal and rectal pain. An abdominal radiograph is obtained (Figure. 49-2). An accompanying upright radiograph indicates free air under the diaphragm. How should this object be removed?
    A. Air insufflation via Foley catheter to reverse vacuum effect
    B. Instrumental extraction sigmoidoscopy
    C. Manual extraction after digital examination
    D. Surgical approach in the operating room
    E. Visualization by proctoscope and ring forceps grasp

11. A 35-year-old woman comes to the ED with a gunshot wound to the right leg. On physical examination, vital signs are stable. There is an entrance wound in the right popliteal fossa, but no exit wound. There are palpable pulses distally and sensory motor testing is intact. What imaging study is required?
    A. Arteriogram
    B. Computerized tomography
    C. Soft tissue radiograph
    D. Sonogram
    E. Xeroradiogram

12. A 25-year-old man fell 40 feet at a construction site and was impaled on a 6-foot metal spike, which passed completely through his left thigh. He is tachycardic but otherwise stable. Paramedics are on the scene but cannot get the patient into their helicopter because of the protruding spike. What should the emergency physician acting as medical director recommend?
    A. Await special transport such as a flatbed truck
    B. Await the on-scene arrival of a specially trained trauma team
    C. Cut off the spike close to the patient, stabilize it, and transport the patient
    D. Immediately extract the spike and transport the patient to the nearest hospital
    E. Push the spike through because a track is already established

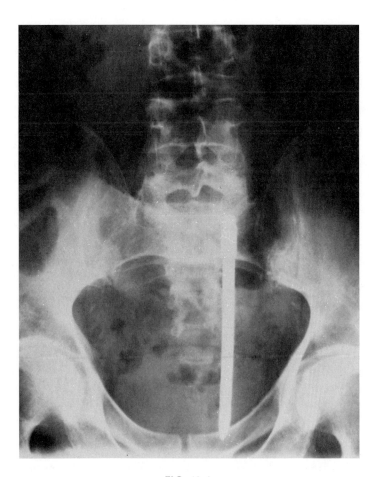

FIG. 49-2

13. A 30-year-old man comes to the ED with severe left hand pain after he accidentally triggered a high-pressure grease gun, injecting his left palm. Physical examination shows a pinpoint puncture wound to the left palm. The hand is slightly edematous and erythematous and is very dirty with grease and oil. What is the most important intervention by the emergency physician?
   A. Antibiotic administration covering skin flora, especially *Staphylococcus*
   B. Careful history concerning tetanus immunity status
   C. Elevating the hand to reduce swelling and pressure on neurovascular structures
   D. Emergency surgical referral for decompression and debridement
   E. Thorough cleansing with degreasers and surgical scrub

14. A 32-year-old female is brought to the ED by police after she swallowed several condoms filled with cocaine to avoid arrest. The police have a court order for recovery of evidence. The patient is stable and has an unremarkable examination. All of the following are appropriate actions except which one?
   A. Administration of ipecac to induce vomiting
   B. Admission to hospital or jail infirmary for observation
   C. Consultation with general surgeon for emergency laparotomy
   D. Gut decontamination with charcoal if signs of drug intoxication occur
   E. Request for clarification of the court order while treating

# 50 ▼ Soft-Tissue Spine Injuries and Back Pain

*Barbara N. Wynn*

Select the appropriate letter that correctly answers the question or completes the statement.

1. Which of the following best describes the evaluation of neck injuries?
   A. Appropriate radiographs can definitively diagnose cervical strain
   B. CT scan is safer than MRI in pregnant women
   C. CT scan with and without contrast is the radiographic modality of choice in cervical disk disease
   D. Radiographs are not indicated in acute torticollis
   E. When attempting to exclude a cervical fracture, lateral AP odontoid and flexion extension films are the initial required studies

2. Which of the following is most characteristic of cervical strain?
   A. Complaints of numbness, weakness or paresthesias in the arms are rare
   B. Head rests have significantly reduced the incidence of cervical hyperextension injuries

C. Most patients develop pain immediately after an accident
   D. Patients should be advised to expect a prolonged treatment period
   E. Use of soft collars is controversial and probably not indicated

3. In which of the following are plain radiographs believed to be important?
   A. Cervical disk herniation
   B. Lumbar disk herniation
   C. Lumbosacral strain
   D. Thoracic disk herniation
   E. Thoracic muscle strain

4. Which of the following best describes the epidemiology of back pain?
   A. Disk herniation is least common in 30 to 40 year olds
   B. Eighty percent of the population will undergo back pain at some point
   C. Incidence of disk herniation increases in pregnancy
   D. It is unique to the industrialized world
   E. Sex, age younger than 45 to 50 years, posture, congenital differences in leg length, and mild scoliosis are associated with an increased incidence of back pain

5. In which of the following patients presenting with back pain is a lumbar x-ray indicated?
   A. 6-year-old boy with no history of trauma
   B. 30-year-old attorney with pain for 10 days
   C. 36-year-old accountant with no history of trauma
   D. 40-year-old teacher with pain for 3 weeks
   E. 45-year-old manager with pain after moving a television set

6. A 19-year-old college gymnast presents with low back pain after falling from the uneven parallel bars. Lumbar x-rays show 25% slippage of L5 on S1. What condition does this describe?
   A. Scheuermann's disease
   B. Spondylolisthesis
   C. Spondylolysis
   D. Spondylosis
   E. Transitional vertebrae

7. What is the most accurate neurologic examination?
   A. Foot dorsiflexion tests L4 motor function
   B. Knee reflexes test L3-4 motor function
   C. L5 motor function is tested by having the patient walk on toes
   D. Positive straight leg test is back pain without leg pain
   E. S1 dermatome involves the medial foot and web space of the great toe

8. Which of the following is least indicative of disk pain?
   A. Back pain greater than leg pain
   B. Leg pain distal to the knee
   C. Motor and deep tendon reflex deficit
   D. Positive straight leg rare
   E. Sharp shooting pain

9. Which of the following admission criteria for back pain is suggestive of a spinal tumor?

A. Cauda equina syndrome
B. Multiple nerve root involvement
C. Progressive neurologic deficit
D. Severe neurologic deficit
E. Severe unremitting pain

10. All of the following describe appropriate management of acute back pain except:
    A. Advising the patient with mechanical back pain to expect improvement within 2 months
    B. Emergent neurosurgical consultation in the case of absent saddle area sensation and anal sphincter tone
    C. Increased activity starting in the first week
    D. Strict bed rest with bathroom and meal privileges only for the next 3 days
    E. Use of analgesia in the emergency department

# 51 Animal Bites and Rabies

*Barbara N. Wynn*

Select the appropriate letter that correctly answers the question or completes the statement.

1. Which of the following is the least appropriate wound management for animal bites?
   A. Careful exploration and debridement of even small pig bites
   B. CT or skull films for all children younger than 2 years old with scalp bites
   C. Immediate wound cleansing for 20 minutes for primate bites
   D. Suturing of bite wounds to the face from any species except for the monkey
   E. Use of cephalexin as prophylactic drug of choice with cat bites

2. Which of the following has the highest risk for infection?
   A. Cat bite to arm
   B. Cat bite to lower leg
   C. Cat bite to neck
   D. Dog bite to face
   E. Dog bite to hand

3. Regarding sepsis caused by *Capnocytophaga canimorsus*, which of the following is most accurate?
   A. Associated with gangrene at the bite site
   B. History of animal bite necessary to make diagnosis
   C. Most cases occur after cat bites
   D. Purpura and petechiae are rare findings
   E. Symptoms are present 1 to 2 weeks after contact

4. Which of the following is most characteristic of human bites?
   A. Antibiotic of choice with a clenched fist injury is cefuroxime
   B. Carry a high risk for transmission of HIV
   C. Location anywhere on the body is associated with a high incidence of infection

D. Tetanus booster within the past 7 years provides immunity
E. Usually a single organism causes the infection

5. Which of the following best describes the management of human bites?
   A. Antibiotic prophylaxis may eliminate the need for wound irrigation and debridement
   B. Hand wounds that involve infection of deeper structures require parenteral antibiotics
   C. Lacerations should not be closed primarily
   D. Penicillin is the prophylactic drug of choice
   E. Self-inflicted mucosal lacerations require antibiotics

6. A 25-year-old man states, "I'm worried I might get rabies." The physician should be worried also if which of the following occurred?
   A. Awakened to find a bat in the bedroom
   B. Bite from neighbor's cat
   C. Bite from a rat
   D. Bite from a squirrel
   E. Contact with blood of an animal found to be rabid

7. Which of the following is most characteristic of rabies?
   A. Incubation period does not vary with the bite site
   B. Initial symptom is inability to swallow
   C. Postexposure prophylaxis costs about $300.00 per series
   D. Specific and effective treatment is available at designated centers
   E. Treatment decisions may be modified if the animal is available for testing or observation

8. Which of the following is most characteristic of an animal thought to be rabid?
   A. Can infect equally well from bites, scratches, or abrasions
   B. Dogs are more likely to have the disease than cats are
   C. Location may be anywhere in the United States
   D. Will become sick and die within 10 days
   E. Will exhibit aggressive behavior

**PART THREE    ENVIRONMENTAL DISORDERS**

## 52 ▼ Venomous Animal Injuries

*Gwen L. Hoffman*

Select the appropriate letter that correctly answers the question or completes the statement.

1. Which of the following has resulted in the most fatalities in the United States?
   A. Bees
   B. Coral snakes
   C. Rattlesnakes
   D. Spiders
   E. Wasps
2. Which of the following identifies a snake as venomous?
   A. Double row of subcaudal plates
   B. No fangs
   C. Pits
   D. Round head
   E. Round pupils
3. What is the best pre-hospital management of a venomous snake bite to the lower leg?
   A. Apply suction
   B. Encourage movement of toes
   C. Incise the wound
   D. Pack the extremity in ice
   E. Place a tourniquet tightly around the thigh
4. Which of the following best describes a Grade II envenomation?
   A. Muscle fasciculation; painful muscular cramping; cold, clammy skin; tachycardia; and convulsions
   B. 1-5 inches of edema and erythema surround a fang wound; no systemic involvement after 12 hours of observation
   C. Rapidly progressing course with development of shock and edema and generalized petechiae over the entire extremity
   D. Sudden pain and rapidly progressive swelling that may reach and involve the trunk within a few hours; ecchymosis, bleb formation, and necrosis in the extremity. Systemic manifestations begin within 15 minutes
   E. Widely distributed pain with edema spreading toward the trunk; petechiae and ecchymosis in the area of edema; nausea, vomiting, and mild temperature elevation
5. Which of the following best describe antivenin administration?
   A. Children require a more diluted dose
   B. It is contraindicated in pregnancy
   C. Serum sickness is common if more than 10 vials are given

D. Skin testing before administration is no longer needed
   E. Small amount should be injected at the site of the wound
6. A 20-year-old man presents with a generalized urticarial rash after being stung on the arm by a bee. Lungs are clear to auscultation and vital signs are stable. What is the best management?
   A. Diphenhydramine 50 mg PO
   B. Diphenhydramine 50 mg IM and cimetidine 150 mg IV
   C. Diphenhydramine 50 mg IM and epinephrine 0.3 ml of 1:1000 SQ
   D. Epinephrine 5 ml of 1:10,000 dilution slowly IV and diphenhydramine 50 mg IM
   E. Epinephrine 0.3 ml of 1:1000 SQ, diphenhydramine 50 mg IM, and methylprednisolone 100 mg IV
7. A 25-year-old woman who is 7 months pregnant presents with a black widow spider bite to her lower leg. What is the best management?
   A. Administer antivenin after testing for hypersensitivity
   B. Apply heat directly over the bite
   C. Give normal saline boluses for hypotension
   D. Order dapsone to apply to the area of the bite
   E. Use meperidine for pain control
8. Which of the following best describes brown recluse spider envenomation and treatment?
   A. Give antivenin
   B. Excise the wound locally
   C. If no evidence of envenomation in 4 hours, discharge the patient with follow-up
   D. In children, death occurs most often from intravascular hemolysis
   E. Systemic reactions are rare
9. Which of the following best describes treatment of venomous marine animal envenomation?
   A. Antivenin should be given in most cases
   B. Deaths are usually a direct result of the envenomation
   C. Ice should be applied to the area of a stingray wound
   D. Nematocysts should be washed in sea water, then "fixed" with vinegar
   E. Tetanus prophylaxis is not needed because it is a clean wound

## 53 ▼ Thermal Burns

*Dale J. Ray*

Select the appropriate letter that correctly answers the question or completes the statement.

1. A 16-month-old boy has been sent to the emergency department by a public health nurse for evaluation of a burn she considered suspicious. The mother states the

burn occurred when the child pulled over a hot pan of water from the stove. Which of the following is most suggestive of such an accidental burn injury?
A. Anterior trunk burns
B. Bilateral burns of the feet that extend to the upper ankle
C. Burns with sharply demarcated edges
D. Dorsal hand burns
E. Posterior leg burns

2. A 23-year-old motorcycle rider struck a wall and the gas tank exploded, catching fire. After initial stabilization and secondary evaluation, his right leg is noted to have visible blisters, areas of charred skin, and subcutaneous tissues with areas of thrombosed vessels under a translucent surface. What degree burn is this?
A. First
B. Second
C. Third
D. Fourth

3. What is the immediate cardiovascular response to a burn?
A. Decrease in cardiac output and decrease in peripheral vascular resistance
B. Decrease in cardiac output and increase in peripheral vascular resistance
C. Increase in cardiac output and decrease in peripheral vascular resistance
D. Increase in cardiac output and increase in peripheral vascular resistance
E. Increase in cardiac output and no change in peripheral vascular resistance

4. Which of the following is contraindicated in pre-hospital care of a burn?
A. Assessment of the airway, breathing, and circulation
B. Covering the burn with clean sheets or sterile dressings
C. Initiation of normal saline IV
D. Placement of high-flow humidified oxygen on the patient
E. Placement of ice on the burn to decrease the pain

5. A 35-year-old man is burned in an accident in an illegal methamphetamine laboratory. He presents with extensive burns over his entire right upper extremity and the front of his abdomen and chest. What is the estimated total percent body surface area burn?
A. 9
B. 18
C. 27
D. 36
E. 45

6. A 70-kg, 25-year-old male sustained second-degree burns to his anterior chest and entire anterior legs while spraying lighter fluid onto a grill. According to the Parkland formula, what is the closest approximation of the cc/hr of IV lactated Ringer's needed for fluid resuscitation over the first 8 hours?

A. 150
B. 300
C. 400
D. 650
E. 950

7. Which of the following is most correct in considering the fluid resuscitation of burn patients?
A. Burns >20% BSA typically require IV fluid resuscitation
B. Children typically have lesser fluid needs per percent of BSA burned than adults do
C. During resuscitation, the most common error is insufficient rehydration
D. Hypertonic saline resuscitation has been found to lead to the need for fewer escharotomies and lower incidence of ileus
E. When using the Parkland formula for calculating fluid losses, calculation is from the time of the initiation of fluid resuscitation

8. Which of the following patients can be discharged from the emergency department?
A. 3-year-old boy with burns to his buttock and thighs
B. 24-year-old man with second-degree circumferential burns to both hands
C. 28-year-old woman with second-degree burns to one half of her back
D. 45-year-old man with electrical burns to his upper body
E. 65-year-old woman with IDDM and 10% TBSA, second-degree burns

9. A 43-year-old laborer arrives with tar burns on his hands and forearms. He has 6% TBSA second-degree burns and is admitted. What is the best agent for tar removal?
A. Acetone
B. Alcohol
C. Kerosene
D. Neosporin ointment
E. Silvadene cream

# 54 ▼ Frostbite

*Scott A. Carlson*

Select the appropriate letter that correctly answers the question or completes the statement.

1. Which statement regarding the physiology of human cold stress is most accurate?
   A. Acral skin structures (fingers, toes, ears, nose) contain a large number of arteriovenous anastomoses, which facilitate shunting and subsequent adaptive increases in blood flow to these areas
   B. At about 20° C and below, extremities undergo recurring 5- to 10-minute cycles of vasodilation that interrupt vasoconstriction and serve to protect the extremity ("the hunting response"), but this response disappears as the temperature drops below 10° C
   C. Cutaneous blood flow, in response to cold stress, can be reduced ten-fold to below 50 ml/min
   D. The human "central thermostat" is located in the preoptic posterior hypothalamus
   E. Thyroid stimulation and shivering thermogenesis are critical to the body's attempt to prevent frostbite

2. What best describes the process involved in the pathophysiology of frostbite?
   A. Blister formation with fluid that is protective of underlying dermis
   B. Edema progression, causing ultimate tissue death
   C. Ice-crystal formation in the intracellular fluid space
   D. Intracellular fluid shift causing cell ballooning and disruption
   E. Vasospasticity with sludging, stasis, and cessation of flow

3. Which of the following regarding chilblains (pernio) and trench foot (immersion foot) is most accurate?
   A. After rewarming of patients with trench foot, the skin typically is erythematous, dry, and very painful to touch
   B. If ulcerations over the affected area develop, the diagnosis of chilblains is ruled out
   C. Patients with trench foot typically have hypersensitive, painful feet on presentation
   D. Trench foot and chilblains occur when the temperature drops below freezing
   E. Trench foot results from exposure to dry cold; chilblains is from wet cold

4. What is thought to be the cause of frostbite sequelae such as pain, dysesthesias, squamous/epidermoid carcinoma, and premature epiphyseal closure?
   A. Direct neuronal damage and residual abnormalities in sympathetic tone
   B. Irreversible damage to epidermal structures
   C. Long-term extracellular fluid crystalline deposits
   D. Permanent small vessel damage
   E. All of the above

5. What is the most common presenting symptom of frostbite?
   A. Clumsiness and "chunk of wood" sensation
   B. Numbness
   C. Pain
   D. Paresthesias
   E. Ulcerations

*The following paragraph applies to Questions 6 through 9.*

A group of cross-country skiers call 9-1-1 using their cellular phone. They report a 28-year-old member of their party has an insensate, apparently "frozen" hand after losing one of her mittens. They have been successful at starting a small campfire. Because of poor weather and remote location, rescue teams (on snowmobiles) will need at least 3 hours to get her back to the ED. What is the best pre-hospital management?

6. A. Cover and insulate the exposed hand; keep the patient warm but make no attempts at warming the hand directly
   B. Gently massage the hand with snow, thereby allowing gradual thawing
   C. Gently massage the hand with warm hands from other members of the group
   D. Start rewarming the hand immediately by immersing it in warm (40° to 42° C) water
   E. Warm the hand by the fire

7. The patient arrives in the ED approximately 4 hours after the initial call. Earlier instructions have been followed. At this point it is determined that the patient has suffered frostbite of her hand, and her core temperature is 35.9° C. The rest of the physical examination is unremarkable. What is the most appropriate management?
   A. Apply dry, forced air (40°-42° C) to the hand
   B. Gently massage the hand while applying dry, forced air (40°-42° C)
   C. Gently massage the hand while it is in warm water (40°-42° C)
   D. Place the hand in gently circulating warm water (40°-42° C)
   E. Rewarm the patient because she has life-threatening hypothermia and this represents a life-over-limb issue

8. Which of the following may also be appropriate for this patient?
   A. Dependent position for the hand to promote increased blood flow
   B. Immobilization of the hand with a splint
   C. Massage of the hand to increase circulation
   D. Oral ibuprofen administration
   E. Topical application of silver sulfadiazine (Silvadene)

9. After discharge from the hospital 2 days later, the patient returns to the ED to express her thanks. She asks when she will know how much of her extremity will be nonviable and is told it will be apparent in:
   A. 3-5 days
   B. 7-14 days
   C. 21-28 days

D. 28-56 days

E. 60-90 days

10. A 33-year-old man has a frostbitten hand that has been adequately rewarmed. There are several large, tense, intact hemorrhagic blisters present. What is the most appropriate management?

A. Aspiration of the hemorrhagic fluid

B. Compressive dressings

C. Debridement

D. Direct application of aloe vera

E. Splinting in a position of function

# 55 Accidental Hypothermia

*Scott A. Carlson*

Select the appropriate letter that correctly answers the question or completes the statement.

1. Heat loss occurs by five mechanisms, with the rate of loss varying depending on environmental conditions. Which of the following best describes heat loss?

A. Conductive loss, normally only 2%-3% of total loss, can be increased 25 times by body contact with cold, dry objects

B. Convective heat losses are increased by shivering

C. Insensible losses from respiration and evaporation from skin account for <5% of total heat loss

D. Radiation is the greatest source of loss under normal conditions but is minimized in cloudy, non-windy conditions

E. "Wind chill" makes one feel colder but does not account for greater heat loss

2. Which of the following best describes cardiac effects that occur in hypothermia?

A. Atrial fibrillation usually converts spontaneously during rewarming

B. J or Osborn wave, best seen in leads II or $V_6$, is pathognomonic of hypothermia

C. Prolonged PR interval is the most characteristic feature of the rhythm strip

B. Reentrant dysrhythmias are uncommon

E. Spontaneous asystole below 25° C is common, whereas ventricular fibrillation is iatrogenic in nature

3. Which of the following temperature associations in hypothermia is incorrectly paired?

A. 35° C: defined onset of hypothermia

B. 28° C: 50% decline in pulse rate

C. 26° C: shivering ceases

D. 24° C: loss of endocrine and autonomic mechanisms for heat preservation

E. 20° C: EEG silence

4. Which of the following patients is least likely to develop hypothermia?

A. Elderly male with Parkinson's disease

B. Mature female with Addison's disease

C. 4-year-old child suffering from malnutrition

D. 55-year-old male with myxedema

E. 67-year-old female with Grave's disease

5. Which of the following statements best describes pharmacologic issues in the patient with accidental hypothermia?

A. Because of the common association with hypothyroidism, patients should receive an initial dose of levothyroxine (250-500 µg)

B. Because of the high incidence of thromboembolism, prophylactic heparinization should be administered

C. Bretylium tosylate dose necessary for treatment of ventricular fibrillation is at least twice that of a normothermic patient

D. Routine use of steroids should be withheld, unless a definite suspicion of hypoadrenocorticism exists

E. Since the hypotension is potentially treatable, low-dose (2-5 µg/kg/min) dopamine infusion should be utilized

6. Which of the following statements best describes treatment of dysrhythmias associated with hypothermia?

A. Asystole is a more ominous rhythm than ventricular fibrillation

B. Atrial fibrillation is a particularly malignant rhythm because of the associated rapid ventricular rate

C. Bretylium appears to be the drug of choice for both the prophylaxis and treatment of ventricular fibrillation

D. Definitive pharmacotherapy is required for conversion of dysrhythmias induced by hypothermia

E. Lidocaine is useful in facilitating defibrillation

7. What is the last peripheral reflex to disappear and the first to reappear during rewarming of the hypothermia patient?

A. Biceps

B. Cremasteric

C. Jaw-jerk

D. Knee-jerk

E. Plantar

8. With regard to acid-base balance in the hypothermic patient, which of the following is most correct?

A. A "corrected ABG" is given when the blood gas analyzer warms the blood to 37° C for its results

B. Correction of ABG values for the patient's temperature is necessary to guide therapy

C. Maintaining a corrected pH at 7.4 and $PCO_2$ at 40 mm Hg minimizes adverse cardiac events

D. Neutral pH of water lowers with cooling, in parallel with that of blood, maintaining a 0.6 unit pH offset

E. Relative alkalinity offers myocardial protection and electrical stability

9. Which of the following best describes common laboratory abnormalities in hypothermia?
   A. BUN is more accurate than hematocrit in determining a patient's fluid status
   B. Glucose levels are typically depressed, especially in the acute phase
   C. Hematocrit decreases because of venous pooling, with fluid shifts causing hemodilution
   D. Hypokalemia is commonly seen, resulting from potassium entering muscle
   E. Rhabdomyolysis affects potassium balance and can contribute to hyperkalemia

10. A physiologic increase in coagulation occurs with hypothermia, and a DIC-type syndrome has been reported. In hypothermia patients with clinically evident coagulopathies, which of the following is most correct?
    A. Enzymatic nature of activated clotting factors is depressed by the cold
    B. Fresh frozen plasma is preferred to specific factor replacement because several factors can be depressed
    B. Laboratory prothrombin and partial thromboplastin times are necessary to determine the degree of coagulopathy present
    D. Normal laboratory prothrombin and partial thromboplastin times can be used to rule out DIC
    E. Platelets are unaffected by the cold and do not generally contribute to the coagulopathy

11. A patient has been found after a night alone in the woods. His clothes are wet and he has had no means of warming himself. He is alert and neurologically intact although somewhat confused. Paramedics are asking advice on immediate therapy. What is the most appropriate advice?
    A. Allow the patient to walk to stimulate thermogenesis
    B. Intubate the patient and supply warmed oxygen
    C. Massage the extremities to stimulate circulation
    D. Remove the wet clothing and protect the patient with a blanket
    E. Supply the patient with heated oral fluids

12. Which of the following is a recognized indication for active rewarming?
    A. Extensive areas of frostbite
    B. Moderate or severe hypothermia (temperature less than 34° C)
    C. Pharmacologically induced peripheral vasodilation
    D. Sinus tachycardia
    E. Uncontrolled shivering

13. Which of the following statements best describes methods of active rewarming in the hypothermic patient?
    A. Airway rewarming should be reserved for mild and moderate cases because its rewarming rate is insufficient for more severe cases
    B. By applying heat to the thorax and extremities, active external rewarming has been successfully combined with core rewarming
    C. Cardiopulmonary bypass rewarming should be reserved for patients in cardiac arrest undergoing CPR

D. Heated irrigation fluids (e.g., lavage of peritoneum, thorax) provide the most rapid means of core rewarming
E. Warm dry air is preferred for airway rewarming because heat is lost via evaporation with more humidification

14. Which of the following best describes endotracheal intubation in the hypothermia patient?
    A. Can often be avoided since protective airway reflexes quickly return with rewarming
    B. Even when trismus is present, nasotracheal intubation should be avoided
    C. Its performance can precipitate cardiac dysrhythmias
    D. Nasogastric tube placement should typically follow it
    E. Pulmonary edema is the most common reason it is necessary

# 56 Heat Illness

### *Dale E. McNinch*

Select the appropriate letter that correctly answers the question or completes the statement.

1. Which of the following is most characteristic of the thermoregulation mechanisms in humans?
   A. Apocrine sweat glands are more important than eccrine glands
   B. Average basal metabolic rate for a 70-kg person is 70 Kcal/hour
   C. Persons exercising in hot environments lose 1 liter of sweat per hour
   D. Respiratory mechanisms are less important than conduction, convection, or evaporation as sources of heat loss
   E. Vascular responses to heat stress include cutaneous vasoconstriction and vasodilation of the splanchnic and renal beds

2. Which of the following is a physiologic adaptation of acclimatization to a high-temperature environment?
   A. Contraction of plasma volume by 10%-25%
   B. Decreased baseline heart rate
   C. Decreased sweat volume
   D. Increased sweat electrolyte concentration
   E. Onset of sweating at a higher core temperature

3. A 28-year-old woman recently discharged from a psychiatric hospital presents complaining of dysarthria and torticollis. She appears dyspneic but has clear breath sounds. Neurologic examination reveals extreme spasm of the left sternocleidomastoid muscle and increased muscle tonicity in general. Vital signs are BP, 120/80; P, 134; R, 24; and T, 40.3° C. What is the best drug to administer?
   A. Acetaminophen
   B. Dantrolene
   C. Diazepam

D. Diphenhydramine
E. Erythromycin
4. A 17-year-old football player arrives at the emergency department after becoming very weak during practice on an unseasonably hot August afternoon. He is vomiting and complaining of severe headache but is alert and oriented. Vital signs are BP, 124/78; P, 126; R, 20; and T, 38.4° C. What condition does he have?
   A. Classic heat stroke
   B. Exertional heat stroke
   C. Heat edema
   D. Heat exhaustion
   E. Heat syncope
5. Which of the following is least likely to be seen in heat stroke?
   A. Anhidrosis
   B. Core temperature greater than 40.0° C
   C. Elevation of hepatic transaminase level
   D. Profound CNS dysfunction
   E. Sudden onset
6. In a patient with heat stroke, which of the following is least likely to be directly affected?
   A. Brain
   B. Heart
   C. Kidney
   D. Liver
   E. Pancreas
7. Which of the following is most likely to seek treatment for heat stroke on a hot, humid late summer day with laboratory values showing lactic acidosis, myoglobinuria, acute renal failure, elevated LFTs and coagulopathy?
   A. Chronic alcoholic found passed out in the city park
   B. Elderly patient who lives alone in an upstairs apartment
   C. Employee in a fast-food restaurant kitchen
   D. High school football player beginning two-a-day practices
   E. Infant left in an enclosed car too long
8. Heat stroke is a multisystemic disease. Which of the following laboratory findings is least likely to be seen?
   A. Decreased fibrinogen, elevated prothrombin, and elevated fibrin split products
   B. Elevated CPK
   C. Elevated liver function tests
   D. Metabolic alkalosis and respiratory acidosis
   E. Proteinuria, granular casts, and RBCs on urinalysis
9. An 18-year-old army recruit collapses during a training drill in July and is very confused. Vital signs are BP, 93/45; P, 112; R, 28; and T, 41.5° C. What should be done first?
   A. EKG
   B. Glucose determination
   C. Ice water immersion
   D. Intubation
   E. Lumbar puncture
10. What is the most efficient method to treat a patient presenting with heat stroke?

A. Cooling blanket
B. Gastric and peritoneal lavage with cold water
C. Ice packs
D. Immersion in cold water
E. Mist water spray and fan
11. Which of the following is most accurate regarding the treatment of heat stroke complications?
   A. Chlorpromazine should not be used to treat the shivering associated with rapid core cooling
   B. Bretylium, lidocaine, or defibrillation is rarely needed
   C. Mannitol is contraindicated in the treatment of myoglobinuria
   D. Phenobarbital may be dangerous to use for seizures
   E. Potassium replacement is frequently required because of renal injury
12. Which of the following is most likely to be used for effective pharmacologic treatment of heat stroke?
   A. Acetaminophen
   B. Dantrolene
   C. Dexamethasone
   D. Diphenhydramine
   E. Mannitol and bicarbonate

 **57 Chemical Injuries**

*Warren F. Lanphear*

Select the appropriate letter that correctly answers the question or completes the statement.
1. Most chemical agents damage the skin by producing which of the following?
   A. Cellulitis
   B. Chemical reaction
   C. Hypersensitivity reaction
   D. Hyperthermic injury
   E. Secondary response after absorption
2. What is one key element of an appropriate HAZMAT response?
   A. Containing and cleaning up the exposure site
   B. Delay of thorough decontamination until emergency department arrival
   C. Establishment of a command post at the exposure site of a large incident
   D. Identification of the specific hazardous material in the emergency department after evacuation
   E. Rapid, high-pressure irrigation of dry chemical that is adherent to victims
3. What is the most appropriate pre-hospital management for the majority of chemical exposures to the skin?
   A. Application of wet gauze to exposed skin
   B. Copious lavage with water
   C. Establishment of two large-bore IVs
   D. Immediate transport to the emergency department
   E. Removal of clothing

4. Treatment with water lavage is absolutely contraindicated for exposure to which of the following?
   A. Acids
   B. Alkalis
   C. Elemental metals
   D. Hydrofluoric acid
   E. Phosphorus

5. When comparing acid burns of the eye with alkali burns, what is more characteristic of acid burns?
   A. Central cornea burns often heal uneventfully
   B. Damage to deep endothelial cells is common
   C. Injury to the periphery of the cornea and conjunctiva often lead to neovascularization and scarring
   D. Perforation, endophthalmitis, and loss of the eye are common
   E. Rapidly neutralized by tears and conjunctival epithelium

6. What is the recommended treatment for deep hydrofluoric acid burns?
   A. Calcium gluconate infiltration
   B. Copious irrigation with a dilute calcium gluconate solution
   C. Intravenous calcium gluconate
   D. Leaving intact blisters alone
   E. Topical calcium gluconate gel

7. Which of the following may spontaneously combust when exposed to air?
   A. Calcium
   B. Elemental potassium
   C. Elemental sodium
   D. Lithium
   E. White phosphorus

8. Which of the following measures is appropriate treatment for a phenol exposure?
   A. Irrigation with low volumes of water under high pressure
   B. Rinsing the skin with 5% sodium bicarbonate
   C. Rinsing the skin with resorcinol
   D. Swabbing the skin with an undiluted polyethylene glycol solution
   E. Swabbing the skin with water-soaked sponges

## 58 Electrical and Lightning Injuries

*Scott A. Carlson*

Select the appropriate letter that correctly answers the question or completes the statement.

1. Which of the following body tissues has the most resistance to an electrical current?
   A. Blood
   B. Bone
   C. Muscle
   D. Nerve
   E. Skin

2. Which of the following is the "let-go" current range in adults?
   A. 1-4 mA
   B. 6-9 mA
   C. 10-20 mA
   D. 20-50 mA
   E. 60-70 mA

3. Skin is the primary resistor to the flow of current into the body. Which of the following can significantly increase its resistance?
   A. Areas of blistering
   B. Heavy callousing
   C. Increased local vascularity
   D. Perspiration
   E. Prolonged duration of contact with electrical current

4. A 30-year-old lineman presents after being involved in an electrical accident that leaves him with superficial partial-thickness burns on his right upper extremity. Based on the mechanisms of electrical injury, which of the following best describes his injury?
   A. Based on the initial history and physical examination alone, the patient's superficial partial thickness burns are indicative of an electrical flash burn
   B. Blunt traumatic injury can be excluded with a reliable history of not falling or being thrown
   C. Periosteal muscle damage can occur even though the overlying muscle appears normal
   D. Signs of neural injury should not be apparent yet, because they generally take several days to develop
   E. Vascular damage will be apparent with careful examination of distal pulses, color, and capillary refill

5. Which of the following best describes the different mechanisms of injury from lightning?
   A. Arc burns cause very deep burns from the arc of current between the cloud and an object near the victim
   B. Contact refers to the lightning current directly contacting the victim
   C. Implosion refers to the current causing ionization changes and structural damage as it traverses the body
   D. Side splash occurs as lightning jumps from its pathway to a nearby person on its way to the ground
   E. Step voltage is the progressive lessening of current as the lightning steps from one object to another

6. Which of the following best describes specific injuries in electrical and lightning victims?
   A. Cataracts develop in as many as 30% of victims of high-voltage injuries
   B. Lightning strike victims frequently have intraabdominal injuries from the remarkable implosive force
   C. Shoulder dislocations from tetanic muscle contractions are probably more common than most sources report

D. The most common ground or exit point burns seen in electrical injuries are the hands

E. Tympanic membrane rupture is seen more commonly in lightning victims than high-voltage electrical injuries

7. Which of the following best describes oral commissure injuries?

A. Although significant mucous membrane damage can occur, teeth and muscle are typically spared

B. Cosmesis is not usually a major concern

C. May be associated with delayed bleeding from the labial artery

D. Most commonly involve children over the age of four

E. Sometimes called the "kissing burn"

8. Which of the following best describes pre-hospital scene evaluation of electrical and lightning injuries?

A. Electrical injury victims should be encouraged to walk from the scene to EMS personnel waiting just outside of the danger area

B. EMS personnel should wear insulated electrical gloves for protection at the scene of high-voltage incidents

C. For high-voltage incidents, paramedics should turn off the power source before approaching victims

D. In triaging multiple victims from a lightning strike(s), care and resources should concentrate on those with signs of life present, as arrest victims can rarely be resuscitated

E. Proper oxygenation and ventilation of lightning strike victims can help avoid secondary cardiac arrests

9. Caution must be used in interpreting which of the following relationships in electrical injuries?

A. Cervical spine fractures showing a spinous process fracture

B. Elevated CK-MB fraction indicating an acute myocardial infarction

C. Head CT showing a subdural hematoma

D. Technetium pyrophosphate scanning showing viable muscle

E. Urine dipstick examination positive for blood but with no RBCs, indicating myoglobinuria

10. A 40-year-old plumber is brought to the ED after suffering an electrical injury while working on a water heater. He is unresponsive, with a blood pressure of 80 palpable and labored respirations. What would the best estimation of necessary fluid resuscitation in this patient be based on?

A. Brooke formula

B. Fluid bolus of crystalloid of 10-20 ml/kg

C. Parkland formula

D. Systolic blood pressure

E. Urine output

11. Which of the following best describes lightning injuries and their management?

A. Cold, blue, mottled, pulseless extremities are usually secondary to vasospasm that clears within a few hours

B. Mental status changes are uncommon. A head CT should be done if changes are present

C. Signs of peripheral nerve dysfunction seen early after injury have a good prognosis for complete recovery

D. Superficial feathering burns are pathognomonic and should be treated with topical antibiotics

E. Urine output should be maintained at 0.5-1.0 ml/kg/hr with intravenous crystalloid to avoid myoglobinuric renal failure

12. A 26-year-old man presents after suffering an electrical injury while placing a television antenna on his roof. He has an entrance wound on his right hand and an exit wound on his left heel. There are no other injuries identified. After the second day in the hospital it is noticed that his BUN and creatinine are steadily rising. What is the most likely cause?

A. Direct electrical trauma to his kidneys

B. Hypovolemic shock and acute tubular necrosis

C. Myoglobinuria

D. Rising levels of a renal depressant factor

E. Thrombosis of his renal veins

13. A 21-year-old woman in her second trimester of pregnancy is involved in a low-voltage accident. She is asymptomatic, with good fetal heart tones noted. What is the most appropriate disposition for her?

A. Admit to a general bed for observation

B. Admit to a telemetry bed

C. Discharge with reassurance

D. Give IV crystalloids to ensure good urine output

E. Obtain an obstetric consultation

 **59 Diving Injuries**

*Dale E. McNinch*

Select the appropriate letter that correctly answers the question or completes the statement.

1. For physicians treating diving injuries, which of the following is the most unique and valuable service provided by the Divers Alert Network (DAN)?

A. Collects and publishes data on diving accidents and injuries

B. Enhances diving safety and injury prevention as its mission

C. Gives instructional programs on management of diving emergencies

D. Has a 24-hour medical emergency hotline for diving-related problems

E. Provides assistance when injuries occur

2. What is the most common complaint of scuba divers?
   A. Bends (joints)
   B. Chokes (lungs)
   C. Hearing loss (ears)
   D. Squeeze (ears)
   E. Vertigo (ears)

3. A mountain climber would need to ascend to 18,000 feet to reduce the atmospheric pressure by 50%. How many feet does a diver need to descend to double the atmospheric pressure?
   A. 5
   B. 15
   C. 35
   D. 55
   E. 65

4. If the eustachian tubes fail to equalize middle ear pressures, at what diving depths (in feet) is tympanic membrane rupture most likely to occur?
   A. 1-5
   B. 10-15
   C. 25-30
   D. 35-45
   E. 50-60

5. A diver currently has a significant upper respiratory infection. What is the best medical advice?
   A. Avoid diving for up to 2 weeks
   B. Begin taking erythromycin
   C. Drink plenty of fluids and take Vitamin C
   D. Take an oral decongestant (pseudoephedrine)
   E. Use a nasal decongestant (phenylephrine)

6. Because of its biochemical content, which of the following is particularly susceptible to decompression illness?
   A. CNS
   B. Heart
   C. Inner ear
   D. Lungs
   E. Skin and joints

7. Following a dive of 2 hours or less, how many hours does it take at sea level for the body's nitrogen stores to return to normal?
   A. 6
   B. 12
   C. 18
   D. 24
   E. 36

8. Which of the following is most accurate regarding decompression sickness (DCS) and arterial gas embolism (AGE)?
   A. Cardiac arrhythmias respond well to standard medical therapy
   B. Intravenous fluids should be run at KO only
   C. May be prevented by prophylactic use of pseudoephedrine or aspirin
   D. Recompression is the only definitive treatment
   E. Transportation by air to a hyperbaric chamber is all right if cabin pressure can be maintained at 2500 feet

9. Which of the following would suggest a diagnosis of arterial gas embolism (AGE) rather than decompression sickness (DCS)?
   A. Cardiac arrest or seizures are rare complications
   B. History of a routine, controlled, "no problem" dive
   C. Mild or vague peripheral neurologic symptoms
   D. Precipitated by dehydration, fatigue, hypothermia
   E. Rapid onset of symptoms or problems following the dive

10. Which of the following increases the risk for development of arterial gas embolism (AGE) during a dive?
    A. Heavy exertion or fatigue
    B. Hypothermia
    C. Obesity
    D. Panic or inexperience
    E. Tobacco and alcohol use

11. A 22-year-old sports diver just returned by air from a diving trip to the Caribbean and complains of headache, weakness, nausea, and tingling in his arms and legs. What is the most appropriate management?
    A. Contact the nearest hyperbaric chamber and arrange transport
    B. Give lidocaine or benzodiazepines to prevent seizures
    C. Intubate prophylactically for oxygenation and hyperventilation and start intravenous fluids
    D. Observe for 12-24 hours, give 100% oxygen, intravenous fluids, and narcotics prn for pain
    E. Reassure, give acetaminophen or ibuprofen for headache, and apply nasal oxygen

12. Most authorities recommend that flying be delayed for a minimum of how many hours after diving?
    A. 6
    B. 12
    C. 18
    D. 24
    E. 48

13. What is the second leading cause of mortality for sports divers?
    A. Arterial gas embolism (AGE)
    B. Cardiac arrest
    C. Decompression sickness (DCS)
    D. Drowning
    E. Rhabdomyolysis

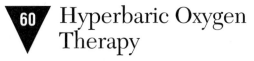

# 60 ▼ Hyperbaric Oxygen Therapy

### *Warren F. Lanphear*

Select the appropriate letter that correctly answers the question or completes the statement.

1. Which of the following is an absolute contraindication to hyperbaric oxygen (HBO) therapy?
   A. COPD

B. History of an oxygen seizure

C. Otitis media

D. Pregnancy

E. Untreated simple pneumothorax

2. What is the most common side effect of HBO therapy?

A. Claustrophobia

B. Ear squeeze

C. Seizures

D. Sinus squeeze

E. Visual refraction

3. A 25-year-old woman who is 8 months pregnant presents with headache and vomiting. Her carboxyhemoglobin level is 20 because of a faulty furnace. What is the best management?

A. Arrange for immediate HBO therapy

B. Call an obstetrician for emergency C-section, then send the mother for HBO therapy

C. Give 100% oxygen, monitor fetal heart tones, and recheck her carboxyhemoglobin level in 1 hour

D. The carboxyhemoglobin level is not high enough for HBO therapy; give oxygen and monitor the fetus

E. Treat with 100% oxygen via mask and monitor the fetus

4. Which of the following is the standard protocol for HBO therapy in the treatment of CO poisoning?

A. 1.5-2.0 ATA for 60-75 minutes

B. 2.4-3 ATA for 60-90 minutes

C. 24 hours of oxygen by mask following HBO therapy

D. Routine retreatment in 12 hours

E. Usage of multiple chambers compressed with 100% oxygen

5. Which of the following best describes HBO therapy for necrotizing soft tissue infections?

A. Bactericidal to clostridia

B. Beneficial even with late presentations

C. Inhibits polymorphonuclear leukocyte function

D. Inhibits production of lethal clostridial alpha toxin

E. Negates the need for antibiotics and surgery

6. Which of the following is not an approved indication for HBO therapy?

A. Crush injury

B. Gas embolism

C. Intracranial abscess

D. Osteomyelitis

E. Thermal burns

 **61** High-Altitude Illness

*Dale E. McNinch*

Select the appropriate letter that correctly answers the question or completes the statement.

1. Which of the following is least likely to affect the development of high altitude illness?

A. Age

B. Duration of stay at any altitude

C. Final altitude achieved

D. Gender

E. Rate of ascent

2. Which of the following is characteristic of the hypoxic ventilatory response (HVR)?

A. Causes respiratory acidosis

B. Correlates directly to acclimatization

C. Not affected by medications

D. Stimulates retention of bicarbonate

E. Ventilation maximizes in 2 to 3 days

3. Which of the following best describes the physiologic response to hypoxemia?

A. Diffuse cerebral vasoconstriction

B. Diffuse pulmonary vasodilation

C. Increases in 2-3 DPG resulting in a rightward shift of the oxyhemoglobin dissociation curve

D. Initial drop in the hemoglobin concentration followed by slow erythropoietin-induced RBC production

E. Retention of bicarbonate by the kidney

4. Which of the following is faulty advice to give an expedition team planning to climb to 16,000 feet?

A. Allow for slow ascent, spending the first night below 8000 feet and ascending no more than 1000 feet per night above 10,000 feet

B. Avoid smoking and alcohol to optimize acclimatization

C. Descend 1500 feet or use oxygen to resolve developing symptoms of AMS

D. Eat a high-carbohydrate diet

E. Sleep at the highest altitude achieved for the day

5. A 38-year-old hiker develops an isolated mild bitemporal headache at 9000 feet. What is the most appropriate treatment?

A. Acetaminophen with codeine

B. Caffeine and a low-carbohydrate diet

C. Furosemide

D. Immediately descending to lower altitude

E. Remaining at this altitude as long as further symptoms do not develop

6. Acute Mountain Sickness (AMS) is common above 10,000 to 12,000 feet elevation. Which of the following indicates a more serious altitude illness?

A. Ataxia

B. Decreased urine output

C. Dyspnea on exertion

D. "Hangover" symptoms (fatigue, headache, nausea)

E. Periodic breathing or apnea episodes while sleeping

7. Which of the following may be deleterious to someone suffering from AMS?

A. Acetaminophen

B. Acetazolamide

C. Benzodiazepine

D. Dexamethasone

E. Prochlorperazine

8. What is the most common adverse reaction to taking acetazolamide?
   A. Altered taste (especially with carbonated beverages and beer)
   B. Blood dyscrasia
   C. Drowsiness
   D. Paresthesias and polyuria
   E. Tinnitus

9. Which of the following is not typical for the syndromes of high-altitude pulmonary edema (HAPE) and high-altitude cerebral edema (HACE)?
   A. Develops quickly (within 12 hours) upon arrival at "critical altitude"
   B. Failure to treat immediately may have life-threatening consequences
   C. Hyperbaric therapy may be beneficial
   D. They rarely occur at altitudes below 12,000 feet
   E. Treatment is oxygen or immediate descent

10. A 40-year-old skier develops cough and mild dyspnea at rest during his second day at 10,000 feet elevation. Which of the following best describes his assessment?
    A. Bed rest and supplemental oxygen are indicated
    B. Bradycardia is present
    C. Chest x-ray reveals cardiomegaly and Kerley B lines
    D. Descent to sea level is indicated
    E. ECG has ischemic changes

11. A 27-year-old trekker develops headache, confusion, and ataxia while mountain climbing. What is the best management?
    A. Acetaminophen or aspirin with codeine
    B. Benzodiazepine
    C. Dexamethasone
    D. Halt ascent and rest until symptoms subside
    E. Oxygen and immediate descent

12. Which of the following is most characteristic of high-altitude retinal hemorrhages?
    A. Generally related to the presence of mild AMS
    B. Often result in permanent residual visual field deficits
    C. Rarely occur above 17,000 feet elevation
    D. Treated with immediate descent of 1500 to 3000 feet
    E. Usually are benign and resolve without treatment

13. A 24-year-old man with sickle cell anemia is planning an ascent of Mt. Denali (above 20,000 feet). What is the most appropriate advice?
    A. Do not make the trip
    B. Get transfused to a pre-trip hematocrit above 40%
    C. Have supplemental oxygen available
    D. Start taking acetazolamide before ascent
    E. Take dexamethasone for 1 week before the trip

# 62 ▼ Near-Drowning

*Michael D. Brown*

Select the appropriate letter that correctly answers the question or completes the statement.

1. A 2-year-old boy is found by his parents floating upside down in the backyard pool. The boy has vital signs when the paramedics arrive but arrests in transit and does not respond to resuscitative efforts. What is this event called?
   A. Drowning
   B. Drowning syndrome
   C. Immersion syndrome
   D. Near-drowning
   E. Secondary drowning

2. Which of the following best describes the effect of water aspirated during drowning?
   A. Lysis of red cells is likely with salt water
   B. Pulmonary edema often occurs with fresh water
   C. Pulmonary surfactant is damaged by fresh and salt water
   D. Serum electrolytes are significantly altered
   E. 10 ml/kg is needed for pulmonary injury

3. A 19-year-old man hit in the head by his surfboard is submerged in the ocean for 2 minutes before being rescued. Witnesses report he aspirated a large amount of sea water. What is the most appropriate initial prehospital management?
   A. Evaluate airway, breathing, and circulation
   B. Give 100% oxygen
   C. Immobilize cervical spine
   D. Position to drain water from lungs
   E. Remove his wet clothes, dry his skin, and cover him with a warm blanket

4. Which of the following is uncommon in near-drowning?
   A. Acidosis
   B. Hypoxemia
   C. Intrapulmonary shunting
   D. Pulmonary edema
   E. Shock

5. An 11-year-old girl with epilepsy is brought in by ambulance after having a seizure while swimming in a pool. She was under water for 5 minutes and was lethargic at the scene. She is now alert with normal vital signs, negative physical examination, and normal chest radiograph. Her ABGs show a significantly increased A-a gradient. What is the most appropriate management?
   A. Admit for observation
   B. Discharge with close follow-up
   C. Give intravenous broad-spectrum antibiotics and admit
   D. Give intravenous steroids and admit
   E. Perform pulmonary lavage to drain aspirated water

6. In a near-drowning victim with possible pulmonary complications, what is the best initial management?
   A. Draw blood for ABGs
   B. Initiate steroid therapy
   C. Order a chest x-ray
   D. Start a broad-spectrum antibiotic
   E. Supply 100% oxygen via non-rebreather mask
7. A 6-year-old boy fell through the ice while skating. He is pulseless and apneic after being in the water for 45 minutes. Which of the following best describes his prognosis?
   A. Chances of surviving neurologically intact are greater than those for an adult with an equally prolonged period of submersion
   B. Mammalian diving reflex may help preserve neurologic and cardiac function by facilitating the release of oxygen from hemoglobin at the tissue level
   C. Prolonged resuscitation efforts are not indicated because survival with neurologic recovery following extended cold-water submersion is unlikely
   D. Severe hypothermia may have a cardioprotective effect by preventing ventricular fibrillation
   E. Severe hypothermia may increase metabolic demands, resulting in severe cerebral hypoxia

# 63 Radiation Injuries

*Dale J. Ray*

Select the appropriate letter that correctly answers the question or completes the statement.

1. Which of the following is characteristic of alpha particles?
   A. Emitted by radiation therapy machines
   B. Emitted by uranium decay
   C. Emitted only by particle accelerators
   D. Readily penetrate the skin
   E. Travel farther and faster than beta particles
2. A 22-year-old graduate student seeks treatment after an accidental exposure from a linear accelerator at the university. He appears healthy and was decontaminated at the scene. His clothes have been removed and properly disposed of. He takes another shower, but his skin still shows high levels of radioactivity. What is the most likely type of radiation involved?
   A. Alpha particles
   B. Beta particles
   C. Gamma rays
   D. Neutrons
   E. X-rays
3. The dose of radiation received is measured in radiation absorbed doses (rad) or Grays (Gy). One Gy is equal to how many rads?

A. 0.1
B. 1
C. 10
D. 100
E. 1000

4. A 50-year-old nuclear technician presents 30 minutes after an intense radiation exposure. He has headache, tinnitus, and vertigo; he complains of numbness in his legs and is quite confused. What is the minimum dose in rads that will produce these symptoms after 30 minutes?
   A. 50
   B. 600
   C. 2000
   D. 4800
   E. 12,000
5. What is the immediate lethal dose of rads for humans in a non–mass casualty radiation exposure?
   A. 50
   B. 150
   C. 250
   D. 450
   E. 750
6. Death resulting from radiation exposure is most likely caused by failure of which of the following systems?
   A. Cardiovascular
   B. Central nervous
   C. Gastrointestinal
   D. Hematopoietic
   E. Respiratory
7. A 40-year-old power plant worker is accidentally exposed to high levels of radiation. He has no symptoms when transported to the ED 1 hour after exposure. What should be done first?
   A. Administration of ipecac to rid the stomach of radioactive material
   B. Connection to cardiac monitor and placement of two large-bore IV lines
   C. Gastric lavage to rid the stomach of radioactive material
   D. Placement of protective face mask on the patient to protect staff
   E. Removal of all clothes and cleansing of hair and skin
8. What is the best laboratory test to determine a patient's prognosis for survival after high-level radiation exposure?
   A. Absolute lymphocyte count 48 hours after exposure
   B. Platelet count 24 hours after exposure
   C. Qualitative prothrombin time 72 hours after exposure
   D. Total red blood cell count 48 hours after exposure
   E. Total white blood cell count 24 hours after exposure

# 64  The Pediatric Patient: General Approach And Unique Concerns

### Sandra K. Dettmann and Gwen L. Hoffman

Select the appropriate letter that correctly answers the question or completes the statement.

1. Which of the following best describes pediatric patients?
   A. All vital signs, except for temperature, change with age
   B. Compared with adults, more rib fractures, sternal fractures, and flail chests occur
   C. Livers and spleens are less susceptible to injury than those of adults
   D. Meningitis is most likely caused by *Haemophilus influenzae* in a 1 month old
   E. Most cardiac arrests are the result of dysrhythmias

2. A 3-year-old boy presents after falling six feet to the ground from a deck. He states his neck hurts and his arms and legs "feel funny." On examination his neck is slightly tender but he is neurologically intact. Cervical spine films are negative. What is the most appropriate management?
   A. Admit for observation
   B. Discharge home with follow-up
   C. Keep in the emergency department for 2 hours and re-evaluate
   D. Obtain neurosurgery consultation
   E. Order CT imaging of the cervical spine

3. Which of the following must be taken into consideration when interpreting plain films of the pediatric cervical spine?
   A. Decreased preodontoid space
   B. Incomplete ossification
   C. Narrowed prevertebral spaces
   D. Pseudosubluxation of C4 on C5
   E. Rounder and less horizontal facet joints

4. What is the chief complaint of pediatric patients transported by EMS?
   A. Cardiorespiratory
   B. CNS (mainly seizures)
   C. Medical arrest
   D. Metabolic/toxicologic
   E. Trauma

5. When evaluating a child utilizing the Yale Observation Scale, what is considered severe impairment?
   A. Acrocyanosis
   B. Brief smile
   C. Doughy skin
   D. Intermittent crying when held by parents
   E. Whimpering cry

6. A 12 year old presents with an extensive knee laceration that occurred while he was climbing over a chain-link fence. He is accompanied by his 16-year-old sister, but their parents cannot be reached. What is the most appropriate management?
   A. Bandage the wound appropriately and ask him to return with his parents
   B. Cleanse the wound but do not suture until the parents are located and provide consent to treat
   C. Refuse to even perform examination of the child until parental permission to treat is obtained
   D. Notify the police of possible parental neglect
   E. Treat the child as per standard protocols even though permission cannot be obtained to treat

7. A 14-year-old sexually active girl presents with vaginal discharge. Her boyfriend was recently diagnosed with gonorrhea. She does not want her parents contacted. What is the most appropriate management?
   A. Call her home and attempt to obtain permission to treat
   B. Examine and treat her appropriately while making no attempts to contact her family
   C. Examine her but refuse to prescribe medication without parental consent
   D. Notify protective services
   E. Refer her to Planned Parenthood for evaluation and treatment

8. What age in months is a child that can sit unsupported, has a unilateral reach, babbles, and can recognize strangers?
   A. 2
   B. 3
   C. 4
   D. 5
   E. 6

# 65  Fever in Children

### Sandra K. Dettmann

Select the appropriate letter that correctly answers the question or completes the statement.

1. Which of the following best describes occult bacteremia in children younger than 36 months of age?
   A. Children 24 to 36 months of age are more likely than those under 24 months of age to be bacteremic
   B. Children under 36 months of age with a rectal temperature of 39° C and no obvious source of fever have an incidence of bacteremia of over 20%
   C. Most common pathogen is *H. influenzae* type b
   D. Presence or absence of a drop in temperature after administration of acetaminophen does not influence the risk of bacteremia

E.  With *H. influenzae* type b bacteremia, most children become afebrile in 3 or 4 days with or without antibiotic coverage

2. Which of the following best describes an uncomplicated febrile seizure?
   A.  Affects approximately 10% of all children
   B.  Greatest risk of meningitis is at 36 months of age
   C.  Lumbar puncture is not required in a well appearing 12- to 18-month-old child
   D.  Peak incidence is between 24 and 36 months of age
   E.  Usual occurrence is at the peak of the fever

3. Which of the following is not a major diagnostic criterion for Kawasaki disease?
   A.  Cervical lymph nodes larger than 1.5 cm
   B.  Erythematous polymorphous skin rash
   C.  Fever above 38.5° C for at least 5 days
   D.  Oral inflammatory changes including fissuring, erythema, and crusting of the lips
   E.  Unilateral, exudative conjunctivitis

4. Which of the following is the most accurate method of temperature determination in a 3 year old?
   A.  Axillary
   B.  Forehead
   C.  Oral
   D.  Rectal
   E.  Tympanic

5. In the emergency department, which of the following is the most appropriate antibiotic to use for a febrile 5 week old?
   A.  Ampicillin 100 mg/kg IM
   B.  Ampicillin 50 mg/kg and cefotaxime 50 mg/kg IV
   C.  Cefotaxime 50 mg/kg IM
   D.  Cefotaxime 50 mg/kg IV and gentamycin 2.5 mg/kg IM
   E.  Ceftriaxone 50 mg/kg IM

6. A 20-month-old boy has been pulling on his left ear and has a rectal temperature of 39.2° C. Physical examination is normal, except for a nonmoving, red, bulgy left tympanic membrane. What is the most appropriate management?
   A.  CBC, blood culture, and cefotaxime IM
   B.  CBC, blood culture, lumbar puncture, and antibiotic IM or IV
   C.  CBC, blood culture, and oral antibiotic
   D.  CBC and oral antibiotic
   E.  Oral antibiotic

7. An 18-month-old boy has a normal physical examination and has been acting normally, but his rectal temperature is 39.2° C. What is the most appropriate management?
   A.  CBC and blood culture
   B.  CBC with the addition of a blood culture if the WBC is 15,000/mm³ or more
   C.  CBC with the addition of a blood culture if the WBC is 15,000/mm³ or more and urinalysis
   D.  Fever instructions with next-day follow-up
   E.  Fever instructions and urinalysis

8. A 3-year-old boy with leukemia presents with a fever. His last chemotherapy was 10 days ago. He has a Broviac catheter in place. What is the best management?
   A.  Flush the Broviac line to ensure patency
   B.  Obtain all blood work from the Broviac
   C.  Obtain a rectal temperature
   D.  Order CBC with differential and blood cultures
   E.  Prescribe oral antibiotics if tolerated

9. A 4-year-old boy with a history of sickle cell disease is febrile and has right hip pain. Following appropriate diagnostic studies, what antibiotic should be started before admission?
   A.  Ceftriaxone
   B.  Cefuroxime
   C.  Mezlocillin
   D.  Tobramycin
   E.  Vancomycin

10. What is the most common bacterium in cases of ventriculoperitoneal shunt infections?
    A.  *Haemophilus influenzae*
    B.  *Neisseria meningitidis*
    C.  *Staphylococcus aureus*
    D.  *Staphylococcus epidermidis*
    E.  *Streptococcus pneumoniae*

---

 **66** Sudden Infant Death Syndrome

*Scott A. Carlson*

Select the appropriate letter that correctly answers the question or completes the statement.

1. Which of the following increases the risk of sudden infant death syndrome (SIDS)?
   A.  Being a sibling of a SIDS victim
   B.  Maternal age less than 25 years
   C.  Maternal alcohol use
   D.  Maternal cigarette smoking
   E.  Recent diphtheria-pertussis-tetanus (DPT) vaccine

2. SIDS most commonly occurs at which of the following ages?
   A.  2-4 months
   B.  6-18 months
   C.  12-24 months
   D.  18-36 months
   E.  Under 1 month of age

3. Avoidance of which of the following has led to a decline in the incidence of SIDS in some countries?
   A.  Inadequately heated rooms during winter months
   B.  Respiratory syncytial virus (RSV) exposure
   C.  Sleeping in the prone position
   D.  Sleeping with a parent
   E.  Soft pillows and bedding materials

4. An afebrile 3-month-old infant comes to the ED after an apparent life-threatening event (ALTE). He stopped breathing for 20 to 30 seconds and had some circumoral and peripheral cyanosis but is now fine. Which of the following is the most appropriate management?
   A. Admit for further observation and testing
   B. Arrange for an apnea monitor at home and discharge
   C. Observe for 2 hours and discharge
   D. Observe for 6 hours and discharge
   E. Observe for 6 hours and discharge with a home apnea monitor

5. Which of the following best describes the use of theophylline in infants?
   A. Acts as a cardiac stimulant
   B. Helps in managing apnea of prematurity
   C. Improves the pneumogram in approximately 50% of users
   D. Therapeutic levels range from 20 to 25 μg/ml
   E. Useful in preventing SIDS

6. Which of the following infants may benefit from home monitoring?
   A. One recently infected with RSV
   B. One with heavy smokers living in the home
   C. One with repeated episodes of periodic breathing
   D. One with severe bronchopulmonary dysplasia (BPD)
   E. Sibling of SIDS victim

7. Which of the following suggestions is appropriate for the physician dealing with the parents of an infant who has just died?
   A. Explain that the cause of death is unknown (SIDS)
   B. Fully explain the details of complete resuscitative efforts before telling them the child has died
   C. Lack of an emotional response should be a red flag to probe the possibility of abuse
   D. No matter how seemingly inappropriate, allow the family to vocalize their feelings
   E. Realize that use of the word "dead" can be overly traumatic and should be avoided

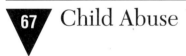

# 67 ▼ Child Abuse

*Sandra K. Dettmann*

Select the appropriate letter that correctly answers the question or completes the statement.

1. All of the following are true of suspected abuse in a 10 month old except:
   A. Epidural hematomas are common with shaken baby syndrome
   B. Homicide is rarely seen in this age-group
   C. Nutritional neglect is not often the cause of failure to thrive

D. The younger the child, the greater the potential for abuse
E. Up to 50% of fractures will be secondary to physical abuse

2. Which of the following best describes child abuse?
   A. Families of abuse usually have adequate support systems
   B. Poisoning accounts for a small number of abuse cases and carries a relatively low mortality rate
   C. The majority of abused children are younger than 4 years of age
   D. The main perpetrators are male
   E. Victims of shaken baby syndrome are usually younger than 3 months of age

3. Which of the following best describes the caretaker in Polle's syndrome (Munchausen's syndrome by proxy)?
   A. Has a past history of depression
   B. Has had similar symptoms within the past 5 years
   C. Has little medical education or expertise
   D. Is overly concerned about the child
   E. Pays little attention to the child

4. Which of the following bruised areas is most consistent with an accidental injury?
   A. Ear lobe
   B. Floor of mouth
   C. Forehead
   D. Frenulum
   E. Lower back

5. Which of the following is most correct regarding skeletal trauma in child abuse?
   A. Epiphyseal, metaphyseal, and periosteal injuries are the most common lesions
   B. Fewer than 20% of abused children exhibit skeletal injuries
   C. Joint dislocations are common in small children
   D. Nuclear scanning is useful for diagnosis but picks up injuries only at least 1 week old
   E. Radiographic changes are typically apparent

6. Which of the following is the most important physical sign indicating shaken baby syndrome?
   A. Apnea
   B. Bradycardia
   C. Full fontanelle
   D. Lethargy
   E. Retinal hemorrhage

7. Which of the following best describes child sexual abuse?
   A. Gonorrhea is the most commonly encountered infection
   B. Incest is uncommon
   C. False accusations by children of sexual abuse are not uncommon
   D. The offender is seldom known by the child
   E. Violence is often a factor

8. On physical examination, which of the following is most diagnostic of sexual abuse in a 4-year-old girl?
   A. Decreased rectal tone

B. Fimbriated hymen

C. Labial fusion

D. Torn hymen

E. Vaginal opening larger than 8 mm

2. In an asthma patient, what is an unreliable physical finding in evaluating the degree of respiratory distress?
   A. Agitation
   B. Dyspnea
   C. Tachycardia
   D. Use of accessory muscles
   E. Wheezing
3. A 6-year-old 25-kg boy with a long-standing history of asthma is having an acute attack. He has been taking theophylline, and his serum level is 4 µg/ml. What mg dose of aminophylline would raise his level to 12 µg/ml?
   A. 50
   B. 100
   C. 150
   D. 200
   E. 250
4. An 8-year-old known asthmatic boy presents with an acute attack. At home he uses an albuterol inhaler. Pulse oximetry is 92%. He is on 2 L nasal oxygen and receiving albuterol nebulization. Vital signs are BP, 120/80; P, 130; R, 36; and T, 37.4° C . What is the best additional management?
   A. Arterial blood gases and chest x-ray
   B. Arterial blood gases and theophylline
   C. Chest x-ray and corticosteroids
   D. Peak flow and corticosteroids
   E. Peak flow and theophylline
5. Which of the following best describes bronchiolitis?
   A. Bacterial etiology
   B. Disease of childhood
   C. Improvement with corticosteroids
   D. Risk for apnea
   E. Upper airway disease
6. A previously healthy 10-month-old boy presents with wheezing. A diagnosis of bronchiolitis is made. What is the best treatment?
   A. Antibiotics
   B. Bronchodilator
   C. Corticosteroids
   D. Oxygen
   E. Theophylline
   *Match the following items with the appropriate question.*
   A. Adrenergic agonist
   B. Antiinflammatory agent
   C. Blocks muscarinic receptors
   D. Increases diaphragmatic contractility
   E. Stabilizes mast cells
7. Ipratropium _____
8. Cromolyn _____
9. Nedocromil _____
10. Terbutaline _____
11. Theophylline _____

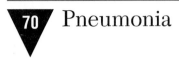

# 70 Pneumonia

*Gwen L. Hoffman*

Select the appropriate letter that correctly answers the question or completes the statement.
1. Beyond the newborn period, what is the leading bacterial cause of pneumonia in all age-groups?
   A. Group A streptococci
   B. *Haemophilus influenzae*
   C. *Neisseria meningitidis*
   D. *Staphylococcus aureus*
   E. *Streptococcus pneumoniae*
2. What is the best single indicator of pneumonia?
   A. Cough
   B. Nasal flaring
   C. Retractions
   D. Tachypnea
   E. Wheezing
3. What is the most common systemic complication of childhood pneumonia?
   A. Dehydration
   B. Epiglottitis
   C. Meningitis
   D. Pericarditis
   E. Soft tissue infections
4. An afebrile 4-month-old infant presents with coughing episode. His mother states he coughs until he turns red and at times he appears to quit breathing. He has a normal physical examination and a pulse oximetry of 98%. His WBC is 20,000/mm³ with a marked lymphocytosis. What is the most appropriate management?
   A. Admit for monitoring and start erythromycin
   B. Admit for observation
   C. Begin a septic work-up including a lumbar puncture
   D. Give ceftriaxone and discharge with follow-up
   E. Observe for 6 hours and if stable, discharge
5. A 7-year-old girl has a history of sore throat, headache, and malaise for 3 days. She now has a nonproductive, hacking cough. Rales are present on physical examination. What is the most likely etiology of her pneumonia?
   A. Bacteria
   B. Chlamydia
   C. Mycoplasma
   D. Pertussis
   E. Virus
6. What is the most appropriate management for mycoplasma pneumonia in a 7 year old?
   A. Amoxicillin
   B. Amoxicillin/clavulanate
   C. Cefaclor
   D. Erythromycin
   E. Tetracycline
7. A 3-year-old previously healthy boy has viral pneumonia. What is the most appropriate management?

A. Admit to an observation bed

B. Give ceftriaxone 50 mg/kg as a precaution

C. Instruct parents on supportive measures and discharge

D. Observe for 6 hours and discharge if no change in condition

E. Prescribe erythromycin to prevent superinfection

8. What is the most likely etiology of conjunctivitis and a staccato cough in an afebrile 6-week-old infant?

A. *Bordetella pertussis*

B. *Chlamydia trachomatis*

C. *Mycoplasma pneumoniae*

D. Respiratory syncytial virus (RSV)

E. *Streptococcus pneumoniae*

# 71 Cardiac Disorders

### *Gwen L. Hoffman*

Select the appropriate letter that correctly answers the question or completes the statement.

1. Which of the following best describes an innocent flow murmur?

A. Continuous

B. Grade III/VI late systolic

C. Pansystolic

D. Short ejection systolic

E. Short II/IV diastolic

2. In which of the following might there be increased pulmonary vasculature on chest x-ray?

A. Aortic stenosis

B. Coarctation of the aorta

C. Pulmonary stenosis

D. Tetralogy of Fallot

E. Ventricular septal defect

3. A neonate with central cyanosis breathes 100% oxygen for 15 minutes and has a $PaO_2$ of 99 mm Hg. What condition does this most likely represent?

A. Congenital heart disease

B. Hyaline membrane disease

C. Meconium aspiration syndrome

D. Persistent fetal circulation

E. Pneumonia

4. Central cyanosis is present in which of the following?

A. Aortic stenosis

B. Coarctation of the aorta

C. Patent ductus arteriosus

D. Transposition of the great vessels

E. Ventricular septal defect

5. What is the outstanding clinical feature of tetralogy of Fallot?

A. Clubbing of the nails

B. Cyanosis

C. Exertional dyspnea

D. Hemoptysis

E. Jugular venous distention

6. An infant presents with cool, pale skin, diaphoresis, and pulmonary congestion. Congestive heart failure is suspected. What would support this diagnosis?

A. Bradycardia

B. Hepatomegaly

C. Jugular venous distention

D. Pedal edema

E. Splenomegaly

7. In an infant with congestive heart failure, what is the mainstay of medical management?

A. Bed rest

B. Digoxin

C. Furosemide

D. Low-sodium formula

E. Oxygen

8. A 14-year-old girl has congestive heart failure. She has been in good health except for a recent upper respiratory infection and sore throat. What is the most likely diagnosis?

A. Acute rheumatic fever

B. Endocarditis

C. Kawasaki syndrome

D. Myocarditis

E. Pericarditis

9. What is the most common dysrhythmia in the pediatric age-group?

A. Atrial flutter/fibrillation

B. Complete AV block (congenital and acquired)

C. First- and second-degree AV blocks

D. Supraventricular tachycardia

E. Ventricular tachycardia

10. A stable 1 year old is in supraventricular tachycardia. What is the most widely accepted vagal maneuver?

A. Carotid massage

B. Ice bag to the face

C. Nasogastric tube placement

D. Ocular pressure

E. Rectal examination

11. A 10-month-old boy presents with supraventricular tachycardia. What treatment is contraindicated?

A. Adenosine

B. Cardioversion

C. Ice bag to the face

D. Propranolol

E. Verapamil

# 72  Gastrointestinal Disorders

*Sandra K. Dettmann*

Select the appropriate letter that correctly answers the question or completes the statement.

1. Which of the following best describes GI bleeding in the pediatric age-group?
   A. An Apt test should be utilized on the neonate's specimen to determine the presence of maternal blood
   B. Bleeding is most often painful
   C. For melena to exist, a blood loss of 25 ml is needed
   D. Hematochezia is the hallmark of upper GI bleeding
   E. Most children with a Meckel's diverticulum eventually become symptomatic

2. A 10-year-old afebrile boy presents with a history of abdominal pain for 2 days. It is spasmodic, intermittent, usually periumbilical, and occasionally severe, but he has not been vomiting. He thinks his last bowel movement was yesterday. His mother states he has had similar episodes of pain on and off over the last 6 months. On physical examination a tender mass is palpated in the left lower quadrant. There is no rigidity or guarding, and firm stool is palpable on rectal examination. What is the most appropriate management?
   A. Administration of enemas
   B. CAT scan to rule out malignancy
   C. Discharge home with follow-up
   D. Immediate surgical consultation
   E. Plain radiograph of the abdomen

3. In the pediatric age-group, which of the following is least likely to be an esophageal foreign body?
   A. Aluminum pull-tabs
   B. Buttons
   C. Coins
   D. Crayons
   E. Food

4. An 18-month-old asymptomatic toddler presents after swallowing a disc battery an hour ago. His mother brought in an identical battery from home; it measures 15 mm in diameter. An x-ray shows the battery to be lying in the stomach. What is the most appropriate management?
   A. Administration of a cathartic
   B. Administration of an emetic
   C. Endoscopic removal if the battery does not pass the pylorus within 3-7 days
   D. Immediate endoscopic removal
   E. Surgical exploration

5. What is the most reliable method for diagnosing pediatric appendicitis?
   A. Abdominal radiographs
   B. Clinical judgment
   C. C-reactive protein (CRP)
   D. Elevated white blood cell count with left shift
   E. Ultrasonography

6. In suspected appendiceal perforation, what antibiotic regimen should be instituted?
   A. Ampicillin and gentamycin
   B. Ampicillin, gentamycin, and clindamycin
   C. Ceftriaxone
   D. Cephalexin, metronidazole, and gentamycin
   E. Ciprofloxacin

7. Which of the following best describes pediatric biliary tract disease?
   A. Children receiving ceftriaxone have been reported to develop gallbladder sludge
   B. CT scan is the most sensitive and safest method for identifying gallstones
   C. Gallstones in younger children are usually the result of an obstructive process
   D. Hydrops of the gallbladder results from bacterial infection
   E. Virtually all children with gallstones are symptomatic

8. Which of the following best describes Hirschsprung's disease?
   A. Dilated, feces-filled rectum
   B. More frequently seen in females
   C. Most common cause of partial intestinal obstruction in early infancy
   D. Passage of large amounts of stool, but infrequently
   E. Pharmacologic management is the mainstay of treatment

9. Where is the most common location of intussusception?
   A. Colocolic
   B. Ileocolic
   C. Ileoileal
   D. Ileoileocolic
   E. Jejunoileal

10. Which of the following is least likely to be found in a patient with intussusception?
    A. Intermittent severe abdominal pain
    B. Left upper quadrant sausage-shaped mass
    C. Lethargy
    D. Rectal bleeding
    E. Vomiting

11. Which of the following is consistent with a diagnosis of pyloric stenosis?
    A. Age 2-6 weeks
    B. Bilious vomiting
    C. Female predominance
    D. Maternal age greater than 30
    E. More common in fall and winter births

12. Which of the following is the study of choice for diagnosing pyloric stenosis?
    A. Abdominal CT scan
    B. Abdominal radiograph
    C. Barium swallow
    D. Ultrasonography
    E. Upper Gl series

13. Which of the following abnormalities is often seen with pyloric stenosis?
    A. Hyperchloremia and hypokalemia alkalosis
    B. Hyperkalemia and hypoglycemia acidosis
    C. Hypernatremia and hypokalemia acidosis
    D. Hypochloremia and hypokalemia alkalosis
    E. Hypochloremia and hyponatremia acidosis

14. Which of the following is an important metabolic derangement often seen in Reye's syndrome?
    A. Hypercalcemia
    B. Hyperkalemia
    C. Hypoglycemia
    D. Hypomagnesemia
    E. Hyponatremia

15. A 2-month-old infant presents with bilious vomiting, abdominal distension, and palpable abdominal mass. What is the most likely diagnosis?
    A. Appendicitis
    B. Meckel's diverticulum
    C. Pyloric stenosis
    D. Reye's syndrome
    E. Volvulus

## 73 ▼ Acute Infectious Diarrhea Disease and Dehydration

### Sandra K. Dettmann

Select the appropriate letter that correctly answers the question or completes the statement.

1. In the United States, what is the most common bacterium causing acute diarrhea?
   A. *Campylobacter jejuni*
   B. *Salmonella* species
   C. *Shigella* species
   D. *Staphylococcus aureus*
   E. *Yersinia enterocolitica*

2. What best describes rotavirus?
   A. Causes an acute afebrile illness with vomiting and diarrhea
   B. Causes no significant intravascular volume compromise
   C. Has an incubation period of 10-14 days
   D. Mainstay of treatment is oral antibiotic therapy
   E. May involve symptoms of an upper respiratory tract infection

3. A 3-year-old with a fever of 39° C presents with cramping abdominal pain and watery, bloody, odorless diarrhea. What is the most likely cause?
   A. *Giardia*
   B. Norwalk agent
   C. Rotavirus
   D. *Salmonella*
   E. *Shigella*

4. In an older child what characteristic distinguishes *Yersinia* enteritis from other types of bacterial gastroenteritis?
   A. Color of stools
   B. Location of pain
   C. Presence of fever
   D. Presence of vomiting
   E. Type of onset

5. Vancomycin is recommended for treatment for which of the following?
   A. *Campylobacter*
   B. *Clostridium difficile*
   C. *Giardia*
   D. *Salmonella*
   E. *Shigella*

6. A 10-month-old boy presents with diarrhea. He is approximately 15% dehydrated and is hypotensive, tachycardic, and lethargic. Serum sodium is 140 mEq/L. What is the most appropriate dehydration management?
   A. 20 ml/kg 0.2% normal saline
   B. 20 ml/kg 0.45% normal saline
   C. 20 ml/kg 0.9% normal saline
   D. Pedialyte
   E. Rehydralyte

7. Which of the following best describes oral rehydration therapy?
   A. Desired volume is 20 ml/kg for mild dehydration
   B. Even children with significant sodium derangements may be candidates
   C. May be administered even if the patient continues to vomit or has diarrhea
   D. Patient needs to be monitored for 2 hours to determine success or failure of the treatment
   E. Should not be used in infants with acute gastroenteritis and volume depletion

8. A 4-week-old infant weighing 4 kg presents with a 2-day history of vomiting and diarrhea. He appears severely dehydrated, and his blood sugar is 30 mg/dl on Accucheck. What is the most appropriate dose of intravenous glucose?
   A. 4 ml of D10
   B. 4 ml of D25
   C. 8 ml of D10
   D. 8 ml of D25
   E. 8 ml of D50

9. In a 14-kg child, what best represents normal maintenance fluid requirements over 24 hours?
   A. 800 ml
   B. 1200 ml
   C. 1400 ml
   D. 1600 ml
   E. 2000 ml

# 74 Neurologic Disorders

### Dale J. Ray

Select the appropriate letter that correctly answers the question or completes the statement.

1. An 8-day-old infant, born at term, presents with lethargy and a temperature of 38.4° C. A spinal tap demonstrates cloudy fluid and is sent for analysis. What is the most likely bacterial organism?
   A. Group B streptococcus
   B. *Escherichia coli*
   C. *Haemophilus influenzae* type B
   D. *Haemophilus influenzae,* nontypeable strain
   E. *Streptococcus pneumoniae*

2. Which of the following best describes children older than 1 year of age with meningitis?
   A. Approximately 40% will present with coma on admission
   B. Focal neurologic findings occur in 15%-20%
   C. Most will present with septic shock
   D. Only a small percentage will complain of headache
   E. Trochlear nerve impairment is the most frequently seen cranial nerve neuropathy

3. Which of the following is most helpful in distinguishing brain abscess from viral meningitis?
   A. CSF glucose
   B. CSF Gram stain
   C. CSF India ink stain
   D. CSF white cell count
   E. Focal neurologic findings

4. A 4-year-old girl presents with a 36 hour history of fever associated with declining mental status. On physical examination she reacts minimally to pain, has left-sided weakness, a dilated right pupil, and nuchal rigidity. An intravenous line has been started and blood drawn for analysis. What is the most appropriate next step?
   A. Brain CT scan with contrast
   B. Brain CT scan without contrast
   C. Cefotaxime 50 mg/kg IV
   D. Lumbar puncture
   E. Phenobarbital 18 mg/kg IV

5. A 21-month-old girl has a spinal tap done for possible meningitis in the evaluation of a temperature of 40.3° C. Her blood work reveals a white blood cell count of 14,300 and a serum glucose of 110. Which of the following best describes evaluation of her CSF?
   A. CSF glucose of 58 is normal
   B. High percentage of polymorphonuclear leukocytes is often present in early viral meningitis
   C. If bacterial meningitis is caused by one of the most common organisms for her age-group, the likelihood of a positive blood culture is approximately 50%

D. If partially treated meningitis is considered, counter-current immunoelectrophoresis (CIE) is of little use
E. Spinal fluid C-reactive protein is a useful and sensitive method of distinguishing bacterial from viral meningitis in the emergency department

6. Which of the following best describes the treatment of childhood bacterial meningitis?
   A. Ceftazidime is the preferred third-generation cephalosporin
   B. Dexamethasone dosage for the treatment of *H. influenzae* meningitis is 0.15 mg/kg
   C. High-dose gentamycin (7 mg/kg) may be used as the only drug in the 1- to 3-month-old age-group
   D. Rifampin chemoprophylaxis is recommended for all health care workers if exposed to a child with meningococcal meningitis before the initiation of the child's intravenous antibiotics
   E. Treatment of bacterial meningitis for children up to the age of 1 year should include ampicillin

7. Which of the following best describes West's syndrome (infantile spasms)?
   A. Peak onset is before 3 months of age
   B. Responds to phenobarbital or carbamazepine
   C. Suggested by repetitive phenomenon
   D. Typically unilateral or asymmetric
   E. Vast majority have no associated CNS pathology

8. Which of the following is least consistent with a benign febrile seizure?
   A. Age of 4½ years
   B. Family history of epilepsy
   C. Roseola infantum
   D. Seizure duration of 12 minutes
   E. *Shigella* gastroenteritis

9. A 16-month-old boy with an unremarkable past medical history presents with a febrile seizure but is now doing well. His parents ask about the likelihood of recurrence. What is the most accurate percentage estimate of overall risk of recurrence?
   A. 1
   B. 10
   C. 20
   D. 33
   E. 66

10. A 14-year-old girl presents with her friends who state she had a "seizure." She has no seizure disorder history. Which of the following historical features would most support that her attack was a seizure rather than another type of "attack"?
    A. Confusion for 5 minutes after the episode
    B. Lightheadedness and diaphoresis before the episode
    C. Loss of motor tone
    D. Opisthotonic movements
    E. Suddenly frightened by another child

11. A 4-year-old, 15-kg boy presents in generalized status epilepticus. He has a seizure disorder but has not had any medication for 3 months. What is the most correct initial medication and dosage?

A. Diazepam 8 mg IV
B. Diazepam 15 mg rectal
C. Lorazepam 1 mg IV
D. Phenytoin 150 mg IV
E. Phenobarbital 150 mg IV

12. A 9-year-old boy presents after his first unprovoked seizure. Which of the following factors is most supportive in deciding to withhold anticonvulsant therapy at this time?
A. Blood chemistry results are normal
B. EEG is normal
C. Encephalemia is seen on CT related to prior head injury
D. He is a competitive swimmer
E. The seizure occurred while he was playing in the yard

13. In which of the following patients is emergent head CT scan indicated?
A. 12-year-old girl with vomiting and a throbbing unilateral headache that was preceded by seeing "zigzagging" lines
B. 14-year-old girl with recurrent headaches associated with unilateral blindness and flashes of bright light
C. 16-year-old boy with an occipital headache that began while weightlifting and intensity was worse at onset
D. 17-year-old boy with 2-week history of recurring unilateral severe orbital headache lasting approximately 45 minutes at a time and during attacks has a reddened, watery eye
E. 18-year-old boy with photophobia and a right frontal throbbing headache

14. A 4-year-old child presents with a recurrent unresponsive episode. What is most consistent with the diagnosis of breath-holding spell?
A. Body jerking and urinary incontinence
B. Loss of motor tone and posture followed by cyanosis
C. Onset of episodes 8 months ago
D. Post-episode confusion
E. Resolution of symptoms once the patient lies down

## PART FIVE   TOXICOLOGIC PROBLEMS

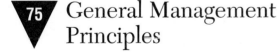

# 75 ▼ General Management Principles

### Greg Ledbetter

1. Which of the following is false regarding toxidromes?
A. A toxidrome is a classic constellation of symptoms associated with a particular poison.
B. Sedative-hypnotic poisoning may occur with clonus, rigidity, and hyperreflexia.
C. SLUDGE (salivation, lacrimation, urination, defecation, GI upset, emesis) is used to describe cholinergic poisoning.
D. The classic triad for opiate poisoning is coma, respiratory depression, and mydriasis.

2. Which of the following combinations can be safely used on a patient who arrives comatose and in respiratory depression?
A. Dextrostik, flumazenil, naloxone
B. Dextrostik, naloxone, thiamine
C. Flumazenil, glucose, naloxone
D. Flumazenil, glucose, thiamine
E. Glucose, naloxone, thiamine

3. Identify the false statement regarding laboratory data and the overdose patient.
A. Urine microscopic examination is of low yield and as such is unnecessary in suspected overdoses
B. An initial baseline CBC is often helpful, especially if the patient is to be admitted
C. Normal arterial blood gas values do not rule out methanol and ethylene glycol ingestions
D. Serum and urine toxicologic screens often do not provide the definitive answer in overdose cases

4. Which of the following is true regarding toxicologic screening tests?
A. Cocaine metabolites are rapidly eliminated and therefore significant if found
B. Drugs found on the screen may not be responsible for the symptoms seen
C. Drugs not routinely screened for are rarely involved in critical overdoses
D. They rarely if ever fail to identify the offending substance

5. Which of the following statements regarding gastrointestinal decontamination is correct?
A. Activated charcoal prevents absorption throughout the GI tract
B. All oral overdose patients should have either ipecac or lavage
C. Ipecac has an advantage over lavage in that it will not move drugs from the stomach into the intestine
D. All of the above are correct

6. A 25-year-old female presents after an unknown ingestion. The patient has the smell of garlic on her breath. Which is a possible intoxicant?
A. Alcohol
B. Arsenic
C. Cyanide
D. Organophosphates

7. A 30-year-old male presents 2 hours after an unknown ingestion. The patient is tachycardic and has mydriasis, decreased bowel sounds, and hot, dry, flushed skin. Which is the most likely intoxicant?
A. Ativan
B. Benadryl
C. Cocaine
D. Insecticide

8. A 40-year-old female presents with altered mental status, hyperreflexia, fever, and shivering. The family reports that her only medications are an unknown antidepressant and a decongestant she has been taking for a head cold. This history is most typical of which syndrome?
   A. Anticholinergic syndrome
   B. Cholinergic syndrome
   C. Serotonin syndrome
   D. Sympathomimetic syndrome

9. Which of the following does not correctly match toxin and antidote?
   A. Acetaminophen: acetylcysteine
   B. Beta blockers: glucagon
   C. Isoniazid: pyridoxine
   D. Lead: deferoxamine

# 76 ▼ Aspirin, Acetaminophen, and Nonsteroidal Agents

*Greg Ledbetter*

Select the appropriate letter that correctly answers the question or completes the statement.

1. All of the following statements are true regarding absorption of salicylates after an acute overdose except which one?
   A. Absorption of enteric-coated aspirin occurs in the small intestine, and peak serum levels may be reached 6 to 9 hours after ingestion
   B. Absorption of most aspirin products (non-enteric-coated) occurs in the stomach
   C. Approximately two thirds of the ingested dose is absorbed within 1 hour
   D. In most aspirin preparations, peak levels occur 2 to 4 hours after ingestion
   E. Large oral doses cause pylorospasm and delay gastric emptying

2. All of the following are typical metabolic consequences of salicylate overdose except which one?
   A. Hyperglycemia
   B. Hypothermia
   C. Metabolic acidosis
   D. Respiratory alkalosis
   E. Uncoupling of oxidative phosphorylation

3. What is the predominant acid-base disturbance seen in infants with acute salicylate overdose?
   A. Metabolic acidosis
   B. Metabolic alkalosis
   C. Respiratory acidosis
   D. Respiratory alkalosis

4. Common signs and symptoms of salicylism may include which of the following?

A. Lethargy or coma
B. Nausea and vomiting
C. Pulmonary edema
D. Tinnitus
E. All of the above

5. Which are the potentially toxic and lethal doses of salicylates?
   A. 50 mg/kg and 100 mg/kg, respectively
   B. 100 mg/kg and 300 mg/kg, respectively
   C. 100 mg/kg and 500 mg/kg, respectively
   D. 200 mg/kg and 500 mg/kg, respectively
   E. None of the above

6. The Done nomogram is useful in predicting salicylate toxicity in which of the following patients?
   A. A depressed patient who ingested a bottle of aspirin 6 hours earlier
   B. An elderly patient on chronic aspirin therapy for rheumatoid arthritis who has signs of salicylism
   C. A patient who took Alka-Seltzer and Pepto Bismol in the morning for an upset stomach, then attempted suicide at bedtime by ingesting a bottle of aspirin
   D. A patient with an acute fracture who ingested two bottles of aspirin over the last 12 hours in an attempt to relieve the pain
   E. A 2-year-old child who ingested an unknown quantity of enteric-coated aspirin tablets

7. All of the following are potentially helpful in the treatment of a salicylate overdose except which one?
   A. Alkalinization of urine with intravenous sodium bicarbonate
   B. Correction of potassium deficit
   C. Forced diuresis with normal saline
   D. Hemodialysis
   E. Multidose activated charcoal

8. Which of the following statements regarding chronic salicylate ingestion is true?
   A. Most overdoses are unintentional
   B. Symptoms of toxicity may mimic myocardial infarction, encephalitis, diabetic ketoacidosis, or alcoholic ketoacidosis
   C. Serum salicylate levels correlate poorly with the severity of intoxication
   D. The most common problem is gastric intolerance, which appears as epigastric pain, nausea, and anorexia
   E. All of the above

9. A patient arrives at the ED 12 hours after an acetaminophen (APAP) overdose. His signs and symptoms may include which of the following?
   A. Anorexia, nausea, and vomiting
   B. CNS depression and/or coma
   C. Right upper quadrant pain
   D. Possibly none
   E. Both A and D

10. What is the initial dose of N-acetylcysteine (NAC or Mucomyst) for a presumed APAP overdose?

A. 70 mg/kg

B. 140 mg/kg

C. 210 mg/kg

D. NAC should never be given until a toxic ingestion is confirmed with a serum APAP level

11. A 25-year-old woman comes to the ED 2 hours after ingesting an unknown quantity of APAP tablets. Her initial APAP level is 45 µg/ml. What is the most appropriate next step in this patient's management?

A. Administer N-acetylcysteine at 140 mg/kg PO

B. Continue to monitor and recheck serum APAP level in 2 hours

C. Initiate gastric lavage and activated charcoal

D. Start forced diuresis

E. Transfer to a psychiatric facility for evaluation of her suicide attempt

12. All of the following are true regarding APAP-induced hepatotoxicity except:

A. Acute ethanol ingestion decreases the toxicity of APAP.

B. Barbiturates increase the toxicity of APAP.

C. Children are more susceptible to APAP hepatotoxicity.

D. The actual hepatotoxin is a metabolite produced when APAP is metabolized by the cytochrome P-450 system.

E. All of the statements are true.

13. Which of the following statements about nonsteroidal antiinflammatory drug (NSAID) toxicity is not true?

A. Drug levels are useful only in acute NSAID ingestions

B. Most frequent symptoms with NSAID overdose are nausea and vomiting

C. NSAID overdose can cause acute renal failure

D. Most patients with NSAID overdose do well with no long-term sequelae

14. N-acetylcysteine should be administered up to how many hours after acetaminophen ingestion?

A. 8

B. 12

C. 16

D. 24

15. Indications for hemodialysis in salicylate overdose include all of the following except which one?

A. Coma, hepatic failure, or renal failure

B. Failure to respond to the more conservative treatments of charcoal and urinary alkalinization

C. Serum salicylate levels >100 mg/dl

D. Rising serum salicylate levels in toxic patients

E. All of the above

# 77 Alcohol-Related Disease

*Greg Ledbetter*

Select the appropriate letter that correctly answers the question or completes the statement.

1. Which of the following statements is not true of alcohol use in the United States?

A. There are an estimated 20 million alcoholics

B. Mortality from alcoholism is exceeded only by that from heart disease and cancer

C. It is the most common recreational drug taken by Americans

D. Alcoholism costs the nation more than $130 billion annually

E. All of the above are true

2. Which of the following statements is true of alcohol metabolism?

A. Alcohol dehydrogenase is located in the gastric mucosa

B. Alcohol is eliminated at a rate of 15-20 mg/dl/hr in the alcoholic

C. Alcohol metabolism is increased in women

D. Alcohol oxidation is a complex process involving a single-enzyme system

E. All of the above are true

3. A nonalcoholic has been drinking steadily through the evening. He exhibits impaired coordination and difficulty with gait and balance. Which of the following is his probable blood alcohol concentration?

A. 20-50 mg/dl

B. 50-100 mg/dl

C. 100-150 mg/dl

D. 150-250 mg/dl

E. 250-300 mg/dl

4. In most states, what is the acceptable legal level of intoxication?

A. 50-80 mg/dl (0.05%-0.08%)

B. 80-100 mg/dl (0.08%-0.1%)

C. 100-150 mg/dl (0.1%-0.15%)

D. 150-200 mg/dl (0.15%-0.2%)

5. An alcoholic woman arrives at the ED approximately 24 hours after attempting to quit drinking alcohol. She is complaining of nausea and anxiety and exhibits a gross tremor. At this time, what is she suffering from?

A. Delirium tremens

B. Major alcohol withdrawal

C. Minor alcohol withdrawal

D. Wernicke's encephalopathy

E. Withdrawal seizures

6. What is the most appropriate single treatment regimen for the patient described in Question 5?
   A. Atenolol
   B. Haloperidol
   C. Lorazepam
   D. Naloxone
   E. Phenytoin

7. All of the following disease manifestations may be similar to those of alcohol withdrawal syndrome except which one?
   A. Acute schizophrenia
   B. Alcohol-induced hypoglycemia
   C. Anticholinergic poisoning
   D. Narcotic ingestion
   E. Thyrotoxicosis

8. Which of the following is the best laboratory test to assess the severity of alcoholic hepatitis?
   A. Bilirubin
   B. Blood urea nitrogen (BUN)
   C. Prothrombin time (PT)
   D. Aspartate aminotransferase (AST) (formerly SGOT)

9. A 44-year-old alcoholic man has eaten poorly for the past 12 days but has continued to drink. He is brought in by friends. On neurologic examination, he is confused but otherwise normal. Blood glucose is 50 mg/dl by dipstick. Intravenous administration of 50% dextrose is given. His confusion increases, and he develops ataxia, horizontal nystagmus, and a heart rate of 130 beats per minute. At this point, which of the following should be ordered?
   A. Folic acid 5 mg IV
   B. Immediate CT of the head
   C. Lorazepam 2 mg IV
   D. Repeat bolus of 50% dextrose
   E. Thiamine 100 mg IV

10. What is the most common cause of bacterial pneumonia in alcoholics?
    A. Gram-negative rods
    B. *Klebsiella pneumoniae*
    C. Mixed flora
    D. *Streptococcus pneumoniae*
    E. Tuberculosis

11. Iron deficiency anemia is common in alcoholics and is usually secondary to which of the following?
    A. Blood loss from the gastrointestinal tract
    B. Malnutrition
    C. Severe liver disease
    D. Small bowel absorption
    E. All of the above

*The following paragraph applies to Questions 12 through 15.*

A 58-year-old alcoholic arrives at the ED with vomiting and shortness of breath. Laboratory analysis reveals an increased anion-gap metabolic acidosis. Match the urinalysis results below with the appropriate question.
    A. Alcoholic ketoacidosis
    B. Diabetic ketoacidosis

   C. Ethylene glycol poisoning
   D. Uremia
_____ 12. Elevated glucose and ketone levels
_____ 13. Ketonuria without glucosuria
_____ 14. Oxalate crystals
_____ 15. Proteinuria, cellular casts, and low specific gravity

16. Which of the following is a true statement about delirium tremens?
    A. Characterized by mild autonomic hyperactivity, tachycardia, and nausea
    B. A relatively common manifestation of alcohol withdrawal
    C. The death rate from delirium tremens is greater than 20%
    D. Delirium tremens seldom occurs before the third post-abstinence day
    E. All of the above are true

17. A 59-year-old white man with a history of chronic alcohol abuse comes to the ED inebriated but awake and oriented. Physical examination shows no focal abnormalities. The blood alcohol level is 350 mg/dl (0.35%). Six hours later while "sleeping off" his binge, the patient becomes hypertensive, tachycardic, and hallucinatory. He also develops a rapid tremor, which is more pronounced when his arms are extended. Treatment considerations include all of the following except which one?
    A. Benzodiazepines
    B. Hydration
    C. Phenothiazines
    D. Thiamine
    E. All of the above

18. A 60-year-old white male with known alcohol abuse presents after having a generalized seizure. The patient had documented alcohol withdrawal seizures in the past. He reports that he has not had any alcohol in the past 2 days. Blood alcohol level is less than 100 mg/dl (0.10%). Vital signs and physical examination findings are normal. What is the most appropriate next step for the emergency physician?
    A. Full seizure work-up including head CT and lumbar puncture
    B. Patient should be started on an anticonvulsant, preferably phenytoin
    C. Nothing other than ensuring appropriate follow-up with primary care doctor
    D. Patient should be treated only for alcohol withdrawal

19. Which of the following is not a characteristic of Wernicke's encephalopathy?
    A. Ascending paralysis
    B. Ataxia
    C. Global confusion
    D. Oculomotor disturbances
    E. All of the above

# 78 ▼ Other Alcohols

*Greg Ledbetter*

Select the appropriate letter that correctly answers the question or completes the statement.

1. Which of the following is characteristic of isopropyl alcohol ingestion?
   A. Decreased serum osmolal gap
   B. Hypertension
   C. Ketosis
   D. Metabolic acidosis
2. Treatment of methanol and/or ethylene glycol ingestion includes all of the following except which one?
   A. Bicarbonate
   B. Dialysis
   C. Ethanol administration
   D. Gastric lavage up to 4 to 6 hours after ingestion
   E. IV folate 50 mg every 4 hours
3. Which of the following statements about methanol ingestion is not true?
   A. Formic acid is the methanol metabolite that causes serious toxicity
   B. Methanol can be found in antifreeze, windshield washer fluid, and glass cleaners
   C. Methanol has no serious sequelae with proper treatment
   D. Folate deficiency can prolong the half-life of formic acid
   E. All of the above are true
4. What is the neurologic effect unique to methanol toxicity?
   A. Ascending paralysis
   B. Dizziness
   C. Ocular toxicity
   D. Sixth nerve palsy
5. What are the classic laboratory findings in methanol/ethylene glycol ingestion?
   A. Increased anion gap metabolic acidosis, elevated osmolal gap
   B. Normal anion gap metabolic acidosis, elevated osmolal gap
   C. Increased anion gap metabolic acidosis, normal osmolal gap
   D. Normal anion gap metabolic acidosis, normal osmolal gap
6. A 30-year-old male is brought into the ED obtunded. The family reports he has a history of drinking antifreeze as an alcohol substitute. What should the physician obtain for a prompt confirmation of ethylene glycol poisoning?
   A. Blood sample for ethylene glycol level
   B. Head CT
   C. Lumbar puncture
   D. Urine sample

# 79 ▼ Anticholinergics

*David Hughes*

Select the appropriate letter that correctly answers the question or completes the statement.

1. Which of the following drugs or classes of drugs exhibits anticholinergic properties?
   A. Benztropine (Cogentin)
   B. Carbamazepine (Tegretol)
   C. Cyclobenzaprine (Flexeril)
   D. Phenothiazines
   E. All of the above
2. Signs and symptoms of an anticholinergic overdose include all of the following except which one?
   A. Diarrhea
   B. Dry, hot skin
   C. Mydriasis
   D. Tachycardia
   E. Urinary retention
3. A patient presents after taking a bottle of pills and is found to have mydriasis, tachycardia, diaphoresis, and increased bowel sounds on physical examination. Which of the following is the most likely agent responsible for the physical findings?
   A. Diphenhydramine
   B. Seldane
   C. Organophosphate
   D. Ritalin
4. Which of the following EKG changes is frequently seen with anticholinergic toxicity?
   A. Wide QRS complex
   B. Prolonged QT interval
   C. PR depression
   D. None of the above
5. A 35-year-old man comes to the ED after taking a massive overdose of diphenhydramine. He is extremely agitated, and performing an examination is difficult. The nursing staff manages to obtain a temperature and places the patient on a cardiac monitor. His temperature is 40.6° C, and the monitor shows sinus tachycardia at a rate of 136. The patient's eyes are widely dilated, and his skin is hot and flushed. What is the most appropriate initial treatment for this patient?
   A. Aggressive sedation and cooling measures
   B. Gastric lavage followed by multidose activated charcoal
   C. Intravenous hydration
   D. Multidose activated charcoal without lavage
   E. Both A and C

6. A 25-year-old woman arrives at the ED after ingesting a "handful" of jimson weed seeds. She is agitated and combative. What is the most appropriate medication for sedating this patient?
   A. Chlorpromazine (Thorazine)
   B. Droperidol (Inapsine)
   C. Haloperidol (Haldol)
   D. Midazolam (Versed)
   E. All of the above

7. When physostigmine is used to treat anticholinergic overdoses in adults, what are the appropriate dose and route of administration?
   A. 1-2 mg rapid IV push
   B. 1-2 mg slow IV push over 2-4 minutes
   C. 5 mg IM
   D. 5 mg rapid IV push
   E. 5 mg slow IV push over 2-4 minutes

*Match the appropriate treatment sequence below with the appropriate question.*
   A. Gastric lavage, multidose activated charcoal in sorbitol, monitor, admit
   B. Initiate gastric lavage and multidose activated charcoal in water, monitor, admit
   C. Intubate, initiate gastric lavage and activated charcoal in water, monitor, admit
   D. Administer multi-dose activated charcoal in sorbitol, monitor, observe.
   E. Administer physostigmine, midazolam, gastric lavage, and multidose activated charcoal in sorbitol, monitor, admit.

8. A 25-year-old male who ingested 20 diphenhydramine (Benadryl) tablets 2 hours ago, is asymptomatic and has bowel sounds  _____

9. An 18-year-old female who ingested an unknown quantity of multiple drugs including a tricyclic antidepressant 4 hours ago is comatose with agonal respirations; bowel sounds are absent.  _____

10. A 12-year-old boy who ingested a bottle of chlorpromazine (Thorazine) 1 hour ago and has dilated pupils, dry skin, and a tachycardia of 110; bowel sounds are present.  _____

11. A patient presents 3 hours after a moderate overdose of meclizine and is found to be agitated and have markedly decreased bowel sounds, mydriasis and slight tachycardia. Which is the best method of initial decontamination?
    A. Gastric lavage
    B. Charcoal with sorbitol via nasogastric tube
    C. Charcoal with water via nasogastric tube
    D. Charcoal with water via enema

# 80 Common Cardiovascular Drugs

### *David Hughes*

Select the appropriate letter that correctly answers the question or completes the statement.

1. In chronic digoxin overdose, which of the following will not increase the risk of toxicity?
   A. Congestive heart failure
   B. Hypomagnesemia
   C. Hypothyroidism
   D. Renal insufficiency
   E. All of the above may increase toxicity

2. Which of the following digitalis toxicities has the highest mortality rate?
   A. Acute toxicity in adults
   B. Acute toxicity in children
   C. Chronic toxicity
   D. All have same mortality

3. Which of the following is not an indication for the administration of digitalis antibody fragments?
   A. Potassium less than 4 mEq/L
   B. Severe ventricular dysrhythmias
   C. Worsening hemodynamics secondary to bradydysrhythmias unresponsive to atropine
   D. All are indications for treatment

4. Which of the following is not true of beta-blocker overdoses in general?
   A. Atropine, glucagon, and catecholamines may be useful in treatment
   B. Bradycardia is the most common manifestation
   C. Extracorporeal elimination may have a role in some instances
   D. Ventricular dysrhythmias are characteristic and do not respond well to cardioversion and defibrillation

5. Which of the calcium channel blockers has the deadliest profile combining severe myocardial depression and peripheral vasodilation?
   A. Diltiazem
   B. Nifedipine
   C. Verapamil
   D. All have the same toxicity

6. After an acute ingestion, which of the following merits admission to the hospital for monitoring despite being asymptomatic after 6 hours?
   A. Atenolol toxicity
   B. Digoxin toxicity
   C. Diltiazem toxicity
   D. All need to be admitted for observation

7. A 60-kg diabetic teenage girl is brought to the ED after having locked herself in her grandmother's bathroom for an hour. At the scene, she was comatose and had bradycardia and weak pulses. An overdose is suspected. Bottles of prescription medications in the bathroom at the

scene included conjugated estrogens (Premarin), propranolol, digoxin, gemfibrozil, and aspirin. All of the following would be appropriate measures in the management of this patient except which one?

A. 10 ml calcium chloride 10% solution IV over 5 minutes

B. Glucagon 5 mg IV bolus every 5 minutes for a total of 15 mg

C. 100 g activated charcoal by NG tube

D. Atropine 0.5 mg IV bolus

E. All of the above

 # 81 Corrosives

### David Hughes

Select the appropriate letter that correctly answers the question or completes the statement.

1. Which statement below is false concerning corrosive ingestions?

A. Alkalis produce a rapidly penetrating liquefactive necrosis

B. Early complications of both acid and alkali ingestions are perforation and infection

C. Strong acids produce a coagulative necrosis with formation of an eschar

D. The stomach is spared in acid burns because acids usually are diluted in the oropharynx and esophagus

2. A 2-year-old boy was observed swallowing a small disk battery. A chest radiograph performed in the ED shows the battery is lodged in the esophagus. Which statement is true concerning the management of this patient?

A. If the battery reaches the stomach, then gastric aspiration should be promptly performed

B. Ipecac should be administered to dislodge the battery

C. The alkali of the battery is best neutralized with a weak acid

D. The disc battery should be removed promptly

3. Treatment considerations for an ingestion of a strong acid such as sulfuric acid, found in battery acid and commercial drain cleaners, include which of the following?

A. Antibiotics

B. Corticosteroids

C. Dilution with water

D. Gastric aspiration

4. Which of the following ingestions is associated with the highest morbidity and mortality?

A. Acid ingestion

B. Alkali ingestion

C. Oxidant ingestion

D. All have an equivalent profile

 # 82 Antidepressants and Monoamine Oxidase Inhibitors

### David Hughes

Select the appropriate letter that correctly answers the question or completes the statement.

1. Which of the following electrocardiographic abnormalities is not seen with cyclic antidepressant overdose?

A. Prolonged QT interval

B. QRS interval >0.10 seconds

C. Right axis deviation

D. Shortened PR interval

E. All may be seen

2. A 16-year-old girl who stated that she took "a handful" of amitriptyline tablets 2 hours before arrival has been observed for 6 hours in the ED. Which of the following should preclude her discharge or release for psychiatric evaluation?

A. Absence of major CNS signs

B. Absent bowel sounds

C. Heart rate of 110 beats per minute

D. QRS vector <120 degrees

E. Any of the above preclude discharge

3. Which of the following is the drug of choice for protracted seizures caused by cyclic antidepressants?

A. Diazepam

B. Phenobarbital

C. Phenytoin

D. Physostigmine

E. Sodium bicarbonate

4. First-line management of cardiac disturbances includes which of these?

A. Alkalinization by hyperventilation or sodium bicarbonate IV

B. Bretylium 5 mg/kg IV

C. Lidocaine 1 mg/kg IV bolus, then infusion of 2 to 4 mg/min

D. Phenytoin 500-1000 mg slow IV

E. Physostigmine 2 mg slow IV push

5. Which of the following statements is true of monoamine oxidase inhibitor (MAOI) overdose?

A. Bradycardia is a near-terminal event and should be treated with atropine

B. Most patients should be admitted to a monitored bed for 24 hours

C. Phase one consists of symptoms of catecholamine excess, which may be mistaken for anticholinergic overdose

D. Prolonged hypertension occurs, and a long-acting antihypertensive should be used

E. Tachycardias should be treated with beta blockers

6. Which of the following statements is true of drug and food interactions with MAOIs?
   A. Activated charcoal is not indicated
   B. "Fava beans and a nice Chianti," as well as aged cheese, may provoke a tyramine-based reaction
   C. Symptoms are usually delayed for hours
   D. Syrup of ipecac is useful early
   E. They produce the same basic symptoms seen in MAOI overdose

7. Which of the following is not one of four major effects of cyclic antidepressant overdose?
   A. Alpha-adrenoceptor blockade
   B. Anticholinergic effects
   C. Calcium channel blockade
   D. Inhibition of reuptake of serotonin and norepinephrine
   E. Sodium channel blockade

8. Which of the following is the treatment of choice for ventricular tachycardia in cyclic antidepressant overdose?
   A. Lidocaine
   B. Phenytoin
   C. Procainamide
   D. Sodium bicarbonate

9. All of the following are indicated in cyclic antidepressant overdose with significant EKG changes except which one?
   A. Hypertonic saline
   B. Hyperventilation
   C. Physostigmine
   D. Sodium bicarbonate
   E. All may be indicated

10. Which of the following is not considered one of the criteria defined by Sternbach (1991) for serotonin syndrome?
    A. Agitation
    B. Ataxia
    C. Diaphoresis
    D. Diarrhea
    E. Nausea and vomiting

# 83 Hallucinogens

*David Hughes*

Select the appropriate letter that correctly answers the question or completes the statement.

1. A 34-year-old man goes to a neighbor who hears him screaming, "They're going to get me" and other paranoid-type delusional statements. No history of ingestions or exposures is known, no empty medication bottles are found, and the neighbor knows no past medical history. Vital signs are blood pressure, 170/100; pulse, 126; respirations, 28; and oral temperature, 99° F. The patient is extremely agitated and frightened. All of the following are differential diagnoses except which one?
   A. Acute psychotic break
   B. Buspirone overdose
   C. Cocaine intoxication
   D. LSD intoxication
   E. Mixed-drug intoxication

2. A 5-year-old boy who became ill after ingesting some wild mushrooms is brought to the ED by his parents. The time of ingestion was approximately 2 hours before arrival, and the parents note that the child is "not acting quite right." The child complains only of abdominal pain. A sample mushroom brought in is identified as *Amanita muscaria*. What treatment is indicated?
   A. Admission to pediatric ICU
   B. Atropine 1 mg IV
   C. Diazepam 5 mg PO or IV
   D. Intubation and gastric lavage
   E. Observation for 6-12 hours and then discharge if not worse

3. Which of the following is true of marijuana intoxications?
   A. Intravenous use is associated with high mortality
   B. The most frequently seen adverse reaction is panic
   C. "Toxic psychosis" can occur with ingestion as well as inhalation
   D. Schizophrenics commonly use the drug because it lessens subjective symptoms of their illness

4. A 19-year-old man is brought to the ED by police officers who believe the patient to have taken phencyclidine. Initially, the patient is agitated and requires restraint. He calms down after being given droperidol 5 mg IM. Five minutes later, he becomes stuporous, then comatose. All of the following are indicated except which one?
   A. Gastric lavage, then gastric suction
   B. Intubation and establishment of intravenous access
   C. Removal or cleansing of clothing or any possibly contaminated materials
   D. Thiamine 100 mg IV, 50% dextrose 50 gm IV, naloxone 2 mg IV
   E. Urine acidification to enhance renal elimination

5. Complications of phencyclidine intoxications include all of the following except which one?
   A. Bradycardia (<60 beats/min)
   B. Bronchospasm
   C. Hypertension (diastolic >115 mm Hg)
   D. Hyperthermia (>40° C or 104° F)
   E. Myoglobinuric renal failure

6. The highest morbidity and mortality caused by hallucinogens is as a result of which of the following ingestions?
   A. Cannabinoids
   B. LSD
   C. MDMA
   D. PCP

7. Which of the following is true regarding LSD?
   A. Extremely potent with high margin of physical safety
   B. Extremely potent with low margin of physical safety
   C. Weak hallucinogenic with high margin of safety
   D. Weak hallucinogenic with low margin of safety
8. Which of the following is not considered to be a major clinical pattern of PCP intoxication?
   A. Acute brain syndrome
   B. Bizarre behavior
   C. Catatonic syndrome
   D. Toxic psychosis

## 84 Hydrocarbons

### David Hughes

Select the appropriate letter that correctly answers the question or completes the statement.

1. A 40-year-old refinery worker arrives at the ED after being exposed to a high-toxicity volatile hydrocarbon. He is in moderate respiratory distress. Vital signs are pulse, 120 and regular; blood pressure, 90/60; respirations, 30. Which of the following is indicated in the treatment of this patient?
   A. Chest radiography if respiratory status declines
   B. Epinephrine 1-4 μg/min IV, titrate to systolic blood pressure >100
   C. Gastric emptying with ipecac
   D. Normal saline 1-2 L wide open
   E. Removal of clothing and skin decontamination
2. Which of the following patients with acute hydrocarbon exposure may be discharged with follow-up?
   A. Patient asymptomatic on arrival and 6 hours after exposure to an unknown quantity of hydrocarbon
   B. Patient asymptomatic on arrival who later develops mild symptoms
   C. Patient symptomatic on arrival
   D. Patient with history of intentional ingestion
   E. All of the above
3. Which of the following is not considered a target organ system for hydrocarbon toxicity?
   A. Central nervous system
   B. Gastrointestinal tract
   C. Heart
   D. Lungs
   E. All are target organ systems
4. Which of the following characteristics of hydrocarbons is associated with potential toxicity?
   A. Chemical side chains
   B. Surface tension
   C. Viscosity
   D. Volatility
   E. All of the above
5. Which of the following situations would warrant GI decontamination?

A. A 2 year old who drank 5 ml of gasoline and is asymptomatic
B. A 10 year old who drank 1 ounce of camphor accidentally and is asymptomatic
C. A 30 year old who drank 6 ounces of kerosene in a suicide attempt and is asymptomatic
D. A 42 year old who presents obtunded after inhaling paint fumes
E. All of the above

## 85 Acute Iron and Lead Poisoning

### David Hughes

Select the appropriate letter that correctly answers the question or completes the statement.

1. Which of the following statements regarding iron poisoning in children is false?
   A. Maternal prenatal vitamins, because of their lack of added flavoring, are not often implicated in iron poisoning
   B. Parental counseling is mandatory because a child suffering an ingestion has a 25% chance of suffering another ingestion within 1 year
   C. The average age for iron poisoning is about 24 months
   D. The average bottle of children's chewable vitamins contains 5 to 10 times the possible lethal dose of iron
   E. The body has no organized mechanism for iron excretion
2. Which of the following statements is true of toxic iron ingestion?
   A. Causes indirect cardiac toxicity
   B. Has five phases, the first and third of which include gastrointestinal hemorrhage
   C. Is significant only if the iron level exceeds the measured total iron binding capacity (TIBC)
   D. Produces mild symptoms in ingestions exceeding 60 mg/kg of elemental iron
   E. Usually produces hyperglycemia and a depressed white blood cell count
3. A 2-year-old child arrives at the ED 30 minutes after ingestion of an unknown number of chewable multivitamins. The child has vomited once. There is no blood in the vomitus. His mental status is age appropriate. All of the following would be correct treatment procedures except:
   A. Abdominal radiograph after gastric emptying
   B. Deferoxamine challenge by intramuscular injection of 50 mg/kg with 6-hour observation for "vin rose" urine
   C. Gastric lavage with bicarbonate-containing solution
   D. Serum iron level and TIBC 4 hours after ingestion
   E. Whole-bowel irrigation at 0.5 L/hr

4. Which of the following is the most useful laboratory test for acute iron toxicity?
   A. Acute abdominal series
   B. Peak serum iron level
   C. Total iron binding capacity
   D. White blood cell count
   E. None of the above

5. Which of the following methods of decontamination is not indicated in acute iron poisoning?
   A. Activated charcoal
   B. Gastric lavage
   C. Intravenous deferoxamine
   D. Oral deferoxamine
   E. All are effective

6. A 6-year-old child presents after swallowing his father's lead fishing weight. Which of the following would be the most appropriate ED course?
   A. Admit for chelation therapy despite lead level
   B. Draw lead level; if less than 25 μg/dl, discharge to home for follow-up in 1 week
   C. Draw lead level, then remove endoscopically
   D. Induce emesis immediately
   E. Whole-bowel irrigation immediately

# 86  Opioids

### David Hughes

Select the appropriate letter that correctly answers the question or completes the statement.

1. Which of the following is false regarding opioid pharmacology?
   A. Diphenoxylate is known as the opioid with the most rapid onset
   B. If patients are asymptomatic for 2-3 hours after ingestion, the dose is considered nontoxic
   C. Maximum toxic and therapeutic effects are seen in 10 minutes if by IV, 30 minutes if by IM injection, and 90 minutes if given PO or SQ
   D. Most GI absorption occurs within 1-2 hours, principally in the small intestine
   E. All of the above are true

2. Identify the true statement regarding narcotics.
   A. Hemodialysis is very effective if less than 2 hours have elapsed since ingestion
   B. No narcotics are fat soluble, and thus little storage in fatty tissues is noted
   C. Increased metabolism is seen with hepatic disease and selected agents
   D. The significant dosing difference between parenteral and oral administration is because of a first-pass effect through the hepatic circulation for orally administered narcotics

3. Which of the following is false regarding narcotic antagonists?

A. Nalorphine was once the antagonist of choice despite its agonist activity
B. Naloxone is currently the antagonist most favored because it acts at the three major opioid receptors, mu, kappa, and sigma
C. Naltrexone, a new antagonist, has demonstrated longer lasting effects
D. All of the above are true

4. All of the following statements are true regarding narcotic overdose except which one?
   A. Miosis may be absent in meperidine intoxication
   B. Narcotics produce orthostatic hypotension through vasodilation with no direct effects on the heart
   C. Opioids produce analgesia and significant respiratory depression before producing decreased consciousness
   D. Respiratory depression occurs by decreasing the rate, with little change in the tidal volume
   E. Tolerance in addicts develops to all symptoms

5. All the following regarding noncardiogenic pulmonary edema are true except which one?
   A. It is common and present in virtually all fatal cases
   B. Physical examination findings vary from normal to coarse rales and rhonchi
   C. Pulmonary edema may be found in therapeutic as well as toxic dosages
   D. The edema clears rapidly (24-36 hours) with simple oxygen therapy
   E. All of the above are true

6. All the following occur with narcotic overdose except which one?
   A. Convulsions are routinely seen in children and adults
   B. Nausea and vomiting may occur spontaneously, but are often difficult to induce
   C. Opioids decrease GI transit time, allowing removal of narcotics from the stomach hours later
   D. Some agents (such as fentanyl) will cause widespread increase in neuromuscular tone
   E. All of the above occur

7. Which of the following is true regarding parenteral narcotic overdose?
   A. During reversal, hyperventilation, nausea, and vomiting are commonly seen
   B. Naloxone can be administered by IV infusion at a rate of 0.4-0.8 mg/hr
   C. Naloxone lasts 30-60 minutes; repeat dosing may be necessary to prevent recurrent toxic symptoms
   D. The dose of naloxone is 0.4 mg, IV test dose, followed by 2 mg IV every 5 minutes to a total of 10 mg
   E. All the above are true

8. Which of the following is true regarding oral narcotic overdoses?
   A. Activated charcoal is useful only if less than 3 hours have elapsed since ingestion
   B. Following oral ingestion, discharge is acceptable after lavage regardless of symptoms

C. Most toxic ingestions involve pure opioid analgesics

D. Naloxone should be given in any known narcotic overdose, even if the patient is asymptomatic

E. All of the above

9. Which of the following requires higher doses of naloxone to precipitate reversal?

A. Codeine

B. Pentazocine

C. Propoxyphene

D. All require higher doses

10. Which is incorrect?

A. Dextromethorphan: no respiratory depression

B. Diphenoxylate: not for use in children younger than age 5

C. Methadone: relatively short acting

D. Propoxyphene: rapid onset, psychosis

11. Which of the following statements is true regarding opioid withdrawal and treatment?

A. Failure to treat opioid withdrawal is likely to have significant morbidity and mortality

B. Opioid withdrawal should be treated aggressively in the ED with long-acting opioid agonists

C. The minimum sustained use period for opioids before withdrawal will be noted on abstinence is 90 days

D. There is no clear indication for an emergency physician to administer opioids to an addict claiming to be in withdrawal

E. None of the above

12. The treatment of noncardiogenic pulmonary edema secondary to heroin overdose includes which of the following?

A. Digitalis loading

B. High-dose diuretics

C. High-dose steroids

D. Naloxone infusion

E. All of the above

13. A 30-year-old man has taken 50 Darvocet (propoxyphene) tablets in a suicide attempt. Which of the following is true?

A. Adverse effects of propoxyphene overdose usually do not occur until 4-6 hours after ingestion

B. Propoxyphene is relatively benign, and co-ingestants must be ruled out before medical clearance

C. Relatively small doses of naloxone may be required to reverse respiratory depression

D. This patient could suffer a catastrophic collapse within 15 minutes of ingestion

E. None of the above

# 87 Lithium Intoxication

*David Hughes*

Select the appropriate letter that correctly answers the question or completes the statement.

1. All of the following statements regarding the use of lithium are true except which one?

A. Acute intentional overdose tends to be less severe than chronic therapeutic overdose

B. Despite a small volume of distribution and lack of protein binding, the serum half-life of lithium can be more than 50 hours with chronic therapy

C. Effects of overdose are primarily to the central nervous system, and irreversible brain dysfunction may result from toxicity

D. Lithium is widely used as an antidepressant despite an unclear mechanism of action and a very narrow therapeutic index

E. Weakness, difficulty with attention and memory, and gastrointestinal distress indicate mild to moderate intoxication

2. Which of the following statements is true of lithium toxicity?

A. Activated charcoal should be used for mild, recent ingestion

B. In severe toxicity, prolonged dialysis is the appropriate treatment

C. Levels >4 mEq/L without signs of severe toxicity can be managed expectantly

D. Mild hypokalemia with an ECG demonstrating hypokalemia is common

E. With normal renal function, forced saline diuresis is very effective in moderate overdose

3. Which of the following situations is likely to lead to lithium toxicity in a patient receiving lithium for bipolar disorder?

A. A 20 year old with hepatitis B and mild liver failure

B. A 25 year old who recently took up smoking

C. A 30 year old with gastroenteritis

D. A 35 year old started on phenytoin for an unrelated seizure disorder

E. All of the above

4. ECG changes that occur during lithium intoxication may mimic which electrolyte disturbance?

A. Hypercalcemia

B. Hyperkalemia

C. Hypocalcemia

D. Hypokalemia

E. None of the above

5. Which of the following has been found to increase lithium toxicity when taken concomitantly?
   A. Fluoxetine
   B. Ibuprofen
   C. Lasix
   D. Phenothiazines
   E. All of the above

6. Which of the following is not considered an effective means of GI decontamination in acute lithium overdose?
   A. Activated charcoal
   B. Gastric lavage
   C. Kayexalate
   D. Whole-bowel irrigation
   E. All are effective

# 88 Neuroleptics

## David Hughes

Select the appropriate letter that correctly answers the question or completes the statement.

1. Which of the following statements is true of the side effects of neuroleptics?
   A. Life-threatening dysrhythmias due to neuroleptics are not produced at therapeutic levels
   B. Orthostatic hypotension is produced by alpha-adrenergic blockade
   C. Phenothiazines lower the seizure threshold and often cause seizure activity
   D. Tardive dyskinesia is most likely to result from neuroleptics with the lowest anticholinergic activity
   E. The potential for acute dystonia can be predicted by knowing only the dopaminergic activity of the drug

2. Which of the following statements is true of neuroleptic overdose?
   A. Anticholinergic effects produce mydriasis
   B. Class 1A antidysrhythmics are the drugs of choice for ventricular dysrhythmias
   C. Hyperthermia as well as hypothermia may result
   D. Neuroleptic malignant syndrome is dose related and frequently accompanies severe overdoses
   E. Respiratory depression is common

3. Which of the following is a result of long-term neuroleptic use rather than acute overdose?
   A. Akathisia
   B. Dystonia
   C. Neuromuscular malignant syndrome
   D. Tardive dyskinesia

4. All of the following may predispose patients to NMS except which one?
   A. Dehydration
   B. Increase in drug dosage
   C. Rapid drug loading
   D. Rapid withdrawal of drug therapy

5. A 30-year-old male presents to the emergency department complaining of tremors 2 weeks after beginning haloperidol therapy. He is found to have normal vital signs and on physical examination is rigid and dystonic and has a course tremor. Which is the appropriate ED disposition?
   A. Admission for IV anticholinergics
   B. Emergent psychiatry consult
   C. Oral anticholinergics and discharge to home
   D. Withdrawal of haloperidol, IV anticholinergics, and discharge to home on oral anticholinergics if improved

# 89 Pesticides

## Lars Blomberg

Select the appropriate letter that correctly answers the question or completes the statement.

1. Which of the following is false regarding organophosphates?
   A. Common causes of morbidity and mortality include bronchorrhea and respiratory insufficiency
   B. They are noncompetitive inhibitors of acetylcholinesterase
   C. They cause a classic cholinergic syndrome
   D. They have a very high lipid solubility
   E. All of the above are true

2. Which of the following should be included in the diagnosis and treatment of organophosphate poisonings?
   A. Atropine until secretion control occurs
   B. Cholinesterase levels in both serum and RBCs
   C. Pralidoxime chloride (2-PAM)
   D. All the above

3. Identify the correct statement associated with carbamate insecticides.
   A. Mechanism differs from the organophosphates in that they are parasympathomimetic agents
   B. They closely resemble organophosphates but have shorter duration of effects
   C. Treatment is similar to that for organophosphate poisoning, with large doses of atropine and pralidoxime
   D. None of the above

4. Which of the following is not related to chlorinated hydrocarbon pesticide poisoning?
   A. Central and peripheral neuronal excitation
   B. Excessive use of lindane (Kwell)
   C. High lipid solubility and storage in fatty tissue
   D. Ventricular dysrhythmias
   E. All are related to chlorinated hydrocarbons

5. Which of the following is true regarding the diagnosis and treatment of chlorinated hydrocarbon poisoning?
   A. With very high doses, hemodialysis should be considered

B. The course of treatment relies heavily on the plasma level

C. Ventricular dysrhythmias are best treated with class Ia antiarrhythmic agents

D. None of the above

6. Concerns in the treatment of chlorinated hydrocarbon poisonings include all of the following except which one?

A. Continuous cardiac monitoring is essential

B. Pralidoxime is an effective reversal agent

C. Renal failure should always be considered

D. Seizure control is achieved with benzodiazepines or barbiturates

E. All of the above are concerns

7. All the following statements are true regarding the substituted phenols except which one?

A. One of the most obvious symptoms is hypothermia

B. They are widely used in currently available insecticides, including over-the-counter preparations

C. Toxicity is related to uncoupling of oxidative phosphorylation and methemoglobinemia

D. Treatment is directed toward controlling body temperature and metabolism while watching for possible complications

E. All of the above are true

8. Identify the false statement regarding chlorophenoxy pesticides.

A. Discharge after 6 hours of observation is possible if symptom development is minimal

B. Skeletal muscle is the primary target organ

C. They were used in Vietnam and are most commonly known as "agent orange"

D. There are few identifying symptoms, so diagnosis relies heavily on laboratory evaluation

E. All of the above are true

9. Which of the following is not a common finding in paraquat poisoning?

A. Chemical burns of the oropharynx

B. Esophageal perforation as a frequent cause of death

C. Pulmonary involvement

D. Rapid onset leading to death within a few hours from florid respiratory failure

E. All of the above are common findings

10. Cumulative toxicity following repeated exposure is common with all of the following pesticides except which one?

A. Chlorinated hydrocarbons

B. Chlorophenoxy compounds

C. Phenols

D. Organophosphates

E. All of the above cause cumulative toxicity

11. A 2-year-old child presents with seizure and ventricular tachycardia following exposure to lindane for treatment of presumed scabies. Which of the following is the most appropriate antiarrhythmic to treat the patient's dysrhythmia?

A. Lidocaine

B. Phenytoin

C. Procainamide

D. Propranolol

E. None of the above. The dysrhythmia is self-limited

12. Choose the correct statement concerning pyrethrins and pyrethroid insecticides.

A. Both the natural pyrethrins and the synthetic pyrethroids may potentiate allergic reactions

B. Cumulative toxicity may be a problem

C. Dermal exposure is most common

D. The most severe complication is an acute asthmatic reaction

E. None of the above

 **90** Sedative-Hypnotics

### *Lars Blomberg*

Select the appropriate letter that correctly answers the question or completes the statement.

1. Which statement is false concerning barbiturates?

A. Short-acting barbiturates are more lipid soluble than long-acting preparations

B. They cross the placenta, and they are excreted in breast milk

C. They inhibit hepatic microsomal enzymes, decreasing the metabolism of other drugs

D. They work at the GABA receptor in the central nervous system

E. All of the above are true

2. A 35-year-old man comes to the ED after taking an overdose of "yellow jackets" or pentobarbital (a short-acting barbiturate). On arrival, the patient responds only to painful stimuli, deep-tendon reflexes are absent, and he appears hypoxic. After securing an airway, management considerations include all of the following except which one?

A. Forced alkaline diuresis

B. Hemodialysis

C. Late gastric lavage

D. Oral activated charcoal

E. All of the above are appropriate

3. Which statement below is a distinguishing feature of methaqualone (Quaalude) ingestion, as compared with barbiturate ingestion?

A. Abstinence syndrome occurs only in chronic barbiturate abuse

B. Diazepam may be necessary to treat severe muscular hyperactivity in methaqualone ingestion

C. Forced alkaline diuresis is an effective elimination technique in methaqualone ingestion

D. Methaqualone ingestion causes a much more severe cardiovascular and respiratory depression

E. None of the above

4. Which of the following drugs belonging to the broad classification of sedative-hypnotics is distinguished by its combination with codeine as an oral substitute for heroin, called a "load," "hit," or "set"? (This drug also has a potent anticholinergic effect, creating fixed and dilated pupils on physical examination.)
   A. Chloral hydrate (Noctec)
   B. Glutethimide (Doriden)
   C. Methaqualone (Quaalude)
   D. Methyprylon (Noludar)

5. Chloral hydrate is a sedative-hypnotic agent used especially in pediatric and elderly patients. Which statement below is false concerning the use of this medication?
   A. Chloral hydrate has a corrosive effect on the GI tract
   B. Chloral hydrate sensitizes the myocardium to catecholamines, producing arrhythmias
   C. Large doses of chloral hydrate inhibit the action of ethanol by increasing the activity of alcohol dehydrogenase
   D. The action of chloral hydrate depends on the rapid production of an active metabolite
   E. None of the above

6. A 23-year-old woman with a psychiatric history comes to the ED by way of EMS, with decreased mental status, dilated and unreactive pupils, flushed dry skin, dry mucous membranes, and absent bowel sounds. Two empty bottles of Nytol, an over-the-counter nighttime sleep aid (OTC-NSA) were found beside the patient by the paramedics. Which of the following statements is true concerning OTC-NSA overdoses?
   A. Children are more likely to have CNS excitation, usually agitation, delirium, and convulsions
   B. Dantrolene is the treatment of choice if hyperthermia is present
   C. Most OTC-NSAs contain diphenhydramine, which is unlikely to cause this condition
   D. Physostigmine (Antilirium) administered as an IV bolus followed by continuous IV infusion is the recommended treatment
   E. None of the above

7. Bromides, once used as over-the-counter sleep aids, are still popular in other countries. Acetylcarbromal (Paxarel) is an organic bromide prescribed in the United States. What side effect is unique to bromide ingestion compared to other sedative-hypnotics?
   A. Elevated serum chloride level
   B. GI irritation
   C. Hyperthermia
   D. Neuropsychiatric symptoms
   E. None of the above

8. Neonatal withdrawal syndrome secondary to phenobarbital use during pregnancy is characterized by all of the following except which one?
   A. Appearance of symptoms 1-4 days after birth
   B. Frantic fist sucking
   C. High-pitched cry

D. Seizures
E. All of the above are characteristics

9. Which of the following statements concerning the presentation of antihistamine toxicity is correct?
   A. Cardiac toxicity associated with diphenhydramine poisoning is common
   B. Children are more likely to present with severe CNS depression
   C. Conduction abnormalities with diphenhydramine are thought to be secondary to quinidine like membrane stabilizing effects
   D. Severe toxicity is more common with H1 blockers than with OTC preparations containing scopolamine or methapyrilene
   E. None of the above

10. Which of the following barbiturates has the lowest lipid solubility?
    A. Methohexital
    B. Pentobarbital
    C. Phenobarbital
    D. Thiopental

---

 **91** ## Cocaine, Amphetamines, and Other Sympathomimetics

*Lars Blomberg*

Select the appropriate letter that correctly answers the question or completes the statement.

1. Which of the following is not recommended for treatment of amphetamine or cocaine overdoses?
   A. Ammonium chloride to acidify urine
   B. Benzodiazepines for psychiatric manifestations
   C. External cooling for hyperthermia
   D. Lidocaine for ventricular dysrhythmias
   E. Mannitol or furosemide for rhabdomyolysis

2. What is the most common complaint in the patient with an acute overdose of sympathometics?
   A. Altered mental status
   B. Chest pain
   C. Palpitations
   D. Seizures
   E. Syncope

3. Which of the following is true about laboratory testing in a patient with suspected cocaine toxicity?
   A. ECG may show multifocal atrial tachycardia, which in younger patients is pathognomonic for cocaine toxicity
   B. Cocaine will give a positive urine test for 5 to 7 days
   C. In acute toxicity a serum cocaine level should be used to guide therapy
   D. Plain films of the abdomen will confirm the presence of cocaine-filled condoms in the GI tract of a "body packer"

E. Urinalysis other than for a toxicology screen is not helpful

4. Which of the following statements is true regarding chest pain in a patient using cocaine?
   A. An elevated CPK indicates an acute infarction
   B. If cardiac ischemia is excluded, the patient can safely be discharged
   C. It is most often caused by myocardial ischemia
   D. It may have an infarct with normal coronary arteries
   E. Thrombolytics should be used if an infarct is definitely established

5. Which of the following hallucinogenic amphetamines is considered to have a low abuse potential?
   A. DMA (dimethoxyamphetamine)
   B. MDA (methylenedioxyamphetamine), "the love pill"
   C. MDEA (methylenedioxyethamphetamine), "eve"
   D. MDMA (methylenedioxymethamphetamine), "ecstasy"
   E. All have high abuse potential

6. A 21-year-old male presents to the emergency department after taking an overdose of an unknown sympathomimetic. He complains of persistent emesis and significant abdominal pain. Which of the following drugs is the most likely etiologic agent?
   A. Caffeine
   B. Cocaine
   C. Methamphetamines
   D. Phenylpropanolamine

7. A 30-year-old female arrives at the emergency department with ventricular tachycardia 6 hours after a large cocaine binge. Which of the following antiarrhythmics is the most appropriate in this setting?
   A. Diazepam
   B. Esmolol
   C. Lidocaine
   D. Sodium bicarbonate
   E. None of the above; the dysrhythmia is self-limited

---

# 92 Toxic Inhalations

### Lars Blomberg

Select the appropriate letter that correctly answers the question or completes the statement.

1. The half-life of carboxyhemoglobin in hyperbaric oxygen chambers is _____ the half-life of carboxyhemoglobin when breathing room air.
   A. Equal to
   B. One eighth
   C. One half
   D. One twentieth
   E. Twice

2. A 30-year-old man comes to the ED after being trapped inside his burning home. His carboxyhemoglobin level is 50%. Which of the following statements is true?

A. Both $Po_2$ and pulse oximetry readings are likely to be normal
B. Carboxyhemoglobin causes a shift of the oxygen dissociation curve to the right and therefore interferes with delivery of oxygen to the tissues
C. Serum carboxyhemoglobin levels correlate well with toxicity
D. Symptoms would be expected to be equivalent to those of a patient with a 50% blood loss
E. None of the above

3. A 27-year-old woman who is 24 weeks pregnant was exposed to carbon monoxide. She is relatively asymptomatic. The institution has a hyperbaric oxygen facility, and the department standard is that patients with a carboxyhemoglobin level of 25% require hyperbaric oxygen treatment. Which of the following statements will help guide further therapy while waiting for the carboxyhemoglobin level results?
   A. Fetal hemoglobin has a higher affinity for carboxyhemoglobin, so dropping the standard for hyperbaric therapy should be considered
   B. Hyperbaric therapy is absolutely contraindicated in pregnancy except for the most dire situations
   C. The standard for hyperbaric therapy should be raised because fetal hemoglobin is better able to tolerate carboxyhemoglobin
   D. The patient should be treated exactly the same as the nonpregnant patient

4. An adult patient arrives at the ED in a coma with metabolic acidosis after smoke inhalation. After ABCs and 100% oxygen, what would be the next most appropriate step?
   A. Amyl nitrite
   B. Carboxyhemoglobin level; if low, treat with Lilly cyanide antidote kit
   C. Sodium nitrite
   D. Sodium thiosulfate
   E. None of the above

5. Which of the following findings on history and physical examination would place a patient at very low risk for delayed noncardiogenic pulmonary edema?
   A. Ammonia exposure
   B. Laryngeal edema
   C. Ozone exposure
   D. Phosgene exposure
   E. Respiratory arrest

6. A 24-year-old man is comatose. His skin and nails are cherry red, and his skin has a number of bullae. On high-flow oxygen, initial arterial blood gas readings are pH, 7.30; $Pco_2$, 30; $Po_2$, 300; and oxygen saturation, 99%. This clinical presentation is most consistent with which of the following toxic inhalations?
   A. Amyl nitrate
   B. Carbon monoxide
   C. Cyanide
   D. Hydrogen sulfide
   E. Phosgene

7. A 35-year-old construction worker is brought to the emergency department after a significant exposure to carbon tetrachloride. Choose the incorrect statement.
   A. Acute complications are generally related to hypoxia
   B. Arterial blood gas determination may reveal a respiratory acidosis with an increased A-a gradient
   C. Extreme caution should be observed if epinephrine administration is required
   D. Treatment involves supportive ventilation and oxygenation
   E. All of the above are true

8. A 24-year-old female seeks treatment in the ED after a brief exposure to hydrogen chloride gas. Which of the following is true?
   A. Corticosteroids are indicated if the patient develops noncardiogenic pulmonary edema
   B. Immediate symptoms are usually absent, although significant pulmonary sequelae may develop 2-24 hours after exposure
   C. Inhaled β-agonists are ineffective for treating bronchospasm in such patients
   D. Nebulized 2% sodium bicarbonate may provide symptomatic relief
   E. None of the above

9. A 60-year-old victim of a house fire arrives in the emergency department in cardiopulmonary arrest. CPR has been initiated and IV access obtained. When the IV was placed it was noted that the patient's venous blood was bright red. Which of the following is an unnecessary ED action?
   A. ABG analysis with co-oximeter
   B. Treatment for presumed cyanide poisoning with amyl nitrite
   C. Chest radiograph
   D. ECG

## 93 Benzodiazepines

### Lars Blomberg

Select the appropriate letter that correctly answers the question or completes the statement.

1. The duration of the benzodiazepines' drug effect is not significantly affected by which of the following?
   A. Distribution of drug from blood to fatty tissue
   B. Drugs inhibiting hepatic cytochrome P-450 oxidation
   C. Presence of active metabolites
   D. Presence of free drug in the blood

2. Which of the following is a common physical sign in pure benzodiazepine overdose?
   A. Areflexia
   B. Hypotension

C. Profound coma
D. Tachycardia
E. All of the above

3. A 35 year old is known to have overdosed on a benzodiazepine and a large quantity of ethanol. Which of the following would be an unusual finding in this setting?
   A. Failure of a response to flumazenil
   B. Hypotension
   C. Marked respiratory depression
   D. Profound coma unresponsive to pain
   E. All of the above are common

4. Which of the following is true when using flumazenil to treat benzodiazepine overdose?
   A. Is difficult to evaluate because of the slow recovery time
   B. May cause a withdrawal reaction
   C. Protects against precipitating seizures
   D. Works best when given in a large bolus rather than incrementally
   E. None of the above

5. The symptoms of benzodiazepine withdrawal are:
   A. Delayed in onset, typically 1 to 2 weeks after discontinuation of the drug
   B. Inevitable, even with gradual discontinuation of the drug
   C. Very different from a rebound effect precipitated by drug discontinuation
   D. Similar to those of a patient's original anxiety disorder

6. Which of the following best describes the similarity of buspirone to benzodiazepines?
   A. Has muscle relaxant and anticonvulsant properties
   B. Interacts with ethanol significantly
   C. Is rapidly absorbed orally and is metabolized in the liver
   D. Leads to tolerance and withdrawal symptoms with discontinuation after long-term use
   E. None of the above

7. Cimetidine is known to alter the pharmacokinetics of all of the following benzodiazepines except which one?
   A. Alprazolam
   B. Diazepam
   C. Lorazepam
   D. Midazolam

8. Which of the following benzodiazepines is most likely to precipitate significant withdrawal symptoms?
   A. Clonazepam
   B. Diazepam
   C. Lorazepam
   D. Midazolam
   E. None of the above

9. A 23-year-old female presents to the ED with severe respiratory depression following a suicide attempt. An empty bottle of Ativan was found along with the patient. All of the following are absolute or relative contraindications to flumazenil administration except which one?

A. Cocaine intoxication
B. Concomitant cyclic antidepressant overdose
C. Known seizure disorder
D. Significant alcohol consumption
E. All of the above are contraindications

# 94 ▼ Dyspnea

### Michael S. Buchsbaum and Leonard A. Nitowski

Select the appropriate letter that correctly answers the question or completes the statement.

1. The nerve that transmits afferent information from the airways in the lungs to the brain is the:
   A. Glossopharyngeal
   B. Phrenic
   C. Spinal accessory nerve
   D. Vagus

2. A 72-year-old woman with lung cancer and severe COPD is seeking treatment for acute onset of dyspnea 1 hour ago. She appears to be in severe respiratory distress and denies any trauma. All of the following may be responsible for her acute decline except which one?
   A. Acute MI with mitral valve rupture
   B. Pleural effusion
   C. Pulmonary embolus
   D. Reactive airway disease
   E. Spontaneous pneumothorax

3. A 60-year-old man arrives at the ED with progressive dyspnea over the past 24 hours. He also complains of orthopnea, malaise, and a minimally productive cough. Examination reveals RR, 36; HR, 106; BP, 180/95; bilateral wheezing, poor air movement, and a paradoxical split second heart sound. What is the most likely diagnosis?
   A. Aspiration pneumonia
   B. Asthma
   C. Cardiomyopathy
   D. Chronic obstructive pulmonary disease
   E. Pulmonary embolism

*Match the conditions below with the appropriate sign or symptom.*

   A. Carbon monoxide poisoning
   B. Chronic obstructive pulmonary disease
   C. Congestive heart failure
   D. Psychogenic dyspnea
   E. Pulmonary embolus

4. Cor pulmonale _____
5. Headache _____
6. Perioral tingling _____
7. S3 gallop _____
8. Syncope _____

9. High-altitude pulmonary edema has occurred as low as:
   A. 3000 meters
   B. 5000 meters
   C. 7000 meters
   D. 10,000 meters
   E. 12,000 meters

10. A 65-year-old man comes to the ED complaining of increasing dyspnea, cough, orthopnea, and malaise. Examination reveals equally decreased breath sounds bilaterally with no rales, rhonchi, or wheezing. He also has jugular venous distention while sitting and pretibial edema. Given these findings, what is the most likely diagnosis?
    A. Asthma
    B. Cardiomyopathy
    C. Chronic obstructive pulmonary disease
    D. Pneumonia
    E. Toxic gas exposure

# 95 ▼ Adult Acute Asthma

### Kenneth D. Katz and Gordon D. Reed

Select the appropriate letter that correctly answers the question or completes the statement.

1. Which of the following factors is associated with increased mortality from asthma?
   A. Frequent emergency department visits for acute exacerbations of asthma
   B. Low socioeconomic status
   C. Overuse of prescribed or over-the-counter medications leading to delays in seeking treatment
   D. Prior history of intensive care unit stays
   E. All of the above

2. The immunologic mechanisms of extrinsic (allergic) asthma can best be characterized by which of the following?
   A. Extrinsic (allergic) asthma is characterized by a well-defined sensitivity to a specific allergen, a family history of multiple allergic diseases, increased IgE levels, and positive skin tests
   B. The early asthmatic response has been shown to be associated with cellular inflammation with neutrophils, eosinophils, and mononuclear cells
   C. The late asthmatic response is characterized by bronchoconstriction beginning as early as 10 minutes from exposure to an antigen
   D. The late response in allergic asthma is mast-cell dependent
   E. The late response may be best treated with beta-agonist therapy

3. A 35-year-old woman with a history of recent referral to an ENT specialist for persistent nasal congestion and rhinorrhea presents to the emergency department with wheezing and dyspnea after taking aspirin for a headache. A physical examination reveals nasal polyps and scattered wheezes throughout both lung fields. The emergency physician may suspect which of the following concerning this patient:
   A. A male predominance is common
   B. Cross-reactivity with other NSAIDs will not occur in this patient
   C. Shock may occur with as little as 300 mg of aspirin ingestion
   D. The pathogenesis is due to an IgE mechanism
   E. This patient may take acetaminophen for headaches without risk of bronchospasm

4. The majority of patients with asthma have which of the following collection of symptoms?
   A. Cough, dyspnea, and wheezing
   B. Cough, sputum production, and dyspnea
   C. Orthopnea, dyspnea on exertion, and cough
   D. Wheezing, sputum production, and paroxysmal nocturnal dyspnea
   E. Wheezing, stridor, and cough

5. Which of the following parameters is most important concerning mechanical ventilation of the asthmatic patient?
   A. High respiratory rates
   B. High tidal volumes
   C. Hypercarbia should be corrected immediately
   D. Muscle paralysis should be avoided
   E. Prolonged inspiratory to expiratory ratio

6. The correct dose of epinephrine given to an adult asthma patient is:
   A. 2-10 cc of 1:10,000 solution IV
   B. 2-10 cc of 1:1000 solution IV
   C. 2-10 cc of 1:1000 solution SQ
   D. 2-5 cc of 1:1000 solution SQ
   E. 0.2-0.5 cc of 1:1000 solution IV

7. Which of the following may herald the need for mechanical ventilation?
   A. Clinical and subjective response to nebulized bronchodilators
   B. $FEV_1$ approximately 60% expected
   C. Normalization of arterial blood gas despite tachypnea
   D. Presence of wheezing
   E. Respiratory alkalosis

8. According to U.S. and Canadian guidelines, in asthmatic patients with a good response to initial therapy (PEFR, $FEV_1 > 70\%$ predicted) which of the following is true concerning treatment and disposition?
   A. Administer magnesium sulfate
   B. Administer subcutaneous epinephrine or terbutaline
   C. Continue beta-agonist therapy hourly, with clinical and objective monitoring every 30-60 minutes and reassess at 4 hours

   D. Hospitalize for further observation
   E. Observe for 30-60 minutes and discharge with close medical follow-up on appropriate outpatient medications

9. Which of the following is true concerning corticosteroid therapy in asthma?
   A. Hydrocortisone is five times more potent than methylprednisolone as an antiinflammatory agent
   B. Hydrocortisone is the steroid of choice for IV therapy
   C. Prednisone requires hepatic conversion to prednisolone
   D. Steroids have not been shown to reduce relapse rates after treatment of acute exacerbations of asthma
   E. There is clinical evidence that IV steroids are more effective than oral agents

10. Which of the following statements concerning methylxanthines is correct?
    A. Drugs that may increase serum theophylline levels include carbamazepine, phenytoin, and rifampin
    B. Every 1 mg/kg loading dose of aminophylline will increase the theophylline level by approximately 5 $\mu g/ml$
    C. The IV aminophylline dose is 0.80 times the PO theophylline dose, since the oral form is only 80% as potent
    D. The loading doses of IV aminophylline is 5-6 mg/kg actual body weight over 20 minutes
    E. The optimal serum theophylline level is approximately 20-30 $\mu g/ml$

11. The correct sequence for metered-dose inhaler use is:
    (1) Hold breath for at least 10 seconds
    (2) Shake canister
    (3) Exhale fully
    (4) Actuate the inhaler at the beginning of a slow, full inhalation
    (5) Assemble the MDI
    (6) Place the mouthpiece between the teeth
       A. 2, 6, 3, 5, 4, 1
       B. 2, 6, 5, 3, 4, 1
       C. 5, 2, 6, 3, 4, 1
       D. 5, 2, 6, 4, 1, 3
       E. 5, 2, 6, 3, 1, 4

12. Which of the following statements is true regarding the pregnant patient?
    A. Epinephrine is considered safe in pregnancy
    B. Most asthmatics become worse
    C. Steroids are unsafe in pregnancy
    D. Terbutaline can inhibit uterine contractions
    E. Theophylline can cause fetal abnormalities

13. Which of the following statements concerning ipratropium bromide is correct?
    A. Ipratropium bromide nebulization should not be performed as part of the initial treatment for the severe asthmatic

B. Nebulization with ipratropium bromide and a beta-agonist results in a greater bronchodilatory effect than with a beta-agonist alone

C. Its clinical effects relate to its alpha receptor stimulation

D. The correct dose for nebulized ipratropium bromide is 1 mg

E. Its potency as a bronchodilator is greater than that of a beta-agonist, and it can be used as a sole agent in the treatment of an asthma attack

14. A 35-year-old pregnant woman comes to the emergency department with an asthma attack. Which of the following therapeutic agents should be avoided?
A. Albuterol
B. Epinephrine
C. Ipratropium bromide
D. Prednisone
E. Terbutaline

15. Which of the following statements is true regarding asthma therapy?
A. Increased medication doses are required for nebulized therapy
B. Inhaled beta-agonist therapy should be avoided in severe bronchospasm
C. Subcutaneous terbutaline is more effective than nebulized albuterol as initial therapy for asthma
D. Subcutaneous terbutaline is the drug of choice if asthma is suspected to be related to an allergic reaction with bronchospasm
E. Terbutaline has similar bronchodilating effects as epinephrine with less adverse cardiac effects

16. A 50-year-old woman presents with wheezing after taking propranolol. Her initial peak flow is 60. She states she cannot tolerate albuterol. What is the best choice for treatment?
A. Albuterol
B. Hydrocortisone
C. Ipratropium bromide
D. Magnesium sulfate
E. Theophylline

17. Which of the following conditions will decrease the clearance of theophylline and thus require a lower dose?
A. Diabetes mellitus
B. Liver dysfunction
C. Renal failure
D. Smoking
E. Younger age

18. Which of the following is a pharmacologic action of theophylline?
A. Decreases cardiac output
B. Decreases contractility of the diaphragm
C. Increases systemic and pulmonary resistance
D. Inhibits airway inflammation
E. Potentates histamine release

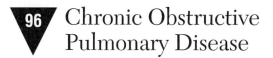

# 96 ▼ Chronic Obstructive Pulmonary Disease

*Janice K. Balas and Gordon D. Reed*

Select the appropriate letter that correctly answers the question or completes the statement.

1. When examining the COPD patient in the ED, which of the following findings is most worrisome?
A. Able to speak in only short sentences
B. High-pitched wheezes on auscultation
C. Chest silent to auscultation
D. Visible retractions

2. Which of the following is associated more commonly in a patient with emphysema (pink puffer) than in a patient with bronchitis (blue bloater)?
A. Cor pulmonale
B. Heat intolerance
C. Hyperviscosity
D. Normal or slightly increased blood pressure
E. Peripheral edema

3. The chest radiograph in an emphysema patient, as compared with that in a patient with bronchitis, shows:
A. Coarse reticulations of the lower lung fields
B. Elevation of the diaphragm
C. Increased anteroposterior diameter of the thorax
D. On the lateral film, right ventricle impingement on the retrosternal airspace
E. Slightly enlarged cardiac silhouette

4. A 50-year-old, 70-kg man who does not smoke but has chronic obstructive pulmonary disease (COPD) arrives at the ED with an acute COPD exacerbation. He has no other underlying disease. There is no prior history of aminophylline use. What would the approximate loading dose in milligrams be?
A. 70
B. 140
C. 210
D. 280
E. 350

5. A patient of the same age and weight presents but is not critically ill. The aminophylline level is 6 mg/ml. How much aminophylline, in mg, should be given to raise the blood level to approximately 10 mg/ml?
A. 70
B. 140
C. 280
D. 420

6. What is the maintenance infusion dose of aminophylline in mg/hr for adults without impaired liver function?
A. 0.25
B. 0.5
C. 1.0
D. 1.5
E. 2.0

*Match the possible adverse effect in COPD patients below with the appropriate question.*

    A. Can increase blood aminophylline levels

    B. Can induce bronchospasm

    C. Interferes with motor end-plate function

    D. Can cause respiratory depression

7. Neomycin     _____

8. Aspirin     _____

9. Alcohol     _____

10. Acetylcysteine     _____

11. Ciprofloxacin     _____

12. What is the appropriate management of multifocal atrial tachycardia (MAT) in the setting of COPD?

    A. Cardioversion

    B. Digoxin

    C. Propranolol

    D. Verapamil

13. Which of the following may be useful in treating cor pulmonale in COPD patients?

    A. ACE inhibitors

    B. Alpha blockers

    C. Calcium channel blockers

    D. Theophylline

*Match the diseases below with the appropriate question.*

    A. Emphysema

    B. Chronic bronchitis

    C. Both

    D. Neither

14. Cough is the hallmark     _____

15. Dyspnea is the hallmark     _____

16. Wheeze is the hallmark     _____

17. Hypoxia     _____

18. Hyperviscosity     _____

19. Pursed lips     _____

20. Tends to be sedentary     _____

21. Irreversible     _____

22. Cor pulmonale may occur     _____

23. May see tanning and induration of the skin just proximal to the knees     _____

24. Electrocardiogram changes are specific     _____

25. Anxiety     _____

 # Pleural Disease

*Martin A. Bennett and Robert A. Rosenbaum*

Select the appropriate letter that correctly answers the question or completes the statement.

1. A 40-year-old man with acquired immunodeficiency syndrome (AIDS) presents to the emergency department complaining of shortness of breath and pleuritic chest pain. He was treated for *Pneumocystis carinii* pneumonia 6 months ago and is currently taking prophylactic pentamidine. A chest x-ray on this admission shows a small right pneumothorax. His pulse oximetry is 95% on room air. Which of the following statements is true?

    A. Bilateral pneumothorax almost never occurs in AIDS patients taking pentamidine

    B. Delayed re-expansion often complicates the clinical course

    C. The incidence of pneumothorax in AIDS patients taking pentamidine exceeds 10%

    D. The mechanism of his pneumothorax most likely involves lung necrosis secondary to pentamidine therapy

    E. Treatment of choice for this patient is needle aspiration

2. A 16-year-old boy comes to the emergency department complaining of sharp pleuritic chest pain and shortness of breath. Pneumothorax (probably spontaneous) is confirmed by chest x-ray. What is the likelihood of a recurrence?

    A. 5%

    B. 10%

    C. 30%

    D. 45%

    E. 60%

3. Of the following, which is the most common cause of secondary spontaneous pneumothorax?

    A. Acute bronchitis

    B. Emphysema

    C. Lung cancer

    D. Pneumonia

    E. Tuberculosis

4. Which period of life is associated with the greatest frequency of spontaneous pneumothorax?

    A. Elderly

    B. Neonate

    C. School age

    D. Toddler

    E. Young adult

5. During the history, what is the most common complaint of patients with suspected spontaneous pneumothorax?

    A. Anxiety

    B. Chest pain

    C. Cough

    D. Dyspnea

    E. Weakness

6. What percentage pneumothorax is considered the limit beyond which significant hypoxia from arterial shunting is likely to occur?

    A. 5%

    B. 20%

    C. 35%

    D. 50%

    E. 70%

7. Which of the following statements is true regarding pneumothorax in the COPD patient?

    A. Absent breath sounds and hyperresonance to percussion are virtually diagnostic

    B. Dyspnea is not a prominent feature

C. Mortality ranges from 1% to 16%

D. Pain is often out of proportion to the degree of collapse

E. The diagnosis of tension pneumothorax often depends on x-ray findings

8. A 68-year-old woman with a history of congestive heart failure presents to the emergency department with shortness of breath, a non-productive cough, and pleural effusion on chest x-ray. She denies fevers, chills, or chest pain but describes progressive orthopnea over the past 2 weeks. Her primary care physician recently stopped her furosemide. Which of the following is true?

A. A transudative pleural effusion makes pulmonary embolism unlikely in this setting

B. Fluid-to-blood LDH ratio is likely to be <0.6

C. Fluid-to-blood protein ratio is likely to be >0.5

D. The chest x-ray most likely shows unilateral pleural effusion

E. The effusion is most likely exudative

9. Which is the correct statement concerning pleuritis?

A. Bornholm disease (pleurodynia) is usually associated with a bacterial infection

B. Idiopathic pleuritis is best treated with opiate analgesics

C. If the pleura overlying the central diaphragm is involved, pain may be referred to the neck

D. Pulmonary embolism rarely causes pleuritic chest pain

E. The visceral pleura, when inflamed, causes localized pain directly over the affected area

10. Which of the following is most helpful in distinguishing between idiopathic (viral) pleuritis and pulmonary embolism?

A. Abrupt onset pleuritic chest pain

B. Decreased $PO_2$

C. Low-grade fever

D. Pleural effusions on chest x-ray

E. Tachypnea

11. Which of the following organisms is most likely to cause a large exudative pleural effusion?

A. Adenovirus

B. Anaerobes

C. *Escherichia coli*

D. *Mycoplasma* species

E. Parainfluenza

# 98 ▼ Upper Respiratory Tract Infections

### Dana A. Ger and Robert A. Rosenbaum

Select the appropriate letter that correctly answers the question or completes the statement.

1. The age distribution of patients with epiglottitis is best described as:

A. 1-4 years old

B. 5-7 years old

C. Bimodal: 1-4 and 20-40 years old

D. Bimodal: 5-7 and 15-25 years old

2. The most commonly isolated bacterial pathogen causing epiglottitis is:

A. *Haemophilus influenzae*

B. *Neisseria* species

C. *Staphylococcus aureus*

D. *Streptococcus pneumoniae*

3. Adult epiglottitis usually presents with which of the following?

A. Cough and cervical lymphadenopathy

B. Dysphagia and sore throat

C. Hoarseness and fever

D. Prodrome lasting 10-12 days

4. A 28-year-old male is brought into the emergency department complaining of a sore throat and difficulty swallowing. He is speaking softly but without hoarseness and is spitting into a cup. The patient denies abdominal pain, nausea, and vomiting. He does have mild stridor. What is the first step in treatment?

A. Direct laryngoscopy and antibiotics

B. Discharge the patient with throat lozenges and recommend an air dehumidifier

C. Lateral soft tissue neck x-ray, antibiotics, and IV hydration

D. Monospot and two sets of blood cultures

5. Acute pharyngitis:

A. Involves the tonsillar crypts rather than the tonsils themselves

B. Is caused by the same agents in adults as in children

C. Is most commonly caused by mycoplasma pneumonia

D. Is most commonly caused by respiratory viruses

*Match the following types of pharyngitis with the associated symptoms.*

A. Temperature above 38.3° C, tonsillar exudates, tender cervical lymphadenopathy, absence of cough or rhinorrhea

B. Follicular, unilateral conjunctivitis

C. Cough, rhinorrhea, myalgia, headache, odynophagia

D. Pharyngeal erythema with gray-green adherent pseudomembrane

E. Epidemics, high fever, myalgia, headache

F. Tonsillar exudate, generalized lymphadenopathy, splenomegaly

G. Painful superficial vesicles on an erythematous base

6. Adenovirus _____

7. Diphtheria _____

8. Herpes _____

9. Influenza _____

10. Mononucleosis _____

11. Streptococcal infection _____

12. Viral infection _____

13. Rapid Strep tests are useful because:
    A. Sensitivity is 31%-100%
    B. Specificity is 70%-100%
    C. The test is positive only in those patients who need treatment for active infection
    D. The test obliterates the need for confirming *Streptococcus* culture

14. Which is true for treatment for streptococcal pharyngitis?
    A. Can be delayed 9 days and still will prevent rheumatic fever
    B. Greatly decreases the incidence and improves the course of poststreptococcal glomerulonephritis
    C. Has little effect on the rapidity of resolution of pharyngitis
    D. Should not be initiated without a positive confirming test for *Streptococcus* organisms

15. Treatment for diphtheria includes antitoxin, which:
    A. Has a standard dose of 20,000 units
    B. May cause an allergic reaction to horse serum
    C. Should be given as soon as diphtheria infection has been proven
    D. Should be given over 5 minutes

16. Which is true of patients with deep space infections?
    A. Blind nasopharyngeal intubation is safe
    B. Intubation should be simple due to the depth of infection, allowing more space for intubation
    C. Neuromuscular blockade may worsen the airway obstruction
    D. Tracheostomy is the surgical airway of choice

17. Peritonsillitis:
    A. Has a high recurrence rate
    B. Is less common in smokers
    C. Is not found in patients who have undergone complete tonsillectomies
    D. Usually occurs in patients younger than 15 years old

18. Which is used for the diagnosis of peritonsillitis?
    A. Biopsy
    B. Clinical observation
    C. Gram's stain and culture
    D. X-ray studies

19. Which of the following statements is true regarding Ludwig's angina?
    A. It is a progressive cellulitis that begins in the submandibular space
    B. It is caused by dental disease in 40%-60% of the cases
    C. It is usually seen in very ill patients
    D. It is, by definition, a deep space infection

20. A hoarse voice would be expected in all of the following except which one?
    A. Lingual tonsillitis
    B. Ludwig's angina
    C. Peritonsillitis
    D. Viral pharyngitis

21. Retropharyngeal abscess:
    A. Is equally common in patients with and without underlying systemic disorders
    B. Is usually seen in children 6-8 years old
    C. May be diagnosed by palpation of the fluctuant mass
    D. May present with the tracheal "rock" sign

22. A 6-year-old girl presents with a 3-day history of sore throat, dysphagia, odynophagia, drooling, fever, and dysphonia that sounds like a duck's quack (cri du canard), stating that she feels like there is a lump in her throat. She most likely has
    A. Epiglottitis
    B. Laryngitis
    C. Peritonsillitis
    D. Retropharyngeal abscess

23. Pathologic widths for the retrotracheal space are
    A. 3.4 mm in children and 3.5 mm in adults
    B. 3.5 mm in children and 3.4 mm in adults
    C. 14 mm in children and 22 mm in adults
    D. 22 mm in children and 14 mm in adults

24. Which applies to Lemierre syndrome?
    A. May involve metastatic infections affecting the lung
    B. Presents with elevated amylase and lipase levels with normal liver enzymes
    C. Should be treated with oral antibiotics
    D. Usually follows chronic pharyngitis

25. Sinusitis:
    A. Can be diagnosed with facial x-rays, which are the gold standard of sinus imaging
    B. Can be treated on an outpatient basis with amoxicillin and topical and systemic decongestants
    C. Should be treated with oral antibiotics and an antihistamine
    D. Usually causes a clear to slightly yellowish nasal discharge

---

 # Pneumonia

*Robert D. Hagan and Donnita M. Scott*

Select the appropriate letter that correctly answers the question or completes the statement.

1. The most common cause of community-acquired pneumonia among adults is:
   A. *H. influenzae*
   B. *K. pneumoniae*
   C. *M. catarrhalis*
   D. *M. pneumoniae*
   E. *S. pneumoniae*

2. A 37-year-old male has suffered from a persistent cough since his return from a mountain biking vacation in Nevada 1 month ago. A chest x-ray showed numerous

granulomas as well as hilar adenopathy. What is the most likely pathogen?

A. *Blastomyces dermatitides*
B. *Coccidioides immitis*
C. Hantavirus
D. *Histoplasma capsulatum*
E. Influenza

3. A 47-year-old male presents to the emergency department with sudden onset of fever, myalgias, severe headache and a nonproductive cough. The physical exam is unremarkable except for a fever and coarse rhonchi that are auscultated in the right lung base. A chest x-ray demonstrates an infiltrate in the right lung base. A social history reveals that the patient raises exotic birds as a hobby. What is the most likely cause of this patient's pneumonia?

A. *C. pneumoniae*
B. *C. psittaci*
C. *H. influenza*
D. *L. pneumoniae*
E. *M. pneumoniae*

4. A 74-year-old man with an history of diabetes and alcoholism presents with dyspnea, chest pain, fever, and a cough productive with currant-jelly–like sputum. On physical examination the patient appears toxic, with fever and tachypnea. Coarse breath sounds are auscultated bilaterally. A sputum Gram stain shows numerous gram-negative rods. What is the most likely pathogen?

A. *H. influenzae*
B. *K. pneumoniae*
C. *L. pneumoniae*
D. *M. catarrhalis*
E. *S. pneumoniae*

5. A 54-year-old woman with a 40-pack-year history of smoking presents to the emergency department with symptoms of a dry, nonproductive cough; fever; pleuritic chest pain; and severe diarrhea. The patient appears toxic and is very confused. What is the drug of choice?

A. Cephalexin
B. Clindamycin
C. Erythromycin
D. Penicillin
E. Trimethoprim-sulfamethoxazole

6. Which of the following diagnostic studies most accurately defines the causative agent in pneumonia?

A. Chest radiograph
B. Cold hemagglutinins
C. Positive blood cultures
D. Sputum Gram stain
E. Sputum cultures

7. Patients with HIV rarely develop *Pneumocystis carinii* pneumonia (PCP) until their CD4 count drops below what level?

A. 50
B. 100
C. 200
D. 300
E. 400

8. Which of the following laboratory studies might be valuable in diagnosis as well as in assessing the prognosis of a patient with PCP?

A. CBC
B. CPK
C. Electrolytes
D. Liver function tests
E. LDH

9. Which of the following is not associated with PCP in an HIV-positive patient?

A. Diffuse or perihilar infiltrates on chest radiograph
B. Productive cough
C. ESR >50 mm/hr
D. LDH >220 IU
E. Thrush or hairy leukoplakia

10. A patient who was found unresponsive is brought into the emergency department. In order to protect the airway, the patient is intubated. During the intubation the patient regurgitates and subsequently aspirates his stomach contents. What is the most appropriate treatment for this patient after intubation?

A. Broad-spectrum antibiotics
B. Systemic corticosteroids
C. Antibiotics and systemic corticosteroids
D. Bronchodilator therapy
E. Supportive care only

11. Which of the following drugs is thought to have utility in the treatment of Hantavirus?

A. Acyclovir
B. Amantadine
C. Foscarnet
D. Interferon alpha-2b
E. Ribavirin

12. A patient with cystic fibrosis presents to the emergency department with a history and physical examination consistent with pneumonia. The diagnosis is confirmed on radiograph. What would the best choice be for initial antibiotic therapy?

A. Ceftazidime and gentamycin
B. Cefuroxime and erythromycin
C. Erythromycin
D. Penicillin
E. Trimethoprim-sulfamethoxazole

13. Which is an appropriate choice for outpatient antibiotic therapy for pneumonia in an otherwise healthy individual?

A. Amoxicillin
B. Ampicillin
C. Azithromycin
D. Ciprofloxacin
E. Trimethoprim-sulfamethoxazole

14. In an AIDS patient with pneumonia that is presumed to be PCP but is not yet confirmed, an appropriate empiric regimen of antibiotics would be:
    A. Pentamidine
    B. Pentamidine plus erythromycin
    C. Dapsone
    D. Clindamycin plus primaquine
    E. Trimethoprim-sulfamethoxazole

15. Which of the following drugs used in the treatment of TB can cause peripheral neuritis?
    A. Ethambutol
    B. Isoniazid
    C. Pyrazinamide
    D. Rifampin
    E. Streptomycin

---

## SECTION 2  CARDIAC DISORDERS

## 100 Syncope

### *Richard S. Hartoch*

Select the appropriate letter that correctly answers the question or completes the statement.

1. The ECG of a patient with syncope is found to have a prolonged QT interval. This condition may be:
    A. A precipitant of ventricular tachycardia
    B. A result of hypocalcemia, hypomagnesemia, or hypokalemia
    C. A result of medication
    D. Inherited
    E. All of the above

2. A 65-year-old man is brought to the ED following an episode of syncope while chasing a bus. Which valvular lesion is most likely to be responsible?
    A. Aortic insufficiency
    B. Aortic stenosis
    C. Mitral regurgitation
    D. Mitral stenosis
    E. Pulmonary stenosis

3. Vagal stimulation is generally believed to be involved in which of the following syncopal syndromes?
    A. Carbon monoxide toxicity
    B. Glossopharyngeal neuralgia
    C. Massive pulmonary embolus
    D. Subclavian steal syndrome
    E. Ventricular tachycardia

4. A 50-year-old patient is noted to have several seconds of clonic motion during a brief unconscious period. Which is true of this finding?
    A. Is diagnostic of an underlying seizure disorder
    B. May be seen in cough syncope

C. Suggests prolonged QT syndrome
D. Requires immediate EEG
E. All of the above

5. A 75-year-old woman with multiple medical conditions arrives at the ED after a brief episode of syncope. Evaluation reveals no specific etiology. What should the emergency physician do next?
    A. ED evaluation should be extended to include an EEG
    B. If ECG is normal and no murmurs are detected, patient should be discharged home
    C. Patient should be admitted for observation
    D. Any medications that inhibit the SA or AV node should be discontinued and the patient discharged

6. A woman in her thirty-fourth week of pregnancy arrives at the ED following a syncopal episode. Evaluation reveals a prominent systolic murmur, systolic blood pressure of 90, and a hematocrit of 28%. At this time, the patient should:
    A. Be prescribed bed rest for the remainder of her pregnancy
    B. Be placed in the left lateral decubitus position
    C. Undergo echocardiography
    D. Undergo pelvic ultrasound
    E. Undergo an immediate C-section

7. Which of the following statements is true of a 3-year-old boy who comes to the ED with syncope?
    A. An ECG is not part of the initial ED evaluation in a patient of this age
    B. If "blue" or cyanotic breath-holding syncope is diagnosed, the patient should be given atropine
    C. Pressure applied to the optic globe may be useful for diagnosis
    D. All of the above

8. An otherwise healthy 28-year-old male experiences syncope immediately following micturition. ED evaluation is essentially unrevealing. The patient should:
    A. Be admitted to the telemetry unit for overnight observation
    B. Be discharged home
    C. Be scheduled for an outpatient EEG
    D. Be started on a low-dose beta-blocker if mitral valve prolapse is suspected
    E. Have a drug toxicity screen performed

9. An 80-year-old woman with a history of syncope and the recent onset of back pain is found to have cannon A waves in the neck on examination. The patient:
    A. May be in paroxysmal supraventricular tachycardia (PSVT)
    B. May benefit from an abdominal ultrasound
    C. Should be given a trial of adenosine
    D. All of the above

10. Which of the following statements is true of carotid sinus hypersensitivity?
    A. It is seen in 50% of the adult population
    B. May be inhibited by beta-blockers, digitalis, and alpha-methyldopa

C. May be demonstrable on physical examination
D. May result in ventricular slowing, but never asystole
E. All of the above

 ## 101 Dysrhythmias

*Richard J. Harper*

Select the appropriate letter that correctly answers the question or completes the statement.

1. The underlying disease most often associated with multifocal atrial tachycardia is:
   A. Accessory pathway
   B. Coronary artery disease
   C. Chronic obstructive pulmonary disease
   D. Mitral valve stenosis
   E. Myocarditis

2. What does the arrhythmia depicted in Figure 101-1 represent?
   A. Nonconducted premature atrial contractions
   B. Second-degree AV block Type I
   C. Second-degree AV block Type II
   D. Sinus node block
   E. Third-degree AV block

3. What is the best way to differentiate a PVC from a PAC on an electrocardiogram?
   A. A PVC should be associated with a fully compensatory pause
   B. Fusion beats are present
   C. The PAC may demonstrate an ectopic P wave buried in the preceding T wave
   D. The QRS axis is bizarre, with QRS duration often greater than 0.14 seconds
   E. There is widening and deepening of T wave changes opposite the main QRS deflection (secondary T wave abnormalities)

4. All of the following are true regarding atrial fibrillation except:

A. Atrial fibrillation of more than 72 hours' duration is associated with a significant risk of embolic events when cardioverted
B. Ibutilide, if successful, will produce cardioversion within 20 minutes
C. "Holiday heart" atrial fibrillation typically spontaneously reverts to sinus rhythm in 24-48 hours
D. Magnesium sulfate, 2 gm over 2 minutes given IV, will usually cause reversion to sinus rhythm
E. Pharmacologic cardioversion can be attempted with procainamide at 50 mg/min to a total dose of 20 μg/kg

5. A patient arrives at the ED with a narrow complex regular tachycardia. What is the best way to distinguish AV nodal reentry tachycardia from one with an accessory pathway?
   A. Adenosine will convert atrioventricular nodal reentrant tachycardia (AVNRT) but not tachycardia based on an accessory pathway
   B. Delta waves are present with an accessory pathway.
   C. Inverted P waves 0.07 seconds after the QRS are present with an accessory pathway.
   D. Secondary P-wave changes are associated with an accessory pathway
   E. The patient with an accessory pathway is more likely to be symptomatic

6. Which of the following is a common side effect of adenosine?
   A. Drug effects augmented by aminophylline
   B. Palpitations
   C. Pressure-like chest pain
   D. Transient hypertension
   E. Visual halos and blurred vision

7. What electrolyte is most responsible for maintaining cellular electrical charge?
   A. Ca++
   B. Cl
   C. K+
   D. Mg++
   E. Na+

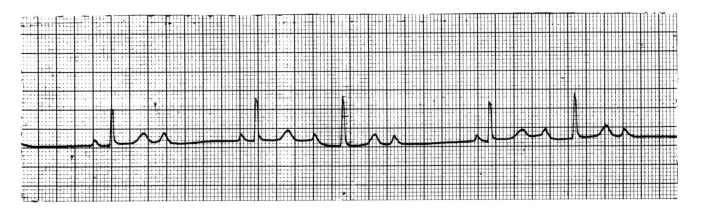

**FIG. 101-1**

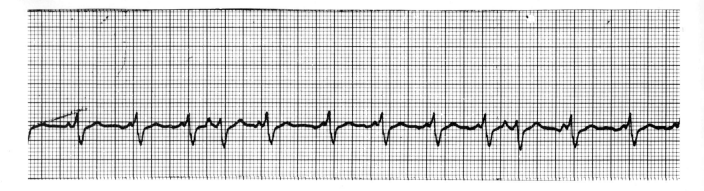

FIG. 101-2

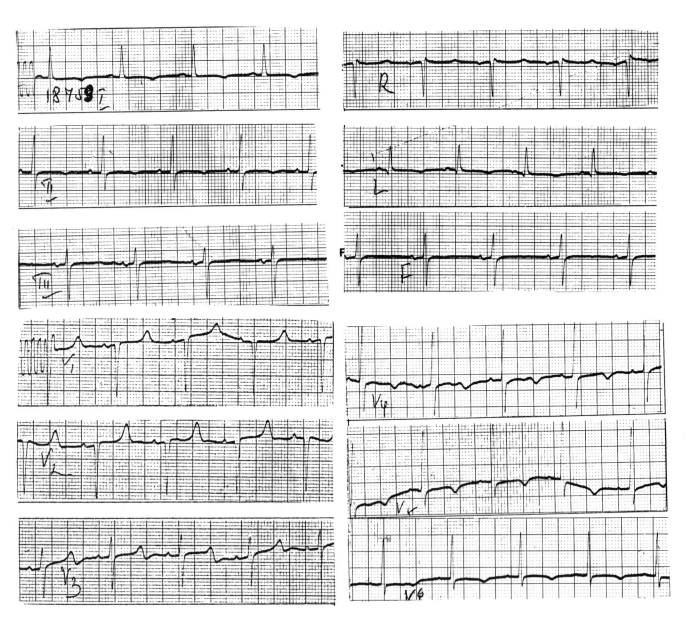

FIG. 101-3

8. The phase of the action potential in which pacemaker cells differ from other cardiac cells is:
   A. Phase 0
   B. Phase 1
   C. Phase 2
   D. Phase 3
   E. Phase 4

9. Magnesium is considered the drug of choice for which of the following dysrhythmias?
   A. Ischemia-induced ventricular fibrillation
   B. Multifocal atrial tachycardia
   C. Premature atrial contractions
   D. Premature ventricular contractions associated with ischemia
   E. Polymorphic ventricular tachycardia

10. A 65-year-old man complains of palpitations and short-ness of breath. He has a history of both cardiac and pulmonary diseases and is taking multiple medications (he cannot name any of them). Vital signs are blood pressure 140/90 and pulse irregular at 98 beats per minute. His rhythm is shown in Figure 101-2. Which of the following is the best ED treatment for this arrhythmia?
    A. Adenosine
    B. Digitalis
    C. Magnesium
    D. Oxygen
    E. Verapamil

11. A 70-year-old man comes to the ED with a 3-hour history of chest pain. After initial assessment and treatment with oxygen and nitrates, he is pain free. He has a pulse of 54 and a blood pressure of 110/70. His ECG shows anterior ischemic changes with a Mobitz type II second-degree AV block. The best therapy at this point would be:
    A. Atropine
    B. Isoproterenol drip
    C. Lidocaine
    D. Observation in CCU
    E. Transcutaneous pacemaker

12. All of the following are differences between type I and type II second-degree AV blocks except which one?
    A. Atropine would be expected to worsen type I but improve type II
    B. Carotid massage should worsen type I but improve type II
    C. Type I involves the AV node, while type II is infranodal
    D. Type I is acute, while type II is often chronic
    E. Type I is associated with a prolonged PR interval, while type II has a normal PR interval

13. Which dysrhythmia is the patient with the rhythm shown in Figure 101-3 at particular risk for?
    A. Atrial fibrillation
    B. Multifocal atrial tachycardia
    C. Second-degree AV block
    D. Torsade de pointes
    E. Ventricular fibrillation

14. Select the agent which is a class 1C antidysrhythmic.
    A. Lidocaine
    B. Mexiletine
    C. Phenytoin
    D. Propafenone
    E. Quinidine

# 102 Heart Failure

*J. Leibovitz*

Select the appropriate letter that correctly answers the question or completes the statement.

1. What are the two leading causes of heart failure in adults?
   A. Endocarditis and alcoholism
   B. Ischemic heart disease and dilated cardiomyopathy
   C. Thiamine deficiency and anemia
   D. Valvular heart disease and hypertension

2. All of the following are risk factors for developing heart failure except which one?
   A. Advanced age
   B. Cardiac dysrhythmias
   C. Smoking
   D. Systemic infection
   E. Thyroid disease

3. All of the following are true regarding the epidemiology of heart failure except which one?
   A. ACE inhibitors have decreased the death rate due to heart failure
   B. Approximately 40% of the deaths in patients with heart failure are caused by out-of-hospital ventricular dysrhythmias
   C. Deaths due to dysrhythmia in heart failure patients have decreased with the use of current antidysrhythmic medications
   D. Fifty percent of heart failure patients die within 5 years of initial diagnosis
   E. Heart failure secondary to ischemic heart disease has a poorer prognosis than heart failure secondary to valvular disease

4. Knowledge of cardiovascular anatomy and physiology is important in understanding the concepts involved in heart failure. Which is false regarding cardiac physiology?
   A. Cardiac cell performance is a function of contractility and fiber length
   B. Cardiac output will increase as heart rate increases up to 200 beats per minute
   C. Preload is a stretching force that determines cardiac muscle fiber length
   D. Pulsatile flow from the heart is converted to continuous flow in blood vessels
   E. Vascular resistance is directly related to the fourth power of the vessel's radius

5. Heart failure can result from a primary dysfunction of which of the following?
   A. Cardiac valves
   B. Coronary arteries
   C. Lungs
   D. Peripheral blood vessels
   E. All of the above

*Match the patient characteristics below with the appropriate question.*
   A. 17-year-old patient with syncope during strenuous exertion
   B. 29-year-old female 1 week postpartum
   C. 43-year-old female with sarcoidosis

6. Dilated cardiomyopathy          _____
7. Hypertrophic cardiomyopathy     _____
8. Restrictive cardiomyopathy      _____
9. All of the following are causes of myocarditis except which one?
   A. Cocaine
   B. Coxsackie virus
   C. Lyme disease
   D. Thyroid disease
   E. Transplant rejection
10. Which is not true of valvular heart disease in adults?
    A. Aortic dissection can lead to aortic insufficiency
    B. Complete rupture of the papillary muscle can complicate myocardial infarction
    C. It is the third leading cause of heart failure
    D. Mitral and aortic valves are most commonly affected
    E. Prosthetic valves can fail because of acute valvular insufficiency
11. All of the following can cause high-output heart failure except:
    A. Anemia
    B. Beriberi (thiamine deficiency)
    C. Hyperthermia
    D. Hyperthyroidism
    E. All of the above are causes
12. All of the following are cardiac compensatory responses that occur in heart failure except:
    A. Cardiac muscle-fiber stretching
    B. Chamber hypertrophy
    C. Decreased heart rate
    D. Increased vasopressin levels
    E. None of the above
13. Which of the following is the most common cause of acute cardiogenic pulmonary edema?
    A. Acute dysrhythmia
    B. Coronary insufficiency
    C. Medication noncompliance
    D. Subendocardial infarct
    E. Worsening of underlying heart failure
14. All of the following are true of patients coming to the ED with acute cardiogenic pulmonary edema except which one?
    A. Elevated systolic blood pressure >160 mm Hg is a poor prognostic sign

B. Fifty percent will have jugular venous distention
C. The typical acid base disturbance is a metabolic acidosis with respiratory compensation
D. Thirty-three percent will have peripheral edema
E. Twenty-five percent have an audible $S_3$

15. Which of the following may cause acute pulmonary edema in patients with preexisting heart disease?
    A. Hypertensive crisis
    B. Medication noncompliance
    C. Pneumonia
    D. Pulmonary emboli
    E. All of the above
16. A 69-year-old man with a history of heart disease comes to the ED complaining of increasing shortness of breath. He is in moderate respiratory distress with a blood pressure of 105/60 and a heart rate of 120 beats per minute. Pulmonary examination reveals bibasilar rales, and an $S_3$ gallop is found on heart examination. His extremities are cool to touch with decreased capillary refill. Chest radiograph is consistent with pulmonary edema. All of the following therapeutic interventions used in the emergency department may be effective except which one?
    A. Combination therapy using nitrates and dopamine at middle ranges (5-15 µg/kg/min)
    B. Combination therapy using nitroprusside and dobutamine
    C. Dopamine administration as a single agent to reduce pulmonary congestion
    D. Preload reduction with nitrates, morphine, and diuretics
    E. None of the above

*Match the mechanism of action below with the appropriate question.*
   A. Beta-1 agonist with slight beta-2 and alpha effects
   B. Central sympatholytic effect causing peripheral vasodilation
   C. Mixed venous and arteriolar dilator
   D. Precursor of norepinephrine with dose-dependent effects

17. Dopamine        _____
18. Dobutamine      _____
19. Nitroprusside   _____
20. Morphine        _____
21. A 63-year-old woman comes to the ED complaining of chest pain. On physical examination, the patient is anxious and diaphoretic. Her vital signs reveal a blood pressure of 85/52 mm Hg and a pulse of 65 beats per minute. Jugular venous distention is noted, and lungs are clear to auscultation. Electrocardiogram reveals a 3 mm ST elevation in leads II, III, and $a_{VF}$. Which of the following is the best initial treatment of this patient's hypotension?
    A. Combination therapy of nitroprusside and dopamine
    B. Intraaortic balloon pump
    C. Nitroglycerin drip
    D. Normal saline bolus
    E. None of the above

22. All of the following are true of cardiac glycosides (digoxin) except:
    A. Heart failure accompanied by atrial fibrillation responds well to glycosides
    B. Patients with chronic ischemic heart failure and diastolic dysfunction respond poorly to glycosides
    C. They have a high toxic-to-therapeutic ratio
    D. They inhibit sodium-potassium ATPase
    E. Toxicity is enhanced by hypokalemia
23. Which is not true regarding the use of beta blockers in a patient with congestive heart failure?
    A. Beta-1 selective agents are preferable to nonselective agents
    B. Beta blockers enhance long-term neurohormonal regulatory mechanisms and result in improvement in functional class
    C. They are contraindicated in acute heart failure
    D. They have been shown to be beneficial in selected patients with heart failure
    E. They may be most beneficial in patients with preexisting hypertension, angina, or arrhythmias
24. All of the following are true regarding heart failure in the presence of end-stage renal disease (ESRD) except which one?
    A. Excess fluid removal can be accomplished by oral administration of sorbitol
    B. Fifty percent of ESRD heart failure patients have dilated cardiomyopathy
    C. Furosemide is ineffective in anuric patients
    D. Precipitating factors of heart failure include fluid overload, drug toxicity, and uremic pericardial effusion
    E. The prevalence of heart failure in ESRD is 10%-20%

# ▼ 103 Acute Ischemic Coronary Syndromes

*Richard J. Harper*

Select the appropriate letter that correctly answers the question or completes the statement.

1. Which is true regarding the epidemiology of acute ischemic coronary syndromes (AICS)?
    A. About 25% of heart attacks occur in people younger than 65 years of age
    B. Approximately two thirds of sudden deaths from coronary disease occur within 2 hours of onset of symptoms
    C. Ischemic heart disease accounts for about one third of all deaths in the U.S.
    D. More men than women die of cardiovascular disease
    E. The cost of treating AMI is falling
2. Select the patient with Canadian class II angina.
    A. A man who usually runs 2 miles a day runs 4 miles and develops chest pain
    B. A man who usually has chest pain after walking about a mile develops chest pain after an argument
    C. A woman who can do most routine activities knows that if she walks up three flights of stairs she will develop chest pain
    D. A woman who can walk one or two blocks or climb a flight of stairs before developing chest pain
    E. A woman who states she is unable to wash dishes without chest pain
3. Select the correct characterization for these patients with unstable angina.
    A. A man whose chest pain began 3 weeks ago and occurs with extreme exertion is diagnosed with new-onset angina
    B. A patient complains that his chest pain used to be limited to instances when he walked more than a mile but over the last month it occurs with walking two blocks; he is diagnosed with increasing angina
    C. A patient with 2 weeks of chest pain occurring at rest and lasting less than 10 minutes is diagnosed with rest angina
    D. A woman with 1 week of class II angina is diagnosed with new-onset angina
    E. A woman with several months of angina while attempting to perform routine daily activities is diagnosed with increasing angina
4. Which is true regarding delays in treatment of AMI?
    A. Influenced by race and gender but not age
    B. Mortality could be reduced to less than 1.5% if treatment begins <60 minutes after onset
    C. Due primarily to health care providers
    D. Rarely result from patient self-treatment of symptoms
    E. Result in a 50% reduction in potential benefit at 4 hours
5. Select the symptom more likely to represent angina.
    A. Lasting 2-5 minutes
    B. Rapid onset
    C. Reproducible with deep respiration
    D. Sharp, stabbing pain
    E. All the above
6. Up to 25% of acute myocardial infarctions have atypical presentations. Select the correct statement regarding atypical presentations:
    A. Dyspnea is the most common complaint in atypical infarction
    B. Less than one third of atypical presentations are "silent" infarctions
    C. Most patients older than age 85 have typical symptoms of infarction
    D. Patients with atypical presentations are usually older smokers with no history of angina
    E. The prognosis for patients with atypical symptoms is better than that for patients with typical symptoms

7. Regarding AMI patients released unintentionally from the emergency department:
   A. Almost 5% have missed ECG findings or obvious angina at rest
   B. Approximately 20,000 per year are released from emergency departments
   C. Missed myocardial infarctions account for 30% of malpractice dollars awarded
   D. Patients with previous hospitalizations for cardiac disease are more likely to be sent home
   E. Younger men (ages 30-45) make up a small fraction of these patients

8. Select the correct statement regarding emergency department ECGs:
   A. Comparison to old ECGs reduces under-diagnosis of acute myocardial infarction
   B. Five percent of patients who are admitted for chest pain and have completely normal ECGs are diagnosed with AICS
   C. Short-term but not long-term mortality is proportional to the degree of abnormality on the initial ECG
   D. Significant discrepancies between the readings of cardiologists, emergency medicine staff physicians, and emergency medicine residents are common
   E. The ECG has a sensitivity of >60% in acute myocardial infarction

9. A specific and sensitive sign of right ventricular infarction is:
   A. Delay in the intrinsicoid deflection in $V_{4R}$
   B. Hyperacute T wave in III
   C. ST depression in $V_{4R}$
   D. ST elevation in $V_{4R}$
   E. T wave inversion in III

10. A 32-year-old man arrives at the ED with a 3-day history of chest pain localized to the xiphisternal junction. His ECG (Fig. 103-1) is most consistent with which of the following diagnoses?
    A. Acute myocardial infarction
    B. Acute pericarditis
    C. Benign early repolarization
    D. Hyperkalemia
    E. Pericardial tamponade

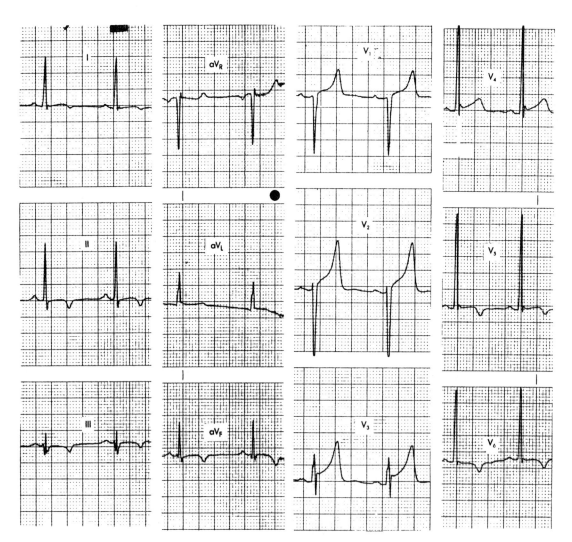

FIG. 103-1

11. Electrical alternans is virtually pathognomonic of which of the following entities?
    A. Digitalis toxicity
    B. Hyperkalemia
    C. Hypokalemia
    D. Pericardial effusion with tamponade
    E. Quinidine toxicity

12. The ECG in Figure 103-2 demonstrates changes consistent with what disease entity?
    A. Acute pericardial effusion
    B. Hyperkalemia
    C. Hypokalemia
    D. Myocardial contusion
    E. Quinidine toxicity

13. A 67-year-old woman with a history of chronic congestive heart failure caused by cardiomyopathy has the ECG tracing in Figure 103-3. What is the diagnosis?
    A. Acute myocardial infarction (AMI)
    B. Left anterior fascicular block (LAFB)
    C. Left bundle branch block (LBBB)
    D. Right bundle branch block (RBBB)
    E. Left posterior fascicular block (LPFB)

14. Regarding bundle branch block, which of the following statements is true?
    A. A diagnosis of LAFB is made if the QRS axis is more positive than 120 degrees
    B. Left posterior fascicular block is associated with left axis deviation
    C. ST elevation in $V_1$ or the inferior leads is a characteristic finding in RBBB
    D. The characteristic signature of RBBB is that the terminal forces are directed rightward and posterior
    E. The preservation of the initial QRS complex permits the recognition of pathologic Q waves in LBBB

15. Which of the following conditions produces the Osborne wave, an elevation of the initial portion of the ST segment contiguous with the J point?
    A. Inferior myocardial infarct
    B. Hyperthyroidism
    C. Hypothermia
    D. Pericarditis
    E. Tricyclic antidepressant overdose

16. All of the following are true of pathologic Q waves found on electrocardiograms except which one?
    A. Are directed away from an infarcted area
    B. Commonly develop 24 hours after infarct
    C. Indicate an septal infarct if found in leads $V_3$-$V_4$
    D. May be normal in leads $aV_R$ and $V_1$
    E. May not occur in up to 50% of patients with acute myocardial infarct

17. All of following are true of the ECG in Figure 103-4 except which one?
    A. It represents an acute inferior myocardial infarct
    B. Diagnostic Q waves are not present
    C. ST depression in the precordial leads likely represents left anterior descending coronary artery disease
    D. The R wave in lead $V_1$ is considered normal
    E. All of the above

18. Select the correct statement regarding bundle branch block in myocardial infarction.
    A. Left bundle branch block is not associated with anterior infarction
    B. New right bundle branch block has a higher associated mortality than left bundle branch block
    C. New right bundle branch block is less likely than left to progress to complete heart block
    D. Right and left bundle branch blocks obscure signs of myocardial infarction
    E. Right bundle branch block is not associated with anterior infarction

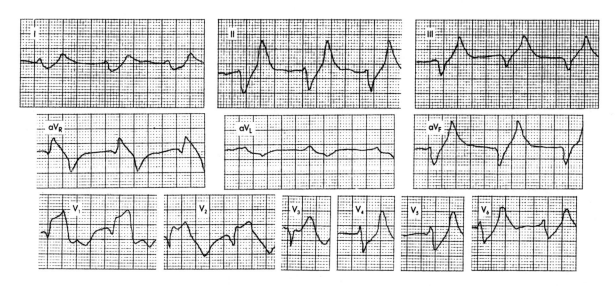

FIG. 103-2

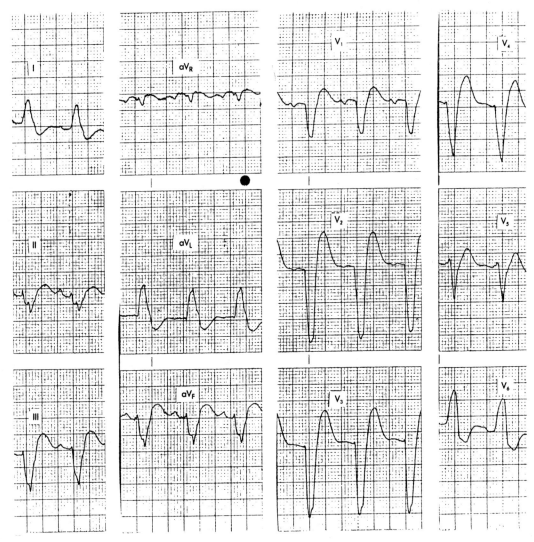

**FIG. 103-3**

19. Select the correct ischemia mimic.
    A. Digitalis-related convex ST depression
    B. Q waves in leads II, III, and aV_F due to pulmonary embolism
    C. ST depression in V_1-V_2 due to pulmonary embolism
    D. CK-MB elevation due to cerebrovascular accident
    E. CK-MB elevation due to pulmonary embolism

20. Select the correct statement regarding CK-MB.
    A. CK-MB has a sensitivity and specificity of greater than 90% within 3 hours of ED presentation
    B. The negative predictive value of CK-MB assays ranges from 75% to 85% at the time of initial ED presentation
    C. The positive predictive value of various CK-MB assays are in the range of 90%-95% at 3 hours from presentation
    D. The sensitivity of CK-MB approaches 100% in about 3 hours
    E. The specificity of the CK-MB assay increases significantly from initial presentation to 3 hours later

21. Select the correct statement regarding myoglobin.
    A. Myoglobin has a negative predictive value of nearly 100%
    B. Myoglobin has a specificity about the same as CK-MB at 3 hours from presentation
    C. Myoglobin levels peak within 2-3 hours after symptom onset
    D. Renal failure does not raise myoglobin levels
    E. Skeletal muscle contains little myoglobin

22. Which statement is true regarding troponins?
    A. Troponin I and T are similar-sized molecules
    B. Troponin levels remain elevated for up to 72 hours
    C. Troponins have initial-release kinetics similar to CK-MB
    D. Troponins may be falsely elevated in skeletal muscle injury
    E. Troponin T is highly specific for acute myocardial infarction

23. Select the correct statement regarding ECG exercise testing.

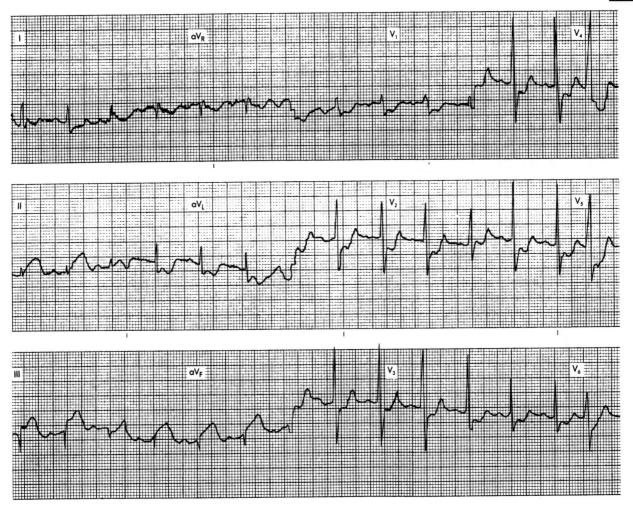

FIG. 103-4

A. Exercise testing requires a normal resting ECG
B. Fixed lesions of the circumflex artery are particularly difficult to identify
C. Safety of emergency department exercise testing is well documented
D. The sensitivity for exercise-induced ischemia is approximately 90%
E. Young women are particularly good candidates for exercise testing

24. A patient presents with chest pain. Which is the correct statement?
    A. An ECG should be obtained and interpreted within 20 minutes
    B. Average time to treatment is now 90-120 minutes
    C. If admitted to a chest pain evaluation and treatment unit, charges and cost may be decreased by 25%-50%
    D. Protocol-driven treatment is inferior to individualized therapy
    E. The goal for initiation of treatment of ischemic chest pain is 30 minutes

25. Select the event that does not result in increased myocardial damage during a typical ischemic episode.
    A. Coronary artery vasospasm
    B. Platelet aggregation
    C. Reperfusion
    D. Spontaneous thrombolysis
    E. Thrombus formation

26. Select the agent that does not work by platelet inhibition.
    A. Argatroban
    B. Clopidogrel
    C. Glycoprotein IIb-IIIa inhibitors
    D. Ticlopidine
    E. All the above work primarily by platelet inhibition

27. Which is an absolute contraindication to the use of thrombolytic therapy?
    A. Diabetic retinopathy
    B. History of ischemic CVA
    C. Menstruation
    D. Previous coronary artery bypass graft
    E. Prolonged CPR

28. Select the therapy inappropriate for cocaine-induced myocardial infarction.
    A. Beta blockers
    B. Morphine
    C. Nitroglycerin
    D. Sodium bicarbonate
    E. Thrombolytic therapy

---

## 104 ▼ Pericardial and Myocardial Disease

### *Richard S. Hartoch*

Select the appropriate letter that correctly answers the question or completes the statement.

1. All of the following are potential causes of pericarditis except which one?
    A. Cancer
    B. Collagen vascular disease
    C. Esophageal rupture (Boerhaave's syndrome)
    D. Infection
    E. Myocardial infarction

2. Which is true of chest pain associated with pericarditis?
    A. Is typically relieved by sitting up and leaning forward
    B. Is usually substernal and may not be distinguishable from the pain associated with a myocardial infarction
    C. May be associated with anxiety and anorexia
    D. May cause isolated shoulder pain
    E. All of the above

3. Classic ECG findings in early acute pericarditis include:
    A. A normal ECG
    B. Deep, symmetrical T wave inversions throughout the tracing
    C. Diffuse PR and ST segment depression
    D. Diffuse ST elevation and PR depression
    E. Q waves in the inferior and precordial leads

4. Which one is true regarding pericarditis related to myocardial infarction?
    A. Dressler syndrome, which may occur after an MI, consists of pericarditis associated with fever, leukocytosis, and pleuritis
    B. Pericarditis usually resolves within 3 days with nonsteroidal antiinflammatory therapy only
    C. The pattern of diffuse ST elevation on the ECG is rarely seen
    D. All of the above

5. Which of the following ECG findings provides the best way to differentiate acute pericarditis from myocardial infarction?
    A. Absence of Q waves
    B. Diffuse PR segment depression
    C. ST segment morphology
    D. T wave morphology
    E. U wave morphology

6. What is the earliest sign of cardiac tamponade?
    A. Hypotension
    B. Jugular venous distention
    C. Pulsus paradoxus
    D. Tachycardia
    E. Postural hypotension

7. Beck's triad of signs of pericardial tamponade includes all of the following except which one?
    A. Hypotension
    B. Jugular venous distention
    C. Muffled heart sounds
    D. Tachycardia
    E. All of the above are included

8. Electrical alternans on the ECG is pathognomonic of:
    A. Acute myocardial infarction in the presence of a bundle branch block
    B. Early pericardial effusion
    C. Pericardial tamponade
    D. Pericarditis
    E. Pulmonary emboli

9. What is the treatment of choice for suspected cardiac tamponade in a patient who is steadily deteriorating?
    A. Afterload reduction with nitroprusside
    B. Inotropic support with dobutamine or isoproterenol
    C. Pericardiocentesis
    D. Volume expansion with crystalloids or blood
    E. Emergent thoracotomy

10. Signs and symptoms of constrictive pericarditis are most often confused with:
    A. Acute myocardial infarction
    B. Congestive heart failure
    C. Myocarditis
    D. Pericardial tamponade
    E. All of the above

11. All of the following are characteristic of hypertrophic cardiomyopathy (HCM) except which one?
    A. A normal ECG
    B. Diastolic dysfunction
    C. Dyspnea
    D. Ischemic chest pain
    E. Syncope or near syncope

12. Which of the following statements is true of HCM?
    A. Characterized by a hypertrophied, non-dilated left ventricle
    B. Inherited as an autosomal-dominant trait with variable penetration
    C. Recognized as the most common cause of sudden death among young athletes
    D. Treated preferentially with beta-blockers
    E. All of the above

13. Which of the following statements is true regarding myocardial sarcoidosis?
    A. It is most common in blacks
    B. It is most common in whites

C. It is usually a benign disease with few clinical sequelae

D. The highest incidence is in males over 40 years of
age

E. None of the above

## 105 Infective Endocarditis and Acquired Valvular Heart Disease

*Brian Hoyt*

Select the appropriate letter that correctly answers the question or completes the statement.

1. Prolapse of the mitral valve is a common, usually benign, disorder. All of the following are serious complications of this condition except which one?
   A. Bacterial endocarditis
   B. Cerebral ischemia
   C. Paroxysmal supraventricular tachycardia
   D. Syncope and/or sudden death
   E. Third-degree heart block

2. Which organism is the most common cause of native valve bacterial endocarditis:
   A. Coagulase-negative *Staphylococcus*
   B. *Enterococcus* sp.
   C. *Staphylococcus aureus*
   D. *Streptococcus pneumoniae*
   E. *Streptococcus viridans*

3. Several skin lesions may be found in patients with endocarditis. Select the incorrect association from the list below.
   A. Janeway lesions: tender erythematous maculopapular lesions of finger pulp
   B. Osler nodes: painful, tender, erythematous nodules on the palmar surface of the finger tip
   C. Petechiae: nonblanching, nontender lesions usually of conjunctiva or mucous membranes
   D. Roth spots: retinal flame hemorrhages with pale centers
   E. Splinter hemorrhages: linear hemorrhages beneath the nails

4. Which ancillary evaluation for suspected endocarditis is incorrect?
   A. Echocardiogram
   B. ECG
   C. Erythrocyte sedimentation rate
   D. One blood culture
   E. Urinalysis looking for microscopic hematuria

5. Which is a common procedure for which antibiotic prophylaxis is not indicated in an individual with valvular or congenital heart disease?
   A. Cleaning and repair of a dirty laceration
   B. Dental procedures that cause gingival bleeding
   C. Incision and drainage of an abscess
   D. Insertion of a Foley catheter in a patient without a urinary tract infection
   E. Hemorrhoidal thrombectomy

6. Regarding the diagnosis of rheumatic fever, which of the following represents a major diagnostic criterion? (The others are minor criteria.)
   A. Arthralgia
   B. Elevated erythrocyte sedimentation rate
   C. Erythema marginatum
   D. Fever
   E. Prolonged PR interval

7. Which of the following is true regarding mitral valve disease?
   A. Atrial fibrillation is the most common complication of mitral stenosis
   B. Chronic and acute mitral regurgitation have the same etiology but their treatment differs
   C. Infectious endocarditis is a frequent complication of isolated mitral stenosis
   D. Left atrial enlargement and left ventricular hypertrophy are common ECG findings in acute mitral regurgitation
   E. The most common cause of both mitral stenosis and acute mitral regurgitation is rheumatic heart disease

8. All of the following statements are true of aortic stenosis except which one?
   A. Dyspnea on exertion, angina, and exertional syncope, once present, are associated with a 5-year survival of <50% without surgical intervention
   B. Hypotension secondary to acute decompensation usually responds to gentle fluid resuscitation
   C. In persons under age 65, bicuspid aortic valve is the most common cause
   D. Significant obstruction is defined as a valve orifice <25% of its normal size
   E. Typical ECG findings include left ventricular hypertrophy and left atrial enlargement

9. Select the correct statement regarding aortic regurgitation.
   A. Acute aortic regurgitation is a surgical emergency, whereas chronic regurgitation without overt left ventricular failure is amenable to medical management
   B. Connective tissue diseases such as Takayasu's aortitis and rheumatoid arthritis are the leading cause of chronic aortic regurgitation
   C. In acute aortic regurgitation the systolic pressure is normal to elevated and the pulse pressure is widened
   D. Pressors are used in the initial medical management of acute aortic regurgitation
   E. Water-hammer pulse is a finding in acute aortic regurgitation

10. Which statement is false regarding the patient with a prosthetic valve?
   A. Chronic hemolysis is abnormal and indicates valvular dysfunction
   B. On physical examination, signs of mechanical valvular failure include absence of a closure sound and a loud (3/6 or greater) regurgitant murmur
   C. Soft regurgitant and systolic murmurs are a normal finding regardless of valve type
   D. The risk of endocarditis is approximately 0.5% per year
   E. Thromboembolic events are the most serious complications of prosthetic valves

11. All of the following are true regarding hypertrophic cardiomyopathy except which one?
   A. Beta-blockers are an effective treatment and may have an antidysrhythmic effect
   B. ECG changes are rare
   C. Some patients have no symptoms
   D. Sudden death is the most serious complication
   E. Valsalva maneuver may help with the diagnosis

---

**SECTION 3  VASCULAR DISORDERS**

 **106 Hypertension**

*Richard S. Hartoch*

Select the appropriate letter that correctly answers the question or completes the statement.

1. The emergency provider's primary role in the management of hypertension includes all of the following except which one?
   A. To arrange appropriate follow-up for long-term treatment
   B. To begin antihypertensive therapy on an outpatient basis on newly diagnosed cases of hypertension
   C. To evaluate and manage complications that arise from long-standing hypertension
   D. To identify new cases of hypertension
   E. To recognize and treat hypertensive emergencies

2. All of the following are true regarding the renin-angiotensin system except which one?
   A. Angiotensin I is acted upon by a converting enzyme in the liver to form angiotensin II
   B. Angiotensin II is a potent vasoconstrictor that also stimulates aldosterone production
   C. Angiotensin inhibition has minimal effects on blood pressure in hypertensive patients with normal total body sodium
   D. Patients with high plasma renin levels will have a better therapeutic response to beta-blockers and an-

giotensin converting enzyme (ACE) inhibitors than patients with low plasma renin levels
   E. All of the above

3. Most cases of hypertension are considered to be essential (i.e., no specific etiology is identified). Which of the following is the most prevalent cause of secondary hypertension?
   A. Coarctation of the aorta
   B. Pheochromocytoma
   C. Renal disease
   D. Steroid therapy
   E. Thyroid disease

4. Which of the following is not considered a hypertensive emergency?
   A. A 21-year-old G2P1 female at 34 weeks' gestation with a blood pressure of 160/90 who comes to the ED with seizures
   B. A 35-year-old female with a blood pressure of 210/105 involved in a motor vehicle collision with a brief loss of consciousness who arrives with decreasing level of consciousness
   C. A 55-year-old male with a blood pressure of 260/130 and a normal physical examination and laboratory evaluation
   D. A 60-year-old female with a blood pressure of 190/110 complaining of a headache, nausea, vomiting, and confusion
   E. A 62-year-old male with a blood pressure of 220/110 and ECG revealing 3 mm ST elevation in leads $V_1$-$V_3$

5. All of the following statements are true regarding nitroprusside therapy, except which one?
   A. Extravasation can cause skin necrosis
   B. It is unstable in ultraviolet light
   C. It may lead to thiocyanate toxicity
   D. It may worsen angina
   E. It should be avoided in pregnancy

6. A 34-year-old G6P5 woman comes to the ED at 32 weeks' gestation with a blood pressure of 200/105 and a normal physical examination and laboratory evaluation. What is the agent of choice for blood pressure reduction?
   A. IV hydralazine
   B. IV magnesium sulfate
   C. IV nitroprusside
   D. PO hydralazine
   E. None of the above

7. A 15-year-old G1P0 female at 33 weeks' gestation complains of blurred vision, headache, and epigastric pain. On physical examination, blood pressure is 160/100, the patient is anxious, edema of the face is noted, DTRs are 3+ equal. The funduscopic exam is positive for bilateral retinal hemorrhages. Which of the following is the best initial agent to use in the treatment of this patient?
   A. Diazoxide PO
   B. Hydralazine IV
   C. Magnesium sulfate IV

D. Phenobarbital IV

E. Propranolol IV

8. A 67-year-old man with a long-standing history of hypertension comes to the ED after a reported syncopal episode. He complains of severe, tearing chest pain radiating to his back and shortness of breath. Physical examination reveals a diaphoretic male with a BP of 180/110 mm Hg and a pulse of 110. Lung examination reveals bibasilar rales, and cardiac examination reveals a blowing diastolic murmur. Neurologic examination reveals a left-sided hemiplegia. All of the following are true regarding the management of this patient except which one?

A. A cardiothoracic surgeon should be consulted

B. Computed tomography, MRI, or aortography is needed to confirm the diagnosis

C. Nitroprusside and/or trimethaphan is the antihypertensive agent of choice

D. Systolic blood pressure should be lowered to 100-120 mm Hg

E. The patient could be managed with medical treatment alone

*Match the precaution or complication below with the appropriate antihypertensive agent.*

A. Bladder atony, ileus, gastric atony, cycloplegia, and severe postural hypotension

B. Contraindicated in patients with CHF, heart block, asthma

C. Extravasation leads to skin necrosis and thiocyanate toxicity

D. Hyperuricemia, hyperglycemia, contraindicated in congestive heart failure

E. Rebound hypertension

9. Clonidine _____

10. Diazoxide _____

11. Labetalol _____

12. Nitroprusside _____

13. Trimethaphan _____

*The following paragraph applies to Questions 14 and 15.*

A 40-year-old man comes to the ED after a wine and cheese party, complaining of headache, blurred vision, and palpitations. He is noted to be anxious and diaphoretic with facial flushing. He reports similar episodes in the past 3 months since he started taking a medicine for depression. Physical examination reveals a blood pressure of 220/110, normal funduscopic findings, clear lungs, normal heart examination, and a nonfocal neurologic examination.

14. The most likely cause of this patient's symptoms would be:

A. Clonidine withdrawal

B. Hyperthyroidism

C. Pheochromocytoma

D. Propranolol withdrawal

E. Tyramine-induced hypertension

15. Treatment would best be accomplished using which of the following agents?

A. Clonidine

B. Nifedipine

C. Phentolamine

D. Phenylephrine

E. Propranolol

16. Which of the following is not true of malignant hypertension?

A. A patient with a normal physical examination and laboratory evaluation and a diastolic blood pressure of >130 has malignant hypertension

B. It is usually associated with a diastolic blood pressure >130

C. Patients with malignant hypertension usually have marked retinal findings, such as cotton-wool spots and linear hemorrhages

D. The pathologic change found in end organs that are damaged is fibrinoid necrosis of small arterioles

E. Treatment consists of lowering the blood pressure by 30%-40% of pretreatment level within 1 hour

17. Hypertensive urgency is defined as a severe elevation of blood pressure (diastolic pressure of 115 mm Hg or greater) without evidence of end-organ disease. Which of the following statements is true regarding the management of hypertensive urgencies?

A. Blood pressure should be reduced within 48 hours to reduce the potential risks to the patient

B. Evaluation should comprise a history and physical and laboratory tests including BUN, creatinine, electrolytes, ECG, and urinalysis

C. Rapid reduction of blood pressure may be beneficial

D. The agent of choice for treatment is nitroprusside

E. Trial of sublingual nifedipine is indicated

*Match the mechanism of action below with the appropriate antihypertensive agent.*

A. Alpha-adrenergic blocker at postsynaptic receptors

B. Beta-blocker

C. Calcium channel blocker

D. Central sympathomimetic inhibitor

E. Competitive inhibitor of angiotensin I converting enzyme

F. Sodium reabsorption inhibitor at the ascending loop of Henle

18. Captopril _____

19. Clonidine _____

20. Furosemide _____

21. Nifedipine _____

22. Prazosin _____

23. Propranolol _____

# 107 Pulmonary Embolism

*James E. Thompson*

Select the appropriate letter that correctly answers the question or completes the statement.

1. Which of the following is the most common source of thromboembolism leading to pulmonary emboli?
   A. Deep veins below the knee
   B. Deep veins of the pelvis and thigh
   C. Right side of the heart
   D. Superficial veins of the lower extremities
   E. Upper extremity veins

2. Which of the following substances can cause pulmonary emboli?
   A. Air
   B. Fat
   C. Amniotic fluid
   D. All of the above
   E. A and B only

3. All of the following are true of amniotic fluid pulmonary emboli except which one?
   A. Disseminated intravascular coagulation is a frequent complication
   B. It most frequently occurs near the end of the first stage of labor
   C. It may occur in the setting of abortion
   D. Treatment includes delivery of the fetus
   E. Treatment involves administration of thrombolytic agents when circulatory collapse occurs

*The following paragraph applies to Questions 4 and 5.*

A 23-year-old female who is 6 months pregnant comes to the ED after an automobile collision in which she sustained a closed commuted fracture of her tibia. She subsequently becomes confused, disoriented, and severely short of breath. Physical examination reveals petechial hemorrhages on her chest and neck.

4. Which of the following is most likely to account for this?
   A. Air embolism
   B. Amniotic fluid pulmonary embolism
   C. Fat embolism
   D. Pulmonary thromboembolism
   E. None of the above

5. Which of the following therapeutic interventions would be the most beneficial for this patient?
   A. High-dose heparin therapy
   B. High-dose steroid therapy
   C. Immediate evacuation of the fetus
   D. Placement in left lateral position
   E. None of the above

6. Sources of pulmonary air embolism include which of the following?
   A. Air-powered surgical drills
   B. Iatrogenic vaginal insufflation
   C. Orogenital sex during pregnancy

D. Underwater pressurized breathing apparatus
   E. All of the above have been described as sources of air emboli

7. All of the following may be effective in the management of air emboli except which one?
   A. Aspiration of air through right heart catheter
   B. Emergency thoracotomy and direct needle aspiration
   C. Hyperbaric oxygen therapy
   D. Placing the patient with right side up
   E. All of the above may be effective

8. Which of the following is the most common clinical symptom in patients with pulmonary emboli?
   A. Cough
   B. Dyspnea
   C. Hemoptysis
   D. Pleuritic chest pain
   E. Syncope

9. Which of the following is the most common clinical sign associated with pulmonary emboli?
   A. Cyanosis
   B. Fever above 37° C
   C. Lower extremity edema
   D. Rales
   E. Tachypnea

10. The classic clinical triad of dyspnea, hemoptysis, and pleuritic chest pain is found in what percentage of patients with proven pulmonary emboli?
    A. 5%
    B. 20%
    C. 50%
    D. 75%
    E. 90%

11. All of the following are risk factors for pulmonary emboli except which one?
    A. Advanced age
    B. Current deep vein thrombosis
    C. Malignancy
    D. Obesity
    E. Pregnancy

12. Which of the following does not cause a hypercoagulable state?
    A. Cigarette smoking
    B. Polycythemia
    C. Pregnancy
    D. Protein S deficiency
    E. All of the above can cause a hypercoagulable state

13. All of the following statements are true regarding antithrombin III deficiency except which one?
    A. It is a familial disease
    B. It should be suspected in a young patient with recurrent thromboembolism
    C. Onset usually occurs in the third decade of life
    D. Patients must be anticoagulated with warfarin
    E. Treatment involves high-dose heparin therapy

14. Which of the following should be avoided in patients with protein C deficiency?

A. Warfarin
B. Heparin
C. High-dose steroids
D. Low molecular weight dextran

15. All of the following statements are true regarding pulmonary function tests and diagnosis of pulmonary emboli except which one?
   A. A ratio of dead space to tidal volume (Vd/Vt) >40% with a normal spirometry indicates a high probability for pulmonary emboli
   B. An increased A-a gradient and a decreased $PaO_2$ is common in patients with pulmonary emboli
   C. 50% of patients with pulmonary emboli have a $PaO_2$ >80 mm Hg
   D. Normal ABG results can be seen in up to 50% of patients with pulmonary emboli
   E. Pulse oximetry is a good diagnostic aid for pulmonary emboli

16. Which of the following is (are) the most common ECG finding(s) in pulmonary emboli?
   A. Atrial fibrillation and left axis deviation
   B. Nonspecific ST and T wave changes and tachycardia
   C. Peaked T waves and right axis deviation
   D. Right bundle branch block and S1-S2-S3
   E. S1-Q3-T3

17. Which of the following statements is true regarding chest radiography in pulmonary emboli?
   A. A focal infiltrate that develops 3 days after symptoms of pulmonary emboli is meaningless
   B. Eighty percent of patients with submassive pulmonary emboli will have a normal chest radiograph
   C. Hampton's hump is a dilation of pulmonary vessels proximal to the emboli
   D. Westermark's sign, if present, is the earliest detectable chest radiograph abnormality
   E. Westermark's sign is a wedge-shaped infiltrate with the apex toward the hilum

18. Which of the following may cause decreased ventilation on a V/Q scan?
   A. Atelectasis
   B. Bronchospasm
   C. Pulmonary infiltrates
   D. A and B only
   E. All of the above

*Questions 19 to 26 refer to the Prospective Investigation of Pulmonary Emboli Diagnosis (PIOPED) study coordinated by the National Heart, Lung, and Blood Institute of the NIH and published in 1990.*

19. All of the following are considered high-probability V/Q scans except:
   A. Four subsegmental perfusion defects with a normal chest radiograph and normal ventilation
   B. Non-segmental perfusion defect
   C. Two or more segmental perfusion defects with a normal chest radiograph and normal ventilation

D. Two segmental perfusion defects with an abnormal chest radiograph and a ventilation defect smaller than the perfusion defect
   E. Two subsegmental defects and one segmental perfusion defect with a normal chest radiograph and normal ventilation

20. A 60-year-old obese woman with a history of breast cancer comes to the ED complaining of pleuritic chest pain and shortness of breath. She has recently been traveling several hours in an automobile. According to the PIOPED study, which of the following would be an acceptable end-point to the work-up of pulmonary emboli in this patient?
   A. A high-probability V/Q scan
   B. A low-probability V/Q scan
   C. A normal V/Q scan
   D. An intermediate-probability V/Q scan
   E. None of the above

21. All of the following statements are true of intermediate V/Q scans except which one?
   A. If this pattern is presumed to be positive for pulmonary emboli, it will be wrong 70% of the time
   B. If presumed negative, it will miss pulmonary emboli 41% of the time
   C. This pattern does not change the prior clinical likelihood of pulmonary emboli
   D. With a high clinical suspicion of pulmonary emboli, this pattern is an acceptable end-point for work-up
   E. All of the above are true

22. According to the PIOPED study, a normal V/Q pattern will miss what percentage of pulmonary emboli?
   A. 2%
   B. 10%
   C. 15%
   D. 20%
   E. 25%

23. Which of the following is a complication of pulmonary angiogram?
   A. Anaphylactoid reaction
   B. Cardiac arrest
   C. Dysrhythmia
   D. Vessel perforation
   E. All of the above

24. All of the following statements are true of pulmonary angiography except which one?
   A. A false-positive test may occur in the presence of lung cancer
   B. Angiographic evidence of pulmonary emboli may persist up to 1 week after anticoagulation
   C. Complications are increased in patients with primary pulmonary hypertension
   D. Delayed angiography may be performed after thrombolytic therapy
   E. It has mortality rates of up to 0.4%

25. All of the following are treatment options for pulmonary embolism except which one?
    A. Anticoagulation
    B. Catheter embolectomy
    C. Open embolectomy
    D. Thrombolytic agents
    E. All of the above

26. Which of the following cardiotropic agents is preferred for the patient with pulmonary emboli?
    A. Dobutamine
    B. Dopamine
    C. Epinephrine
    D. Isoproterenol
    E. None of the above

27. Which of the following is not true of heparin therapy in the treatment of pulmonary emboli?
    A. Acts to dissolve the clot
    B. Can be used in pregnancy
    C. May induce an immune thrombocytopenia
    D. Prevents progression of clot
    E. Reduces the mortality from pulmonary emboli to <10%

28. All of the following are benefits of thrombolytic therapy over heparin therapy in the treatment of pulmonary emboli and deep vein thrombosis except which one?
    A. Improved postphlebitic syndrome
    B. Lower risk of bleeding complications
    C. Pulmonary hypertension prevention
    D. Rapid clot resolution
    E. Rapid normalization of hemodynamic instability

29. All of the following are absolute contraindications to the use of thrombolytic therapy except which one?
    A. Active internal bleeding
    B. Active major external bleeding
    C. Neurosurgery in the past 8 weeks
    D. Recent renal biopsy
    E. Recent stroke

30. A 69-year-old man comes to the ED with leg pain and swelling. Work-up is positive for deep vein thrombosis. Before treatment, the patient suddenly gasps for air and collapses; full cardiac arrest ensues. The best treatment approach for this patient with suspected pulmonary embolus would be:
    A. CPR and high-dose heparin
    B. CPR and immediate administration of a thrombolytic agent
    C. Emergent cardiothoracic surgery consult for surgical thromboembolectomy
    D. Immediate bilateral thoracotomy with pulmonary vessel massage
    E. Immediate consultation for a catheter embolectomy

# 108 Abdominal Aortic Aneurysm

### James E. Thompson

Select the appropriate letter that correctly answers the question or completes the statement.

1. All of the following statements regarding abdominal aortic aneurysm (AAA) are true except which one?
    A. AAAs can be intact, leaking, or ruptured
    B. Appropriate referral can be made for follow-up and elective repair in asymptomatic patients
    C. The distinction between leaking and ruptured AAA is made on the basis of volume and rapidity of blood loss, integrity of the remaining aorta, and the patient's general condition
    D. The mortality rate for repair of ruptured aneurysms is about 20%
    E. All of the above are true

2. The goal for emergency physicians with respect to the diagnosis and management of AAAs is:
    A. Earlier diagnosis in the symptomatic patient
    B. Early involvement of the vascular surgeon
    C. Improved management of the unstable patient
    D. More frequent diagnosis of the asymptomatic patient
    E. All of the above

3. All of the following statements regarding the pathophysiology of AAAs are true except which one?
    A. Most AAAs are suprarenal, and the majority involve the renal arteries
    B. True aneurysms of the abdominal aorta are localized dilations of the wall that are >3 cm in diameter and involve all three layers of the vessel
    C. The mean diameter of abdominal aortas is 1.9 cm in women and 2.4 cm in men
    D. The natural course of AAA is to enlarge gradually at a mean rate of expansion of 0.5 cm per year
    E. All of the above are true

4. Comparing aortic aneurysms with aortic dissections, which of the following statements is false?
    A. Aneurysms occur almost exclusively in the abdomen
    B. Congenital cardiovascular lesions in pregnancy are commonly associated with isolated aortic dissections
    C. Dissections occur predominantly in the thoracic aorta
    D. Isolated abdominal aortic dissections occur in middle age, affect more men than women, and occur more in hypertensive patients
    E. Most dissections that involve the abdominal aorta are actually extensions of dissections of the thoracic aorta

5. Which of the following statements is false?
    A. Collagen content in an AAA is usually increased
    B. Collagen provides the aortic wall with tensile strength

C. Elastin contributes to blood vessel compliance

D. Most patients with atherosclerosis in other blood vessels have aneurysms

E. The current concept of the etiology of AAA is that loss or failure of elastin leads to aneurysm formation

6. What is the most common misdiagnosis in patients with ruptured AAA?

A. Acute MI

B. Musculoskeletal back pain

C. Pancreatitis

D. Perforated viscus

E. Renal colic

7. Which of the following is not a risk factor for the development of AAA?

A. Age

B. Black race

C. Family history

D. Male gender

E. Smoking history

8. Regarding findings on physical examination of the patient with AAA, which of the following statements is true?

A. Most aneurysms are palpated below the navel

B. Most patients have significant abdominal tenderness and guarding

C. Most patients with AAA have full and equal femoral pulses

D. Tenderness with palpation is not suggestive of ruptured AAA

9. Regarding imaging modalities for AAA, all of the following statements are true except which one?

A. AAAs are detected on plain films in 55% to 75% of cases

B. Angiography can overestimate the size of an aneurysm

C. CT scan is more accurate than ultrasound in determining size and detecting thrombus

D. The accuracy of ultrasound detection approaches 100%

E. All of the above are true

10. The single most significant preoperative factor associated with increased mortality is:

A. Age

B. Co-morbid disease

C. Hypotension

D. Gender

 ## 109  Aortic Dissection

### *James E. Thompson*

Select the appropriate letter that correctly answers the question or completes the statement.

1. Regarding the epidemiology of aortic dissection, all of the following statements are true except which one?

A. It is the most common and the most lethal catastrophe involving the aorta

B. One half of the aortic dissections in women under the age of 40 occur in association with pregnancy

C. The incidence of aortic dissection is higher in patients with a bicuspid aortic valve

D. The majority of cases occur in patients between 50 and 70 years of age

E. The type of trauma that is usually associated with aortic dissection is blunt

2. Predisposing syndromes associated with an increased risk of aortic dissection include which of the following?

A. Coarctation of the aorta

B. Congenital heart disease

C. Marfan syndrome

D. All of the above

E. None of the above

3. Aortic dissection occurs in which layer of the aortic wall?

A. Adventitia

B. External elastic lamina

C. Intima

D. Media

E. Can occur in any layer

4. Regarding the Stanford classification of aortic dissections, which of the following statements is true?

A. About two thirds of patients have type A dissections

B. Patients with type B dissections tend to be older, heavy smokers with chronic lung disease, generalized atherosclerosis, and/or hypertension

C. Type A dissections are much more lethal

D. All of the above

E. None of the above

5. Regarding diagnostic findings, which of the following statements is not true?

A. Aortic regurgitation occurs in about 50% of patients with type A dissection

B. In about 20% of patients, neurologic deficit is the presenting manifestation

C. Pain is the most common presenting complaint

D. Pulse deficit, a unilaterally weakened or absent pulse, occurs in almost 50% of patients with proximal dissections

E. The most common neurologic abnormality is ischemic paraparesis

6. Comparing the DeBakey classification to the Stanford, which of the following is correct?
   A. I = A
   B. II = A
   C. III = B
   D. I = II + III
   E. All of the above

7. A 66-year-old white man with a history of hypertension and a known patent foramen ovale has sudden onset of ripping chest pain radiating to his back, a blood pressure of 210/120, and a heart rate of 110. Regarding his initial treatment, which of the following would not be a wise choice?
   A. Labetalol
   B. Nitroprusside alone
   C. Nitroprusside and propranolol
   D. Trimethaphan

8. Which of the following patients with an acute dissection requires immediate surgery?
   A. 40-year-old pregnant female with a type A dissection
   B. 68-year-old black male with a progressive stroke
   C. 77-year-old hypertensive white male with a type B dissection
   D. All of the above
   E. None of the above

9. Which of the following statements regarding laboratory and radiographic evaluation in the work-up of aortic dissection is true?
   A. Cardiac enzymes are usually elevated
   B. Chest x-rays will be abnormal in 80%-90% of cases
   C. CT scanning requires arterial catheterization for delivery of contrast dye
   D. Aortography is no longer the gold standard
   E. Transthoracic echocardiography has a sensitivity approaching 96%

## 110 ▼ Peripheral Arteriovascular Disease

### Hans Notenboom

Select the appropriate letter that correctly answers the question or completes the statement.

1. Atherosclerosis is least common in the:
   A. Abdominal aorta
   B. Axillary artery
   C. Circle of Willis
   D. Popliteal artery
   E. Thoracic aorta

2. All of the following statements are true of arterial thromboembolism except which one?
   A. Arterial emboli result much more commonly from the left ventricle than from the atria
   B. Atrial fibrillation is present in more than half of patients with arterial embolization
   C. More than three fourths of arterial emboli originate in the heart
   D. The bifurcation of the common femoral artery is the most common site of embolism
   E. The iliac artery is a more common site for embolism than the popliteal artery

3. Which of the following statements is true of Raynaud's disease?
   A. Ergot preparations are the treatment of choice
   B. Histologic changes of the arterial wall are pathognomonic
   C. Sympathectomy is indicated for severe, progressive symptoms
   D. Symptoms are typically unilateral
   E. Tissue loss is common

4. All the following statements are true of chronic arterial insufficiency except which one?
   A. Aortoiliac disease producing bilateral claudication almost always results in impotence
   B. Calf pain is more severe than hip and buttock pain
   C. Patients with resting pain often dangle their feet over the bedside for relief
   D. Resting pain is usually located in the calf
   E. The level of occlusion and the location of symptoms of claudication are well correlated

5. In differentiating thrombosis from embolism, which of the following is characteristic of embolus?
   A. Arteriography reveals diffuse atherosclerosis with well-developed collaterals
   B. History of severe claudication is commonly present
   C. Source is identified
   D. Proximal or contralateral limb pulses are diminished or absent
   E. There is no sharp demarcation of ischemia

6. Which of the following would be least typical of a patient with thromboangiitis obliterans (Buerger's disease)?
   A. Age older than 50 at onset
   B. History of smoking
   C. Hand claudication or fingertip ulcers
   D. Instep claudication
   E. Involvement of both the upper and lower extremities

7. Which of the following is true of popliteal artery aneurysms?
   A. Not associated with abdominal aortic aneurysms
   B. Not associated with limb-threatening thromboembolic events, claudication, or atherosclerotic events
   C. Often bilateral
   D. Second most common form of peripheral aneurysm
   E. Do not result in deep venous thrombosis formation

8. Which of the following statements is not true of the patient with an infected aneurysm?
   A. About 25% of patients do not require surgery
   B. Antibiotic treatment usually lasts 6 to 8 weeks
   C. Mycotic aneurysms (secondary to endocarditis) commonly occur in the superior mesenteric and intracranial arteries

D. Organisms associated with infected atherosclerotic arteries include *Salmonella, Escherichia,* and *Staphylococcus* species

E. The most common site of posttraumatic infected aneurysm is the femoral artery

9. All of the following statements are true of temporal arteritis except which one?

A. It classically includes fevers with a high erythrocyte sedimentation rate

B. It may involve arteries in any location

C. Temporal artery biopsies should be completed within 48 hours

D. Visual loss may be reversed with appropriate therapy

E. 90% of patients are older than age 60

10. Which of the following statements is true of thoracic outlet syndrome?

A. Can reliably be assessed by bedside testing of positional compression of the subclavian artery

B. Cervical ribs are associated with neurologic rather than arterial compression

C. Is detected by the elevated arm stress test (EAST) only if due to brachial plexus compression

D. Is caused by compression of vascular structures in about 50% of patients

E. Often mimics ulnar nerve compression

11. Which of the following statements is true regarding possible arterial injury from intravenous drug abuse?

A. Anticoagulant therapy has documented benefit

B. Distal ischemia caused by arterial injection is associated with loss of pulse

C. Methamphetamine users are at higher risk for necrotizing vasculitis

D. Most infected pseudoaneurysms are found in the upper extremities

E. Ultrasound is useful to distinguish abscess from aneurysm

12. A patient arrives at the ED with a central venous catheter problem. All of the following statements are true except which one?

A. A chest roentgenogram is needed in all cases of persistent catheter occlusion

B. A laceration or fracture of a Hickman-Broviac catheter greater than 4 cm from the insertion site may safely be repaired

C. Fibrin sheath formation is a cause of withdrawal occlusion

D. The Groshong catheter, although it contains a terminal valve, should still allow withdrawal of blood samples

E. The possibility of subclavian vein thrombosis may be safely discounted because of lack of extremity swelling

# 111 Peripheral Venous Disease of the Extremities

*Hans Notenboom*

Select the appropriate letter that correctly answers the question or completes the statement.

1. Most DVT of the lower extremities begin in the:

A. Deep calf veins

B. External iliac vein

C. Femoral vein in the midthigh

D. Femoral vein near the inguinal ligament

E. Popliteal vein near the popliteal fossa

2. All of the following statements regarding deep calf vein thrombi are true except which one?

A. Anticoagulation for deep calf vein thrombi is appropriate

B. Approximately 20% of deep calf vein thrombi propagate

C. Calf vein thrombi do not directly result in pulmonary embolism

D. Postphlebitic syndrome may be a sequela of deep calf vein thrombi

E. The majority of small calf vein thrombi dissolve completely and spontaneously

3. All of the following are risk factors for thrombosis except which one?

A. Diabetes

B. Heparin therapy

C. Polycythemia rubra vera

D. Protein C deficiency

E. Varicose veins

4. Which is not true regarding diagnostic testing for DVT?

A. Contrast venography is a reliable but invasive test

B. Doppler studies are the gold standard for ruling out DVT

C. Duplex scanning is highly operator-dependent and therefore lacks reproducibility

D. MRI offers reliable diagnosis of DVT or other anatomic abnormality causing similar symptoms

E. Venograms using $^{99m}$Tc are poor for ruling out DVT

5. A search for underlying disorders of the coagulation system is suggested by a DVT patient with all the following factors except which one?

A. Age less than 35

B. Anticoagulation difficulty

C. DVT in early pregnancy

D. Mesenteric or portal vein thrombosis

E. Recurrent DVT in a leg with a history of fracture and casting

6. Which is false regarding axillary/subclavian venous thrombosis?
   A. Associated with Swan-Ganz catheterization
   B. Seen in up to 40% of patients receiving chemotherapy or hyperalimentation through subclavian catheters
   C. More commonly seen in IV drug users.
   D. Subclavian and axillary DVTs are becoming more common
   E. Subclavian and axillary DVTs are not associated with morbidity

7. Which of the following statements is false concerning treatment of DVT with heparin?
   A. An aPTT 1.5 times the control value is needed for therapeutic heparin effect
   B. Heparin dissolves thrombi but does not prevent further clots from forming
   C. Heparin is the most commonly used drug in the treatment of acute venous thrombosis
   D. Heparin works by activating antithrombin III
   E. Sub-therapeutic aPTT levels require rebolus rather than higher infusion rate

8. Which of the following statements is false regarding superficial thrombophlebitis?
   A. Clinical examination cannot always distinguish superficial from deep venous thrombophlebitis
   B. Lifetime incidence in those with untreated varicose vein is 20%-50%
   C. Risk of DVT is three times higher in those with varicose veins
   D. Superficial thrombophlebitis is a benign condition
   E. Unrecognized DVT is present in nearly half of all patients with superficial thrombophlebitis

---

**SECTION 4  GASTROINTESTINAL DISORDERS**

 **112** Acute Abdominal Pain

*Craig Lauder and Donnita M. Scott*

Select the appropriate letter that correctly answers the question or completes the statement.

1. What is the most common diagnosis documented for a patient seen in the ED with acute abdominal pain?
   A. Abdominal pain of unknown cause
   B. Acute cholecystitis
   C. Appendicitis
   D. Gastroenteritis
   E. Ureteral stone

2. What two factors modify the ED physician's diagnosis for patients who present with acute abdominal pain?
   A. Age and ethnic race
   B. Age and past medical history

C. Gender and age
D. Gender and past medical history
E. Vital signs and age

3. Which of the following conditions, other than pancreatitis, cause an elevation in the serum amylase level?
   A. Bowel infarction
   B. Diabetic ketoacidosis
   C. Ectopic pregnancy
   D. Liver disease
   E. All of the above

4. Which type of abdominal pain is accompanied by autonomic responses that cause symptoms such as nausea, vomiting, pallor, and diaphoresis?
   A. Referred pain
   B. Somatic pain
   C. Visceral pain
   D. None of the above

5. Which of the following is the most common cause of acute abdominal pain that requires emergency surgery?
   A. Acute appendicitis
   B. Acute cholecystitis
   C. Diverticulitis
   D. Intestinal obstruction
   E. Perforated ulcer

6. Which of the following physical signs is helpful in diagnosing acute cholecystitis?
   A. Iliopsoas sign
   B. Kehr's sign
   C. Murphy's sign
   D. Obturator sign
   E. Rovsing's sign

7. Of the following vital signs, which is most often examined by the emergency physician in evaluating a patient with acute abdominal pain?
   A. Blood pressure
   B. Oxygenation (pulse oximetry)
   C. Pulse
   D. Respiration
   E. Temperature

8. In children, 95% of the diagnoses of acute abdominal pain fall into what two categories?
   A. Acute appendicitis and toxic ingestion
   B. Constipation and acute appendicitis
   C. Nonspecific abdominal pain and acute appendicitis
   D. Nonspecific abdominal pain and intussusception
   E. Urinary infection and constipation

9. In the early development of acute intestinal ischemia, which of the following serum levels is consistently elevated?
   A. Alkaline phosphate
   B. Creatine phosphokinase
   C. Lactic acid
   D. Phosphate
   E. White blood cell count

10. Of the following imaging studies, which is the primary modality for a patient with right upper quadrant abdominal pain?

A. CT scan
B. Endoscopy
C. Laparoscopy
D. Ultrasonography
E. Upper gastrointestinal series

11. A 55-year-old female presents to the ED complaining of nausea, vomiting, and generalized colicky abdominal pain for the past 36 hours. Her past medical history is significant for a cholecystectomy 3 years ago. The obstruction found is shown in Figure 112-1. What is the next appropriate step in management of this patient?

   A. Analgesia, laxatives, and discharge the patient home with careful follow-up in the next 24 hours with a surgeon
   B. Give antiemetics and antibiotics and if the abdominal pain subsides over the next 2-6 hours, discharge the patient home with follow-up with the primary care physician
   C. Observe the patient and perform multiple abdominal examinations over the next 6 hours
   D. Obtain immediate surgical consultation
   E. Secure IV access, place a nasogastric tube, administer analgesia, and obtain surgical consultation

12. An 18-month-old boy presents to the ED with a 2-day history of vomiting, diarrhea, and colicky abdominal pain described as intermittent with asymptomatic intervals. The mother states the child seems more comfort-able in the knee-chest position, and before bringing the child to the ED she noticed some blood in the stool. What is the preferred diagnostic and therapeutic imaging study?

   A. Barium enema
   B. CT scan
   C. Endoscopy
   D. MRI
   E. Radionuclide scanning

# 113 ▾ Gastrointestinal Bleeding

*John R. Leisey and Thomas A. Sweeney*

Select the appropriate letter that correctly answers the question or completes the statement

1. The most common presentation of upper gastrointestinal bleeding (UGIB) in patients with peptic ulcer disease is:
   A. Abdominal pain
   B. Hematemesis
   C. Hematochezia
   D. Melena
   E. Syncope

2. Re-bleeding occurs most commonly with which cause of UGIB?
   A. Esophagitis
   B. Gastritis
   C. Mallory-Weiss tear
   D. Peptic ulcer disease
   E. Varices

3. An 18-month-old infant presents with painless rectal bleeding without passage of stool. The most likely cause of lower gastrointestinal bleeding (LGIB) in this patient is:
   A. Angiodysplasia
   B. Henoch-Schonlein purpura
   C. Incarcerated hernia
   D. Intussusception
   E. Meckel's diverticulum

4. Which is true regarding examination of gastric contents in the evaluation of GI hemorrhage?
   A. A clear gastric aspirate excludes hemorrhage from the duodenum
   B. Anoscopy should be performed before gastric aspiration in patients with hematochezia
   C. Gastric tube placement will aggravate hemorrhage from varices or Mallory-Weiss tears
   D. Nasal trauma from NG tube placement is a rare cause of a false-positive finding of gastric aspirate for blood
   E. The presence of bile in an otherwise clear nasogastric aspirate excludes the possibility of active bleeding above the ligament of Treitz

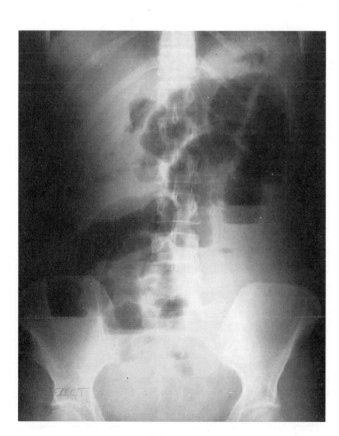

**FIG. 112-1**

5. A 50-year-old man with a 15-year history of daily alcohol use presents to the ED with acute onset of hematemesis. Following initial volume resuscitation with 2 liters normal saline, vital signs are temperature, 37° C (98.6° F); respirations, 16; heart rate, 85; and blood pressure, 115/60. The patient continues to vomit blood. What is the diagnostic procedure of choice?
   A. Angiography
   B. Endoscopy
   C. Gastric aspiration
   D. Radionuclide imaging (bleeding scan)
   E. Upright chest radiograph

6. A 55-year-old woman with a history of diverticulosis presents to the ED with massive bright red hematochezia. Vital signs are temperature, 37° C (98.6° F); respirations, 26; heart rate, 140; and blood pressure, 75/40. What should initial fluid resuscitation consist of?
   A. 10 cc/Kg O-negative whole blood
   B. 10 cc/Kg type-specific whole blood
   C. 20 cc/Kg D5 0.45% normal saline solution
   D. 20 cc/Kg normal saline solution
   E. 20 cc/Kg type-specific packed red blood cells

7. Which of the following is an indication for emergency surgery in a patient with GI bleeding?
   A. Hepatic disease with coagulopathy
   B. Initial presentation in hypovolemic shock
   C. More than 2 units of blood required within the first 4-6 hours
   D. Red gastric aspirate
   E. Unstable vital signs unresponsive to resuscitation

8. The most common cause of UGIB is:
   A. Esophageal varices
   B. Gastric erosions
   C. Gastric varices
   D. Mallory-Weiss tear
   E. Peptic ulcer disease

9. Approximately what percentage of gastrointestinal bleeding will stop spontaneously?
   A. 10%
   B. 20%
   C. 40%
   D. 60%
   E. 80%

10. The most common cause of significant LGIB in the adult is:
    A. Cancer
    B. Diverticulosis
    C. Infectious diarrhea
    D. Meckel's diverticulum
    E. Undiagnosed

11. In the young adult, the most likely cause of massive LGIB is:
    A. Angiodysplasia
    B. Diverticulosis
    C. Hemorrhoids
    D. Infectious diarrhea
    E. Ulcerative colitis

# 114 Acute Gastroenteritis and Constipation

*David M. Morrison and Thomas A. Sweeney*

Select the appropriate letter that correctly answers the question or completes the statement.

1. Which of the following is most commonly associated with acute diarrhea?
   A. Antibiotic therapy
   B. Bacterial infection
   C. Occupational exposure
   D. Protozoal infection
   E. Viral infection

2. Which of the following statements is true regarding typical characteristics of invasive diarrhea?
   A. Duration is typically less than 24 hours
   B. Fecal leukocytes are absent
   C. Incubation period of infectious diarrhea is typically less than 24 hours
   D. Onset is typically gradual
   E. Patients rarely have abdominal pain

3. Which of the following is an indication for obtaining a stool culture in the ED?
   A. Absence of fecal leukocytes
   B. Age greater than 65 years old
   C. Age less than 6 years old
   D. Clinical suspicion of toxigenic diarrhea
   E. Employment in a daycare center

4. Which is the most important aspect of acute management of diarrhea?
   A. Antimicrobial treatment
   B. Identification of causative organism
   C. Fluid and electrolyte replacement
   D. Prevention of further spread of the organism
   E. Symptomatic relief

5. What is the best empiric antibiotic therapy for infectious diarrhea?
   A. Ampicillin
   B. Cefazolin
   C. Ciprofloxacin
   D. Erythromycin
   E. Trimethoprim-sulfamethoxazole

6. Which of the following conditions is alone an indication for admission?
   A. Age less than 6 years old
   B. Inability to keep up with fluid losses via oral intake
   C. Mild dehydration
   D. Need for antibiotic treatment
   E. Sickle cell disease

7. A 6-year-old boy presents to the ED 3 days after returning from a hiking trip with the rapid onset of fever, cramping abdominal pain, and flu-like symptoms for 1 day and bloody diarrhea, starting the day of presentation. What is the most likely organism?

A. *Campylobacter* sp.

B. *E. coli*

C. *Giardia* sp.

D. *Salmonella* sp.

E. *Shigella* sp.

8. What is the most likely source from which to acquire infection with *Salmonella* sp.?

A. Direct person-to-person contact

B. Green leafy vegetables

C. Aerosolized droplets

D. Unbroken eggs

E. Unpeeled fruits

9. A 6-year-old boy presents with cramping abdominal pain, vomiting, and bloody diarrhea 7 days after eating an undercooked hamburger. Low numbers of fecal leukocytes are seen on smear. What is the most serious complication to be concerned about?

A. Chronic inflammatory bowel

B. Hemolytic uremic syndrome

C. Ischemic bowel

D. Osteomyelitis

E. Pancreatitis

10. A 25-year-old man presents to the ED with abdominal cramping, loose stools, and throbbing headache that started 30 minutes after he ate spicy seafood chowder. Vital signs are blood pressure, 150/90; pulse, 120/min; respiration, 24/min; temperature, 38° C. Examination reveals anxiety with facial flushing, dry mucous membranes, and light erythematous papules on the chest. He denies any history of similar reaction. What is the most likely etiology?

A. Anxiety disorder

B. Chowder tainted with an anticholinergic agent

C. Reaction to the spice

D. Scombroid fish poisoning

E. Seafood allergy

11. What is the first step in managing *Clostridium difficile* enterocolitis associated with antibiotic use?

A. Abdominal CT

B. Cessation of all antibiotic therapy

C. Ciprofloxacin

D. Clindamycin

E. Symptomatic relief

12. A 40-year-old factory worker presents to the ED with abdominal cramps and foul, explosive stools. She had been in Leningrad the previous month. Her two sons, one of whom is a chef, live with her but did not go on the trip. Neither of them has similar symptoms. Three days later, the mother's stool examination is found to be positive for *Giardia* sp. What further course of action is appropriate?

A. The mother and the chef son should be empirically treated

B. The mother should be treated

C. The mother should be treated and both sons empirically treated

D. The mother should be treated and both sons tested

E. The mother should be treated and the chef son tested

13. A 3-year-old girl presents with itching around the anus, which is worse at night. Cellophane tape pressed against the perianal area shows parasite ova. What is the appropriate course of action?

A. Arrange follow-up and provide reassurance without specific treatment

B. Treat the 3 year old with mebendazole

C. Treat the 3 year old with mebendazole and test other family members

D. Treat the 3 year old and all family members with mebendazole

E. Refer the 3 year old to an infectious disease specialist

14. Which of the following statements regarding diarrhea in a patient with AIDS is true?

A. All such patients need to be admitted

B. Causative agents are rarely identified

C. Causative agents that are identified are rarely treatable

D. It is usually self-limited

E. Stool and blood cultures should be obtained on all patients

15. What is the most common cause of chronic diarrhea in patients with AIDS?

A. *Cryptosporidium* sp. and *Isospora belli*

B. *E. Coli*

C. *Entamoeba histolytica*

D. *Giardia lamblia*

E. *Salmonella* sp.

16. Which of the following is recommended regarding traveler's diarrhea?

A. Avoid bismuth subsalicylate because it may mask symptoms

B. Do not start antibiotics until a causative agent is identified

C. Eat foods that are freshly prepared and served hot

D. *Salmonella* is the most prevalent organism

E. Start prophylactic antibiotics in all cases

17. Which of the following statements regarding constipation is true?

A. Enemas have no role in the treatment of constipation

B. Fluid and fiber are essential in the treatment of constipation

C. Magnesium salts are safe for long-term use

D. Oral mineral oils are useful and of low risk if aspirated

E. Stool softeners have no potential side effects

18. Which of the following statements is true regarding fecal impaction?

A. Complications are uncommon

B. Hemoccult-positive stool need not be investigated with fecal impaction

C. Manual disimpaction is never indicated in the ED

D. Passage of watery stool excludes the diagnosis

E. Urinary symptoms of frequency and retention are common

# 115 Disorders of the Upper Gastrointestinal Tract

*Elizabeth A. Moy and James K. Bouzoukis*

Select the appropriate letter that correctly answers the question or completes the statement.

1. The classic acid-base and electrolyte abnormality seen with protracted vomiting is:
   A. Hyperchloremic, hyperkalemic metabolic alkalosis
   B. Hyperchloremic, hypokalemic, metabolic acidosis
   C. Hypochloremic, hypokalemic, metabolic alkalosis
   D. Increased anion gap acidosis
   E. Normal anion gap acidosis

2. Dysphagia localized to the neck may be referred only from which level of the esophagus?
   A. Any part
   B. Cervical
   C. Lower third
   D. Middle third
   E. Thoracic inlet

3. A thin, 42-year-old male presents with substernal chest pain that occurs with eating and drinking. It is associated with a retrosternal "sticking sensation," and has progressed over the past 4 months, resulting in a 20-pound weight loss. The most likely cause is:
   A. Achalasia
   B. Carcinoma

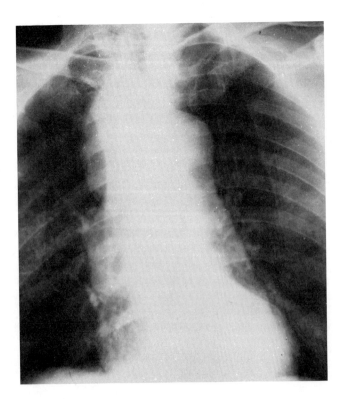

**FIG. 115-1**

C. Esophageal strictures
D. Gastric ulcer
E. Gastroesophageal reflux

4. A 29 year old woman from an inpatient psychiatric facility is transferred to the ED because she states she has swallowed razor blades. She is in no acute distress but does complain of neck pain. A chest x-ray shows a razor in the mid-esophagus. What is the best course of action to remove it?
   A. Administer 0.5 mg of glucagon IV
   B. Endoscopy
   C. Esophagotomy to remove with forceps
   D. Ingestion of effervescent agents (carbonated beverages)
   E. Foley catheter passed into the esophagus, past the razor, then the balloon inflated to pull the razor back out

5. A 50-year-old man with multiple alcohol-related admissions presents with substernal chest pain radiating through to his back. He had several episodes of vomiting before the chest pain started. On physical examination, he is in moderate distress and has decreased breath sounds and epigastric tenderness. Which is the best initial diagnostic study to reveal the diagnosis?
   A. Chest x-ray
   B. CT scan of the thorax/abdomen
   C. Endoscopy
   D. Gastografin swallow
   E. Mediastinoscopy

6. Which of the following findings is most helpful in differentiating esophageal chest pain from that of coronary artery disease?
   A. Pain associated with diaphoresis, pallor, or vomiting
   B. Positional exacerbation
   C. Precipitation of pain with exercise and relief with rest
   D. Radiation of pain into the jaw, shoulders, or arms
   E. Relief of pain with nitroglycerin

7. A 25-year-old male presents with severe intermittent substernal chest pain. It was sudden in onset and occurred while the patient was lying in bed. He describes months of dysphagia with eating and drinking and feels that standing up helps food to pass to his stomach. Physical examination reveals a moderately distressed thin white male, with no abnormal findings. 12-lead ECG is normal, and his chest x-ray is shown (Fig. 115-1). The most likely diagnosis is:
   A. Achalasia
   B. Boerhaave's syndrome
   C. Duodenal ulcer
   D. Gastric ulcer
   E. Gastroesophageal reflux disease

8. Which of the following segments of the upper gastrointestinal tract is correctly matched with the area to which pain is usually referred?
   A. Distal duodenum: midline, low epigastrium
   B. Duodenal bulb: left lower quadrant

C. Gastric pain: jaw, neck

D. Lesser sac penetration: anterior chest

E. Middle duodenum: right lower quadrant

9. Which of the following anti-ulcer medications should not be prescribed for women of childbearing age who are trying to conceive?

A. Antacids

B. Cimetidine (Tagamet)

C. Misoprostol (Cytotec)

D. Omeprazole (Prilosec)

E. Sucralfate (Carafate)

 **116** Disorders of the Liver, Biliary Tract, and Pancreas

*Brent Passarello and James K. Bouzoukis*

Select the appropriate letter that correctly answers the question or completes the statement.

1. In attempting to differentiate patients with cholangitis from patients with cholecystitis, the most helpful clinical marker is:

A. Elevated WBC count

B. Fever

C. Jaundice

D. Murphy's sign

2. What percent of patients that contract hepatitis C go on to develop chronic hepatitis?

A. 10%

B. 25%

C. 50%

D. 75%

3. Sclerosing cholangitis is most commonly associated with what disease?

A. Alcohol-induced cirrhosis

B. Hepatitis B

C. Inflammatory bowel disease

D. Primary biliary cirrhosis

4. Which of the following is true regarding alcoholic liver disease?

A. Compared with viral hepatitis, a relative predominance in elevation of AST compared to ALT is expected

B. Jaundice can usually be detected in patients when their bilirubin level exceeds 1.0 mg/dl

C. Profound elevations in AST and ALT are often seen

D. Steatosis, the most common pathologic change in alcohol-induced liver disease, results from alterations in fatty acid metabolism and, in general, is irreversible

5. Pyogenic liver abscesses are most commonly associated with what disease?

A. Biliary tract obstruction

B. Diverticulitis

C. Inflammatory bowel disease

D. Omphalitis

6. While placing a femoral line in a known intravenous drug abuser, an emergency physician previously immunized against hepatitis B inadvertently receives a needle stick. The physician's preexposure hepatitis panel reveals HBsAg, negative; HBsAb, positive; HBcAb, negative. What does the appropriate treatment to protect against HBV infection include?

A. Administration of both the HB vaccine and hepatitis immunoglobulin (HBIG)

B. Administration of HBIG alone

C. Administration of the hepatitis B vaccine (HB vaccine)

D. No treatment

7. Which of the following etiologic factors has not been incriminated in the development of pancreatic ductal carcinoma?

A. Cigarette smoking

B. Diabetes mellitus

C. High-fat, high-protein diet

D. History of pancreatitis

8. Which of the following organisms is the most common cause of spontaneous bacterial peritonitis (SBP) in a patient with cirrhosis and ascites?

A. *Escherichia coli*

B. *Klebsiella* sp.

C. *Staphylococcus* sp.

D. *Streptococcus pneumoniae*

E. *Streptococcus viridans*

9. A 52-year-old alcoholic with cirrhosis and ascites has had increased confusion and lethargy for 2 days. On physical examination, he is somnolent but arousable and oriented to person with positive asterixis. Abdomen is distended but non-tender. Vital signs are temperature, 99°.8 F; blood pressure, 110/70; and pulse, 96. Laboratory studies reveal a white blood cell count of 9700, blood glucose of 128, and a hemoglobin of 11. The most appropriate therapy at this time would be:

A. IV furosemide

B. Paracentesis of the abdomen

C. Rectal neomycin

D. Transfusion of packed red blood cells

10. Which of the following ancillary tests is the most specific for pancreatic disease?

A. Alkaline phosphatase

B. Amylase

C. Lipase

D. Urinary amylase

11. Which of the following tests would be least helpful in determining the prognosis of a patient with acute pancreatitis?

A. ABG

B. CBC

C. Liver function tests

D. Serum lipase

12. Which of the following statements is true regarding acute cholecystitis?
   A. Acalculous cholecystitis is less common in the elderly and has a relatively chronic clinical course
   B. *E. coli, Klebsiella,* and *Clostridium perfringens* are common causes of emphysematous cholecystitis
   C. Emphysematous cholecystitis is a relatively common variety of cholecystitis that is less common in males
   D. Plain radiographs are valuable in the work-up of cholecystitis because the upper quadrant sentinel loop sign is a common and diagnostic finding

# 117 ▼ Disorders of the Small Intestine

### *Maria C. Vergara and Steven Kushner*

Select the appropriate letter that correctly answers the question or completes the statement.

1. Which of the following is the most likely sequela of gangrenous appendicitis?
   A. Enterocutaneous fistula with sepsis
   B. Localized peritonitis with abscess formation
   C. Perforation followed by septic shock
   D. Pneumoperitoneum with abdominal distension
   E. Small bowel obstruction with ischemia

2. Which of the following statements is true of appendicitis?
   A. Although appendicitis affects people of all ages, the highest incidence is in the fourth and fifth decades of life
   B. Finding an appendicolith on plain film is specific for the disease and indicates the need for immediate surgical intervention
   C. Graded compression ultrasound is an ineffective diagnostic tool to diagnose appendicitis
   D. Pregnant females are more likely to develop appendicitis than are their non-pregnant counterparts
   E. The highest mortality rate is found in the elderly due to delayed diagnosis

3. Which of the following is true about ancillary tests in appendicitis?
   A. A normal white blood cell count excludes the diagnosis of appendicitis
   B. An increase in erythrocyte sedimentation rate and C-reactive protein improves diagnostic accuracy
   C. Confirming radiologic tests are highly recommended for patients with suspected appendicitis
   D. Graded compression ultrasound is an ineffective diagnostic tool to diagnose appendicitis
   E. Sterile pyuria often accompanies appendicitis

4. Which of the following characterizes small bowel obstruction?
   A. As bowel lumen pressure rises, third spacing of fluid occurs secondary to lymphatic stasis and bowel wall edema
   B. Bowel distention stimulates epithelial secretory activity and increases the ability of the bowel to absorb fluid and electrolytes
   C. Even with aggressive treatment, there is little change in the mortality of patients with small bowel obstruction
   D. Peristalsis decreases during early stages of the disease process, increasing fluid accumulation proximal to the site of bowel obstruction
   E. With persistent complete obstruction, increased peristaltic activity occurs in an attempt to overcome the obstruction

5. Which of the following is true regarding small bowel obstruction?
   A. Classic features of small bowel obstruction include abdominal distention and intermittent, severe colicky pain
   B. Early on it is difficult to distinguish small bowel obstruction from adynamic ileus because both result in absent bowel sounds
   C. The absence of rebound tenderness excludes the diagnosis of infarction or strangulation
   D. The presence of large bowel gas on plain film rules out obstruction
   E. Vomiting generally precedes the onset of colicky pain

6. Which of the following most characterizes adynamic ileus?
   A. Adynamic ileus rarely occurs after laparotomy
   B. Amyloidosis is the most common cause of adynamic ileus
   C. Appropriate management is to treat the underlying cause
   D. Hyperkalemia is commonly seen with adynamic ileus
   E. The "coffee bean" sign on abdominal x-ray is characteristic of a segmental ileus

7. How does proximal small bowel obstruction compare with distal small bowel obstruction?
   A. Less likely associated with mild abdominal distention and severe colicky pain
   B. Less likely associated with severe abdominal distention and progressively worsening pain
   C. More likely associated with mild abdominal distention and progressively worsening pain
   D. More likely associated with severe abdominal distention and progressively worsening pain
   E. More likely associated with severe abdominal distention and severe colicky pain

8. Which of the following is true of the radiographic diagnosis of small bowel obstruction?
   A. Abdominal plain films can often distinguish between strangulated and simple small bowel obstruction

B. Abdominal plain films can usually distinguish adynamic ileus from mechanical obstruction

C. Definitive diagnosis of small bowel obstruction by CT scan can be made in more than 80% of cases

D. The "coffee bean" sign is characterized by the presence of a fluid-filled loop of bowel resembling a mass

E. The cause of obstruction is usually demonstrated in plain films

9. Which of the following is appropriate and preferred in the management of small bowel obstruction?

A. Aggressive IV hydration with hypertonic saline

B. Broad-spectrum antibiotics are not necessary in the management of small bowel obstruction

C. Early surgical consultation

D. Immediate surgical intervention

E. IV hydration and use of a long intestinal tube to decompress the bowel

10. Which of the following is true of the pathophysiology of mesenteric ischemia

A. Emboli typically lodge at the origin of the superior mesenteric artery

B. Intestinal infarction secondary to mesenteric venous thrombosis of the portal and superior mesenteric vein junction is common despite patency of the vasa recta

C. Peristalsis slows in response to acute intestinal hypoperfusion decreasing oxygen demand of the bowel

D. The small bowel is extremely sensitive to changes in blood flow, and necrotic changes often occur as soon as 1 hour after the onset of symptoms

E. Vasospasm is responsible for the continued ischemic damage after obstruction has been relieved

11. What is the most common cause of mesenteric ischemia?

A. Atherosclerotic heart disease

B. Hypovolemia

C. Regional splanchnic vasospasm

D. Rheumatic heart disease

E. Sepsis

12. What is true of angiography in mesenteric ischemia?

A. It can distinguish between embolic phenomena and thrombosis

B. It does not permit evaluation of the vascular bed distal to the obstruction

C. It is second to CT scan in diagnosing occlusive mesenteric ischemia

D. Papaverine is a thrombolytic that can be infused through the same catheter used to perform angiography

E. The study can be both diagnostic and therapeutic

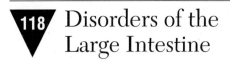

# 118 Disorders of the Large Intestine

### *Tuananh Vu and Steven Kushner*

Select the appropriate letter that correctly answers the question or completes the statement.

1. A 70-year-old man presents to the ED with generalized abdominal pain associated with nausea and vomiting. He also reports fever, malaise, and a history of constipation. Physical examination reveals an obese elderly man in mild distress. Vital signs are temperature, 38.3° C; pulse, 110; blood pressure, 130/80; and respirations, 18. Abdominal examination shows generalized lower abdominal tenderness, distension, and normal active bowel sounds. There is voluntary guarding and rigidity. Rectal examination is heme positive. Obstruction series is negative. Which of the following tests is most useful for diagnosis?

A. Barium enema

B. Colonoscopy

C. Abdominal CT scan

D. Exploratory laparotomy

2. Which of the following fistulas is most commonly seen in diverticulitis?

A. Colorectal

B. Colovaginal

C. Colovesical

D. Rectovaginal

3. Which of the following is not a predisposing factor in the condition depicted in Figure 118-1?

A. Colon cancer

B. Constipation

C. Elderly

D. History of Chagas' disease

E. Psychiatric patient

4. Which of the following is the most common etiology of large bowel obstruction?

A. Adhesions

B. Crohn's disease

C. Diverticulitis

D. Hernias

E. Volvulus

5. Which of the following is the most common age-group seen with intussusception?

A. 3-5 years

B. 5-10 months

C. 6-10 years

D. Newborn-1 month

6. Toxic megacolon is a complication most commonly seen in:

A. Acute amebiasis

B. *C. difficile* colitis

C. Crohn's disease

D. Ulcerative colitis

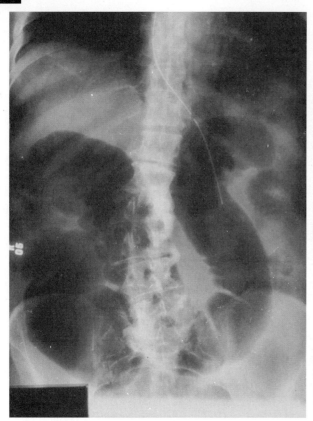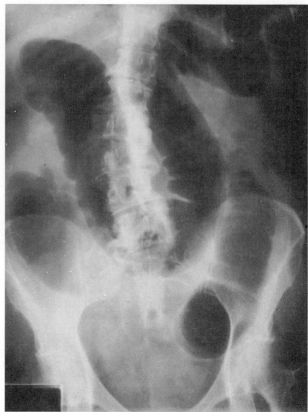

FIG. 118-1

7. Which of the following is the most useful test to diagnose non-fulminating ulcerative colitis?
   A. Abdominal CT scan
   B. Barium enema
   C. Colonoscopy
   D. Plain film radiograph

8. Which part of the GI tract is first involved in ulcerative colitis?
   A. Anus
   B. Cecum
   C. Rectum
   D. Sigmoid colon

9. Marginal "thumbprinting" seen on barium enema is characteristic of which disease?
   A. Crohn's disease
   B. Intussusception
   C. Ischemic colitis
   D. Ulcerative colitis

10. Which of the following symptoms is most commonly seen in ischemic colitis?
    A. Bloody diarrhea
    B. Fever and chills
    C. Nausea and vomiting
    D. Upper abdominal pain

11. A 70-year-old man presents with a 4-day history of diffuse colicky lower abdominal pain, obstipation, and abdominal distension. Physical examination shows an elderly man in severe distress from his abdominal pain. Abdominal examination reveals hypoactive bowel sounds, mild tenderness to palpation, and abdominal distension. Obstruction series shows air-fluid levels in the large bowel. A CBC shows a white blood cell count of 25,000. An electrolyte panel is normal except for a potassium level of 3.0 The urine specific gravity is 1.035. The patient's condition is best managed by:
    A. Administration of broad-spectrum antibiotics
    B. Correction of fluid and electrolyte abnormalities
    C. Exploratory laparotomy with partial bowel resection
    D. Intestinal decompression with nasogastric suction
    E. All of the above

12. The drug of choice for the treatment of fulminating ulcerative colitis in patients who are not already receiving steroids is:
    A. Corticotropin
    B. Cyclosporine
    C. Cytoxan
    D. Methylprednisolone

# 119 ▼ Disorders of the Anorectum

*Henry E. Wang and Howard Rubinstein*

Select the appropriate letter that correctly answers the question or completes the statement.

1. The superior and inferior hemorrhoidal veins drain into which respective systems?
   A. Both drain into the azygous vein
   B. Both drain into the inferior vena cava
   C. Both drain into the portal system
   D. Inferior vena cava and portal system
   E. Portal system and inferior vena cava

2. The superior, middle, and inferior hemorrhoidal arteries arise from which respective systems?
   A. All arise from the internal iliac artery
   B. All arise from the pudendal artery
   C. Aorta, common iliac artery, and pudendal artery
   D. Inferior mesenteric, internal iliac, and pudendal arteries
   E. Internal iliac, pudendal, and inferior mesenteric arteries

3. Which of the following beliefs concerning hemorrhoids is true?
   A. Constipation causes hemorrhoids by direct trauma
   B. Hemorrhoids are rare in pregnant women
   C. Hemorrhoids are varicose veins
   D. Pediatric patients with portal hypertension are not prone to develop hemorrhoids
   E. Portal hypertension in adults does not cause hemorrhoids

4. What is the most common cause of sudden-onset painful rectal bleeding?
   A. Anal fissure
   B. Expanding hemorrhoid
   C. Foreign body
   D. Infectious diarrhea
   E. Rectal prolapse

5. What is the most common location of anal fissures?
   A. Anterior midline
   B. Circumferential
   C. Lateral left
   D. Lateral right
   E. Posterior midline

6. Bacteria that commonly cause anorectal abscesses include the following except:
   A. *Escherichia coli*
   B. *Legionella* sp.
   C. *Proteus* sp.
   D. *Staphylococcus aureus*
   E. *Streptococcus* sp.

7. Anorectal abscesses that can be safely drained in the ED include:
   A. Perianal and horseshoe
   B. Perianal and intersphincteric
   C. Perianal and ischiorectal
   D. Perianal and postanal
   E. Perianal and supralevator

8. What are the components of the WASH regimen for treating anorectal disorders?
   A. Warm water, acetic acid, soap, and hand-washing
   B. Warm water, amoxicillin, soap, and hydrocortisone
   C. Warm water, analgesic agents, stool softeners, high-fiber diet
   D. Warm water, antidepressants, salicylates, and haloperidol
   E. Warm water, atropine, succinylcholine, and heparin

9. Which of the following statements concerning hemorrhoids is true?
   A. Acutely thrombosed external hemorrhoids can be incised and drained in the ED
   B. External hemorrhoids originate below the dentate line and receive blood from the inferior hemorrhoidal plexus
   C. Fourth-degree internal hemorrhoids can be easily reduced in the ED
   D. Internal hemorrhoids originate above the dentate line and receive blood from the inferior hemorrhoidal plexus
   E. Second- and third-degree internal hemorrhoids require surgical reduction

10. The most common cause of pruritus ani is:
    A. Contact dermatitis
    B. Diet
    C. Fecal irritation
    D. Herpes simplex virus
    E. Human papillomavirus

11. All of the following are appropriate techniques for removing rectal foreign bodies except which one?
    A. Administering a light sedative and using manual extraction
    B. Filling of hollow foreign bodies with plaster of Paris and an inset Foley catheter, and applying gentle traction on the catheter
    C. Passing a Foley catheter past the object, inflating the balloon, and applying gentle traction on the catheter
    D. Sending the patient home with stool softeners and a strainer
    E. Using forceps to grasp the foreign body

## 120 Anemia, Polycythemia, and White Blood Cell Disorders

*Michael Baram and Howard Rubinstein*

Select the appropriate letter that correctly answers the question or completes the statement.

1. Which of the following is associated with rapid intravascular red blood cell destruction?
    A. Fevers and mental status changes
    B. Oxidants
    C. Toxins
    D. Transfusions
    E. All of the above

*Match the following anemic states with their corresponding laboratory abnormality*
    A. Combs' positive
    B. Low ferritin with increased total iron binding capacity (TIBC)
    C. Low/normal ferritin and decreased TIBC
    D. Macrocytic anemia
    E. Normal ferritin with normal TIBC

2. Chronic disease          _____
3. Iron deficiency          _____
4. Vitamin B12 deficiency   _____
5. Lead poisoning           _____
6. Transfusion incompatibility _____

7. An elderly woman arrives at the ED with numbness in her hands and feet. Her legs feel very weak, and the emergency physician notes ataxia. Routine CBC shows her to have a hemoglobin and a hematocrit of 10.8 and 31.2, respectively, with a mean corpuscular volume of 112 (normal is <100). Which type of anemia is most likely to be the cause of her symptoms?
    A. Anemia of chronic disease
    B. Folate deficiency
    C. Hemolytic anemia
    D. Iron deficiency
    E. Vitamin B12 deficiency

8. Primary polycythemia, found most commonly in middle-aged or older individuals, usually presents with what symptoms?
    A. Dehydration and rubor
    B. Hematuria and sepsis
    C. Pruritus and jaundice
    D. Syncope and tachycardia
    E. Thrombotic episodes and bleeding

9. With current treatments, survival of chronic myelogenous leukemia is increasing. However, what is considered a poor prognostic indicator of survival?
    A. Anemia
    B. Auer rods
    C. Blast crisis
    D. Pancytopenia
    E. Shift to the right

10. What is the most common malignancy presenting in children younger than 10 years of age?
    A. Acute lymphocytic leukemia
    B. Acute myelogenous leukemia
    C. Chronic lymphocytic leukemia
    D. Chronic myelogenous leukemia

11. In children younger than 2 years of age, what is the lowest WBC level that is highly correlated with bacteremia?
    A. 12,000
    B. 15,000
    C. 18,000
    D. 21,000
    E. 24,000

12. Which of the following would best categorize the laboratory values found in hemolytic anemia?
    A. Decreased haptoglobin, elevated LDH, elevated indirect bilirubin, and decreased reticulocyte count
    B. Decreased haptoglobin, elevated LDH, elevated indirect bilirubin, and elevated reticulocyte count
    C. Elevated haptoglobin, elevated LDH, elevated direct bilirubin, and elevated reticulocyte count
    D. Elevated haptoglobin, elevated LDH, elevated indirect bilirubin, and elevated reticulocyte count

13. Which of the following statements is true concerning emergent anemia?
    A. Folate, B12, TIBC, and reticulocyte count are unaffected by transfusion
    B. Hematocrit may take hours to equilibrate and reflect the degree of blood loss
    C. It is most often caused by hemolytic states
    D. Normal blood pressure and heart rate indicate minimal blood loss
    E. Physical examination is unreliable in assessing emergent anemia

14. Which of the following is the best test to detect a sickle cell vaso-occlusive crisis?
    A. Blood culture
    B. Chest x-ray
    C. Complete blood cell count
    D. Electrolytes
    E. None of the above

## 121 Disorders of Hemostasis

*Brian K. Lentz and George R. Zlupko*

Select the appropriate letter that correctly answers the question or completes the statement.

1. Which of the following statements is true?

A. Epistaxis, menorrhagia, and gastrointestinal bleeding are common presenting signs associated with platelet abnormalities

B. Platelet disorders are less common in women

C. The acute form of idiopathic thrombocytopenic purpura (ITP) is seen primarily in childhood

D. The bleeding time is a test that is independent of the coagulation pathways

E. The platelet count can give a rough estimate of the functional capacity of the platelets

2. The only coagulation protein for which serum levels can be directly measured is:

A. Antihemophilic A factor

B. Fibrinogen

C. Hageman factor

D. Prothrombin

E. Tissue prothrombin

3. Which of the following statements is true of drug-induced thrombocytopenia?

A. After the drug is stopped, improvement occurs slowly over 14-21 days

B. Exchange transfusion is the treatment of choice

C. Implicated drugs, such as quinidine and sulfonamides, are directly toxic to platelets

D. Platelet counts may fall below 10,000/mm$^3$

E. Serious bleeding is seldom associated

4. Which of the following increases bleeding time?

A. Coumadin administration

B. Hemophilia A

C. Hemophilia B (Christmas disease)

D. von Willebrand's disease

5. Which statement is false regarding the use of desmopressin acetate (DDAVP) in the treatment of patients with hemophilia A?

A. Beneficial effects last for only 4-6 hours

B. It is primarily a second-line agent after treatment with danazol fails

C. Its benefits are primarily noted in patients with mild disease

D. The drug is given intravenously in a 0.3 µg/kg/dose

6. Von Willebrand's disease typically exhibits:

A. A decreased factor VIII level

B. A normal bleeding time

C. Disease more severe than hemophilia A

D. Hemarthrosis

E. Thrombocytopenia

7. Which finding is not classically seen in patients with thrombotic thrombocytopenic purpura (TTP)?

A. Acute renal failure

B. Anemia

C. Change in mental status

D. Fever

E. Hepatomegaly

8. An 18-year-old male with a known history of hemophilia A presents as the restrained driver involved in an MVA. The paramedics report that there was moderate front-end damage with spidering of the windshield, and a questionable loss of consciousness as per the patient. In the ED, the primary survey is normal and the neurologic examination is non-focal, but the patient is slow to respond to questions and there is a 2-cm contusion on his mid-forehead. A fingerstick for blood sugar was within normal limits and the patient denies any alcohol or illicit drug use. Which statement best describes the early management and disposition issues of this patient?

A. An emergent CT scan of the head must be ordered. If the CT scan is negative and neurologic status remains stable, the patient may be watched for 4 hours in the ED and discharged.

B. An emergent CT scan of the head should be ordered while prophylactic factor VIII therapy is begun. The patient should be admitted for 24 hours of observation.

C. Emergent coagulation studies and factor VIII:C activity levels must be ordered. A CT scan of the head may be ordered in consultation with a hematologist. If all tests are negative and neurologic status remains stable, the patient may be watched for 4 hours in the ED and discharged.

D. Emergent consultation with a hematologist and neurosurgeon is of paramount importance before any further work-up is done on this patient.

9. In patients with severe von Willebrand's disease, the treatment of choice includes:

A. Cryoprecipitate

B. Desmopressin acetate (DDAVP)

C. Platelet transfusions

D. Ristocetin

E. Vitamin K

10. Hemophilia B is distinguished from hemophilia A by:

A. Clinical presentation of bleeding

B. Factor assay results

C. Genetic pattern of inheritance

D. None of the above

11. How many units of factor VIII:C are assumed in one bag of cryoprecipitate?

A. 1-10 units

B. 11-25 units

C. 26-50 units

D. 80-100 units

E. 125-300 units

12. Which laboratory finding does not support a diagnosis of disseminated intravascular coagulation?

A. High fibrin degradation product level

B. High fibrinogen level

C. Prolonged PT

D. Prolonged PTT

E. Thrombocytopenia

# 122 Oncologic Emergencies

*Jason E. Nace and George R. Zlupko*

Select the appropriate letter that correctly answers the question or completes the statement.

1. Which group of febrile cancer patients is most at risk for serious infection?
   A. It is impossible to differentiate who has infection-induced fever
   B. Patients who have received radiation therapy
   C. Patients with gastrointestinal malignancies
   D. Patients with metastatic disease
   E. The elderly

2. Which is true of infections in patients with cancer?
   A. Incidence of *P. aeruginosa* is on the rise
   B. Lack of physical findings is common
   C. Most bacterial infections are due to gram-positive organisms
   D. Parasitic infections are a common source of infection in patients with solid tumors
   E. *S. epidermidis* is likely a contaminant and seldom pathogenic

3. A 67-year-old man recently diagnosed with lung cancer arrives at the ED with a complaint of shortness of breath and facial and neck swelling that is worse in the morning when he awakens. Which statement regarding this syndrome is true?
   A. Airway obstruction is the usual cause of morbidity in this syndrome
   B. Chest radiograph reveals a mass in approximately 50% of patients
   C. It is a life-threatening emergency
   D. The majority of the cases are caused by thoracic aortic aneurysm
   E. Venous access should be used only when absolutely necessary

4. Which is true about the management of the above condition?
   A. Chemotherapy has little role in treatment
   B. It requires immediate surgical intervention
   C. Overall survival at 1 year is 50%-60%
   D. Prognosis depends on tumor type
   E. Use of diuretics is the treatment of choice

5. Patients with tumor lysis syndrome:
   A. Have a poor prognosis even in the absence of renal failure
   B. Have hyperuricemia, hyperkalemia, hypercalcemia, and hypophosphatemia
   C. Manifest symptoms 7-10 days after receiving chemotherapy
   D. Often have a very high blood lactate dehydrogenase level
   E. Should continue their chemotherapy

6. Which of the following is consistent with hyperviscosity syndrome (HVS)?
   A. Clinical manifestations of HVS become apparent when the serum viscosity is greater than 9-10 times that of water
   B. IgG myeloma has the greatest incidence of dysproteinemias.
   C. Initial therapy should focus on adequate rehydration and diuresis
   D. It is rarely seen with leukemia
   E. Mucosal bleeding is uncommon

7. A 66-year-old man with a 3-year history of metastatic prostate cancer was found by his family to be very lethargic and sleepy. Previously, he had been acting strangely and complaining of nausea, constipation, abdominal pain, and constant thirst. Which of the following statements is most consistent with his diagnosis?
   A. Blood calcium levels >15 mg/dl are necessary for symptoms
   B. ECG shows a prolonged QT interval
   C. Hyperkalemia is also present in 50% of patients
   D. It may be caused by benign conditions such as hyperparathyroidism and Paget's disease
   E. It occurs only with bony metastases

8. Emergency treatment of the above patient includes:
   A. Aggressive saline diuresis along with furosemide 40-80 mg
   B. Calcitonin 3-8 MRC units/kg body weight
   C. Intravenous phosphates
   D. Mithramycin 25 µg/kg every 4 to 5 days
   E. Prednisone 60-80 mg/day

9. A 58-year-old man with a history of Hodgkin's lymphoma presents to the ED ashen and pale, with a clouded sensorium, severe dyspnea, and hypotension. Which of the following statements most likely accompanies this man's clinical condition?
   A. An ECG showing electrical alternans is considered pathognomonic
   B. Imaging studies play no part in the diagnosis of this condition
   C. Long-term prognosis of this condition is excellent
   D. The etiology of this condition is often tumor or radiation fibrosis
   E. True orthopnea and paroxysmal nocturnal dyspnea are common associated features

10. Which is true concerning cerebral herniation?
    A. Abscesses and metastases usually require surgical management
    B. Central herniation usually gives focal neurologic signs
    C. Mannitol and dexamethasone are generally not recommended in managing these patients
    D. Tonsillar herniation results in rapidly decreasing level of consciousness, occipital headache, and vomiting
    E. Uncal herniation usually results in slowly decreasing level of consciousness, small reactive pupils, and Cheyne-Stokes respirations

11. Which is true with regard to epidural spinal cord compression?
    A. After steroids, the next step in treatment is usually surgery
    B. Back pain, although considered to be a common complaint, occurs in only 50% of patients
    C. CT scans are proven diagnostically superior to myelograms in evaluating these patients
    D. Most cases occur in the lumbosacral spine
    E. Plain films will show evidence of tumor in the vertebral body in 90% of patients with vertebral metastases

12. Which is true concerning a patient with head and neck cancer who presents with fever, headache, and altered mental status?
    A. Absence of WBCs in the CSF is sufficient reason to rule out meningitis
    B. Brain abscess can account for more than half of the CNS infections in cancer patients
    C. Encephalitis is rare in cancer patients and is most often caused by herpes zoster and *T. gondii*
    D. Infections with *Haemophilus influenzae* and *Neisseria meningitidis* are quite common and require the appropriate antibiotics
    E. The first step is always a lumbar puncture

## SECTION 6  NEUROLOGIC DISORDERS

 **123** Coma

*Lars Blomberg*

Select the appropriate letter that correctly answers the question or completes the statement.

1. Which of the following is intact in an awake and aware patient with normal cranial nerve test results?
   A. Ascending reticular activating system
   B. Cerebellum
   C. Cerebral hemispheres
   D. Pons and midbrain

2. A 59-year-old alcoholic is brought to the ED in a comatose state. His pupils are midposition and unreactive, reflecting which of the following conditions?
   A. Hyperosmolar state
   B. Hypocalcemia
   C. Hyponatremia
   D. Midbrain hemorrhage

3. Cold caloric testing by instilling ice water into a patient's left ear stimulates the patient to deviate his eyes to the left, where they remain. Which of the following diagnoses is most likely?
   A. Alert wakefulness
   B. Bilateral cerebral hemisphere dysfunction

C. Right medial longitudinal fasciculus dysfunction
D. Right oculomotor nerve dysfunction

4. A 25-year-old woman with normal vital signs has a 6-hour history of unresponsiveness. She is unresponsive to deep pain and resists eye opening, but snaps her eyes shut when the lids are released. Cold-water caloric testing induces bilateral nystagmus. Which of the following is the most likely diagnosis?
   A. Akinetic mutism
   B. Catatonia
   C. Conversion disorder
   D. Locked-in syndrome

5. A 27-year-old white male is brought to the ED. He is conscious but exhibits no spontaneous activity. He will awaken if stimulated, although he has very little verbal or motor activity. What does this description best describe?
   A. Coma
   B. Delirium
   C. Obtundation
   D. Stupor

6. Which of the following is the most likely cause of coma in a patient presenting to the ED whose history does not suggest an obvious cause?
   A. Brain stem infarct
   B. Cerebellar hemorrhage
   C. Intracerebral hemorrhage
   D. Pontine hemorrhage

7. A 49-year-old female is brought to the ED by EMS. She does not open her eyes, nor does she make any sound. Her Glasgow Coma Scale score is calculated to be 5. Which of the following best describes her motor response?
   A. Decerebrate posturing
   B. Decorticate posturing
   C. Localizes noxious stimuli
   D. Moves body but does not localize or remove noxious stimuli

8. Which of the following cause tachypnea through direct CNS effects?
   A. Alcohol intoxication
   B. Diabetic hyperosmolar coma
   C. Hepatic coma
   D. Uremia

9. Normal oculocephalic testing (doll's eyes) requires all of the following to be intact except which one?
   A. CN II
   B. CN III
   C. CN VI
   D. Medial longitudinal fasciculus

10. The empiric use of which of the following drugs is not suggested for the comatose patient?
    A. Glucose
    B. Flumazenil
    C. Naloxone
    D. Thiamine

# 124 ▼ Headache

*Lars Blomberg*

Select the appropriate letter that correctly answers the question or completes the statement.

1. All of the following are pathologic conditions that affect the pain-sensitive structures of the head and neck except which one?
   A. Compression
   B. Inflammation
   C. Tension/traction
   D. Vascular

2. An otherwise healthy 62-year-old woman comes to the ED complaining of left-sided headache, tenderness, and "blurry vision." Which of the following laboratory tests would be most useful?
   A. Arterial blood gases
   B. Complete blood cell count
   C. Erythrocyte sedimentation rate
   D. Serum glucose
   E. None of the above

3. A 55-year-old woman without previous history of headache complains of boring left eye pain, nausea, and decreased vision. On examination, one pupil is midpoint with a hazy cornea. Which of the following is the most likely diagnosis?
   A. Acute glaucoma
   B. Cluster headache
   C. Maxillary sinusitis
   D. Trigeminal neuralgia

4. Which of the following best characterizes ophthalmoplegic migraine?
   A. Extreme pain over involved eye
   B. Middle-aged adult
   C. Miosis, ptosis, and esotropia
   D. Third motor nerve palsy
   E. All of the above

5. All of the following are characteristic of common migraine except which one?
   A. Homonymous hemianopsia
   B. Nausea and vomiting
   C. Photophobia
   D. Sonophobia

6. Which of the following best characterizes cluster headache?
   A. Awakens patient after 2-3 hours of sleep with characteristic prodrome
   B. Has bilateral vascular-type pain
   C. Is triggered by histamine-containing compounds
   D. Occurs predominantly in females
   E. All of the above

7. Which of the following treatment modalities is specific for cluster headaches?

   A. Amitriptyline
   B. Chlorpromazine
   C. Cocaine and oxygen
   D. Ergotamine/belladonna/phenobarbital
   E. None of the above

8. Which of the following is most characteristic of pseudotumor cerebri?
   A. Papilledema
   B. Photophobia
   C. Thin white male
   D. Unilateral throbbing headache
   E. All of the above

9. A 35-year-old man arrives at the ED with "the worst ever" headache. Physical examination reveals diaphoresis, tachypnea, tachycardia, photophobia, and a third nerve palsy. Which of the following is the most likely diagnosis?
   A. Cluster headache
   B. Subarachnoid hemorrhage
   C. Subdural hematoma
   D. Trigeminal neuralgia

10. A 24-year-old white female and her two children present to the emergency department with dizziness, malaise, and worsening headache. Which of the following is the most appropriate diagnostic test?
    A. ABG with COOX
    B. Cranial CT
    C. Lumbar puncture
    D. RMSF titers

11. Pregnancy is an absolute contraindication for migraine treatment with which of the following?
    A. Ergotamine preparations
    B. Meperidine
    C. Naproxen
    D. Prochlorperazine
    E. All are contraindicated

# 125 ▼ Organic Brain Syndrome

*Lars Blomberg*

Select the appropriate letter that correctly answers the question or completes the statement.

1. The majority of cases of delirium are caused by which of the following entities?
   A. Drug use
   B. Electrolyte disturbance
   C. Hepatic failure
   D. Hypoxia
   E. None of the above

2. All of the following would be expected in a delirious patient except which one?
   A. Disorientation
   B. Fluctuation in symptoms

C. Global cognitive impairment

D. Rapid onset of symptoms

E. All are usually present

3. A 21-year-old steroid-dependent, asthmatic woman arrives at the ED acutely delusional. Which of the following would most likely be diagnostic in this setting?

A. Complete blood cell count

B. Determination of anion gap

C. Lumbar puncture

D. Pulse oximetry

4. A tremulous 21-year-old man is agitated, occasionally disoriented and incoherent, and complaining occasionally of "things" in the room with him. His vital signs show mild fever and tachycardia. Which of the following diagnoses is most consistent with this situation?

A. Acute psychosis

B. Delirium

C. Mania

D. Paranoia

5. A gradually progressive deterioration of cognitive function caused by metabolic abnormalities and anomalous drug reactions best describes which of the following diagnoses?

A. Acute psychosis

B. Delirium

C. Dementia

D. Pseudodementia

6. In dementia, all of the following are present except which one?

A. Anxiety, depression, and insomnia

B. Asterixis and myoclonus

C. Clear sensorium

D. Normal electroencephalogram

E. Normal vital signs

7. In cases of hyperactive delirium, which of the following classes of drugs is the preferred treatment?

A. Benzodiazepines

B. Butyrophenones

C. Narcotics

D. Phenothiazines

8. A 72-year-old male presents with symptoms consistent with a progressive dementia. Which of the following suggests a cortical rather than subcortical etiology?

A. Anomia

B. Ataxic gait

C. Choreic movements

D. Dysarthric speech

9. A 39-year-old homeless man is brought to the ED with acute delirium, ataxia ,and nystagmus. The patient was given 1 ampule of D50 before arrival and his symptoms appear to be worsening. He is immediately given 100 mg of thiamine; what other electrolyte abnormality needs to be emergently corrected in the ED?

A. Hypocalcemia

B. Hypokalemia

C. Hypomagnesemia

D. Hyponatremia

10. What percentage of all chronic dementias are reversible?

A. 10%

B. 20%

C. 30%

D. 40 %

E. 50%

11. A 55-year old-woman presents to the ED with progressive dementia, loss of balance, and urinary incontinence. Which of the following heads the list of differential diagnoses?

A. Alzheimer's disease

B. Normal pressure hydrocephalus

C. Pick's disease

D. Slow virus infection

E. Subcortical dementia

 **126** Seizures

*Lars Blomberg*

Select the appropriate letter that correctly answers the question or completes the statement.

1. Which of the following best characterizes a simple febrile seizure?

A. No focal findings

B. Most common between 4 months and 6 years of age

C. Often occur in series

D. Rare to see familial incidence

E. None of the above

2. Which of the following seizure types has little or no alteration of consciousness?

A. Absence (petit mal)

B. Complex partial

C. Psychomotor (temporal lobe)

D. Simple partial

E. All alter consciousness

3. A 2-day-old white female is brought to the ED following a documented 5-minute seizure. She is afebrile. What is the most likely etiology?

A. Drug withdrawal

B. Hypoglycemia

C. Hypoxic-ischemic encephalopathy

D. Infection

4. Which of the following metabolic abnormalities does not commonly cause seizures?

A. Hypercalcemia

B. Hypernatremia

C. Hypocalcemia

D. Hyponatremia

5. What is the most common cause of seizures in the elderly?

A. Arteriovenous malformations

B. CNS neoplasms

C. Stroke

D. Vasculitis

6. Which of the following is not a typical characteristic of pseudoseizures?
   A. Absence of acidemia
   B. Multiple patterns of seizures
   C. Observed post-ictal period
   D. Prolonged seizure activity
   E. All of the above are characteristics
7. An 18-year-old black female presents after a first-time seizure lasting 1 minute. She is afebrile with no persistent focal neurologic deficits. Which of the following diagnostic tests should always be performed?
   A. Blood glucose
   B. CBC
   C. Lumbar puncture
   D. Toxicology screen
8. A 40-year-old male presents to the ED in status epilepticus, presumed secondary to alcohol withdrawal. Which of the following is recommended for initial treatment?
   A. Diazepam
   B. Lorazepam
   C. Midazolam
   D. Phenytoin
9. Anticonvulsant therapy with which of the following drugs may result in aplastic anemia?
   A. Carbamazepine
   B. Phenobarbital
   C. Phenytoin
   D. Valproic acid
   E. All of the above

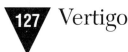

# 127  Vertigo

### Lars Blomberg

Select the appropriate letter that correctly answers the question or completes the statement.
1. A 50-year-old man has sudden, severe vertigo with nausea and vomiting. History and physical examination disclose a low-pitched tinnitus and decreased hearing in his left ear. He states that this has happened before. Which of the following is the most likely diagnosis?
   A. Acoustic neuroma
   B. Ménière's disease
   C. Vertebrobasilar insufficiency
   D. Vestibular neuronitis
2. Which of the following tests screens for conductive hearing loss?
   A. Audiology
   B. Electronystagmography
   C. Rinne test
   D. Weber test
3. A 65-year-old man has nausea, vomiting, and nystagmus. Physical examination discloses left-sided ptosis, miosis, and decreased sensation on the right side of the body

and left side of the face. Which of the following is the most likely diagnosis?
   A. Eaton-Lambert syndrome
   B. Multiple sclerosis
   C. Subclavian steal syndrome
   D. Wallenberg syndrome
4. The presence of true vertigo implies disturbances in which of the following?
   A. Semicircular canals, posterior columns, and eye muscles
   B. Semicircular canals, utricle, and eighth cranial nerve
   C. Tendons, muscles, joints, and posterior columns
   D. Visual system
5. Which of the following drugs is considered extremely effective in quickly stopping peripheral vertigo?
   A. Diazepam
   B. Diphenhydramine
   C. Meclizine hydrochloride
   D. Promethazine
   E. Scopolamine
6. Bilateral internuclear ophthalmoplegia is virtually pathognomonic of what condition?
   A. Cerebellar hemorrhage
   B. Multiple sclerosis
   C. Perilymphatic fistula
   D. Vertebrobasilar insufficiency
7. A 50-year-old female presents with worsening vertigo, nystagmus, and a decreased corneal reflex on the left. Which radiographic study would be most helpful to determine the cause of this patient's symptoms?
   A. Angiography
   B. Audiology
   C. MRI
   D. Uninfused cranial CT
8. A 27-year-old male presents to the ED with sudden onset of severe vertigo and horizontal nystagmus. His symptoms are not positional, nor does he have any associated hearing loss. Which of the following is the most likely diagnosis?
   A. Benign positional vertigo
   B. Labyrinthitis
   C. Ménière's disease
   D. Vestibular neuronitis

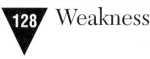

# 128  Weakness

### Greg Harders

Select the appropriate letter that correctly answers the question or completes the statement.
1. A 27-year-old man has noted "weakness" in his legs during his usual bicycle ride over the past 2 days. His physical examination reveals symmetrically diminished deep tendon reflexes in the lower extremities. Which of the following is the most likely diagnosis?

A. Botulism
B. Early myasthenia gravis
C. Eaton-Lambert syndrome
D. Guillain-Barré syndrome

2. Which of the following tests can be most helpful in the initial diagnosis of myasthenia gravis?
A. Atropine
B. Electrocardiogram
C. Ice pack
D. Serologic ELISA

3. Eaton-Lambert syndrome is generally associated with which of the following etiologies?
A. Adherent gravid tick
B. Carcinoma of the lung
C. Erythema chronicum migrans
D. Tick-borne spirochetes

4. All of the following cranial nerves can be affected by Lyme disease except which one?
A. VI
B. VII
C. VIII
D. XI

5. Which of the following is a characteristic of Guillain-Barré syndrome?
A. Asymmetric leg weakness
B. CSF cell count <10/ml (all mononuclear)
C. Decreased CSF protein <400 mg/L
D. Fever
E. Hyperreflexia

6. Which of the following statements about myasthenia gravis is true?
A. Cholinergic crisis is secondary to under-treatment with acetylcholine inhibitors
B. Dysarthria and dysphagia rarely occur
C. Edrophonium IV will improve patients with myasthenic crisis
D. Initial symptoms often involve upper extremity weakness

7. Which of the following statements best characterizes infant botulism?
A. Diarrhea is common
B. Using antitoxin has good results
C. Breast-feeding is less risky
D. Infant has normal mental status with a feeble cry
E. All of the above

8. A 38-year-old male presents approximately 2 hours after eating clams. He is complaining of weakness, respiratory difficulty, and paresthesias. Which of the following statements is true?
A. Atropine administration will reverse the neurotoxin
B. IV antibiotics will likely cause a Jarisch-Herxheimer reaction
C. Treatment is supportive with airway management
D. If the patient's condition is unstable, antitoxin administration is required

9. Which is the most commonly seen electrolyte abnormality in patients with generalized weakness?
A. Calcium

B. Magnesium
C. Potassium
D. Sodium

10. Which of the following is not characteristic of tick paralysis?
A. Ascending paralysis mimicking Guillain-Barré syndrome
B. Fever
C. Limited sensory involvement
D. Rapid recovery with tick removal
E. All of the above are characteristic

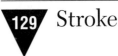

# 129 Stroke

### *Greg Harders*

Select the appropriate letter that correctly answers the question or completes the statement.

1. Which of the following is related to brain dysfunction during stroke?
A. Decreased intracellular calcium
B. Decreased lactate
C. Elevated ATP levels
D. Elevated blood glucose

2. Contralateral paralysis that is more severe in the lower limb than the upper limb is characteristic of a stroke in the distribution of which of the following?
A. Anterior cerebral artery
B. Middle cerebral artery
C. Posterior cerebral artery
D. Vertebrobasilar artery system

3. Lacunar strokes account for what percentage of all strokes?
A. <1%
B. 10%-20%
C. 50%
D. 80%
E. >90%

4. Discovery of a silent myocardial infarction in a stroke victim makes which of the following etiologic groups more likely as a cause for the neurologic deficits?
A. Embolic
B. Hemorrhagic
C. Lacunar
D. Thrombotic
E. None of the above

5. Which of the following statements is true of transient ischemic attacks?
A. An infarct distribution that is different from those seen on CT or MRI scanning may be seen
B. Arterial disease is routinely seen in carotid arterial distribution
C. In 1 month, 90% will have a stroke
D. No infarct is demonstrable by angiography or radiologic scanning

6. Decreased level of consciousness immediately following the onset of an initial ischemic stroke would be caused by which of the following?
    A. Brain stem involvement
    B. Cerebral edema
    C. Dominant hemisphere involvement
    D. Non–stroke-related factors exclusively
    E. None of the above

7. A pure motor deficit from a lacunar stroke can be differentiated from a sensory motor middle cerebral artery deficit by testing for which of the following?
    A. Asymmetric sensation to pain and light touch
    B. Babinski's sign
    C. Graphesthesia
    D. Pronator drift

8. Which of the following is true of a hemorrhagic transformation of an ischemic infarction?
    A. Is heralded by a severe headache
    B. Is not evident radiographically
    C. Occurs acutely most of the time
    D. Occurs for unknown reasons

9. Which of the following is true regarding an arteriovenous malformation that bleeds, causing a subarachnoid hemorrhage?
    A. Becomes symptomatic before the acute hemorrhage
    B. Is more disruptive to cerebral function than a hypertensive bleed
    C. May occur anywhere in the brain
    D. Occurs primarily in the elderly

10. Which of the following is the most important prognostic factor regarding an individual subarachnoid hemorrhage patient?
    A. Age
    B. Clinical condition at time of arrival
    C. Preexisting hypertension
    D. Size of the hemorrhage on CT scan

11. A 40-year-old man has the sudden onset of the worst headache of his life. He is alert without focal neurologic deficits. His CT scan is negative for a bleed. What is the next step in his care?
    A. Careful discharge instructions and reevaluation in 24 hours
    B. Lumbar puncture
    C. MRI
    D. Repeat CT scan in 48 hours

12. Which of the following best describes the surgical management of intracerebral hemorrhage?
    A. Beneficial in most cases
    B. More beneficial than treating any degree of hypertension acutely
    C. Not of benefit to patients with medium to large-sized lobar hemorrhages, despite progressive neurologic deterioration
    D. Recommended in patients with cerebellar hemorrhage

13. A 35-year-old woman has severe headache, meningismus, and altered level of consciousness. Her temperature is 100° F orally (37.8° C). Her condition appears to be deteriorating. Which of the following is the proper order of care?
    A. An immediate lumbar puncture followed by intravenous antibiotics if leukocytosis is present
    B. Intravenous antibiotics followed by CT scanning and then lumbar puncture
    C. Parenteral analgesia with reevaluation in 1 hour
    D. Prompt CT, then lumbar puncture and antibiotics if leukocytosis is present

14. Which of the following is a risk factor for strokes in young adults?
    A. Blood dyscrasias
    B. Cocaine
    C. Pregnancy
    D. All of the above
    E. None of the above

15. All of the following risk factors are classically characteristic of an ischemic stroke except which one?
    A. Aneurysmal disease
    B. History of valvular disease
    C. Hypercoagulable states
    D. Recent myocardial infarction

16. All the following tests assess cerebellar function except which one?
    A. Finger to nose
    B. Gait
    C. Heel to shin
    D. Pronator drift

# 130 Meningitis, Encephalitis, and Central Nervous System Abscess

### Greg Harders

Select the appropriate letter that correctly answers the question or completes the statement.

1. A 48-year-old man comes to the ED with a fever of 102° F and cephalgia. Which of the following is more consistent with meningitis than with brain abscess?
    A. Abnormalities of brain CT scan
    B. Focal neurologic signs
    C. Kernig's sign
    D. Papilledema
    E. Symptoms progressive over 2 weeks

2. A 21-year-old woman has a 16-hour history of severe headache. On examination, the patient's vital signs are temperature, 103° F; blood pressure, 113/70; pulse, 96; and respirations, 18. The fundi are not visible because of roving eye movements; mental status is profoundly depressed, and respiratory effort is adequate. Which of the following is the next most appropriate step?
    A. Administer antibiotics
    B. Obtain CBC

C. Order CT scan of brain

D. Perform lumbar puncture

3. A lumbar puncture is performed on a patient in the left lateral decubitus position. The patient has no significant past medical history. Which of the following results is considered normal?

A. CSF to serum glucose ratio of 0.4 to 1

B. CSF opening pressure of 240 mm $H_2O$

C. CSF PMN count of 2/mm$^3$

D. CSF protein level of 40 mg/dl

E. CSF WBC count of 8/mm$^3$

4. At what CSF cell count will clinically detectable changes in CSF clarity begin to be seen?

A. 10 cells/mm$^3$

B. 50 cells/mm$^3$

C. 150 cells/mm$^3$

D. 200 cells/mm$^3$

E. 350 cells/mm$^3$

5. In interpreting CSF, which of the following statements is true?

A. India ink stain is extremely sensitive and specific for cryptococcal disease

B. In a traumatic tap, the ratio of RBCs to WBCs is approximately 700:1 in a patient with normal peripheral erythrocyte and leukocyte counts

C. Pretreatment with antibiotics substantially decreases the CSF leukocyte count

D. Pretreatment with antibiotics may cause gram-negative bacteria to be identified as gram-positive bacteria

6. What is the recommended treatment in a 55-year-old otherwise healthy adult with suspected bacterial meningitis?

A. Ampicillin

B. Cefazolin

C. Cefotaxime

D. Nafcillin

E. Penicillin G

7. Which of the following is false regarding the use of rifampin in chemoprophylaxis of contacts with patients who have confirmed meningococcal meningitis?

A. Eradicates the organism from the nasopharynx

B. Is ineffective in invasive meningococcal disease

C. Is recommended for household contacts of the patient

D. Is routinely recommended for health care workers who treated the patient before identification of meningococcus

8. The Waterhouse-Friderichsen syndrome is associated with which type of meningitis?

A. Fungal

B. *Haemophilus influenzae*

C. Meningococcal

D. Pneumococcal

E. Tuberculous

9. What is the recommended protocol for a severely ill patient with a high suspicion of bacterial meningitis?

A. Cranial CT, then lumbar puncture followed by IV antibiotics

B. Empiric antibiotics; "too sick to tap"

C. Immediate lumbar puncture then IV antibiotic

D. IV antibiotics then cranial CT and admission

E. None of the above

10. All of the following are characteristics of xanthochromia except which one?

A. Develops within 2 hours

B. Is sometimes seen in normal CSF

C. Lasts up to 30 days

D. Is suggestive of SAH

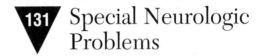

# 131 ▼ Special Neurologic Problems

### *Greg Harders*

Select the appropriate letter that correctly answers the question or completes the statement.

1. A 24-year-old male has a 5-day history of lower leg weakness. The weakness has become much more severe, and he now has weakness of the hips. His legs ache and "feel sort of numb," but there are no objective sensory findings. Lower extremity deep tendon reflexes are markedly diminished. He is afebrile and without meningeal signs. Admission is arranged. Based on the above clinical findings, what inpatient treatment is anticipated?

A. Laminectomy

B. Plasmapheresis

C. Therapeutic lumbar puncture

D. Thymectomy

E. Ventriculoperitoneal shunting

2. Which of the following is inconsistent with a diagnosis of Bell's palsy?

A. Gaze paralysis

B. Hyperacusis

C. Loss of taste

D. Loss of tears

E. Subjective facial numbness

3. Which of the following should be suspected in a patient with bilateral Bell's palsy?

A. Embolic lesion

B. Mercury poisoning

C. Sarcoidosis

D. Syphilis

E. Tuberculosis

4. In considering treatment for varicella zoster virus neuralgia, which of the following statements is true?
    A. Even in patients with more than one dermatome involved, IV acyclovir is rarely indicated
    B. Involvement of the bridge of the nose is a marker for potential corneal involvement
    C. The combination of prednisone and acyclovir has proven effective in decreasing the incidence of postherpetic neuralgia
    D. The incidence of postherpetic neuralgia in patients older than 70 years of age at 1 month following herpes zoster infection is approximately 75%
    E. Treatment for early herpes zoster (within 72 hours of onset of symptoms) with intravenous acyclovir is much more effective in decreasing pain and increasing healing than treatment with oral acyclovir

5. Which of the following is least helpful in distinguishing psychogenic from organic disease?
    A. Lack of response to pin prick
    B. Optokinetic nystagmus
    C. Presence of Bell's phenomenon
    D. Sensation loss at joint line
    E. Vibratory sense only on one side of skull

6. Patients who have multiple sclerosis may have optic neuritis, which may be confused with papilledema. Which of the following is more typical of optic neuritis than papilledema?
    A. Bilateral involvement
    B. Intact vision
    C. Loss of venous pulsations
    D. Pain

7. A 19-year-old woman has a 6-week history of increasing headache that is worse in the morning and increases with coughing. CT of the head is negative. Lumbar puncture opening pressure is 320 with 0 white cells, 2 red cells, glucose of 60 and protein of 35. What would be the appropriate initial treatment?
    A. Carbamazepine
    B. Cyclic antidepressant
    C. Plasmapheresis
    D. Therapeutic lumbar puncture
    E. Ventriculoperitoneal shunting

8. A 70-year-old woman presents to the ED with tinnitus and vertigo. Evaluation of the tympanic membrane reveals herpetic vesicles. What is the likely diagnosis?
    A. Herpes simplex I
    B. Lyme neuroborreliosis
    C. Ménière's disease
    D. Varicella

9. Typical findings in patients with psychogenic coma include all of the following except which one?
    A. Bell's phenomenon (upward deviation of the eyes)
    B. Fast and slow nystagmus with cold caloric testing
    C. Response to "nasal tickle"
    D. Slow eyelid closure after opening

10. A patient presents with several old healing burns in the upper extremities. Physical examination reveals dimin-ished pain and temperature sensation in a "cape-like" distribution. What are these findings most consistent with?
    A. Amyotrophic lateral sclerosis
    B. Pseudotumor cerebri
    C. Parkinson syndrome
    D. Syringomyelia

# 132  Urologic Emergencies

### Greg Harders

Select the appropriate letter that correctly answers the question or completes the statement.

1. A 26-year-old woman has had dysuria for 1 week. She denies any history of fever, nausea, vomiting, or back pain. She does admit to having a new sexual partner over the past month. Physical examination reveals a small amount of whitish discharge from the cervical os but is otherwise normal. Urinalysis shows 10 WBCs, 0 RBCs, no epithelial cells, and no bacteria. Which of the following is the most likely diagnosis?
    A. Cystitis secondary to *E. coli* infection
    B. Pyelonephritis secondary to *E. coli* infection
    C. Urethritis secondary to *Chlamydia* infection
    D. Vaginitis secondary to *Candida* infection

2. A urine culture is recommended in all of the following patients except which one?
    A. Child with positive urinalysis
    B. Neonate with negative urinalysis
    C. Young adult female with classic UTI symptoms and positive urinalysis
    D. Young adult male with classic UTI symptoms and positive urinalysis

3. A 50-year-old man complains of shaking chills, generalized malaise, perineal pain, and urinary urgency. Which of the following statements is true?
    A. The prostate should be massaged
    B. Trimethoprim sulfamethoxazole is adequate treatment
    C. Urethral catheterization is recommended if urinary retention is present
    D. Urine culture is usually negative

4. Which of the following statements is true regarding an elderly nursing home patient with an indwelling Foley catheter?
    A. Bacteriuria is uncommon
    B. If fever develops, outpatient therapy with oral antibiotics is recommended
    C. If fever develops, the catheter must be changed
    D. Long-term antibiotic prophylaxis is of proven benefit

5. Which of the following statements is true regarding testicular torsion?
   A. Loss of the cremasteric reflex is common with torsion
   B. Manual detorsion is curative if successful
   C. Nuclear imaging should be obtained before calling a urologist
   D. Prehn's sign is reliable in differentiating torsion from epididymitis
6. All of the following are indications for admission in a 6-year-old girl with UTI except which one?
   A. Elevated BUN
   B. Fever
   C. Hypertension
   D. Persistent vomiting
7. During pregnancy, which of the following statements is true?
   A. Asymptomatic bacteriuria does not affect the fetus
   B. Asymptomatic bacteriuria may be treated with a 3-day course of antibiotic
   C. There is an increased risk of pyelonephritis if diagnosed with UTI
   D. Trimethoprim-sulfamethoxazole is the agent of choice in treatment of UTI
8. Urine cultures are often obtained when urinary tract infection is suspected. In regard to the urine culture, which of the following statements is true?
   A. Bag specimen is recommended in infants less than 1 year old
   B. Catheterization is recommended in adolescent males
   C. There is often poor correlation between in vitro testing and clinical response
   D. They should be obtained on all patients
9. Acute urinary retention may be caused by all of the following except which one?
   A. Anticholinergic medication
   B. Benign prostatic hypertrophy
   C. Multiple sclerosis
   D. Seizure
   E. Sympathomimetic agents
10. A patient has classic signs of renal colic, and an IVP is ordered. Which of the following statements is not true?
    A. Columnization is often present
    B. Delayed nephrogram is the most reliable sign of obstruction
    C. Renal insufficiency is a contraindication to IVP dye
    D. Repeat films should be obtained every 10 minutes until the study is complete
11. All of the following are features of nephrolithiasis except which one?
    A. Females more commonly affected
    B. May present without hematuria
    C. Recurrence is common
    D. Stones are usually radiopaque
12. Which of the following bacteria are most commonly associated with orchitis?
    A. *Chlamydia* and gonococci
    B. *Klebsiella, E. coli,* and *Pseudomonas*

C. Mumps
D. *Staphylococcus* and *Streptococcus*
13. Which of the following is not a clinical feature of epididymitis?
    A. Gradual onset of symptoms
    B. May have urethral discharge
    C. No associated fever
    D. Pain in the scrotum or groin

---

 ## Renal Function Evaluation and the Approach to the Patient With Acute Renal Failure

*Greg Harders*

Select the appropriate letter that correctly answers the question or completes the statement.

1. A 10-year-old boy recently treated for streptococcal pharyngitis shows evidence of acute renal failure. All of the following may be present except which one?
   A. Edema
   B. Hematuria
   C. Hypertension
   D. Proteinuria
   E. Renal tubular epithelial cells
2. Acute tubular necrosis may be caused by which one of the following?
   A. Henoch-Schönlein purpura
   B. Nonketotic hyperosmolar coma
   C. Prostatitis
   D. Scleroderma
3. Which of the following is the most reliable test in suspected cases of rhabdomyolysis?
   A. Creatine phosphokinase
   B. Low BUN-to-creatinine ratio
   C. Potassium
   D. Urine dip stick
4. A patient who sustained a severe crush injury has evidence of rhabdomyolysis. Which of the following is the least effective in preventing acute renal failure?
   A. Alkalization of urine
   B. Fluid volume repletion
   C. Furosemide
   D. Mannitol
5. A patient is diagnosed with acute renal failure secondary to obstruction. It is suspected that the obstruction has been present for 1 week but has now been corrected. Which of the following statements is correct?
   A. A delay in diagnosis for a few days is acceptable
   B. Full renal recovery will never be possible
   C. Serum creatinine should return to baseline within 24 hours
   D. Ultrasound is only 60% sensitive in detecting obstruction

6. All of the following are indications for dialysis in acute renal failure except which one?
   A. BUN greater than 100 mg/dl
   B. Creatinine greater than 5 mg/dl
   C. Life-threatening hyperkalemia
   D. Intractable volume overload

7. Urinalysis usually reveals red cell casts in which of the following conditions?
   A. Acute tubular necrosis
   B. Glomerulonephritis
   C. Nephrotic syndrome
   D. Prerenal azotemia

8. A 55-year-old woman arrives at the ED with urinary frequency and dysuria. Urinalysis reveals 100 RBCs and no WBCs. Which of the following tests should be obtained?
   A. Coagulation studies
   B. Intravenous pyelogram
   C. Platelet count
   D. Urine culture

9. Which of the following factors is most suggestive of a renal source of hematuria?
   A. Fractional excretion of sodium less than 1%
   B. History of rifampin use within 1 week
   C. Red cell casts
   D. Waxy (hyaline) casts

10. A 38-year-old patient on long-term NSAID therapy presents with weakness. Which of the following findings is not consistent with the diagnosis of acute interstitial nephritis?
    A. Eosinophilia
    B. Fever
    C. Jaundice
    D. Rash

11. Which of the following characteristic electrolyte changes is not expected in patients with end-stage renal disease?
    A. Hyperkalemia
    B. Hyperphosphatemia
    C. Hypocalcemia
    D. Hypomagnesemia

---

## 134 ▼ Chronic Renal Failure and Dialysis

*Greg Harders*

Select the appropriate letter that correctly answers the question or completes the statement.

1. A 72-year-old man with a history of chronic renal failure has a sudden worsening of renal function. He is taking multiple medications. All of the following types of medications could contribute to worsening his renal failure except which one?
   A. Angiotensin converting enzyme inhibitor
   B. Diuretic
   C. Nitrate
   D. Nonsteroidal antiinflammatory drug

2. Increased bleeding tendency in a patient with end-stage renal disease is usually secondary to:
   A. Decreased erythropoietin
   B. Platelet dysfunction
   C. Prolonged prothrombin time
   D. Thrombocytopenia

3. The ECG of a 50-year-old woman with a history of chronic renal failure shows peaked T waves. She is also found to be in acute pulmonary edema. All of the following treatments should be considered except which one?
   A. Calcium gluconate IV
   B. Furosemide IV
   C. Glucose and insulin IV
   D. Inhaled albuterol
   E. Sodium bicarbonate IV

4. A chronic hemodialysis patient has recurrent fevers but on examination has no obvious identifiable source of infection. Which of the following statements is true?
   A. If the access site shows no signs of inflammation, then it is not the source
   B. Outpatient management is an acceptable option for this patient population
   C. *Pseudomonas* is the most common organism responsible for access site infections
   D. Vancomycin should be avoided secondary to renal toxicity

5. A patient on chronic hemodialysis comes to the ED with persistent bleeding from the access site. Which of the following statements is true?
   A. Bleeding is usually not controlled by simple pressure at the site
   B. Cryoprecipitate is of no value
   C. Presence of a thrill after the bleeding has stopped is a true medical emergency
   D. Vigorous compression may occlude the vessel, resulting in thrombosis

6. A 63-year-old man who has just undergone hemodialysis is brought to the ED with persistent hypotension, despite the administration of a fluid bolus at the hemodialysis unit. All of the following should be considered as possible etiologies, except which one?
   A. Hypokalemia
   B. Hypomagnesemia
   C. Myocardial infarction
   D. Pericardial tamponade

7. A 57-year-old woman on chronic hemodialysis has persistent chest pain immediately after a dialysis treatment. Which of the following statements is true?
   A. CPK is useless following hemodialysis
   B. ECG is useless following hemodialysis
   C. Fifty percent narrowing of the coronary artery on a recent catheterization indicates a nonischemic origin for the chest pain
   D. Pericardiocentesis should be performed if the patient arrests shortly after arrival

8. Which of the following is not an indication for emergency dialysis in a patient with chronic renal failure and a history of routine weekly hemodialysis?
   A. pH 7.0
   B. Creatinine 10 mg/dl
   C. Hypermagnesemia
   D. Hypertensive encephalopathy
   E. Pulmonary edema

9. An asymptomatic patient with ESRD on peritoneal dialysis presents with "cloudy fluid" noticed during exchange. Laboratory data shows predominance of eosinophils. All of the following are true except which one?
   A. Cultures should be sent
   B. Requires intraperitoneal vancomycin
   C. This self-limited condition resolves spontaneously
   D. Exchanges should be continued

10. A hemodialysis patient presents with a complaint of loss of thrill at the vascular access site. Management should include which of the following?
    A. Attempt vascular access and if successful, arrange follow-up
    B. Heparin therapy and nephrology consult
    C. Reassurance and early morning follow-up
    D. Vascular surgery consult immediately

11. Which of the following matched problems and treatments associated with end-stage renal disease is incorrect?
    A. Nausea and vomiting: prochlorperazine
    B. Constipation: magnesium citrate
    C. Itching: hydroxyzine
    D. Restless leg syndrome: carbamazepine

---

 **Pelvic Pain**

*Greg Harders*

Select the appropriate letter that correctly answers the question or completes the statement.

1. An 18-year-old woman was jogging yesterday when she developed the sudden onset of severe, sharp, lower abdominal pain. Today the pain has persisted but is less intense. On examination, there is minimal tenderness noted in the right lower quadrant and no adnexal masses palpated on pelvic examination. The patient's last menstrual period was 2 weeks ago, and her pregnancy test is negative. Which one of the following is the most likely diagnosis?
   A. Appendicitis
   B. Ovarian torsion
   C. Ruptured corpus luteum cyst
   D. Ruptured follicular cyst

2. All of the following conditions increase the risk of uterine perforation except which one?
   A. Endometrial curettage and biopsy
   B. IUD
   C. Pregnancy
   D. Youth

3. A 33-year-old woman has a lower abdominal pressure sensation for 4-5 days. She has also noted some mild increased urinary frequency over the past months; however, she has no dysuria. Her last menstrual period was 2 weeks ago and was completely normal. She is currently having no vaginal bleeding. Examination reveals a firm, non-tender, enlarged uterus without adnexal mass. Pregnancy test and urinalysis are negative. Which of the following is the most likely diagnosis?
   A. Dysmenorrhea
   B. Endometriosis
   C. Ovarian torsion
   D. Uterine fibroid

4. What is the most likely etiology for cyclical pelvic pain that coincides with menstrual blood flow in an adolescent?
   A. Adenomyosis
   B. Endometriosis
   C. Pelvic inflammatory disease
   D. Ruptured ectopic pregnancy

5. A 27-year-old woman presents to the ED with sudden onset right-sided lower abdominal pain. She is hemodynamically stable but in severe discomfort. Bimanual examination reveals a large tender adnexal mass on the right and cervical motion tenderness. She had a similar episode 2 weeks previously that resolved spontaneously. Which of the following is the most likely diagnosis?
   A. Adnexal torsion
   B. Ectopic pregnancy
   C. Mittelschmerz
   D. Pelvic inflammatory disease

6. What is the emergency department management of a known acutely ruptured follicular cyst?
   A. Culdocentesis
   B. Immediate consultation
   C. Reassurance and discharge
   D. Ultrasound

---

 **Vaginal Bleeding Unrelated to Pregnancy**

*Greg Harders*

Select the appropriate letter that correctly answers the question or completes the statement.

1. Which of the following is associated with uterine myomas (fibroids)?
   A. Endometriosis
   B. Malignant degeneration
   C. Noncyclic bleeding
   D. Postmenopausal atrophy

2. A 17-year-old woman has a 4-month history of amenor-rhea. She now has vaginal bleeding and clots. The pregnancy test is negative. Which of the following is the most likely diagnosis?
   A. Anovulatory cycles
   B. Corpus luteum cyst
   C. Follicular cyst
   D. Normal menses for age

3. Which of the following is true of normal menstrual bleeding?
   A. Average blood loss is 15 to 30 ml
   B. Cycles from 15 to 45 days are normal
   C. Duration of flow ranges from 3 to 7 days
   D. Small clots are common

4. A 66-year-old woman has a history of irregular vaginal bleeding. External genitalia and vagina are normal, and on bimanual examination, normal cervix, uterus, and ovaries are palpated. Which of the following is the most likely diagnosis?
   A. Adenomyosis
   B. Exogenous dysfunctional uterine bleeding
   C. Non-gynecologic bleeding
   D. Ovarian tumor

5. A patient has vaginal bleeding after missing her last three birth control pills. Which of the following statements is true?
   A. Bleeding episode will likely be severe
   B. Contraceptive measures are indicated
   C. Breakthrough bleeding is probable
   D. Progesterone 100 mg intramuscularly is the appropriate treatment

6. Which of the following is true regarding cervical polyps?
   A. Are a cause of postcoital bleeding
   B. Are diagnosed by colposcopy
   C. Often degenerate to cervical carcinoma
   D. Result in heavy cyclic bleeding

7. Which of the following is not a characteristic of a corpus luteum cyst?
   A. Develops in the contralateral side of ovulation in 15%-35% of all patients
   B. May result in amenorrhea
   C. Produces hormones even in the nonpregnant state
   D. When ruptured will clinically mimic an ectopic pregnancy

8. Treatment strategies for non–pregnancy related dysfunctional uterine bleeding include all of the following except which one?
   A. Hysterectomy
   B. Methotrexate
   C. Nonsteroidal antiinflammatory drugs
   D. Progesterone

*Match the description below with the appropriate question.*

   A. Benign tumor which may cause increased cyclic bleeding
   B. Glandular and stromal infiltration of the myometrium

   C. May cause vaginal bleeding which is characteristically light
   D. Proliferation of endometrial tissue outside the uterus

9. Adenomyosis _____
10. Cervical polyps _____
11. Endometriosis _____
12. Leiomyoma _____

# 137 Genital Infections

### Greg Harders

Select the appropriate letter that correctly answers the question or completes the statement.

1. Which of the following statements regarding genital herpes simplex virus (HSV) is true?
   A. HSV-2 infects only squamous epithelium
   B. Symptoms worsen with each recurrent outbreak
   C. Treatment with oral acyclovir is for 7-10 days initially and for 5 days in recurrences
   D. Tzanck slide preparation is the standard for laboratory diagnosis

2. Which of the following is associated with secondary syphilis?
   A. Condyloma acuminata
   B. False-negative VDRL
   C. Infectious skin lesions
   D. Painless hard chancre

3. A 28-year-old man has large, coalescing, bilateral inguinal lymph nodes that have now formed ulcers. His girlfriend had a chlamydial infection 6 weeks ago. Which of the following is the most likely diagnosis?
   A. Chancroid
   B. Condyloma acuminata
   C. Granuloma inguinale
   D. Lymphogranuloma venereum

4. Which of the following is appropriate therapy for a patient who has a malodorous vaginal discharge showing motile flagellated organisms on wet mount?
   A. Ampicillin
   B. Clotrimazole
   C. Erythromycin
   D. Metronidazole

5. All of the following statements are true of toxic shock syndrome except which one?
   A. An erythematous macular rash with desquamation during recovery is expected
   B. Antistaphylococcal antibiotics shorten the course
   C. Blood cultures are negative
   D. Diagnostic criteria include fever above 38.9° C (102° F) and systolic blood pressure below 90 mm Hg in adults

6. A cervical culture returns positive for *Neisseria gonorrhoeae*. Which of the following statements is true?

A. Acceptable treatment is with ceftriaxone alone

B. Gonorrhea is the most common sexually transmitted disease

C. Gram stain will also be positive 90% of the time

D. The patient may be an asymptomatic carrier

7. A patient arrives at the ED with pelvic pain and tenderness. Which of the following would support a diagnosis of pelvic inflammatory disease?

A. Current pregnancy

B. History of endometriosis

C. Recent menstruation

D. Use of birth control pills

8. All of the following are true of *Candida vaginitis* except which one?

A. "Cottage cheese" consistency of discharge

B. Recent antibiotic use

C. Treatment is fluconazole

D. Typically a malodorous discharge

9. Which of the following sexually transmitted diseases is typically painful?

A. Chancroid

B. Granuloma inguinale

C. Lymphogranuloma venereum

D. Syphilis

10. Which of the following statements regarding herpesvirus is false?

A. Active herpes infections are associated with urinary retention

B. Delivery via cesarean section is indicated for pregnant women with active recurrent infections

C. First-line therapy for primary herpes is IV acyclovir

D. Herpes is the most common genital ulcer

# 138 Sexual Assault

*Greg Harders*

Select the appropriate letter that correctly answers the question or completes the statement.

1. Sperm can remain motile in the vagina for a maximum of how many hours after intercourse?

A. 12 hours

B. 18 hours

C. 24 hours

D. 48 hours

2. External evidence of trauma is shown in what percentage of rape victims?

A. Less than 3%

B. More than 50%

C. Up to 30%

D. Up to 50%

3. Which of the following statements is false?

A. Drug regimens to prevent pregnancy are not useful if given 48 hours after the rape

B. Oral conjugated estrogen (Premarin) can be used for pregnancy prophylaxis

C. Pregnancy caused by rape occurs in up to 25% of rape victims

D. The failure rate using oral norgestrel and ethinyl estradiol (Ovral) for pregnancy prophylaxis is less than 2%

4. When performing the vaginal examination in an adult rape victim, which of the following best describes the use of the speculum?

A. Lubricate with water

B. Lubricate with water-soluble lubricant

C. Use no lubrication

D. Use no lubrication; only swabs

5. Use of the Wood's lamp may assist in evaluating for which of the following?

A. Contusion

B. Rope marks

C. Semen stains

D. All of the above

6. All of the following are true regarding HIV exposure in the setting of rape except which one?

A. HIV prophylaxis has been proven to be safe and effective

B. Patients should be followed for several months

C. Risk of transmission is thought to be minimal

D. The ED is not an appropriate setting for HIV testing

7. Which of the following is true regarding STDs and rape victims?

A. Hepatitis B prophylaxis is rarely if ever indicated

B. Prophylactic treatment should be carried out for gonorrhea and chlamydia

C. Syphilis as a result of rape occurs in 5% of cases

D. Testing for gonorrhea and chlamydia at the time of rape examination is essential

**SECTION 8  PREGNANCY**

# 139 Unique Concerns of Pregnancy

*Barbara N. Wynn*

Select the appropriate letter that correctly answers the question or completes the statement.

1. Which of the following is most accurate?

A. Fertilization occurs within minutes to hours after ovulation

B. HCG (human chorionic gonadotropin) originates in the corpus luteum

C. Implantation occurs 3 days after fertilization

D. Parity is the total number of times the patient has given birth to a live child

E. Premature labor occurs any time before 39 weeks' gestation.

2. Which of the following is abnormal during pregnancy?
   A. Decreased plasma osmolality
   B. Decreased platelet count
   C. Glucosuria
   D. Hemoglobin 9.5 gm/dl
   E. Two times normal alkaline phosphatase
3. Which of the following best describes pregnancy?
   A. Bleeding before the fortieth day is rare and usually pathologic
   B. Braxton-Hicks contractions are reliable diagnostic tools
   C. Chadwick's sign is softening of the lower uterine segment
   D. Fetal heart tones can usually be auscultated with a stethoscope by 14 weeks' gestation
   E. More than 10% of women with a positive pregnancy test report there is no chance they are pregnant
4. Which of the following is most characteristic of HCG?
   A. After an abortion, levels may need 30 days to return to zero
   B. Exogenous HCG for ovulation induction does not affect pregnancy test results
   C. Level of 180,000 IU/L is indicative of a molar pregnancy
   D. Peak levels are reached at 7-10 weeks of pregnancy
   E. Positive urine pregnancy test requires levels to be greater than 100 IU/L
5. Which of the following is an abnormal cardiovascular finding in a pregnant woman?
   A. Diastolic murmur
   B. Grade II/VI systolic murmur
   C. Increased resting heart rate of 10-15 beats per minute
   D. Peripheral edema
   E. S3
6. Which of the following best describes domestic violence?
   A. Abused women are offended by direct questions regarding abuse
   B. Domestic violence occurs in less than 10% of spousal relationships
   C. Most abused women are aware of support services available but chose not to use them
   D. Physical abuse in the pregnant patient is more common in the facial area
   E. Spousal abuse is associated with child abuse

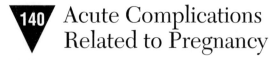

# 140 ▼ Acute Complications Related to Pregnancy

*Barbara N. Wynn*

Select the appropriate letter that correctly answers the question or completes the statement.

1. A woman who is Rh negative with her last menstrual period 8 weeks ago has vaginal bleeding, lower abdominal cramping, and a positive pregnancy test. Physical examination reveals an appropriately enlarged uterus with a closed cervix and a small amount of bright red blood in the vaginal vault. Which of the following best describes this threatened abortion?
   A. Anti-D immunoglobulin is not needed at this point
   B. Bed rest or limited activity is advised until the bleeding stops
   C. Empty gestational sac on ultrasound indicates an embryonic gestation
   D. Patients who miscarry in the first trimester experience minimal psychologic stress
   E. Risk of miscarriage is about 20%
2. A patient with a positive pregnancy test 1 week ago presents with abdominal pain. What findings are indicative of intrauterine pregnancy?
   A. Dry culdocentesis
   B. Double ring sign on ultrasound
   C. Fetal heart activity on ultrasound
   D. History of in vitro fertilization
   E. Progesterone level <25 ng/ml
3. Which of the following best describes ectopic pregnancy?
   A. Always accompanied by pain and heavy bleeding
   B. History of passing tissue excludes diagnosis
   C. Implantation in the uterine horn presents early with severe pain
   D. Occurs simultaneously with intrauterine pregnancy in 1 in 50,000 pregnancies
   E. Very low HCG levels can be present with rupture
4. Which of the following is most characteristic of ultrasound?
   A. Double ring sign is indicative of an ectopic pregnancy
   B. Ectopic gestations are usually visualized
   C. On transvaginal scans, fetal heart activity is visible by 5 weeks
   D. Transabdominal scans have a discriminatory zone of 4500-5000 mIU/ml
   E. Transvaginal scans have a discriminatory zone of 1500 mIU/ml
5. A woman who is 30 weeks pregnant presents with vaginal bleeding. Which of the following is most accurate?
   A. If this is abruptio placentae, the patient will also have pain
   B. If this is abruptio placentae, ultrasound will be diagnostic
   C. If this patient develops pain, the most likely diagnosis is placenta previa
   D. If this is placenta previa, ultrasound will be diagnostic
   E. If this patient had placenta previa diagnosed in the second trimester, it is unlikely her current bleeding could be due to other causes
6. Which of the following is associated with abruptio placentae?
   A. Elevated fibrinogen level
   B. Increased parity

C. Normal abdominal examination

D. Previous cesarean section

E. Smoking history

7. Which of the following best describes pregnancy-induced hypertension (PIH)?

A. Defined by blood pressure greater ≥140/90

B. Eclamptic seizures do not occur postpartum

C. Greatest risk in women older than 20 years of age

D. Proteinuria is always present

E. Severe form is the HELLP syndrome, which is characterized by hemolysis, elevated lipid enzymes, and low potassium

8. Which of the following is least likely to be a complication of pregnancy-induced hypertension?

A. Elevated liver enzymes

B. Hemolysis

C. Low fibrinogen level

D. Normal prothrombin time

E. Thrombocytopenia

9. Which of the following best describes the use of magnesium sulfate for the treatment of eclampsia?

A. Drug levels are the best method to monitor toxicity

B. Hypermagnesemia can be treated with intravenous calcium gluconate

C. Hyperventilation is a sign of toxicity

D. Intramuscular route is preferred over the intravenous route

E. Is an effective antihypertensive and anticonvulsant

10. Which of the following is the most frequently used drug for a patient with eclampsia and a diastolic blood pressure of 114 mm Hg?

A. Furosemide

B. Hydralazine

C. Nifedipine

D. Nitroglycerin

E. Nitroprusside

11. A woman who is 40 weeks pregnant presents hypotensive, hypoxic, and bleeding from needle stick sites. What is the least likely diagnosis?

A. Amniotic fluid embolus

B. Catastrophic pulmonary embolus

C. Drug-induced anaphylaxis

D. Eclampsia

E. Sepsis

12. Which of the following best describes appendicitis in pregnancy?

A. Appendix is in the right upper quadrant by the third month of gestation

B. Leukocytosis is marked

C. Peritoneal signs persist throughout pregnancy

D. Pyuria and bacteriuria are common

E. Ultrasound is very accurate in diagnosing appendicitis in pregnancy

13. Which of the following is most characteristic of a woman 34 weeks pregnant presenting with right upper quadrant pain?

A. Acute fatty liver is a benign process presenting in the third trimester

B. Elevated alkaline phosphatase levels are never normal in pregnancy

C. Has a decreased risk for cholecystitis

D. Hepatitis is the most common cause of liver disease in pregnancy

E. Ultrasound is rarely necessary to diagnose cholecystitis in pregnancy

14. Which of the following best describes thromboembolic disease and pregnancy?

A. Alveolar-arterial gradient up to 30 is normal

B. Doppler ultrasonography is a safe and accurate diagnostic aid

C. Pain and swelling of extremities are good predictors of deep vein thrombosis

D. Right diaphragm remains higher than the left in late pregnancy

E. Technetium-labeled ventilation perfusion scans are contraindicated

15. Which of the following best describes sexually transmitted diseases of the genital tract during pregnancy?

A. *Chlamydia trachomatis* causes preterm labor and neonatal pneumonia

B. Major complication of third-trimester gonococcal infection is chorioamnionitis

C. PID usually occurs after the first trimester

D. Trichomoniasis is more aggressive during pregnancy and should be treated even if the patient is asymptomatic

E. When treating *Candida* infection, vaginal imidazoles are contraindicated during pregnancy

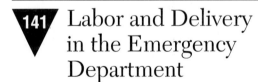

# 141 ▼ Labor and Delivery in the Emergency Department

*Barbara N. Wynn*

Select the appropriate letter that correctly answers the question or completes the statement.

1. Which of the following is most correct?

A. A woman 28-weeks pregnant will have her uterus palpable at the level of the umbilicus

B. Bloody show is a contraindication to vaginal examination in the emergency department

C. Emergency department deliveries are usually in low-risk patients

D. Episiotomy should be performed only for specific indications, not routinely

E. Position is the anatomic part leading through the birth canal

2. Which of the following best describes fetal cardiac activity?
   A. Fetal heart rate accelerations occur during fetal distress
   B. Late decelerations are serious
   C. Sinusoidal tracing is normal
   D. Variability is an indication of fetal distress
   E. Variable and early decelerations are rare

3. Which of the following is most characteristic of preterm labor?
   A. All patients are candidates for medical management
   B. Beta-mimetics are the tocolytics of choice for diabetic mothers
   C. Cardiopulmonary disease is an absolute contraindication for tocolytics
   D. Preterm labor is defined as uterine contractions before 37 weeks' gestation
   E. Use of magnesium sulfate may obscure signs of intrauterine infections

4. Which of the following is most accurate?
   A. Amniotic fluid pH is 3.5-6.0
   B. Clinically significant abruption is diagnosed by electrical fetal monitoring
   C. Concealed bleeding in abruptio placentae occurs 80% of the time
   D. Premature breech infants rarely deliver spontaneously
   E. Shoulder dystocia is not responsive to intrapartum maneuvers

5. Which of the following is least helpful in the management of a prolapsed umbilical cord?
   A. Drainage of the bladder with a Foley catheter
   B. Manual replacement of the cord into the uterus and rapid vaginal delivery
   C. Mother placed in the knee-chest position
   D. Presenting part digitally elevated off the umbilical cord
   E. Tocolysis with ritodrine

6. Which of the following is most accurate?
   A. Grade 3 and 4 vaginal tears are best repaired in an operating room
   B. Hemorrhage caused by retained products of conception is usually delayed
   C. High packing is commonly used to control postpartum hemorrhage
   D. Postpartum hemorrhage is a rare cause of obstetric deaths
   E. Postpartum hemorrhage is defined as blood loss >100 ml

7. A woman presents to the ED having just delivered in the ambulance bay. She is complaining of severe abdominal pain. Which of the following is most correct?
   A. If a uterine inversion exists and the placenta is still inherent, the placenta should be removed quickly
   B. If the patient is hemorrhaging, uterine inversion is unlikely
   C. If the patient has uterine inversion, the initial response is to push the fundus upward

D. If the uterine corpus is not palpable on abdominal examination, uterine rupture is suspected
E. If the uterus is bulging from the vagina, immediate surgery is needed

# 142 Drug Use in Pregnancy

*Bruce W. Nugent*

Select the appropriate letter that correctly answers the question or completes the statement.

1. Which of the following best describes a drug designated "Class C"?
   A. Controlled studies have shown no risk to the human fetus
   B. Is contraindicated in pregnancy
   C. No evidence exists of risk for humans; animal studies demonstrate risk or are negative; no human studies have been done
   D. Positive evidence of risk exists based on studies or post-marketing data
   E. Use may engender risk for the fetus; human studies are lacking; animal studies are positive or lacking

2. What is the most important reason salicylates are generally not recommended as an analgesic in pregnancy?
   A. Chronic ingestion of therapeutic amounts is associated with prematurity
   B. They delay closure of the ductus arteriosus in the neonate
   C. They hasten the onset of labor and decrease its duration
   D. They increase the risk of hemorrhage and blood loss at delivery
   E. They are teratogenic

3. A 24-year-old penicillin-allergic G2P1 woman presents at 10 weeks' gestation with acute cystitis. What is the best treatment?
   A. Amoxicillin
   B. Ciprofloxacin
   C. Doxycycline
   D. Metronidazole
   E. Sulfamethoxazole

4. During evaluation of a patient with a known seizure disorder, a pregnancy test returns positive. The patient is currently taking phenytoin 100 mg tid and phenobarbital 30 mg tid and was unaware of the pregnancy. What is the best management?
   A. Change medications to anticonvulsants without teratogenic effects
   B. Decrease the dose of each drug
   C. Explain risks of anticonvulsants and expedite referral
   D. Measure the level of epoxide hydrolase to determine teratogenic risk
   E. Stop all anticonvulsants until the patient is seen by a neurologist

5. Which of the following anticonvulsants is associated with a 1%-3% risk of spina bifida?
   A. Carbamazepine
   B. Diazepam
   C. Phenobarbital
   D. Phenytoin
   E. Valproic acid

6. A 35-year-old woman presents at 19 weeks' gestation with a history of palpitations and mild shortness of breath over the past 24 hours. Her blood pressure is 90/60 and pulse is 170. On examination she is in no distress but has subtle rales in the lung bases and trace peripheral edema. ECG demonstrates a regular narrow complex supraventricular tachycardia. What is the preferred therapy?
   A. Adenosine
   B. Captopril
   C. Propranolol
   D. Verapamil
   E. Warfarin followed by cardioversion

7. A 26-year-old G4P1Ab2 woman at 9 weeks' gestation is seen for lacerations after a domestic dispute. She has a blood alcohol concentration of 200 mg/dl and admits to alcohol intake of only one drink per day. What best describes her situation?
   A. Benzodiazepines should be avoided if withdrawal occurs
   B. Maternal alcohol concentration is higher than that of the fetus
   C. Risk for fetal congenital abnormalities is less than 1%
   D. There is increased risk for spontaneous abortion
   E. Use of other drugs is unlikely

8. What best describes the result of chronic opiate use during pregnancy?
   A. Equivalent birth weights to non-drug users
   B. Higher incidence of respiratory depression and low Apgar scores
   C. Increased risk of structural birth defects
   D. Shortened fetal exposure because amniotic fluid acts as a reservoir for opiates and metabolites
   E. Signs of withdrawal in up to one third of births

9. One of the most serious complications of chronic opiate use in pregnancy is neonatal withdrawal. What best describes this abstinence syndrome?
   A. Methadone-dependent neonates have less frequent and less severe symptoms than heroin-exposed infants
   B. Often occurs later in the methadone-dependent than in the heroin-dependent neonate
   C. Respiratory depression is common
   D. Symptoms should be seen within the first hour after delivery
   E. Treatment of seizures should be with benzodiazepines

10. What is the most important factor underlying the toxicity of cocaine to the fetus during pregnancy?
    A. Adrenergic vasoconstrictor effect
    B. Hyperthermia

C. Increased frequency of infections
D. Kindling effect
E. Maternal anorexia leading to malnutrition

# 143 ▼ Chronic Medical Illness and Pregnancy

*Bruce W. Nugent*

Select the appropriate letter that correctly answers the question or completes the statement.

1. Which of the following best describes normal respiratory physiology in pregnancy?
   A. Functional residual capacity is increased
   B. Minute ventilation decreases
   C. Resting $P_{CO_2}$ is decreased by an average of 10 mm Hg
   D. Slight respiratory acidosis occurs
   E. Tidal volume decreases

2. A 24-year-old G3P2 afebrile woman presents at 12 weeks' gestation with an acute exacerbation of asthma. Her medications include beclomethasone and albuterol metered-dose inhalers, and today she has required the latter every 2 hours. She is in moderate respiratory distress with BP, 120/60; P, 120; RR, 28; pulse oxymetry, 96%, and PEFR, 200 L/minute. What is the most appropriate management?
   A. Albuterol aerosols, oral steroids, fetal heart tones
   B. Fetal heart tones, $O_2$, albuterol aerosols, inhaled steroids
   C. Fetal heart tones, $O_2$, albuterol aerosols, subcutaneous epinephrine
   D. $O_2$, albuterol aerosols, parenteral steroids
   E. $O_2$, albuterol aerosols, theophylline, inhaled steroids

3. A 41-year-old G2P1 woman presents at 34 weeks' gestation with severe anterior chest pain radiating to the jaw and arms. She has associated symptoms of shortness of breath, diaphoresis, and nausea. Her ECG shows 4-mm ST elevation in the precordial leads with reciprocal changes. Which of the following best describes this situation?
   A. Atypical enzyme changes would be expected
   B. Coronary artery dissection is the most likely cause
   C. Mortality is increased from that of a nonpregnant patient
   D. Nitrates should be avoided due to fetal cyanide toxicity
   E. Thrombolytic therapy is contraindicated.

4. Which of the following valvular heart diseases in pregnancy is most likely to lead to maternal mortality?
   A. Aortic regurgitation
   B. Aortic stenosis
   C. Mitral regurgitation
   D. Mitral stenosis
   E. Mitral valve prolapse

5. Which of the following is most characteristic of nutritional anemia in pregnancy?
   A. Iron deficiency results in an increased incidence of neural tube defects
   B. Maternal anemia has relatively little impact on perinatal mortality until a hemoglobin of 6.0 gm/ml is reached
   C. Megaloblastic anemia is most commonly caused by dietary deficiency of vitamin B12
   D. Microcytic/hypochromic indices are a reliable screening tool for iron deficiency anemia
   E. Without iron supplementation, the incidence of anemia in pregnancy may reach up to 40%

6. Which of the following best describes sickle cell anemia in pregnancy?
   A. Fertility is not affected by sickle cell disease
   B. Hemoglobin SA disease is most serious
   C. Kleihauer-Betke test may be falsely negative
   D. Only 30% of pregnancies result in a live fetus
   E. Painful crises are less common in pregnancy

7. A 19-year-old primigravida presents at 28 weeks' gestation just after a new-onset seizure. Her pregnancy has previously been uncomplicated with no history of fever, drug use, or head trauma. Which of the following would be most helpful in diagnosing eclampsia in this patient?
   A. Disorientation
   B. Hypertension
   C. Papilledema
   D. Peripheral edema
   E. Proteinuria

8. Which of the following is most characteristic of epilepsy in pregnancy?
   A. Anticonvulsant drug toxicity is more frequent
   B. Is the most common neurologic complication of pregnancy
   C. Phenytoin therapy is contraindicated in status epilepticus
   D. Seizure frequency usually decreases
   E. Teratogenic potential of drug therapy outweighs the risk of status epilepticus

9. Which of the following often worsens during pregnancy?
   A. Diabetes mellitus
   B. Grave's disease
   C. Multiple sclerosis
   D. Myasthenia gravis
   E. Rheumatoid arthritis

10. Which of the following is most characteristic of diabetic ketoacidosis in pregnancy?
    A. Fetal mortality is unusual
    B. Hyperemesis is the most common precipitant
    C. Maternal insulin and counter-regulatory hormones cross the placenta
    D. Most commonly seen in gestational diabetes
    E. Serum pH may be deceptively low

11. Which of the following best describes vertical transmission of HIV?
    A. AZT use is associated with the "HIV dysmorphic syndrome"
    B. Breast-feeding is permissible only if the neonate tests HIV positive
    C. Careful monitoring with scalp electrodes is indicated during labor
    D. Occurs at a rate of 60% or higher without antiretroviral treatment
    E. Virtually all neonates will have a positive HIV antibody test

12. What is the first priority when treating a pregnant patient with suspected hyperthyroidism?
    A. Ablation of thyroid with radioactive iodine
    B. Adrenergic blockade with propranolol
    C. Decrease conversion of $T_4$ to $T_3$ with hydrocortisone
    D. Inhibition of thyroid release with iodide
    E. Inhibition of thyroid synthesis with propylthiouracil

13. What is the most important factor contributing to the frequency of vertical transmissions and neonatal morbidity of syphilis and hepatitis B?
    A. Immunosuppression
    B. Inadequate diagnostic tests
    C. Inadequate screening
    D. Ineffective drug therapy
    E. Resistant organisms

14. A woman with a preexisting C7 spinal cord injury presents at 34 weeks' gestation. She is alert but complains of a pulsatile headache and is tachycardic, hypertensive, and diaphoretic, with blotching of the skin. What is most likely?
    A. Distended bladder
    B. Onset of labor
    C. Pulmonary embolism
    D. Subarachnoid hemorrhage
    E. Urinary tract infection with sepsis

---

**SECTION 9    METABOLIC AND ENDOCRINE PROBLEMS**

 **144    Acid-Base Disorders**

*Jeffrey S. Jones*

Select the appropriate letter that correctly answers the question or completes the statement.

1. A young asthmatic patient in respiratory distress presents with the following arterial blood gases: pH, 7.2; $Pco_2$, 70; $PO_2$, 62; $HCO_3$, 26. Which of the following best describes the acid-base status?
   A. Blood pressure and cardiac output are likely to be severely compromised
   B. Initial therapy is directed toward the restoration of pH using $NaHCO_3$ (1 mEq/kg)
   C. Oxygen should be administered carefully to avoid $CO_2$ narcosis

D. Renal compensation is evident

E. Respiratory problem is not chronic in nature

2. Which of the following ingestions is a cause of metabolic alkalosis?

A. Ethylene glycol

B. Licorice

C. Methanol

D. Paraldehyde

E. Salicylate

3. A 54-year-old man presents with acidosis (pH = 7.2). His sodium is 134 mEq/L; chloride is 113 mEq/L; potassium, 4.0 mEq/L; and bicarbonate, 9 mEq/L. What is the most likely cause of his acidosis?

A. Diarrhea

B. Grand mal seizure

C. Rhabdomyolysis

D. Salicylate ingestion

E. Uremia

4. Which of the following complications is associated with the use of sodium bicarbonate therapy in metabolic acidosis?

A. Hypercalcemia

B. Hyperkalemia

C. Hyponatremia

D. Intracellular alkalosis

E. Paradoxical CSF acidosis

5. An elderly male is found comatose following an unknown drug ingestion. Which of the following is the first step in the interpretation of an acid-base disorder?

A. Calculate the anion gap

B. Calculate the expected degree of physiologic compensation

C. Compare the measured and calculated bicarbonate concentrations

D. Ensure that the electrolyte specimen and blood gas sample were obtained at the same time

E. Examine the pH, $Paco_2$, and bicarbonate to determine the predominant acid-base abnormality

6. Which of the following is least likely to be associated with ketoacidosis?

A. Alcoholism

B. Diabetes mellitus

C. Hypoxemia

D. Starvation

E. Stress hormone excess

7. An alcoholic has a pH of 7.1 and a potassium level of 4.0 mEq/L. After correction of the pH, what is his actual serum potassium?

A. 2.8 mEq/L

B. 3.8 mEq/L

C. 4.0 mEq/L

D. 4.8 mEq/L

E. 6.0 mEq/L

8. Which of the following will typically cause a high-anion-gap acidosis?

A. Acetazolamide

B. Isopropyl alcohol ingestion

C. Obstructive uropathy

D. Renal insufficiency

E. Seizures

*Match each of the clinical conditions below with the appropriate acid-base disturbance. Answers may be used once, more than once, or not at all.*

A. Metabolic acidosis

B. Metabolic alkalosis

C. Respiratory acidosis

D. Respiratory alkalosis

9. Cushing's syndrome _____

10. Methanol ingestion _____

11. Thyrotoxicosis _____

12. Heroin overdose _____

 ## 145 Electrolyte Disturbances

*Jeffrey S. Jones*

Select the appropriate letter that correctly answers the question or completes the statement.

1. Which of the following is closest to the kilogram weight of total body water in a 50-kg male?

A. 5

B. 10

C. 20

D. 30

E. 40

2. Infusion of a hypotonic saline solution will immediately cause which of the following fluid shifts?

A. Extracellular fluid (ECF) contraction and intracellular fluid (ICF) contraction

B. ECF contraction and ICF expansion

C. ECF expansion and ICF expansion

D. ECF expansion and ICF contraction

E. ECF expansion and no change of ICF

3. Which of the following is the major intracellular cation?

A. Bicarbonate

B. Calcium

C. Chloride

D. Potassium

E. Sodium

4. Pseudohyponatremia results from the shift of water from the intracellular fluid to the extracellular fluid, which is caused by the presence of osmotically active solutes in the ECF. Which of the following may cause significant fluid shifts?

A. Acetone

B. Alcohol

C. Ethylene glycol

D. Mannitol

E. Urea

5. A 3-year-old boy has been vomiting for 5 days and presents listless with a pulse of 175 and a capillary refill >4 seconds. His weight is 12 kg, and serum sodium is 111 mEq/L. What is the most appropriate fluid regimen?
   A. D5/0.2 normal saline at 20 cc/kg
   B. D5/0.45 normal saline at 250 cc/hr
   C. Hypertonic saline infusion at 1 cc/kg/hr
   D. Hypertonic saline infusion at 1 cc/kg/hr with concomitant administration of parenteral diuretic (e.g., furosemide)
   E. Isotonic saline infusion bolus of 20 cc/kg

6. A 68-year-old man with COPD presents with a serum sodium of 124 mEq/L and concentrated urine (>20 mEq/dl) despite a normal circulating blood volume. What is the most likely diagnosis?
   A. Diabetes insipidus
   B. Hyperaldosteronism
   C. Osmotic diuresis
   D. Psychogenic polydipsia
   E. SIADH

7. A 16-year-old woman with histiocytosis is found to have a sodium level of 122 and a urine concentration of 60 mOsm/L. She is fully alert without other complaints and has stable vital signs. What is the most appropriate treatment?
   A. ADH replacement
   B. Fluid restriction
   C. Hypertonic saline
   D. Hypotonic saline
   E. Normal saline

8. A 96-year-old widow is found unconscious in her non–air-conditioned Chicago apartment in August. Her blood pressure is 55 by palpation and pulse 140. The serum sodium is 180 mEq/L. What is the most appropriate management?
   A. D5/0.45 normal saline at 250 cc/hr
   B. D5W infusion at 500 cc/hr
   C. D5W infusion at 500 cc/hr with concomitant administration of parenteral diuretic (e.g., furosemide)
   D. D5W infusion at 500 cc/hr with concomitant administration of parenteral vasopressin
   E. Isotonic saline infusion, 1 liter in the first hour

9. Which of the following best characterizes diabetes insipidus?
   A. Hypernatremia is a common finding
   B. Intranasal vasopressin may be beneficial
   C. Urine osmolality is high
   D. Urine specific gravity is normal
   E. Water should be withheld

10. Which of the following is a cause of hypernatremia?
    A. Addison's disease
    B. Diarrhea
    C. Hyperglycemia
    D. Psychogenic polydipsia
    E. SIADH

11. A 22-year-old man with a history of schizophrenia is brought to the ED by friends who observed him drinking large amounts of sea water. His only complaints are headache and abdominal cramping. His serum sodium is 158 mEq/L; potassium 4 mEq/L; and urinary sodium 50 mEq/L. Which of the following is the most appropriate treatment?
    A. D5W at 100 ml/hr
    B. Diuretics and water replacement
    C. Fluid restriction
    D. 0.45 normal saline until $Na^+$ is below 150
    E. Normal saline infusion

12. Which of the following can cause a pseudohyponatremia?
    A. Addison's disease
    B. Hyperglycemia
    C. Hyperlipidemia
    D. SIADH
    E. Volume depletion

13. Irritability, disorientation, and confusion are common when the serum sodium mEq/L falls below which of the following levels?
    A. 100
    B. 110
    C. 120
    D. 130
    E. 140

14. A 72-year-old woman presents confused. Vital signs are BP, 105/78; P, 100; and R, 20. Her mucous membranes are dry, but she shows no signs of orthostatic hypotension. Her sodium is 114 mEq/L, and CBC, $K^+$, MG, Ca, and renal function are normal. What is the most appropriate treatment?
    A. Fluid restriction
    B. Furosemide
    C. Hypertonic saline infusion
    D. Normal saline infusion
    E. Oral fluid rehydration

15. Which of the following is least likely to cause hypernatremia?
    A. Administration of carbenicillin
    B. Cushing's disease
    C. Severe burns
    D. SIADH
    E. Vomiting and diarrhea

16. Which of the following will increase $K^+$ excretion by the kidney?
    A. Aldosterone insufficiency
    B. Antibiotics (e.g., carbenicillin)
    C. Discontinuing diuretic therapy
    D. GFR falling below 10 ml per minute
    E. Metabolic acidosis

17. A 35-year-old baseball player presents with chest pain. Incidentally, you find that his potassium is 2.0 mEq/L. He is receiving no prescribed medications. Which of the following would not be among the differential diagnoses for his hypokalemia?
    A. Addison's disease
    B. Chronic laxative abuse

C. Laboratory error

D. Licorice ingestion

E. Tobacco chewing

18. Which of the following electrocardiogram changes would not be present in hypokalemia?

A. Peaked T waves

B. PR-interval prolongation

C. QT-interval prolongation

D. Sinus bradycardia

E. U wave

19. Which of the following may cause hyperkalemia without a change in total body potassium (transcellular shift)?

A. Acute acidosis

B. Hypoaldosteronism

C. Potassium-sparing diuretics

D. Rhabdomyolysis

E. Salt substitute

20. Which of the following is a cause of pseudohyperkalemia?

A. Acidosis

B. Crush injuries

C. Hemolysis of blood sample

D. Mineral corticoid deficiency

E. Transfusions of stored blood

21. Which of the following is least likely to be an effect of hyperkalemia?

A. As $K^+$ levels rise, peaked T waves are the first characteristic manifestation

B. Complete heart block typically occurs at $K^+$ levels above 9 mEq/L

C. Focal neurologic abnormalities (e.g., hemiparesis) have been reported

D. Neuromuscular effects include paresthesias and muscle cramps

E. Paradoxical aciduria may result when kidneys try to excrete $K^+$ at the expense of pH homeostasis

22. A 72-year-old woman presents with weakness and shortness of breath but no chest pain. She is receiving potassium supplementation but is not sure of the dosage. An electrocardiogram reveals an injury pattern and peaked T waves. Serum potassium is 8.6 mEq/L. What is the best initial treatment?

A. Beta-2 agonist

B. Calcium gluconate

C. Glucose and insulin

D. Sodium bicarbonate

E. Sodium polystyrene-sulfonate (Kayexalate)

23. A 55-year-old patient suffering from Addison's disease has diffuse muscle weakness. His potassium is 6.8 mEq/L, and the electrocardiogram is normal. What is the treatment of choice?

A. Aldosterone 10 mg IV

B. Calcium gluconate 10% 10 ml IV

C. Fludrocortisone (Florinef) 0.1 mg IV

D. Hydrocortisone 100 mg IV or IM

E. Normal saline infusion at 250 cc/hr

24. A nursing home resident is suffering from pain secondary to metastatic carcinoma. Her albumin is 1.8 from chronic malnutrition. In light of this albumin level, which of the following choices accurately represents her total $CA^{++}$/ionized $Ca^{++}$ levels?

A. Decreased/decreased

B. Decreased/normal

C. Increased/abnormal

D. Increased/normal

E. Normal/decreased

25. Which of the following is least likely to result in hypocalcemia?

A. Blood transfusions

B. Chronic renal failure

C. Hypermagnesemia

D. Neck surgery

E. Vitamin D toxicity

26. A 61-year-old man presents complaining of weakness, fatigue, and abdominal pain. On examination he has conjunctivitis and diminished deep tendon reflexes. The electrocardiogram reveals shortening of the QT-interval and peculiar notching of the QRS complex. What is the most appropriate treatment?

A. Aldosterone

B. Calcium gluconate

C. Furosemide and normal saline

D. Insulin and dextrose

E. Sodium bicarbonate

27. A 33-year-old man is seen 5 days after thyroidectomy with paresthesia of the distal extremities and perioral area, carpopedal spasm, and laryngeal stridor. What is the most appropriate treatment?

A. Calcium gluconate PO

B. Calcium gluconate 10% IV

C. Furosemide and saline IV

D. Magnesium sulfate 10% IV

E. Potassium chloride 20 mEq/L IV

28. Which of the following does not cause hypercalcemia?

A. Anticonvulsant medication

B. Diuretic therapy

C. Malignancy

D. Sarcoidosis

E. Thyrotoxicosis

29. A 48-year-old man presents complaining of dyspnea. He is taking digoxin for chronic atrial fibrillation. Which of the following could worsen a digitalis-toxicity–induced dysrhythmia?

A. Hypocalcemia

B. Hyperglycemia

C. Hyperkalemia

D. Hypomagnesemia

E. Hypophosphatemia

30. Which of the following best describes magnesium homeostasis?
    A. Both magnesium deficiency and excess cause neuromuscular dysfunction
    B. Hypermagnesemia leads to hypertension via increased vascular tone
    C. Hypomagnesemia from poor nutritional habits is common in the United States
    D. Magnesium elimination occurs mainly in the small intestine and colon
    E. Normal serum levels range from 4.5-5.5 mg/dl

31. Regarding the manifestations of magnesium imbalance, which of the following is incorrect?
    A. Ataxia, nystagmus, and seizures may occur when magnesium levels are <1.2 mg/dl
    B. EKG changes are seen at magnesium levels of 5-6 mg/dl
    C. Loss of deep tendon reflexes occur at magnesium levels <1.2 mg/dl
    D. Nausea, vomiting, weakness, and flushing usually appear at magnesium levels of 3 mg/dl
    E. Respiratory depression is common at magnesium levels >9 mg/dl

32. A healthy 27-year-old woman suffers complete heart block during an infusion of magnesium sulfate for treatment of eclampsia. What is the most appropriate initial treatment?
    A. Calcium chloride IV
    B. Immediate hemodialysis
    C. Loop diuretics and saline IV
    D. Potassium chloride IV
    E. Sodium bicarbonate IV

33. Which of the following is least likely to cause hypophosphatemia?
    A. Alcoholism
    B. Diabetic ketoacidosis
    C. Hypomagnesemia
    D. Hypoparathyroidism
    E. Respiratory alkalosis

34. A 45-year-old man with a history of alcoholism presents with myalgias and weakness. Which of the following is most likely?
    A. Hypercalcemia
    B. Hyperglycemia
    C. Hyperkalemia
    D. Hypokalemia
    E. Hypophosphatemia

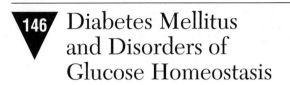

## 146 Diabetes Mellitus and Disorders of Glucose Homeostasis

*Bruce W. Nugent*

Select the appropriate letter that correctly answers the question or completes the statement.

1. Which of the following statements best describes insulin?
   A. Glucose given parenterally evokes more release than oral glucose
   B. Half-life is 1-3 hours in the circulation
   C. Inhibits glucose uptake, storage, and use in fat and muscle
   D. Inhibits hepatic gluconeogenesis and glycogenolysis
   E. Is the major catabolic hormone

2. Which of the following best describes non–insulin-dependent diabetes mellitus (NIDDM)?
   A. Also known as type I diabetes
   B. Associated with islet cell antibodies
   C. Highest prevalence in whites
   D. Varying degrees of pancreatic beta cell dysfunction
   E. Young, lean patient with abrupt onset of clinical disease

3. Which of the following best describes insulin-dependent diabetes mellitus (IDDM)?
   A. Also known as type II diabetes
   B. Highest prevalence in non-whites
   C. Most common form of diabetes
   D. Peak age at onset between 10 and 14 years
   E. Varying degrees of pancreatic beta-cell dysfunction

4. What is the best description of glycogen?
   A. Inhibits gluconeogenesis and glycogenolysis
   B. Major counter-regulatory hormone
   C. Suppresses hepatic ketone production
   D. Unimportant in the pathogenesis of DKA
   E. Works in synergy with insulin

5. Which of the following is most accurate regarding the assessment of diabetic patients?
   A. Diagnosis can be made with a random plasma glucose level >150 mg/dl
   B. Dipstick methods for testing blood glucose are highly accurate
   C. Glycosylated hemoglobin (HBA1C) is an index of glucose concentration in the preceding 6-8 weeks
   D. Most important test is the formal glucose tolerance test
   E. Urine ketone dipsticks do not measure acetoacetate

6. Which of the following is most accurate regarding hypoglycemia in diabetics?
   A. Decreased exercise is a common cause
   B. D50W is appropriate treatment in young children
   C. Glucagon 10 mg IM can be used to treat adults

D. Hypoglycemia unawareness is associated with recurrent episodes

E. Symptoms begin at levels of 30 mg/dl or below

7. A 72-year-old diabetic man with mild renal insufficiency presents with confusion. Blood glucose is 24 mg/dl. He is treated with intravenous dextrose for 24 hours and discharged. Six hours later he returns with hypoglycemic coma. What hypoglycemic agent is the most likely cause of this?

A. Chlorpropamide

B. Glipizide

C. Metformin

E. Tolbutamide

E. Tolazamide

8. A 26-year-old salesman with IDDM presents with abdominal pain, vomiting, sunken eyes, dry tongue, and Kussmaul's respirations. Vital signs are BP, 120/60; P, 120; RR, 28; T, 37° C. Blood glucose via dipstick is 500 mg/dl. What is the most appropriate treatment?

A. D5 normal saline at 500 cc per hour

B. Normal saline at keep-open rate until laboratory results are back

C. Normal saline, 1 L over the first hour

D. Normal saline, 4 L over the first hour

E. 0.45% normal saline 2 L in the first hour, then 500 cc per hour

9. Which of the following best describes diabetic ketoacidosis (DKA)?

A. Acetoacetate is the predominant ketoacid

B. Acute abdominal pain is an uncommon symptom

C. Classically occurs in type 2 diabetics

D. Fever is typical

E. Mental status most closely correlates with osmolarity

10. Laboratory evaluation of the diabetic patient reveals the following: sodium, 132 mEq/L; potassium, 6.0 mEq/L; chloride, 106 mEq/L, bicarbonate, 8 mEq/L; blood glucose, 600 mg/dl; arterial pH, 7.10; and BUN, 48 mg/dl. Which of the following is correct?

A. Anion gap is 10

B. True serum potassium is 2

C. True serum potassium is 8

D. True serum sodium is 125

E. True serum sodium is 139

11. Which of the following is the most appropriate treatment of a patient in diabetic ketoacidosis?

A. Administer bicarbonate when the pH is lower than 7.1

B. Glucose should be added to fluids when the blood glucose is 250 mg/dl

C. Potassium phosphate therapy is routinely needed

D. Start D5.45 saline after 2 liters of normal saline

E. Urine ketone dipsticks accurately reflect the state of ketosis

12. A 5-year-old boy presents in diabetic ketoacidosis with a blood sugar of 620 and a pH of 7.0. He has been improving since receiving fluids and an insulin drip; values just measured are glucose, 150 and pH, 7.3. He complains of a headache and is becoming lethargic. What should be done first?

A. Administer D50W

B. Head CT scan

C. Insulin bolus

D. Intubation

E. Mannitol

13. When comparing diabetic ketoacidosis (DKA) to hyperglycemic hyperosmolar nonketotic coma (HHNC) which of the following best describes DKA?

A. Greater acidosis

B. Greater fluid and electrolyte deficits

C. Higher glucose

D. Higher mortality rate

E. Slower onset

14. What is the most common cause of mortality in diabetes?

A. Cardiovascular

B. Cerebrovascular

C. Diabetic coma

D. Infections

E. Renal failure

15. An elderly patient with decreasing level of consciousness over many days presents from a nursing home after a seizure. On examination she is lethargic and appears dehydrated. Vital signs are BP, 90/60; P, 120; R, 16; and T, 37° C. Laboratory values are sodium, 146 mEq/L; potassium, 5 mEq/L; chloride, 120 mEq/L; $HCO_3$, 22 mEq/L; glucose, 1200 mg/dl; and BUN, 60 mg/dl. Which of the following is most accurate?

A. Associated major infection or illness is likely

B. Focal deficits and seizures are an uncommon presentation

C. High doses of insulin are indicated

D. One half of the fluid deficit should be replaced in the first 2 hours

E. Phenytoin is indicated for treatment of a seizure

16. Which of the following is least likely to have symptoms similar to those of DKA?

A. Child who ingested a large amount of aspirin

B. Chronic alcoholic who has recently abstained from drinking

C. College student with acute renal failure

D. Nursing home resident with blood glucose of 800 mEq/dl

E. Teenager with heroin overdose

17. Which of the following best describes diabetic nephropathy?

A. Angiotensin converting enzyme inhibitors are contraindicated

B. Appearance of microalbuminuria correlates with coronary artery disease and retinopathy

C. Azotemia generally begins within 15 years of diabetes onset

D. Hypertension is associated with but does not accelerate its progression

E. Tight glycemic control has no effect on its progression

18. An elderly patient with long-standing diabetes complains of blurry vision. On ophthalmologic examination a vitreous hemorrhage is noted. What is the most likely associated type of diabetic eye disease?
    A. Background retinopathy
    B. Cataracts
    C. Ischemic optic neuropathy
    D. Maculopathy
    E. Proliferative retinopathy

*Both autonomic and peripheral neuropathy are well known complications of diabetes. Match the clinical presentation with the most appropriate type of neuropathy.*

    A. Diabetic autonomic neuropathy
    B. Diabetic truncal mononeuropathy
    C. Mononeuropathy multiplex
    D. Peripheral sensory neuropathy

19. Altered sympathetic and parasympathetic function _____
20. Manifests bilaterally in the extremities; distal sections of nerves are involved more intensely _____
21. Sensory disorder that may mimic a sympathetic function _____
22. Sudden onset of wrist drop, foot drop, or paralysis of cranial nerves III, IV, or VI _____
23. Which of the following best describes diabetes in pregnancy?
    A. Associated with a regression of retinopathy
    B. Diabetes disease course generally improves
    C. Diabetic ketoacidosis has a 50%-90% maternal mortality
    D. Hypoglycemia is uncommon
    E. Perinatal mortality correlates with glycemic control

    D. Infections
    E. Trauma
3. What is the most likely serious complication of rhabdomyolysis?
    A. Acute renal failure
    B. Compartment syndromes
    C. Disseminated intravascular coagulopathy (DIC)
    D. Hepatic insufficiency
    E. Hyperkalemia
4. What is the most common cause of acute renal failure associated with rhabdomyolysis?
    A. Acute glomerular nephritis (AGN)
    B. Acute intrinsic renal failure (AIRF)
    C. Hyperkalemia
    D. Increased renal vascular resistance
    E. Obstruction of the urinary outflow tract by muscle breakdown products
5. What is the most appropriate initial treatment for rhabdomyolysis?
    A. Acid diuresis
    B. Alkaline diuresis
    C. Dialysis
    D. Frequent monitoring of compartment pressures
    E. Mannitol and furosemide
6. Which of the following is most characteristic of specific metabolic disorders and rhabdomyolysis?
    A. Hypercalcemia occurs early and does not require therapy
    B. Hyperkalemia is a cause
    C. Hyperuricemia is a cause
    D. Hypocalcemia is the most common associated abnormality
    E. Hypophosphatemia is a complication

## Rhabdomyolysis

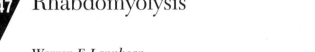

*Warren F. Lanphear*

Select the appropriate letter that correctly answers the question or completes the statement.

1. Which of the following is most characteristic of rhabdomyolysis?
    A. Caused by injury to the smooth muscle
    B. Diagnosis depends on characteristic physical findings
    C. Final common pathway of injury involves damage to the sarcolemma
    D. Measurement of serum myoglobin is a practical way to make the diagnosis
    E. No anion gap
2. Which of the following is least likely to cause rhabdomyolysis?
    A. Alcohol
    B. Drugs
    C. Idiopathic

## Endocrine Disorders

*Jeffrey S. Jones*

Select the appropriate letter that correctly answers the question or completes the statement.

1. Which of the following best describes thyroid storm?
    A. Associated with a sudden increase in serum catecholamine levels
    B. At greatest risk are women in their third and fourth decades
    C. Confirming laboratory tests include serum $T_3$ and $T_4$ levels
    D. Develops in 10%-20% of those with initially uncomplicated hyperthyroidism
    E. Usually preceded by Hashimoto's thyroiditis
2. A 48-year-old woman with a history of Graves' disease presents several hours after outpatient dental surgery. She is delirious and agitated. Vital signs are: BP, 150/70; P, 150; R, 36; T, 39.2° C. Physical examination is other-

wise unremarkable. Which of the following should be given first?
- A. Dexamethasone 2 mg IV
- B. Potassium iodide 3-5 drops PO/NG
- C. Propranolol 1-2 mg slow IV
- D. Propylthiouracil 150 mg PO/NG
- E. Sodium bicarbonate 88 mEq (2 ampules) IV

3. What drug should be avoided in the treatment of thyroid storm and its complications?
- A. Acetaminophen
- B. Aspirin
- C. Corticosteroids
- D. Digitalis
- E. Loop diuretics

4. What is the most common precipitating factor in the development of myxedema coma?
- A. Drugs
- B. Exposure to cold
- C. Hypoxia
- D. Infection
- E. Trauma

5. A 42-year-old woman with a family history of hypothyroidism secondary to Hashimoto's thyroiditis presents with lethargy, cold intolerance, weight gain, and dry skin. What is the best test for confirming the clinical impression of primary hypothyroidism?
- A. Free thyroxine ($FT_4$)
- B. Free thyroxine ($FT_4$) plus triiodothyronine ($T_3$ level)
- C. $FT_4$ index
- D. Serum TSH assay
- E. Triiodothyronine ($T_3$ level)

6. A 65-year-old boarding house tenant is found stuporous in his room by fellow lodgers. An empty thyroxine prescription bottle is found in his room. On examination, the patient is comatose; pulse is 52; and rectal temperature is 30.2° C. There is a midline, transverse scar in the lower neck. Rales are heard at the base of the left lung. What should be the initial management?
- A. Administration of levothyroxine ($T_4$) 300-500 g IV
- B. Determination of glucose
- C. Drawing of arterial blood-gas measurement
- D. Evaluation for infection
- E. Passive rewarming

7. A 33-year-old woman with a history of asthma has symptoms of adrenal insufficiency. What is the most likely etiology of her condition?
- A. Hypoglycemia
- B. Idiopathic
- C. Long-term glucocorticoid therapy
- D. Pituitary insufficiency
- E. Pulmonary infection

8. What laboratory abnormality is typical of primary adrenal insufficiency?
- A. Hypernatremia
- B. Hypocalcemia
- C. Hypoglycemia
- D. Hypokalemia
- E. Hypophosphatemia

9. What test should be selected to differentiate between primary and secondary adrenal insufficiency?
- A. ACTH 48-hour stimulation test
- B. Arterial blood gas
- C. Dexamethasone suppression test
- D. Electrolytes
- E. 24-hour urine for 17-hydroxysteroid determination

10. A 23-year-old diabetic is referred to the ED with undiagnosed but suspected severe adrenocortical insufficiency. What medication should be given without delay?
- A. Cortisone acetate
- B. Dexamethasone phosphate
- C. Florinef
- D. Glucagon
- E. Hydrocortisone hemisuccinate

---

**SECTION 10  SYSTEMIC INFECTIONS**

## 149 Bacterial Infections

*Michael D. Brown*

Select the appropriate letter that correctly answers the question or completes the statement.

1. Which of the following best describes respiratory diphtheria?
- A. Effects of the disease are limited to the respiratory tract
- B. Positive throat culture for group A beta-hemolytic streptococcus essentially excludes the diagnosis
- C. Prevention requires primary immunization plus a booster every 10 years
- D. Transmission is via animal vector to human
- E. Treatment is with erythromycin or penicillin

2. Which of the following characterizes cutaneous diphtheria?
- A. Occurs mostly in the tropics
- B. Often advances to myocarditis
- C. Victims appear ill
- D. Wounds are easily distinguishable from those of other chronic skin conditions
- E. Wounds are not a source of infectious spread

3. Which of the following is least important when administering diphtheria antitoxin?
- A. Duration of illness
- B. Immunization status
- C. Location of the membrane
- D. Overall degree of toxicity
- E. Size of the membrane

4. An infant presents with paroxysmal coughing thought to be caused by pertussis. What is an associated finding?
   A. Expiratory "whoops" during the cough paroxysms
   B. High fever
   C. Lack of preceding upper respiratory infection
   D. Lymphocytosis
   E. Ill appearance between coughing episodes

5. Which of the following best describes pertussis vaccine when it is given according to the recommended schedule?
   A. Causes less adverse reactions than other childhood vaccines
   B. Is 50%-75% effective
   C. Produces life-long immunity
   D. Rarely causes fever and irritability
   E. Severe neurologic complications can occur

6. Which of the following differentiates tetanus from rabies?
   A. Drooling
   B. Dysphagia
   C. Improvement with diphenhydramine
   D. Respiratory muscle dysfunction
   E. Trismus

7. Human tetanus immune globulin (TIG) is utilized to achieve which of the following effects?
   A. Active immunity
   B. Active and passive immunity
   C. Neutralization of toxin already in the nervous system
   D. Neutralization of toxin at the site of toxin production
   E. Treatment of any symptoms already occurring

8. Which of the following best describes the management of suspected tetanus?
   A. Diagnosis is excluded if there is no history of a wound
   B. Local injection of tetanus immune globulin (TIG) is recommended
   C. Nondepolarizing neuromuscular blocking agents are contraindicated
   D. Prognosis worsens with longer incubation period
   E. Repeat dose of TIG is not required

9. Which of the following best describes infant botulism?
   A. Caused by the ingestion of spores
   B. Characterized by fever
   C. Common presentation is diarrhea
   D. Rare form of botulism
   E. Usually occurs in the 1- to 2-year-old age-group

10. Myasthenia gravis can resemble botulism. Which of the following would help distinguish one from the other?
    A. Dysphasia
    B. Extraocular palsies
    C. Fixed, dilated pupils
    D. Peripheral weakness
    E. Ptosis

11. Botulism antitoxin is characterized by which of the following?
    A. Adverse reaction in approximately 50% of patients
    B. Cannot bind circulating neurotoxin
    C. Hypersensitivity testing is not needed
    D. Neutralizes bound toxin
    E. Not beneficial in infant botulism

12. A febrile 18-month-old was placed on amoxicillin for otitis media 24 hours ago. A blood culture drawn at the time was positive but the sensitivity is not yet known. What is the most appropriate follow-up?
    A. Admit for intravenous antibiotics
    B. Change antibiotic for broader spectrum coverage
    C. Contact parents by telephone to reinforce giving amoxicillin as ordered
    D. Return for reevaluation
    E. Wait until sensitivity is available

13. Which of the following is characteristic of overwhelming postsplenectomy infection (OPSI)?
    A. Adrenal hemorrhages and DIC
    B. Decreasing risk of occurrences with increasing time since splenectomy
    C. Fever with maculopapular rash
    D. Occurs rarely
    E. Unchanged incidence in asplenic patients despite pneumococcal vaccination

14. What is the most common initial characteristic of the meningococcemia rash?
    A. Location on the face
    B. Maculopapular
    C. Present only with fever
    D. Pustular
    E. Vesicular

15. Which of the following is predictive of a poor prognosis in meningococcemia?
    A. Absence of fever
    B. Elevated peripheral white blood cell count >15,000
    C. Elevated platelet count
    D. Elevated sedimentation rate
    E. Petechiae within 12 hours of admission

16. An 18-month-old Asian child presents with a 1-week history of fever. He has developed a rash, bilateral conjunctivitis, and cervical adenopathy. Which of the following symptoms would be sufficient to make the diagnosis of Kawasaki disease?
    A. Coryza
    B. Nail bed hemorrhages
    C. Palmar erythema with edema
    D. Petechia
    E. Tonsillar hypertrophy

17. Which of the following is the cornerstone of treatment for Kawasaki disease?
    A. Acetaminophen and gamma globulin
    B. Aspirin and gamma globulin
    C. Ibuprofen
    D. Steroids
    E. Warfarin and heparin

18. In the revised case definition of toxic shock, which of the following is included as diagnostic criteria?
    A. Exclusion of Rocky Mountain spotted fever by titers
    B. Desquamation
    C. Hypertension
    D. Positive *Staphylococcus aureus* blood culture
    E. Vesicular rash

# 150 Viral Infections

*Warren F. Lanphear*

Select the appropriate letter that correctly answers the question or completes the statement.

1. Which of the following best describes immune globulin?
   A. Can transmit HIV
   B. Cannot transmit hepatitis B
   C. Given intramuscularly for active immunization against measles and hepatitis B
   D. Not given intravenously
   E. Prepared from an individual donor

2. Which of the following describes the appropriate use of amantadine?
   A. Contraindicated in the elderly
   B. Contraindicated when the influenza vaccine is also contraindicated
   C. 5-7 days of therapy should be initiated within 2 days of onset of symptoms
   D. Given daily for the entire flu season to high-risk people following the influenza vaccine
   E. Provides prevention and treatment of influenza B

3. Which of the following best describes herpes simplex (HSV) encephalitis?
   A. Acyclovir contraindicated before definite HSV identification
   B. Culture of the CSF generally positive for HSV
   C. Focal neurologic signs often localized to the temporal lobe
   D. Has a distinct clinical picture
   E. Has a seasonal, epidemic occurrence

4. Which of the following statements best describes herpes zoster?
   A. Not highly contagious
   B. Occurs predominantly in younger persons
   C. Oral acyclovir is adequate for multi-dermatome zoster
   D. Post-herpetic neuralgia can be effectively treated
   E. Varicella zoster immune globulin should be given within 72 hours to susceptible immunocompromised patients exposed to infected individuals

5. When comparing cytomegalovirus (CMV) infection to infectious mononucleosis caused by Epstein-Barr virus, what best describes CMV infection?
   A. Heterophile negative
   B. Immunocompetent patients need antiviral chemotherapy
   C. Liver involvement is common
   D. Organ transplant recipients are at risk for lymphoma
   E. Perinatal infection resembles toxoplasmosis

6. Which of the following best describes roseola infantum?
   A. Fever precedes rash by 3-5 days
   B. Most commonly seen in the 5 to 8 year old
   C. Rash initially appears on face and extremities
   D. Treatment is with acyclovir ointment
   E. Vomiting and diarrhea are common

7. Which of the following characterizes erythema infectiosum?
   A. Caused by the same parvovirus responsible for transient aplastic crisis in patients with chronic hemolytic anemia
   B. Causes dramatic prodromal, constitutional symptoms in children
   C. Constitutional symptoms are uncommon in adults
   D. "Slapped cheek" appearance is classic under the age of 2 years
   E. Usually causes a high fever before the rash

8. When comparing parainfluenza virus infections with respiratory syncytial virus (RSV) infections, which of the following is more characteristic of parainfluenza?
   A. Accounts for greatest number of hospitalizations for respiratory infections in infants
   B. Major cause of bronchiolitis
   C. Most common cause of croup
   D. Reinfection does not occur
   E. Results in pneumonia

9. Which of the following best describes the current measles vaccine?
   A. Incidence of measles has not decreased since the two-dose regimen was initiated
   B. Infants should be immunized with it at age 2 months, along with their DPT and OPV
   C. Is an inactivated vaccine
   D. Second dose converts 95% of initial vaccine seroconversion failures
   E. 25% of recipients fail to seroconvert after a single dose

10. Which of the following best describes enterovirus infection?
    A. Chiefly spread by respiratory secretions
    B. Has a distinctive rash
    C. Most common cause of viral meningitis
    D. Most infections are symptomatic
    E. Vomiting and diarrhea are often present

# 151 AIDS and HIV Infection

*Bruce W. Nugent*

Select the appropriate letter that correctly answers the question or completes the statement.

1. Within the United States, in which of the following groups is the proportion of AIDS cases decreasing?
   A. Homosexual/bisexual
   B. Injection drug use
   C. Non-urban (rural) area residents
   D. Socioeconomically disadvantaged and minorities
   E. Women

2. A patient arrives distressed because he has just been notified of a positive EIA HIV test he had for insurance purposes. He is heterosexual, never used intravenous drugs or received blood products, and lives in Wyoming. What best describes appropriate testing procedures?
   A. If a Western blot test is not conclusive, then no further testing is indicated
   B. Initial EIA test should be repeated as it may be falsely positive
   C. Use of the EIA test in an area with high seroprevalence improves the test sensitivity
   D. Use of the EIA test in an area with low seroprevalence improves the test specificity
   E. Western blot test will be done after the EIA since it is more specific but less sensitive

3. An ED staff member sustains a percutaneous puncture from a needle just used in a venous blood draw of an HIV-infected patient. What best describes this situation?
   A. Estimated risk of acquiring HIV is approximately 1 in 500
   B. Maximal benefit of postexposure prophylaxis with antiretroviral therapy is gained when initiated within 72 hours
   C. Negative HIV antibody test at 4 weeks rules out transmission to the staff member
   D. Postexposure prophylaxis with antiretroviral therapy is not indicated unless the source patient is symptomatic
   E. Transmission risk is typically greater than with a suture needle puncture

4. A 26-year-old HIV positive male has a nonproductive cough, hypoxia, and increased serum lactate dehydrogenase. Chest x-ray is normal. Which of the following best describes this patient's condition?
   A. Approximately 30% of patients will respond to treatment
   B. Frequency of adverse reactions to treatment is more common than in the general population
   C. Gallium scanning of the chest is frequently positive, with few false-positive results
   D. Positive Gram stain is expected
   E. Treatment with steroids increases morbidity

5. Which of the following best describes *Mycobacterium tuberculosis* (MTB) in HIV disease?
   A. AIDS patients with tuberculosis should receive a four-drug regimen
   B. Diagnosis is reliably made on chest x-ray
   C. Extrapulmonary disease occurs in up to 25% of cases
   D. Negative PPD rules out infection
   E. Usually occurs late in the course of HIV disease

6. A 28-year-old HIV-positive man presents with 3 days of frontal headache, diminished affect, and memory loss. He has no focal neurologic deficit, fever, or meningismus. Of the following, which is the most likely diagnosis?
   A. Cryptococcal meningitis
   B. Frontal sinusitis

C. Herpes simplex encephalitis
D. HIV-associated depression
E. HIV encephalopathy

7. A 33-year-old HIV-positive female presents with new onset of fever, headache, and right-sided seizure disorder. Which best describes the most common cause of focal encephalitis in AIDS patients?
   A. Characteristic CSF findings are low glucose, high protein, and lymphocytic pleocytosis
   B. Chronic suppressive therapy is usually indicated
   C. Clinical and radiographic features are pathognomonic
   D. Diagnosis is made by CSF India ink preparation
   E. Failure to respond to treatment is common

8. Which of the following best describes oral candidiasis?
   A. Characterized by white plaques that are difficult to scrape away from the base
   B. Involvement usually spares the tongue
   C. It is unrelated to development of other opportunistic infections
   D. Most cases will ultimately require inpatient treatment with systemic ketoconazole
   E. Nystatin suspension is a less effective treatment than clotrimazole troches

9. Diarrhea is the most common gastrointestinal complaint in AIDS patients. Which of the following organisms is most likely to be associated with bacteremia in HIV patients?
   A. *Campylobacter jejuni*
   B. *Cryptosporidium* species
   C. Cytomegalovirus (CMV)
   D. *Isospora* species
   E. *Salmonella* species

10. Herpes infections are common in AIDS patients. Which best describes appropriate treatment?
    A. Herpes simplex infections respond well to standard acyclovir therapy
    B. Intravenous acyclovir treatment is always indicated for herpes zoster in the HIV patient
    C. Ophthalmic zoster does not warrant inpatient treatment
    D. Suppressive therapy for herpes simplex is ineffective in the HIV patient
    E. Varicella immune globulin is indicated in herpes zoster

## 152 Occupational Health in the Emergency Department: Principles and Practice

*No questions*

## 153 Parasitology

*Warren F. Lanphear*

Select the appropriate letter that correctly answers the question or completes the statement.

1. What causes the shaking chills and fever of malaria?
   A. Free sporozoites in the bloodstream after the mosquito's blood meal
   B. Invasion of the spleen by parasitized red blood cells
   C. Lysis of hepatic cells with release of merozoites
   D. Merozoite release from disintegrating red blood cells
   E. White blood cell lysis and release of trophozoites

2. What causes African sleeping sickness?
   A. Freshwater amebas
   B. Hemoflagellates transmitted by the tsetse fly
   C. Larval forms of the pork tapeworm
   D. *Plasmodium falciparum*
   E. *Trypanosoma cruzi*

3. What is the best way to prevent hookworm infection?
   A. Avoiding raw fish
   B. Cooking pork well
   C. Hand washing
   D. Purifying drinking water
   E. Wearing shoes

4. If not treated promptly, swimmer's itch caused by the avian schistosome *Trichobilharzia ocellata* will follow which of the following clinical courses?
   A. Deep scarring
   B. Hepatic abscesses
   C. Retinal invasion
   D. Spontaneous resolution
   E. Suppurative lymphadenitis

5. A patient who recently returned from South America complains of recurrent fevers and has a new right bundle branch block on his ECG. He recalls an insect bite on his face with a lot of local inflammation. What is the most likely diagnosis?
   A. Ascariasis
   B. Chagas' disease
   C. Leishmaniasis
   D. Onchocerciasis
   E. Schistosomiasis

6. A pregnant 21-year-old woman has epigastric pain and malodorous diarrhea after returning from a backpacking trip in the North Country. No cysts, ova, or organisms are seen in her stool, but the history is suspicious for *Giardia* infection. What will be most helpful in making the diagnosis?
   A. Colonoscopy
   B. Duodenal aspiration or fuzzy string retrieval
   C. Giardia toxin assay
   D. Oral metronidazole
   E. Stool culture

7. With no history of travel outside of the United States, which of the following parasitic infections is highly unlikely?
   A. *Ascaris lumbricoides* (roundworm)
   B. *Echinococcus granulosus* (tapeworm causing hydatid cysts)
   C. *Leishmania tropica* (protozoan)
   D. *Taenia saginata* (beef tapeworm)
   E. *Trichinella spiralis* (nematode causing trichinosis)

8. A middle-aged man with bloody diarrhea has multiple negative stool cultures. What parasite is most likely to be responsible for his illness?
   A. *Ascaris lumbricoides* (roundworm)
   B. *Entamoeba histolytica*
   C. *Enterobius vermicularis* (pinworm)
   D. *Giardia lamblia*
   E. *Trichuris trichiura* (whipworm)

9. Which of the following is least likely with a *Trichomonas vaginalis* infection?
   A. Irreversible sterility in males
   B. Pelvic pain in females
   C. Prostatitis
   D. Urethritis
   E. Vulvar pruritus

10. In which of the following diseases is hepatosplenomegaly a frequent finding?
    A. Giardiasis
    B. Intestinal schistosomiasis
    C. Onchocerciasis
    D. Strongyloidiasis
    E. Trichuriasis

Tick-Borne Illnesses

*Michael D. Brown*

Select the appropriate letter that correctly answers the question or completes the statement.

1. Which of the following best describes Lyme disease?
    A. Erythema chronicum migrans is seen in about 75% of cases
    B. Etiologic agent is the rickettsia *Borrelia burgdorferi*
    C. Most commonly affected age-groups are middle-aged and older adults
    D. Nearly two thirds of patients recall a tick bite
    E. Peak incidence of early disease is September to November

2. A 14-year-old boy states that 4 weeks ago he had a 20-cm area of erythema on his lower right leg with central clearing. This was present for 2 weeks, and was associated with flu-like illness. He was then asymptomatic for 2 weeks, and now he has headache and lethargy. Which of the following is most likely present?
    A. Abnormal CSF examination
    B. Abnormal CT of head
    C. Intact cranial nerves
    D. Intact sensory examination results
    E. Positive Kernig's and Brudzinski's signs

3. Which of the following best describes cardiac abnormalities in Lyme disease?
    A. Commonly see asymptomatic AV block
    B. Gradual resolution of AV block
    C. More common than neurologic manifestations
    D. Most common presentation is pericarditis
    E. Results in severe and persistent left ventricular dysfunction

4. A 26-year-old woman who is 3 months pregnant presents with a history of tick bite and the rash of erythema chronicum migrans. She has no medical problems or allergies. What is the treatment of choice?
    A. Amoxicillin
    B. Doxycycline
    C. Erythromycin
    D. None until after delivery
    E. Wait until after delivery, discourage breast-feeding, and treat with tetracycline

5. Which best describes Lyme disease?
    A. Chronic arthritis (stage III) is responsive to antibiotics
    B. Culture of blood and tissue for *Borrelia burgdorferi* is recommended
    C. Pregnant patients with tick exposure should be treated with empiric antibiotics
    D. Secondary skin lesions usually involve the palms and soles
    E. Tick larvae are primarily responsible for disease transmission to humans

6. Which of the following best describes endemic relapsing fever, a tick-borne disease found primarily in the western mountain states of the U.S.?
    A. Drug of choice is penicillin G
    B. Each successive fever relapse is more severe than the last
    C. Jarisch-Herxheimer reaction occurs within a few days of treatment
    D. Responsible organisms are rickettsia
    E. Responsible organisms are visible on routine blood smear

7. A 9-year-old boy has fever, headache, myalgias, and a pink maculopapular rash that started on the wrists, palms, forearms, soles, and ankles following a camping trip 1 week earlier. What is the best rapid diagnostic test?
    A. Blood culture
    B. Complete blood cell count for thrombocytopenia
    C. Latex hemagglutination
    D. Skin biopsy immunofluorescence
    E. Weil-Felix test

8. What percentage of patients with Rocky Mountain spotted fever present within the first 3 days of illness with the triad of rash, fever, and history of tick exposure?
    A. 3
    B. 20
    C. 36
    D. 51
    E. 82

9. What is the antibiotic of choice in a 4 year old with Rocky Mountain spotted fever?
    A. Ceftriaxone
    B. Chloramphenicol
    C. Clindamycin
    D. Erythromycin
    E. Tetracycline

10. What is the recommended method for tick removal?
    A. Grab with bare fingers
    B. Hot match to dorsum of tick
    C. Slow traction with tweezers
    D. Spray with ethyl chloride
    E. "Unscrew" in counterclockwise motion

 Tuberculosis

*Michael D. Brown and Gwen L. Hoffman*

Select the appropriate letter that correctly answers the question or completes the statement.

1. *Mycobacterium tuberculosis* (MTB) is the organism primarily responsible for tuberculosis in the human population. Which one of the following best describes MTB in the United States?
    A. Homeless population is the main reservoir
    B. Mice are the main nonhuman reservoir
    C. Rapid generation time is a critical characteristic

D. Transmission of disease is by fomites, which requires decontamination of clothing and eating utensils

E. Transmission rarely occurs outdoors

2. Which of the following best describes the clinical features of pulmonary tuberculosis?

A. Elderly may have a "brassy" cough

B. Generalized malaise with weight loss is rare

C. Hemoptysis is the most common presenting symptom

D. Initial infection is most often asymptomatic in healthy patients

E. Spiking fever at night frequently occurs

3. What is the most common complication of pulmonary tuberculosis?

A. Empyema

B. Endobronchial spread

C. Pericarditis

D. Pneumothorax

E. Superinfection

4. In a tuberculosis patient, what does this chest x-ray represent? (Figure 155-1).

A. Cavitary lesion

B. Empyema

C. Ghon focus

D. Pneumothorax

E. Superinfection

5. A 23-year-old migrant worker presents with a 2-week history of weight loss, fevers, cough, and mild shortness of breath when working. What best describes an evaluation for possible TB?

A. Elevated erythrocyte sedimentation rate (ESR) is the most useful test result in establishing the diagnosis in the ED

B. Infiltrate with enlarged hilar nodes on chest x-ray is strongly suggestive of the diagnosis

C. Negative acid-fast bacillus (AFB) smear rules out active TB

D. Normal chest x-ray excludes active TB

E. Tuberculin skin testing is an excellent modality to determine the presence of active disease

6. A 5-year-old boy presents with a diagnosis of primary tuberculosis. Which of the following best describes his chest x-ray?

A. Bilateral lower lobe infiltrates

B. Cavitary lesions in the apex

C. Ghon focus

D. Massive hilar adenopathy

E. Small pleural effusion

7. Purified protein derivative (PPD) is an important tool used in the management of tuberculosis. What best describes its use?

A. BCG vaccination may cause a false-negative reaction

B. Extent of erythema is the key measurement for skin testing

C. Healthy individual who remains PPD negative after heavy exposure does not require therapy

D. Induration ≥5 mm in diameter is considered a positive test result in patients with no risk factors for TB

E. Live MMR vaccination may cause a false-positive reaction

8. Which of the following best describes extrapulmonary tuberculosis?

A. Incision and drainage is recommended for the treatment of scrofula

B. Miliary TB is most common in children

C. Spinal TB (Potts' disease) is easily detected on initial plain films

D. Tuberculous lymphadenitis usually consists of a painful red fluctuant mass in the cervical chain

E. Tuberculous meningitis usually requires multiple lumbar punctures to obtain positive culture results

9. A 30-year-old man with a history of right-sided pulmonary TB presents with massive hemoptysis. What management is contraindicated?

A. Intubate with large endotracheal tube (ETT)

B. Obtain consultation for bronchoscopy

C. Place ETT into right mainstem bronchus

D. Position ETT above the carina

E. Position with right side dependent

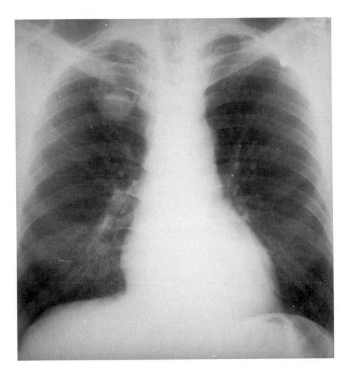

FIG. 155-1
Radiography courtesy John Pearce, M.D.

10. A 26-year-old female presents with weight loss, fatigue, night sweats, and persistent nonproductive cough over the last 3 weeks. The physical examination is normal, but the chest x-ray reveals bilateral upper lobe infiltrates with hilar adenopathy. A sputum sample is negative for AFB. Further history reveals that the patient works at a nursing home that had a recent outbreak of tuberculosis. What is the best treatment?
    A. Ethambutol and INH for 6 months
    B. If the patient is pregnant, supplemental pyridoxine should be given if receiving INH
    C. INH for 8 months
    D. None until a positive AFB smear is obtained
    E. Three-drug regimen for 6 months
11. When describing multiple-drug-resistant tuberculosis (MDRTB), which of the following is least accurate?
    A. Can result when a single drug is added to a failing regimen
    B. Co-infection with HIV is common
    C. Occurs with resistance to two or more first-time antituberculosis agents
    D. Transmission is usually from an MDRTB patient to a person with risk factors for MDRTB
    E. Well-documented spread from patient to patient and from patient to health care worker
12. Which of the following people with active pulmonary tuberculosis may safely be treated as an outpatient?
    A. 25-year-old with active MDRTB
    B. 35-year-old with HIV
    C. 40-year-old health care worker
    D. 60-year-old with fever and vomiting
    E. 80-year-old living alone

# 156 Bone and Joint Infections

*Michael D. Brown*

Select the appropriate letter that correctly answers the question or completes the statement.
1. In which of the following age-groups does the vascular anatomy prevent extension of bone infection from the metaphysis into the joint?
    A. Adult
    B. Child
    C. Elderly
    D. Infant
    E. Newborn
2. Which of the following is at risk for *Pseudomonas* osteomyelitis?
    A. Cat bite of the hand
    B. Child with acute hematogenous osteomyelitis
    C. Fresh-water contaminated wound
    D. Puncture wound through tennis shoe
    E. Sexually active young adult

*Match the conditions below with the appropriate question.*
    A. Gonococcal arthritis
    B. Polymicrobial infection
    C. *Pseudomonas* osteomyelitis
    D. *Salmonella* osteomyelitis
    E. *Staphylococcus aureus* infection
3. A 17-year-old female otherwise healthy just completed her menstrual period. She now presents with 3 days of fever and a hot, swollen, red left index finger PIP joint
4. A 16-year-old presents with a puncture wound sustained 4 days ago when a nail went through his tennis shoe into his foot. He now complains of pain, swelling, and redness of the sole of his foot
5. A 65-year-old woman with diabetes mellitus has a history of foot ulcers. She now complains of increased swelling and redness over the base of her second right toe with minimal pain
6. A 10-year-old black male with a history of sickle cell anemia complains of fever and severe pain in his right hip with no history of trauma
7. This is the leading cause of osteomyelitis in all age-groups except neonates and accounts for more cases of septic arthritis than any other bacterium
8. Which of the following statements is true regarding the diagnosis of osteomyelitis?
    A. Bone scanning with technetium methylene diphosphonate ($^{9m}$Tc MDP) is a very sensitive test for osteomyelitis in patients who have no existing bone abnormalities
    B. Plain radiographs are usually diagnostic early in the course of osteomyelitis and are useful in tracking the response to treatment
    C. Sedimentation rate is less helpful than the WBC count and is an insensitive marker of osteomyelitis
    D. There is usually a significant left shift
    E. WBC count is usually elevated, often greater than 15,000 per mm$^3$
9. Which of the following is characteristic of joint fluid analysis?
    A. Blood culture bottles may be used for joint fluid
    B. Culture from joint fluid is negative in 50% of suspected septic joints
    C. Glucose level is usually increased in the aspirate of a septic joint
    D. Risk of introducing infection during aspiration is 1 in 100
    E. WBC count of greater than 1000 is diagnostic of a septic joint
10. A febrile 3-year-old boy presents with knee pain for the past 2 days. He has a warm, erythematous knee with a joint effusion. He will not flex or extend the knee because of pain. What would be most characteristic of his joint fluid analysis?
    A. High lactic acid level
    B. High synovial fluid-to-blood glucose ratio
    C. Negative culture

D. Negative Gram stain

E. Tight mucin clot

11. Which of the following best describes gonococcal septic arthritis?

A. Joint fluid analysis shows more than 100,000 WBCs

B. Mucosal surface culture is more likely to be positive than joint aspirate culture

C. Polyarticular arthritis is more common than mono-articular arthritis

D. Predominant early complaints are fever, chills, and malaise

E. Tenosynovitis is rare

---

# 157 Soft-Tissue Infections

### Scott A. Carlson

Select the appropriate letter that correctly answers the question or completes the statement.

1. A 2-year-old boy with no significant past medical history presents with facial cellulitis. His temperature is 38.5° C and WBC is 17,000 with a left shift. Blood cultures are drawn and return positive within 48 hours. What is the most likely organism?

A. Beta-hemolytic *Streptococcus*

B. *Haemophilus influenzae B*

C. *Neisseria gonorrhoeae*

D. *Staphylococcus aureus*

E. *Streptococcus pyogenes*

2. A 9-year-old boy with no significant past medical history presents with a "swollen eye." Although the child is afebrile and without signs of infection, his right eye seems to show some mild proptosis with surrounding erythema and edema. His ocular mobility is normal and without discomfort. What is the best management?

A. Admit for broad-spectrum antibiotic therapy

B. Discharge with oral antibiotics and strict instructions to return promptly if eye pain or mobility problems develop

C. Obtain orbital CT scan and admit for IV antibiotics regardless of results because of the concern for orbital cellulitis

D. Obtain orbital CT scan and discharge with oral antibiotics and close follow-up if it is negative

E. Start IV antibiotics immediately and obtain orbital/sinus plain films to look for retro-orbital gas or abscess formation

3. Which of the following best describes toxic shock syndrome (TSS)?

A. Fever above 40° C is necessary to make the diagnosis

B. Hypotension is an absolute criterion for its diagnosis

C. Incidence of TSS appears to be increasing with popularity of tampon use

D. Rash seen on presentation typically is erythematous with skin desquamation

E. Since the clinical manifestations are secondary to a toxin, antibiotic treatment is often not necessary

4. Which of the following best describes staphylococcal scalded skin syndrome?

A. Blister fluid and skin are usually sterile

B. Mucous membranes are usually involved

C. Usual age range is from 3 months to 3 years

D. Usually has a negative Nikolsky's sign

E. Usually not treated with antibiotics since secondary to a toxin

5. Impetigo is a superficial infection of the skin. There are two distinct subtypes: impetigo contagiosa usually caused by beta-hemolytic *Streptococcus* and bullous impetigo caused by *Staphylococcus aureus*. Which of the following best describes this condition?

A. Impetigo contagiosa lesions tend to heal faster than those of bullous impetigo

B. Oral cephalosporins are effective in treating both the contagiosa and bullous forms

C. Poststreptococcal rheumatic fever follows impetigo contagiosa more frequently than streptococcal pharyngitis

D. Systemic and topical antibiotics have been moderately effective in preventing poststreptococcal glomerulonephritis

E. Topical antimicrobial agents in combination with hexachlorophene are effective treatment for impetigo contagiosa

6. A sterile abscess may be found in which of the following?

A. Bartholin cyst

B. Cutaneous abscess secondary to parenteral drug abuse

C. Hidradenitis suppurativa

D. Perirectal abscess

E. Pilonidal abscess

7. Which of the following best describes a Bartholin cyst?

A. Drainage should take place from the mucosal rather than the cutaneous surface

B. *Gonococcus* is cultured 20% of the time

C. Poor hygiene and recurrent STDs are the main etiologies

D. Primary cyst excision is generally preferred because recurrence is so common

E. Systemic symptoms are common

8. Necrotizing fasciitis is the preferred term for soft tissue infections that have several other names (e.g., hemolytic streptococcal gangrene, Meleney's synergistic gangrene, Fournier's syndrome, postoperative progressive bacterial gangrene, clostridial cellulitis). Which of the following best describes this entity?

A. Can occasionally be successfully treated with incision and drainage of the leading edge coupled with broad-spectrum antibiotics

B. Classic radiographic findings are generally necessary to confirm the diagnosis

C. Intense pain and tenderness of the involved area are typical

D. Muscular involvement and dysfunction are common

E. Surgical debridement is always necessary for its successful treatment

## 158 ▼ Dental Disorders

*J. Leibovitz*

Select the appropriate letter that correctly answers the question or completes the statement.

1. In the treatment of traumatic injury to the teeth, which of the following is correct?
   A. An avulsed tooth should be transported in sterile water
   B. Avulsion of the primary teeth requires immediate reimplantation into the socket
   C. Ellis type II fractures involving the dentin require immediate dental consultation in the adult
   D. Subluxation of the tooth may be stabilized using periodontal pack

2. A 2-year-old child has edematous, bluish-red gingivae. The emergency physician must rule out which of the following conditions?
   A. Leukemia
   B. Pyogenic granuloma
   C. Systemic lupus erythematosus
   D. Thrombotic thrombocytopenic purpura

3. Tooth eruption, or teething, is often accompanied by:
   A. Constipation
   B. Dehydration
   C. Temperature above 101° F
   D. Vomiting

4. Which of the following statements is true regarding infections of dental origin?
   A. Ludwig's angina is a form of severe necrotizing gingivitis
   B. Penicillin is the antibiotic of choice in adult gingival infections
   C. Periapical abscess requires incision and drainage
   D. Periodontal abscess has a gray pseudomembrane covering the involved tissue

5. An adult has the sudden onset of excruciating pain 3 days after a tooth extraction. Treatment should include all of the following except which one?
   A. Antibiotics
   B. Medicated dental paste
   C. Nerve block with local anesthesia
   D. Vigorous irrigation of the socket in an attempt to restart bleeding

6. Which of the following statements is false when referring to acute necrotizing ulcerative gingivitis (ANUG)?
   A. ANUG is associated with some systemic symptoms including fever, malaise, and regional lymphadenopathy
   B. Immunologic factors play a role in the pathology of the disease

C. It has been associated with smoking, stress, fatigue, and local trauma
   D. It is the result of an inflammatory response to bacterial plaque and calculus, resulting in widespread extension throughout the gingival tissue
   E. Treatment consists of warm saline rinsing, improving oral hygiene, and systemic antibiotics

## 159 ▼ Ophthalmologic Disorders

*J. Leibovitz*

Select the appropriate letter that correctly answers the question or completes the statement.

1. A pin hole will not correct which of the following?
   A. Astigmatism
   B. Farsightedness
   C. Macular degeneration
   D. Nearsightedness

2. Which of the following is considered an ophthalmologic surgical emergency?
   A. Acutely expanding orbital hematoma with compromise of the retinal circulation
   B. Orbital floor fracture with persistent double vision
   C. Traumatic iridodialysis
   D. Vitreous hemorrhage
   E. All of the above

3. Which of the following is true of cyclopentolate (Cyclogyl)?
   A. Gives complete paralysis of accommodation
   B. Has maximal effect in 15-20 minutes
   C. Lasts 6-8 hours
   D. Provides cycloplegia without mydriasis

4. A healthy automobile mechanic arrives at the ED with a metallic corneal foreign body. After removal, a residual rust ring is seen. Which of the following is recommended?
   A. Complete and immediate removal
   B. Observation as an outpatient until it spontaneously clears
   C. Removal with a cotton-tipped applicator
   D. Removal within 24 hours

5. Which of the following is an indication that an eyelid laceration penetrated the orbital septum?
   A. Presence of Bell's phenomenon
   B. Ptosis
   C. Subconjunctival hemorrhage
   D. Visualization of fat in the wound

6. Which of the following is generally true of allergic conjunctivitis?
   A. Decreased visual acuity
   B. Eye pain
   C. Pruritus
   D. No seasonal variance
   E. Preauricular lymphadenopathy

7. Retina detachment is usually associated with which of the following?
   A. Farsightedness is a risk factor
   B. Flashing lights
   C. Macular involvement is common
   D. More common in males under age 45 with a history of floaters
   E. Severe pain

8. All of the following pharmacologic agents are useful in the treatment of acute angle closure glaucoma except which one?
   A. Acetazolamide
   B. Homatropine methylbromide
   C. Mannitol
   D. Oral glycerol
   E. Pilocarpine

9. Central retinal vein occlusion is characterized by which of the following?
   A. Brief, transient blindness or flickering vision
   B. Pale retina and optic disc with box car segmentation of the retinal veins
   C. Occurs from embolic phenomenon
   D. Treatment includes eye massage, acetazolamide, timolol, and increasing the $P_{CO_2}$
   E. Wide range of clinical symptoms

# 160 Ear, Nose, and Throat Emergencies

*J. Leibovitz*

Select the appropriate letter that correctly answers the question or completes the statement.

1. Which of the following is not associated with the Ramsey-Hunt syndrome?
   A. Ear pain
   B. Facial palsy
   C. Hyperacusis
   D. Treatment with systemic antivirals
   E. Vesicles

2. Which of the following is not a sensorineuronal cause of hearing loss?
   A. Acoustic neuroma
   B. Neurotoxicity secondary to aminoglycoside use
   C. Ischemia
   D. Perforated tympanic membrane
   E. Viral infections

3. A 30-year-old man comes to the ED complaining of decreased hearing in the right ear. His past medical history is significant for recent discharge following a long, complicated hospital course. With the Rinne test, he hears no better when the tuning fork tips are placed next to his ear than when he feels the tuning fork placed on his mastoid. The Weber test lateralizes to the right ear. Which of the following is the most likely cause of his hearing loss?

   A. Acoustic neuroma
   B. Aminoglycoside
   C. Furosemide
   D. Serous otitis media
   E. Viral neuritis

4. Which of the following is not a complication of otitis media?
   A. Brain abscess
   B. Hearing impairment
   C. Labyrinthitis
   D. Meningitis
   E. Trigeminal nerve palsies

5. Which of the following is not true of sialolithiasis?
   A. More common in children
   B. Mumps is the most common viral pathogen
   C. Pain and swelling in the affected gland are the most common presenting symptoms
   D. Staphylococci, streptococci, and pneumococci are prominent bacterial pathogens
   E. Submandibular gland is the most common site

6. Which of the following statements is true about epistaxis?
   A. Anterior epistaxis accounts for 75% of nosebleeds
   B. Anterior epistaxis requires immediate consultation with an otolaryngologist
   C. Anterior epistaxis usually originates from the turbinates of the lateral wall of the nasal cavity
   D. Posterior epistaxis is less likely to require hospitalization than anterior epistaxis
   E. Posterior epistaxis usually occurs from bleeding of the posterior branch of the sphenopalatine artery

**SECTION 12  IMMUNOLOGIC AND INFLAMMATORY DISORDERS**

# 161 Arthritis, Tendinitis, and Bursitis

*Patrick Brunett*

Select the appropriate letter that correctly answers the question or completes the statement.

1. Which of the following usually presents as a monarticular arthritis?
   A. Hepatitis
   B. Lyme disease
   C. Pseudogout
   D. Rheumatoid arthritis
   E. Systemic lupus

2. All of the following are associated with rheumatic fever except which one?
   A. Carditis
   B. Chorea
   C. Erythema marginatum
   D. Monarticular arthritis
   E. Subcutaneous nodules

3. All of the following statements are true of the laboratory evaluation of synovial fluid except which one?
   A. A white cell count >50,000/mm³ is consistent with septic arthritis, gout, and rheumatoid arthritis
   B. Most of the WBCs in severe inflammatory arthritis are PMNs
   C. Synovial fluid glucose of 75% of the serum level is a normal finding
   D. The calcium pyrophosphate crystals of pseudogout are rhomboidal and positively birefringent
   E. Uric acid crystals of gout are needle-like and negatively birefringent

4. Which of the following statements about septic arthritis is not true?
   A. In a patient with a history of gout, the presence of uric acid crystals in the synovial fluid essentially eliminates the diagnosis of septic arthritis
   B. Infants are at risk for *Escherichia coli* infection
   C. *Salmonella* infection is of particular concern in sickle cell patients
   D. *Staphylococcus aureus* is the most common etiology in adults
   E. *Staphylococcus epidermidis* is associated with prosthetic joints

5. All of the following statements about gout are true except which one?
   A. During acute flares, the serum uric acid level is helpful in making the diagnosis
   B. Fever and leukocytosis may both be present during a gouty flare
   C. Gout is less common in women because estrogens increase the renal excretion of uric acid
   D. The great toe MTP is the most common joint involved
   E. Thiazide diuretics increase serum uric acid levels

6. All of the following medications may be useful in the treatment of an acute attack of gout except which one?
   A. Adrenocorticotrophic hormone (ACTH)
   B. Allopurinol
   C. Colchicine
   D. Indomethacin
   E. Prednisone

7. Which of the following statements is true of pseudo-gout?
   A. Colchicine is ineffective in the treatment of pseudogout
   B. NSAIDs and steroids provide little relief during the acute attack
   C. The average attack of pseudogout is usually more severe than an attack of gout

   D. The knee is the most commonly involved joint
   E. None of the statements is true

8. All the following are true of gonococcal arthritis except which one?
   A. A rash of hemorrhagic, necrotic pustules beginning on the distal extremities is present in two thirds of patients
   B. Cervical, urethral, rectal, and pharyngeal cultures are more often positive for *Neisseria gonorrhoeae* than are blood cultures
   C. Most patients are young males
   D. Most patients do not complain of cervicitis or urethritis
   E. The illness begins with fever, chills, and a migratory tenosynovitis and polyarthritis

9. Which of the following statements is true regarding Lyme disease?
   A. Arthralgias, myalgias, and headache are early symptoms of the disease
   B. Arthritis and Bell's palsy occur in the second stage of the disease, approximately 4 weeks after the tick bite
   C. The arthritis is usually symmetric and polyarticular, involving predominantly the distal extremities
   D. The initial illness is seen in the late summer and early fall
   E. All of the statements are true

10. Which of the following statements is true of Reiter's syndrome?
    A. Arthritis is polyarticular and asymmetric and usually involves the weight-bearing joints of the lower extremity
    B. HLA-B27 is positive in most patients
    C. Reactive arthritis is most common in young males and usually follows an episode of urethritis or dysentery
    D. Tetracyclines may improve recovery in some patients
    E. All of the statements are true

11. All of the following statements about rheumatoid arthritis are true except which one?
    A. A prodrome of fatigue, weakness, and musculoskeletal pain may be present for weeks to months
    B. In the hands, the MCP, PIP, and DIP joints are equally involved
    C. Rheumatoid factor is positive in only 70% of the cases
    D. Joint swelling is polyarticular and symmetric and usually begins in the hands, wrists, and elbows
    E. Synovial fluid analysis reveals an inflammatory response, with 75% PMNs and a low glucose

12. Which of the following statements is true regarding bursitis?
    A. Anserine bursitis is a disease of runners that presents with erythema and warmth at the medial aspect of the knee, two inches below the joint line
    B. Bursae are sacs lined by synovium that communicate with the associated joint's synovial cavity

C. Septic prepatellar bursitis is usually caused by *S. aureus,* and most patients require admission for IV antibiotic therapy

D. Primary inflammation of the olecranon bursae may be caused by gout, pseudogout, rheumatoid disease, or uremia

E. Treatment for bursitis includes steroid injection and immobilization for 1-2 weeks

13. All of the following statements regarding tendonitis are true except which one?

A. Supraspinatus tendonitis produces pain at the acromion when passively abducted more than 60 degrees

B. The Yergasons' test (resisting supination at the wrist with the elbow held against the body and flexed at 90 degrees) is used to diagnose bicipital tendonitis

C. Lateral epicondylitis (tennis elbow) is best treated with continued mobilization to prevent stiffness

D. DeQuervain's tendonitis is caused by inflammation of the abductor pollicis longus and extensor pollicis brevis

E. Tendonitis of the shoulder is treated initially with pendulum exercises followed by wall climbing with the hand

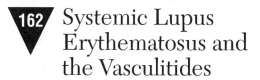

# 162 Systemic Lupus Erythematosus and the Vasculitides

*Michael D. Shertz*

Select the appropriate letter that correctly answers the question or completes the statement.

1. Which of the following is true about systemic lupus erythematosus (SLE)?

A. It has an equal male to female distribution

B. It is has an incidence of 1 in 250 African-American women of child-bearing age

C. It is speculated to be a byproduct of viral infection

D. It is rarely associated with any significant disease states

2. Medications implicated in a lupus-like syndrome include which of the following?

A. Aspirin

B. Hydralazine

C. Penicillin

D. Vancomycin

3. Manifestations of SLE include which one of the following?

A. Arthralgias and myalgias

B. Frequent urinary tract infections

C. Hand inflammation, specifically of the distal interphalangeal joints

D. Mitral valve prolapse

4. Which of the following statements about pericarditis associated with SLE is true?

A. Myocarditis is the most frequent cardiac manifestation of SLE

B. Pericardial effusions are common

C. Purulent pericarditis with *Staphylococcus aureus* and tuberculosis have been reported

D. There is no significant increase in coronary artery disease in SLE patients with hypertension and hypercholesterolemia

5. Which of the following statements is true regarding laboratory testing in SLE?

A. A positive RPR or VDRL test in a patient with SLE can be interpreted as for any other patient with clinical suspicion for syphilis

B. Antibodies to double-stranded DNA (dsDNA) and anti-Smith antibodies are most specific for SLE

C. Antinuclear antibodies are rarely positive except in patients with autoimmune disease

D. The erythrocyte sedimentation rate is an excellent index of disease activity

6. Which of the following statements about drug-induced lupus is true?

A. A positive ANA titer will be found in 90% of patients taking hydralazine or procainamide

B. Full manifestations occur in <1% of patients taking high-risk drugs

C. Most patients manifest rash, whereas arthralgias occur less frequently

D. The condition is irreversible in the majority of cases

7. Which of the following statements about hypersensitivity vasculitis is true?

A. Commonly associated medications include penicillin and sulfa antibiotics

B. Laboratory examination would show a significant reactive leukocytosis and markedly elevated ESR

C. Systemic symptoms are uncommon

D. The fingers are the most frequent site of initial involvement

8. A 6-year-old female is brought to the ED complaining of a new lower-extremity rash and vague arthralgias. Which statement is true about this condition?

A. Gastrointestinal complaints would lead you to doubt the diagnosis

B. Patients with renal involvement should be admitted for IV corticosteroid therapy

C. Renal involvement leads to long-term impairment in only 1% of cases

D. This syndrome occurs most often after a viral upper respiratory tract infection

Allergy, Hypersensitivity, and Anaphylaxis

*Hans Notenboom*

Select the appropriate letter that correctly answers the question or completes the statement.

1. Patients who have experienced severe anaphylaxis may be discharged following an asymptomatic observation period of how many hours?
   A. 1-2
   B. 6-10
   C. 12-18
   D. 24-48
   E. 96-120
2. Which of the following situations represents a correct indication, route, and dosage of epinephrine for anaphylaxis?
   A. 2.0 ml (1:10,000 epinephrine) IV for a 5-year-old weighing 20 kg with shock
   B. 0.2 ml (1:1000 epinephrine) SC for a 5-year-old weighing 20 kg with respiratory failure
   C. 0.3 ml (1:10,000 epinephrine) SC for a 25-year-old with mild bronchospasm
   D. 1 ml (1:10,000 epinephrine) IV for a 25-year-old with angioedema
3. Airway management is a priority in the treatment of life-threatening attacks of hereditary angioedema (HAE). Which of the following should be administered following control of the airway?
   A. Antihistamines
   B. Epinephrine
   C. H2 antagonists
   D. Steroids
   E. Transfusion with fresh frozen plasma
4. Identify the mechanism by which aspirin is postulated to induce bronchospasm.
   A. Direct inhibition of adenylcyclase
   B. Direct stimulation of adenylcyclase
   C. Inhibition of cyclooxygenase
   D. Inhibition of lipoxygenase
   E. Inhibition of phospholipase A2
5. Which of the following is the leading cause of fatal anaphylaxis?
   A. Food-related reactions
   B. Hymenoptera stings
   C. NSAIDs
   D. Oral penicillin
   E. Parenteral penicillin

 Dermatologic Disorders

*Michael D. Shertz*

Select the appropriate letter that correctly answers the question or completes the statement.

1. A 25-year-old man complains of white patches over his chest and back that have not improved over the last month of summer. What is the most likely diagnosis?
   A. Tinea capitis
   B. Tinea cruris
   C. Tinea unguim
   D. Tinea versicolor
2. A first-time mother complains of white patches in the groin of her 1-year-old child. Which of the following features is most suggestive of cutaneous candidiasis?
   A. Fever of 104°
   B. Small satellite papules or pustules peripheral to the main body of a rash
   C. The KOH preparation reveals nothing
   D. The mother states she has recently begun using a new scented diaper
3. A young adult complains of multiple skin eruptions on her back. She states that she had a 2-cm eruption on her chest 1 week before. Other than the presence of the eruptions, her only complaint is of mild itching. Which of the following statements is inconsistent with the tentative diagnosis?
   A. The back eruptions seem to follow dermatomal lines
   B. The lesions will resolve with no intervention
   C. The patient also has oral lesions that appeared with the back eruptions
   D. The patient is not sexually active nor taking any medications
4. A 32-year-old female has a fever and rash consistent with disseminated gonococcal disease. Which of the following statements is true?
   A. All patients require hospitalization
   B. It occurs in 20% of patients with gonorrhea
   C. Lesions are usually positive for the organism if cultured
   D. The arthritis dermatitis syndrome is the most common presentation of disseminated gonococcal disease
5. An infant has multiple erythematous lesions on his face; each is marked by honey-colored crusts and superficial involvement. The child appears otherwise well. Which statement about this condition is true?
   A. Both systemic and topical therapy are equally effective treatment
   B. Group A streptococcus is the most common pathogen
   C. It is rarely contagious among infants
   D. Regional lymphadenopathy is uncommon

6. A 45-year-old male presents complaining of a new rash across his chest. It is red, raised, and intensely pruritic. One week prior he began antibiotics for a dental infection. Which of the following statements is true?
   A. Most drug eruptions occur weeks after the antibiotic is initiated
   B. Penicillin is an infrequent cause of drug eruption
   C. Serum sickness is the most common manifestation of drug eruption
   D. Skin lesions may appear after the drug has been discontinued

7. A 23-year-old female underwent an abortion in Mexico several days ago. Her family is concerned because she has had high fever and a flu-like illness since the procedure. Today she began to experience vomiting and confusion. Her temperature is 39.0° C, systolic blood pressure is 80 mm Hg, and a diffuse skin rash is noted on examination. Which of the following statements is true?
   A. Multisystem organ involvement is not required to meet the diagnostic criteria
   B. Supportive care and high-dose penicillin are the cornerstones of care
   C. Systemic involvement is uncommon
   D. This condition is limited only to tampon use

8. A nonimmunologic mechanism is responsible for urticaria in which of the following etiologies?
   A. Hymenoptera sting
   B. Inhalation of pollen
   C. Mononucleosis
   D. Strawberries

9. A 2-year-old girl had the abrupt onset of headache, nausea, and fever 2 days ago and is now developing a rash. On examination, the patient has an erythematous macular rash over the wrists and ankles, and petechiae noted over both the palms. What is the most likely diagnosis?
   A. Measles
   B. Rocky mountain spotted fever
   C. Roseola
   D. Scarlet fever

10. A 6-year-old female is brought in by her mother over concerns about a rough rash consisting of pinhead-size lesions that began on the child's chest today. In addition, the patient was seen yesterday by her pediatrician for fever and pharyngitis. The throat culture obtained at that time is now growing beta-hemolytic gram-positive cocci in chains. Which of the following statements is true?
    A. Penicillin is of no value since this is likely a viral infection with a positive culture
    B. Penicillin is warranted only to prevent immediate complications like otitis media
    C. Penicillin should be initiated to prevent late complications of this infection
    D. This condition is called erythema infectiosum

11. Which of the following statements about pediculosis is true?
    A. Household contacts require treatment
    B. Involvement of the interdigital web spaces is typical
    C. Nits are seen more frequently than the adult louse form
    D. The organism is a mite

12. Which of the following may be associated with internal malignancy, such as leukemia or Hodgkin's lymphoma?
    A. Contact dermatitis
    B. Erythema nodosum
    C. Pemphigus vulgaris
    D. Scarlet fever

13. Oral acyclovir is recommended for the initial episode of which of the following vesicular conditions?
    A. Genital herpes simplex
    B. Herpes zoster
    C. Oral herpes simplex
    D. Varicella

14. A 20-year-old Army private on leave from basic training presents to the ED worried over a penile ulcer that he noticed several hours before. In addition, he describes a vague "soreness" in his right groin, but denies trauma. Which of the following statements is true?
    A. This could represent either syphilis or genital herpes simplex
    B. The chancre is the principal manifestation of secondary syphilis
    C. The Jarisch-Herxheimer reaction is associated with genital herpes simplex
    D. Without dark-field microscopy, syphilis cannot be established as the diagnosis

15. Which of the following statements is true about serologic syphilis testing?
    A. Once the VDRL test is positive, it rarely returns to negative
    B. The VDRL test can have a false-positive result after some unrelated infections
    C. The VDRL test is positive even early in primary syphilis
    D. The VDRL test is usually negative in secondary syphilis

16. Generalized lymphadenopathy, particularly including the suboccipital and postauricular nodes, with a pinkish maculopapular rash that first appears on the face, is most typical of which illness?
    A. Measles
    B. Rocky Mountain spotted fever
    C. Roseola
    D. Rubella

17. Which of the following statements is true about erythema nodosum?
    A. Birth control pills are the leading cause of drug-induced cases
    B. It is rarely associated with underlying malignancy
    C. It usually occurs on the thighs
    D. Third-generation cephalosporin antibiotics provide prompt relief of symptoms

18. A 30-year-old female presents complaining about an unusual rash on her palms, forearms, and back. She began antibiotics several days ago. Which of the following statements is true?
    A. Mild forms of this disease will resolve in 2 to 3 days
    B. Stevens-Johnson syndrome is a mild form of this disease and as such requires no treatment
    C. Target-shaped lesions with three zones of color are frequently found on the palms in this condition
    D. The appearance of this condition is likely unrelated to the patient's antibiotics

---

**PART SEVEN   BEHAVIORAL AND SOCIETAL PROBLEMS**

---

 ## 165 General Approach to the Psychiatric Patient in the Emergency Department

*Michael D. Shertz*

Select the appropriate letter that correctly answers the question or completes the statement.

1. Which of the following statements is true?
    A. Psychosis is the most common psychiatric presentation in the ED
    B. 10% of typical ED visits are psychiatric emergencies
    C. The majority of ED psychiatric patients are intoxicated
    D. The typical ED psychiatric patient is referred by his or her therapist for acute intervention

2. Which of the following screening laboratory studies should be obtained to assess most psychiatric ED patients?
    A. CBC, PT/PTT, serum electrolytes, BUN, glucose, calcium, chest x ray
    B. CBC, serum electrolytes, BUN, glucose
    C. CBC, serum electrolytes, BUN, glucose, CSF analysis, CT scan
    D. CBC, serum electrolytes, glucose, calcium, blood alcohol level

3. Which of the following statements is true?
    A. A patient experiencing an acute psychosis does not appear to be in touch with reality and may be responding to auditory or visual hallucinations
    B. Family members of the ED psychiatric patient are rarely helpful in the patient's evaluation
    C. Panic attacks are the most common cause of acute anxiety in the ED patient
    D. Symptoms of depression, delusions, or hallucinations are always representations of psychiatric illness

4. Which of the following signs and symptoms is most consistent with psychiatric illness?
    A. A marked personality change
    B. Auditory hallucinations
    C. Heart rate of 140 beats per minute
    D. Urinary incontinence

5. Which of the following is associated with an increased risk of suicide?
    A. History of depression
    B. History of substance abuse
    C. Male gender
    D. Single, divorced or widowed
    E. All of the above

6. Which of the following is false when dealing with the agitated psychiatric patient?
    A. Antipsychotic medications (e.g., haloperidol) can improve psychosis whether organic or psychiatric
    B. Four-point restraints are the safest way to restrain a patient
    C. Neuroleptic medications can be used freely because side effects are minimal
    D. The use of a seclusion or "quiet" room is often helpful

---

 ## 166 Thought Disorders

*James Bryan*

Select the appropriate letter that correctly answers the question or completes the statement.

1. Which symptoms suggest a functional psychosis as the cause of bizarre behavior?
    A. Awake and alert with a flat affect
    B. Disorientation with periods of lucidity
    C. Lethargy and ataxia
    D. Social immodesty and emotional lability
    E. Visual hallucinations and tremor

2. Compared to the newer antipsychotic medications, the earlier, less potent antipsychotic medications such as chlorpromazine produce:
    A. Fewer extrapyramidal symptoms
    B. Less cardiovascular toxicity
    C. Less orthostatic hypotension
    D. Less sedation
    E. All of the above

3. Compared to haloperidol, droperidol:
    A. Causes slightly less sedation
    B. Has a slower onset of action
    C. Has a longer duration of action
    D. Has less antipsychotic activity
    E. Requires higher doses

4. Which of the following ED presentations is most representative of schizophrenia?
    A. A 23-year-old male is brought in by police after his friends called saying he seemed agitated, had not slept for days, and he had been on a shopping spree

for the past 2 days. He is combative, requiring restraints, and perseverating that God has chosen him to save the world.

B. A 28-year-old female is brought in by relatives 3 days after she witnessed the traumatic death of her boyfriend. The patient has a flattened affect, does not make eye contact, and gives only brief, empty replies to questions.

C. A 32-year-old male is brought in by police after being discovered during a social services check on his elderly mother, with whom he lives. He was combative with police at the scene but is now quiet, hiding his face, rocking back and forth, and making vague references to voices that are telling him to hurt himself.

D. A 37-year-old homeless person is brought in by paramedics who were called by the patient's friends because she is acting strange. The patient is hyperactive, disoriented, and experiencing visual hallucinations.

E. A 60-year-old male is brought in by his wife because he has been confused and emotionally labile since yesterday.

5. A 35-year-old woman arrives at the ED with a 5-day history of anxiety, restlessness, and inability to stop moving. Two days ago her doctor increased her haloperidol from 2 mg PO bid to 4 mg PO bid, but her symptoms have not improved. Appropriate therapy at this time would include:

A. Increase haloperidol to 6 mg PO bid, and follow up tomorrow with her primary physician

B. Continue haloperidol 4 mg PO bid, administer diphenhydramine 50 mg IM, prescribe diphenhydramine 50 mg PO qid, and follow up tomorrow with her primary physician

C. Decrease haloperidol to 1 mg PO bid, add lorazepam 1 mg PO tid, and follow up tomorrow with her primary physician

D. Discontinue haloperidol, administer dantrolene 1 mg/kg IV, and admit to the hospital until stable

E. Admit to the hospital for management of her decompensating psychosis

6. Dystonic reactions secondary to neuroleptic medications are characterized by all of the following except which one?

A. Acute torticollis

B. Laryngospasm

C. Motor restlessness

D. Sustained upward deviation of the eyes (oculogyric crisis)

E. Symptoms decrease with voluntary activities and increase with stress

7. After several years of neuroleptic drug therapy, a patient presents to the ED complaining of writhing involuntary movements of his face and tongue. The diagnosis is:

A. Akinesia

B. Dystonia

C. Neuroleptic malignant syndrome

D. Tardive dyskinesia

E. None of the above

# 167 Affective Disorders

### James Bryan

Select the appropriate letter that correctly answers the question or completes the statement.

1. All of the following are implicated in the pathophysiology of depression except which one?

A. Absence of positive role models

B. Altered neurotransmitter metabolism

C. Genetics

D. Hypercritical or abusive parents

E. Insomnia

2. Patients with major depression may exhibit all of the following except:

A. Delusions or hallucinations

B. Diminished self-worth

C. Loss of interest in normal daily activities

D. Poor impulse control

E. Vegetative symptoms such as weight loss or loss of libido

3. Which of the following ED presentations would not raise a suspicion of underlying depression?

A. Accidental wrist laceration

B. Injuries sustained in a multiple vehicle traffic accident

C. Multiple somatic complaints

D. Suicidal ideation

E. Neither B nor C should raise a suspicion of depression

4. Which of the following statements is true regarding drug therapy used for severe depression?

A. In acute overdoses with selective serotonin reuptake inhibitors (SSRIs), patients may develop severe, life-threatening cardiac arrhythmias or neurologic sequelae

B. More than 65% of patients will respond initially to SSRIs or tricyclic antidepressants

C. Patients presenting to the ED with mild to moderate depression and no risk of harming themselves or others should be discharged with a prescription for fluoxetine (Prozac) and follow-up with a psychiatrist the next day

D. Patients who present to the ED and are refractory to SSRIs should have a monoamine oxidase inhibitor (MAOI), such as phenelzine (Nardil), added to their antidepressant regimen

E. Therapeutic response to SSRIs begins in 2-3 days and peaks with a maximal response in 2 weeks

5. Which of the following is not used in the treatment of depression?

A. Bupropion (Wellbutrin)

B. Carbamazepine (Tegretol)

C. Electroconvulsive therapy (ECT)

D. Phenytoin (Dilantin)

E. Trazodone (Desyrel)

6. Which of the following is not characteristic of mania?
   A. Easily distracted
   B. Increased need for sleep
   C. Irritable and argumentative
   D. Preceded or followed by depression in more than 50% of the cases
   E. Reckless driving and spending sprees

7. Which of the following is not used in the acute or long-term management of mania?
   A. Clonazepam
   B. Haloperidol
   C. Lithium
   D. Valproate
   E. All of the above may be used

 ## 168 Anxiety Disorders

### *James Bryan*

Select the appropriate letter that correctly answers the question or completes the statement.

1. A 32-year-old female becomes anxious, diaphoretic, and tachycardic when she sees a spider on her bedroom wall. She is afraid to move because she fears the spider will chase her and jump on her. The diagnosis is:
   A. Agoraphobia
   B. Panic disorder
   C. Posttraumatic stress disorder
   D. Simple phobia
   E. None of the above

2. For the past year, a 12-year-old boy has become increasingly worried about his ability to impress his friends at school. He feels he must be better than anyone else in his classes and in sports. Because of these worries, he has become very anxious. He is restless, irritable, and has trouble concentrating and sleeping. His heart races, he trembles, and he feels hot and sweaty whenever he thinks about his academic or athletic performance. In spite of his fears, he maintains a B+ average and is captain of the football team. The diagnosis is:
   A. Generalized anxiety disorder
   B. Obsessive-compulsive neurosis
   C. Panic disorder
   D. Posttraumatic stress disorder
   E. Simple phobia

3. The fear of public speaking is classified as a(n):
   A. Generalized anxiety disorder
   B. Obsessive-compulsive neurosis
   C. Panic disorder
   D. Simple phobia
   E. None of the above

4. All of the following organic conditions may mimic an anxiety disorder except which one?
   A. Acute myocardial infarction
   B. Hypothyroidism

C. Illicit drug use
D. Pheochromocytoma
E. Pulmonary embolus

5. The drug of choice for the treatment of an acute exogenous anxiety reaction is:
   A. Benzodiazepines
   B. Buspirone
   C. Ethanol
   D. Imipramine
   E. Propranolol

 ## 169 Approach to the Difficult Patient in the Emergency Department

### *Michael D. Shertz*

Select the appropriate letter that correctly answers the question or completes the statement.

1. Which of the following is true of countertransference?
   A. It is the negative reaction that a patient arouses in a physician
   B. It is the negative reaction that a physician arouses in a patient
   C. It rarely comes into play when interacting with the difficult ED patient
   D. The patient's attitude, dress, presenting complaint, or behavior have no bearing

2. Which of the following is true?
   A. Patients' satisfaction correlates with their sense that the physician listened to them and understood their requests
   B. Physicians do not potentiate problems when they refuse or are unable to deviate from their own medical agenda
   C. Physicians spend a significant amount of time educating patients about their illness
   D. Patients file malpractice lawsuits against physicians that they like

3. Which of the following statements is most true of malingering?
   A. It is a mental disorder
   B. It is an easy diagnosis to make in the ED
   C. It is intentional
   D. It is unrelated to external incentives

4. Which of the following statements is most true of somatization?
   A. It is another term for malingering
   B. It is consciously controlled by the patient
   C. It is involuntary
   D. Most patients simply want narcotics

5. Which of the following is representative of borderline personality disorder?
   A. It begins late in life

B. Patients are deceitful to the point of using aliases and lying

C. Patients are overly concerned about abandonment

D. Patients are reluctant to confide in others for fear that the information will be used against them

6. Which is representative of antisocial personality disorder?

A. Unrealistically preoccupied with fears of abandonment

B. Diagnosis that can be made in a person younger than age 15

C. Lack of remorse for actions of stealing or hurting another person

D. Recurrent suicidal behavior

7. Strategies for dealing with the difficult ED patient include which of the following?

A. Be supportive

B. Point out impasses, but agree to disagree

C. Structure the interview, including setting time limits if needed

D. Understand the patient's reason for presenting to the ED

E. All of the above

8. Dependent patients are classified by which of the following?

A. Borderline and histrionic patients infrequently fall into this behavior category

B. Looking for the underlining life stressor that prompted the ED visit is infrequently helpful

C. They rarely make escalating demands for analgesia, reassurance, or affection

D. They see physicians as inexhaustible sources of compassion and understanding

---

# 170 Somatoform Disorders, Factitious Disorders, and Malingering

*Hans Notenboom*

Select the appropriate letter that correctly answers the question or completes the statement.

1. All of the following are true of patients with somatoform disorders except which one?

A. Between the ages of 12-20

B. Fewer than 12 years education

C. Low self esteem

D. Widowed or divorced

E. Women

2. Which of the following is not a characteristic for presentation of conversion disorder?

A. Motivated by external incentive to feign illness (voluntary)

B. Non-painful, usually neurologic complaint

C. Rapid onset

D. Single organ system

E. Without anatomic or physiologic explanation

3. Characteristics of hypochondriasis include all of the following except which one?

A. Fear of disease

B. Lack of true, identifiable symptoms

C. Persistent and unsatisfying pursuit of medical care (doctor shopping)

D. Physical symptoms disproportionate to demonstrable organic disease

E. Preoccupation with one's own body

4. Factors that are associated with a good prognosis in conversion disorder include all of the following except which one?

A. Absence of organic illness or major psychiatric syndromes

B. Acute and recent onset

C. Definite precipitation by a stressful event

D. Poor premorbid health

E. Presenting symptoms of paralysis, aphonia, or blindness

5. Which of the following is not a characteristics of pain in the somatoform pain disorder?

A. It cannot be pathophysiologically explained

B. It involves one or more organ systems

C. It is intentionally feigned

D. It is persistent in nature

E. It limits daily function

6. In which of the following settings would malingering not be strongly suspected?

A. The patient exhibits, or has history of, antisocial behavior

B. The patient is willing to accept possibly painful or dangerous tests and procedures to confirm a diagnosis of physical illness

C. There is marked discrepancy between the person's claimed stress or disability and objective findings

D. There is medicolegal context to the presentation

E. There is poor compliance with previous treatment regimens

---

# 171 Suicide

*Norm Kalbfleisch*

Select the appropriate letter that correctly answers the question or completes the statement.

1. The diagnosis associated with the highest proportional rate of suicide is:

A. Alcoholism

B. Chronic low back pain

C. Bilateral lower extremity amputation

D. Depression

E. Panic disorder

2. In assessing a patient's potential for suicide, which of the following is true?
    A. Asking the depressed patient about suicidal ideation may give the patient the idea of suicide and thus be associated with increased risk
    B. History of schizophrenia is not associated with increased risk of suicide
    C. Intoxication in presence of suicidal ideation increases risk of suicide
    D. Patient history of antisocial personality disorder is associated with suicide attempts but not completed suicides
    E. The ability of a patient to agree to a "no-harm" contract does not decrease the likelihood he or she will attempt suicide

3. Which of the following statements is false regarding the assessment of suicide risk?
    A. Adolescent males are more likely to attempt suicide but less likely to die by suicide than middle-aged adult males
    B. Elderly white males represent less than 7% of the United States population yet account for more than 70% of all suicide deaths
    C. HIV seropositivity even without AIDS-defining conditions is associated with increased risk
    D. Patients and families are sufficiently accurate in reporting the amount and type of medications ingested in their overdose attempts
    E. Remote history of suicide in the patient's immediate family is associated with increased risk of suicide

4. Which of the following statements regarding patients who present to the ED after a suicide attempt or complain of suicidal ideation is true?
    A. Individuals who attempt to elope from the ED after medical clearance but before complete assessment of suicidal risk should be restrained if necessary to prevent their leaving the ED
    B. Intoxicated individuals who recant their initial presenting statement of suicidal thought may be safely discharged with close outpatient follow-up.
    C. Partial-thickness lacerations over the wrists and forearms that do not require suturing are not associated with completed suicide
    D. Suicidal patients typically should undergo involuntary commitment rather than voluntary admission to the hospital because they may change their mind
    E. The SAD PERSONS mnemonic developed to assist in ascertaining risk of suicide has not proven to be clinically reliable

 **172** ## The Violent Patient

*Norm Kalbfleisch*

Select the appropriate letter that correctly answers the question or completes the statement.

1. Features suggesting an organic rather than functional cause for violent behavior include:
    A. Alcohol intoxication
    B. History of psychiatric illness
    C. Onset at 25 years of age
    D. None of the above
    E. All of the above

2. Regarding risk assessment for violence in the ED setting, which of the following statement is true?
    A. Approximately 4% of ED patients carry a weapon
    B. Potentially violent, angry patients rarely allow medications to be given parenterally
    C. Reliable predictors of ED violence include male gender, drug use, ethnicity, and education
    D. The uncooperative, nonverbal patient is likely less physically violent than an angry, verbose patient
    E. When a patient invokes a feeling of fear or trepidation in the emergency provider, the provider should inwardly remember that it is the practitioner who needs to be in control of the situation

3. Regarding a violent adult patient who poses an imminent threat to self or others, which of the following statements is true?
    A. A show of force at a distance of 10-15 feet is an effective and safe way to calm a violent patient with a knife
    B. An ideally designed room for assessment and management of a violent patient is one that is narrow and monitored, with a single door at one end
    C. Once a patient has been physically subdued, the initial minimum number of restraints is four: one on each extremity
    D. Informed consent must be attempted verbally before the restraint of the patient
    E. The ideal number of personnel needed to restrain a violent adult patient safely is four: one on each extremity

4. Regarding utilization of physical restraint of violent, intoxicated patients, which of the following statements is true?
    A. Chemical restraint may be necessary even if the patient is securely held by physical restraints
    B. The patient may be released from physical restraint once he or she has agreed to be nonviolent
    C. The verbally abusive, profane, loud patient who is in physical restraints and is disruptive to patients and staff may be moved safely to a psychiatric evaluation room if the patient is observed every 10 minutes

D. The supine position where the patient's respiration may be observed is safest

E. When properly applied, padded leather restraints will not compromise the patient's circulation distal to the site of application

5. Which of the following statements about management of the violent or agitated patient is true?

A. A show of force rarely helps diffuse or subdue violent impulses in the patient

B. A show of force by hospital security personnel at a distance of 40-50 feet will likely safely subdue a violent patient who has a gun

C. The ideal chemical restraint has a fast onset of action and a long duration of effect

D. The preferred route of administration of a medication utilized for chemical restraint in a violent patient would be intramuscular and/or intravenous

6. A 25-year-old woman is brought to the ED after creating a disturbance at a neighbor's house. On arrival, the patient is shouting and seems paranoid. Which initial response would be most appropriate?

A. Chemically restrain using injectable haloperidol

B. Physically restrain the patient, ideally using five people

C. Perform history, examination, and laboratory studies to rule out an organic medical disorder

D. Place patient in safe environment such as psychiatric evaluation room and attempt to establish rapport by encouraging her to express her feelings

 ## 173 Substance Abuse

*Patrick Brunett*

Select the appropriate letter that correctly answers the question or completes the statement.

1. Which of the follow signs or symptoms is a reliable indicator of sympathetic overload?

A. Absent bowel sounds
B. Dry skin
C. Diaphoresis
D. Flushing
E. Miosis

2. Which of the following is an acute complication of injecting drug use?

A. Botulism sepsis
B. Cotton fever
C. Pulmonary abscess
D. Sacroiliitis
E. Tetanus

3. Acute manifestations of solvent inhalation include all of the following except which one?

A. Cerebellar ataxia
B. Gastrointestinal distress
C. Hypokalemia

D. Ventricular dysrhythmias
E. Wheezing

4. What is the most clinically significant complication seen in patients who abuse nitrites?

A. Hemolytic anemia
B. Hypotension
C. Methemoglobinemia
D. Syncope
E. Tachycardia

5. A 27-year-old man is brought to the ED by the police. He was found naked, driving erratically. En route he became extremely violent and required physical restraint. Examination reveals blood pressure, 180/105; pulse, 110; respirations, 24; temperature, 101° F. He is alert and awake, disoriented, and diaphoretic. He exhibits both horizontal and vertical nystagmus. Which of the following statements is true regarding this patient?

A. Aggressive treatment of the hypertension is indicated

B. Benzodiazepines are effective in controlling violent behavior is such patients

C. Creatine kinase (CK) level will generally be within normal range

D. Haloperidol is not likely to be helpful as a chemical sedation agent

E. Verbal "talk down" therapy should be the first step in suspected PCP intoxication

6. Which statement is true regarding hallucinogen intoxication?

A. Common side effect of LSD ingestion is vomiting

B. Intoxication from LSD, psilocybin, and mescaline are clinically distinct entities

C. Many of the effects of LSD intoxication are due to its parasympathomimetic effects

D. Mydriasis is a common finding in psilocybin ingestion

E. Psilocybin mushrooms provoke vomiting 6 or more hours after ingestion

7. Which statement is true regarding management of hallucinogen intoxication?

A. Activated charcoal is indicated for mushroom ingestion

B. Benzodiazepines are contraindicated for sedation

C. Direct life-threatening complications are fairly common

D. Standard urine toxicologic screens detect most common hallucinogens

E. "Talk down" therapy is not helpful

8. Jimson weed intoxication is characterized by which of the following statements?

A. Droperidol may cause oversedation and respiratory compromise

B. Leaves of the jimson weed contain the greatest amount of toxin

C. Pupillary constriction is the most common peripheral sign

D. Physostigmine should be used only for mild agitation

E. Scopolamine is responsible for CNS excitation and hallucinations

9. With regard to amphetamine intoxication, which statement is most correct?
   A. Hypertension should be managed aggressively with beta blockers
   B. Hallucinogenic amphetamines such as MDMA are closer in effect and safety to traditional hallucinogens such as LSD
   C. Mortality from sympathetic amines is biphasic, with late deaths up to 48 hours after use
   D. Seizures are usually self-limited and require no special therapy
   E. Serotonin syndrome is characterized by hypotension and flaccid paralysis

10. The differential diagnosis of amphetamine overdose includes which of the following?
    A. Alcohol withdrawal
    B. Benzodiazepine withdrawal
    C. Pheochromocytoma
    D. Thyroid storm
    E. All of the above

11. A 26-year-old female who is in the third trimester of pregnancy and has a history of cocaine use presents with chest pain, tachycardia, tachypnea, diaphoresis, agitation, and headache. Which statement is true regarding this patient's presentation?
    A. Computed tomography of the brain should be limited to patients presenting with headache and seizure
    B. Headache is a benign, ubiquitous complaint in patients using cocaine
    C. Preterm labor and precipitous delivery may be induced by cocaine use
    D. Pulmonary hypersensitivity reactions are primarily seen in patients using intravenous cocaine
    E. This patient is at low risk for myocardial ischemia due to her age and gender

12. All of the following mechanisms may be associated with cocaine-induced chest pain except which one?
    A. Accelerated coronary atherosclerosis
    B. Coronary vasospasm
    C. Direct myocardial stimulation
    D. Platelet aggregation
    E. Sodium channel blockade

13. The use of which agent for the management of the cardiovascular effects of cocaine is supported in the medical literature?
    A. Diltiazem
    B. Labetalol
    C. Phentolamine
    D. Tissue plasminogen activator
    E. Verapamil

14. All of the following are correct statements regarding cocaine-induced status epilepticus except which one?
    A. Barbiturates are effective in controlling seizure activity

B. Focal seizures are associated with intracerebral vasculopathy
C. Most generalized seizures are single events and without sequelae
D. Midazolam is effective in controlling seizure activity
E. Phenytoin is effective in controlling seizure activity

# 174 Stress, Wellness, and the Impaired Physician

*James E. Thompson*

Select the appropriate letter that correctly answers the question or completes the statement.

1. Which of the following contribute to stress in the practice of emergency medicine?
   A. Difficult decisions
   B. Difficult patients and professional relationships
   C. Diminished resources
   D. Diversity of practice elements
   E. All of the above

2. All the following are true regarding burnout except which one?
   A. Burnout has not been shown to be a precursor of physician impairment
   B. Burnout is associated with affective changes including hostility, anxiety, and depression
   C. Burnout undermines the relationship between patient and physician
   D. Physicians in the midst of burnout may experience less job satisfaction

3. Regarding physician impairment, which of the following is true?
   A. Chemically dependent physicians are easily spotted by their colleagues
   B. Emergency medicine practitioners are not overrepresented among chemically dependent physicians
   C. Impaired physicians have a higher rate of family difficulties and divorce
   D. Interventions have not been shown to be helpful long-term with the impaired physician

4. Elements in the cultivation of a balanced lifestyle include:
   A. A professional environment that promotes wellness
   B. Cultivation of close family and social relationships
   C. Cultivation of methods of relaxation and personal renewal
   D. Maintaining physical fitness
   E. All of the above

5. Strategies for managing difficult patients include all the following except which one?

A. Accept your own emotional response to the patient
B. Diffuse anger by letting the patient vent verbally, and avoid hostile responses
C. Do not allow difficult patient to "get under your skin"
D. Set limits for patients
E. Set limits for yourself in terms of treatments goals consistent with good medical care

6. Which of the following is true regarding strategies for adjusting to shift work?
   A. Grouping all night shifts in a given month together minimizes circadian disruptions
   B. Having one physician designated to work nights for 1 month or longer while other members of the group fill in isolated nights will facilitate adjustment
   C. Maintaining a day lifestyle when working an isolated night shift helps keep the circadian rhythm on schedule
   D. Twelve-hour shifts with more days off each month is preferable to 8-hour shifts

7. Methods of relaxation and renewal include all of the following except which one?
   A. Autogenic training
   B. Progressive relaxation
   C. Social use of alcohol
   D. Yoga

---

 **175** Domestic Violence

*J. Leibovitz*

Select the appropriate letter that correctly answers the question or completes the statement.

1. What is the lifetime prevalence of female abuse among ED patients?
   A. 10%
   B. 20%
   C. 30%
   D. 40%
   E. 50%

2. Which of the following is true?
   A. Abused women are more likely to have low-birth-weight children
   B. Female children of abused women demonstrate a higher rate of behavioral problems than male children
   C. One million women are victims of domestic violence each year
   D. Ten percent of all homicides are committed by relatives, a spouse, or close friend of the victim
   E. Victim rates peak between the ages of 25-41 for homicide domestic violence

3. Which of the following is false with respect to abused women?
   A. Chronic pelvic pain is a common presenting symptom associated with spousal abuse
   B. Nonspecific somatic complaints are common
   C. She may develop anxiety and depression
   D. There is a higher rate of suicide and alcoholism
   E. Twenty nine percent of all women who attempt suicide have a history of domestic violence that is independent of race

4. All of the following are barriers in the diagnosis of domestic violence except:
   A. Denial
   B. Drug and alcohol use
   C. Fear of repercussions
   D. Inability to volunteer information
   E. All of the above are true

5. What domestic violence situation has the greatest potential for a lethal injury?
   A. An escalating pattern of violence
   B. Evidence of violent behavior outside the home
   C. Escalating drug and alcohol use
   D. The presence of a firearm in the house
   E. When an attempt is made to leave the relationship

6. Which of the following does not indicate a high degree of significant danger from domestic violence?
   A. Assault with a weapon
   B. Attempted strangulation
   C. Hitting with closed fists
   D. Threatening with a weapon
   E. Throwing things or punching a wall

7. An 89-year-old woman is brought to the ED from a nursing home at the insistence of the family, who found her to be much more somnolent than usual. They report that, although bedridden, she is usually very feisty and demanding. A thorough evaluation reveals no evidence of an organic problem, but the nursing home record indicates frequent doses of haloperidol, which is suspected as the cause of the patient's somnolence. This is an example of:
   A. Financial abuse
   B. Medication abuse
   C. Neglect
   D. Physical abuse
   E. Psychologic abuse

## 176 Ethnicity, Culture, and the Delivery of Health Care Services: Enhancing System Outcomes in a Multicultural Environment

*No questions*

## 177 Differential Diagnosis

*Evelyn Kim*

Questions in this chapter come from multiple chapters and are designed to cover a broad differential diagnosis
Select the appropriate letter that correctly answers the question or completes the statement.

1. A 5-month-old female with respiratory distress is brought to the ED with a 3-day history of cough, nasal congestion, and fussiness. Her vital signs are temperature, 100.8° F; respiratory rate, 65; pulse, 160; oxygen saturation, 94%. The child is alert and does not appear seriously ill. She has mild nasal flaring and intercostal retractions, and auscultation of the chest reveals wheezing and diffuse, fine rales. Which of the following is the most likely etiologic agent?
   A. Foreign body
   B. *Haemophilus influenzae* type B
   C. Household allergens
   D. Parainfluenza
   E. Respiratory syncytial virus

2. Which of the following is the most likely complication of the disease in Question 1?
   A. Bacterial superinfection
   B. Death
   C. Pleural effusion
   D. Pulmonary hypertension
   E. Recurrent episodic wheezing

3. A 54-year-old male is brought in to the ED after being found lying on the floor. He has labored breathing and is not speaking. He has no eye opening to command or pain, and he minimally withdraws all four extremities to pain. Pupils are midposition and equally reactive. All of the following are likely possibilities for his presentation except which one?
   A. Acute ethylene glycol intoxication
   B. Infectious meningitis

C. Postictal state
D. Right parietal ischemic stroke
E. Subarachnoid hemorrhage

4. A 78-year-old female is brought to the ED immediately after a fall from a ladder. She complains of right hip pain and on examination has an obvious right femur fracture and multiple large ecchymoses on the right hemithorax and right flank. Her vital signs are temperature, 99.0° F; pulse, 100; respiratory rate, 20; blood pressure, 114/72. She begins acting more agitated and confused and is noted to have increasing respiratory distress. Repeat vital signs are pulse, 120; respiratory rate, 32; blood pressure, 82/50. Oxygen saturation is 92%. Which of the following is the least likely cause of her symptoms at this point?
   A. Acute myocardial infarction
   B. Fat embolism
   C. Hemothorax
   D. Intraabdominal injury
   E. Pneumothorax

5. A 39-year-old woman presents to the ED complaining of vertigo. Subsequent work-up reveals normal orthostatic vital signs, blood glucose, CBC, and 12-lead ECG. The remainder of the examination is entirely within normal limits with the exception of bilateral internuclear ophthalmoplegia. Which of the following is the most likely etiology of her symptoms?
   A. Acoustic neuroma
   B. Acute labyrinthitis
   C. Ménière's disease
   D. Multiple sclerosis
   E. Vertebrobasilar insufficiency

6. A 21-year-old female, 8 months pregnant, comes to the ED complaining of right-sided abdominal pain, anorexia, and nausea. Her vital signs are temperature, 100.4° F; pulse, 96; blood pressure, 128/76. On physical examination, she has tenderness to palpation of the right mid-quadrant of the abdomen and the right flank. White blood cell count is 10 with a normal differential. Which of the following would be the most practical next test?
   A. Abdominal ultrasound
   B. Erythrocyte sedimentation rate
   C. Examination of vaginal/cervical fluid
   D. Quantitative hCG
   E. Urinalysis

*Match the toxicologic syndrome with the appropriate question.*

A. Headache, dizziness, confusion, abdominal pain, nausea, vomiting

B. Hypertension, tachycardia, confusion, tremors, hyperpyrexia

C. Muscular rigidity, tremors, oculogyric crisis

D. Rhinorrhea, perspiration, gooseflesh, mydriasis, nausea

E. Tachycardia, hypertension, tremor, anxiety, visual hallucinations

F. Tachycardia, mydriasis, dry and flushed skin, delirium

G. Violent, agitated behavior, tachycardia, hypertension

7. Alcohol withdrawal _____

8. Cocaine _____

9. Isopropyl alcohol _____

10. Morphine withdrawal _____

11. Over-the-counter nighttime sleep aid _____

12. PCP _____

13. Promethazine _____

# ANSWERS

 Airway Management

*E. David Bailey and Brian E. Burgess*

1. **A,** Page 5.
Difficulty with intubation may be associated with immobilized trauma patients, children, a short neck, prominent upper incisors, a receding mandible, limited jaw opening, limited cervical mobility, facial trauma, laryngeal trauma, or upper airway disease. Edentulousness may facilitate intubation.

2. **E,** Page 7.
Rapid-sequence intubation (RSI) is the cornerstone of emergent airway management. RSI is undertaken with the idea that the intubation is emergently needed, that the patient has a full stomach, that the intubation is predicted to be successful, and if intubation fails, that ventilation will be successful. Resources should be available to provide the patient with a rescue airway if all attempts fail.

3. **D,** Page 9.
Succinylcholine is the only depolarizing neuromuscular blocking agent and has an onset of 60 seconds and a duration of 6-10 minutes, making it a good paralytic for RSI. Short onset allows for rapid intubation while a short half-life means it will wear off quickly in the event that intubation fails. Others such as atracurium, vecuronium, pancuronium, and cisatracurium are all non-depolarizing neuromuscular blocking agents with a slower onset and much longer duration. Although priming doses may shorten the onset of the non-depolarizing neuromuscular blocking agents, their long half-lives make them unfavorable for rapid-sequence intubation in the event that intubation fails. Even with priming, their time to onset and duration of action exceed those of succinylcholine.

4. **D,** Page 9.
Hyperkalemia associated with succinylcholine in burn and trauma patients can be severe but is often delayed several days to a week. Increases in potassium levels usually do not exceed 0.5 mEq/L. Administration of succinylcholine is not contraindicated in patients with renal disease. Succinylcholine should be used with caution in patients with known hyperkalemia. Hyperkalemia is not usually associated with the non-depolarizing neuromuscular blocking agents.

5. **A,** Page 11.
This multiply injured trauma patient has a head injury and is hemodynamically unstable. Ketamine will not affect hemodynamic instability but raises intracranial pressure. Midazo-

lam and thiopental both have cerebroprotective properties but midazolam, thiopental, and fentanyl are negative inotropes and vasodilators with the potential to worsen the patient's hemodynamic status. Etomidate is cerebroprotective without adversely affecting hemodynamic status, making it the induction agent of choice in patients with multiple trauma.

6. **E,** Page 12.
Reflex sympathetic response to laryngoscopy (RSRL) is a catecholamine surge associated with laryngoscopy. Young healthy patients tolerate RSRL well, but it can increase ICP and myocardial oxygen demand. It is of potential concern in patients with head injuries or cardiac or aortic disease. Fentanyl and beta-blockers can blunt RSRL.

7. **D,** Page 12.
Succinylcholine causes an increase in ICP that is not shared by the competitive neuromuscular blockers (NMBs). IV lidocaine can blunt the ICP response to intubation, as do defasciculating doses of competitive NMBs. Blind nasal tracheal intubation causes a dramatic increase in ICP, likely induces hypercarbia, and is associated with a higher complication rate.

8. **B,** Page 5.
The child's airway differs from the adult airway in several crucial ways. The larynx is higher in the neck, and the epiglottis is soft, making the visualization of the cords difficult. A Miller blade may aid in visualization. The prominent occiput of the child's head brings the head too far forward. Elevating the torso slightly may aid in visualization. The cricoid is the narrowest portion of the pediatric airway.

9. **E,** Page 14.
Before airway management, the airway should be assessed for the ease of intubation and bag valve mask ventilation. If both look difficult, an awake method of intubation such as nasal tracheal intubation should be attempted if the patient's condition warrants it. Several alternative airways exist, including the laryngeal mask and esophageal obturator airways. The crucial rescue airway to master is the cricothyrotomy.

10. **D,** Page 14.
Cricothyrotomy is the rescue technique used by trained emergency physicians when intubation and ventilation have failed. Relative contraindications include coagulopathy, distorted anatomy, and infection, but necessity for an airway overrides the relative contraindications. Cricothyrotomy should not be performed on children younger than 10 years of age. Cricothyrotomy is preferred over tracheostomy because of ease, success, and lower complication rate.

# 2 ▼ Mechanical Ventilation and Noninvasive Ventilatory Support

### Greg Ledbetter

1. **D,** Page 25.
Significant respiratory acidosis is the fourth criteria of acute respiratory failure.

2. **D,** Page 26.
Synchronized intermittent ventilation (SIMV) supports a patient's spontaneous breath at a preset rate that prevents a mechanical breath being delivered at the same time as a spontaneous breath (stacking). The other choices are all potential adverse effects of positive-pressure ventilation.

3. **D,** Pages 27-28.
Noninvasive ventilatory support has many advantages over more invasive measures, including likely decreased length of stay in the intensive care unit; preservation of speech, swallowing, and physiologic airway defense mechanisms; ease of weaning, and reduced risk of airway injury and nosocomial infections. There is, however, an increased risk of pulmonary barotrauma, aerophagia, and pressure stress to the face.

4. **C,** Pages 27-28.
Positive end-expiratory pressure (PEEP) is pressure applied during mechanical ventilation. The primary physiologic effect of PEEP is to increase functional residual capacity by maintaining patency of alveoli at the end of exhalation. PEEP increases $PaO_2$, at constant $FiO_2$ by decreasing intrapulmonary shunting and V/Q mismatch. PEEP has minimal effect on $CO_2$ exchange.

5. **B,** Page 29.
Peak inspiratory pressure (PIP) is a very useful measurement of ventilatory function. PIP increases with airway occlusion, acute bronchospasm, pneumothorax, and pulmonary edema. Leaks in the breathing circuit, inadequate volume delivery, and failure of the ventilator cause a decrease in PIP.

6. **A,** Page 31.
In acute chronic obstructive pulmonary disease (COPD) exacerbations, $PaCO_2$ and pH should be corrected gradually to numbers that reflect the steady state expected to be maintained by the patient after extubation. The other goal of mechanical ventilation is the normalization of lung volume. This is accomplished by decreasing intrinsic positive end-expiratory pressure (PEEP) by adding extrinsic PEEP (at levels slightly lower than intrinsic PEEP), administering bronchodilators and steroids, increasing the expiratory time, and minimizing the tidal volume.

# 3 ▼ Cardiopulmonary Arrest

### Kevin Bristowe and Brian Burgess

1. **D,** Page 36.
Cardiopulmonary arrest accounts for up to one third of all non-traumatic arrests in the United States. Approximately 75% are attributed to cardiovascular disease; only 25% have a non-cardiac cause. Up to one third of patients who survive pre-hospital cardiac arrest will have neurologic impairment. Although cardiac arrest has a poor outcome, the type and training of pre-hospital providers has affected patient survival.

2. **E,** Page 36.
Cardiac arrest from a primary cardiac cause typically is seen as ventricular fibrillation (VF) or, less commonly, pulseless ventricular tachycardia (VT). More than 50% of patients with out-of-hospital cardiac arrest have VF. Coronary artery disease is the most common pathologic condition found in patients who die suddenly from VF.

3. **E,** Page 37.
Circulatory obstruction initially presents as tachycardia and hypotension that deteriorates from bradycardia to PEA, VF, or asystole. Drowning produces a bradysystolic cardiac arrest secondary to hypoxia. Hyperkalemia is the most common metabolic cause of cardiac arrest and progressively widens the QRS complex and results in deterioration to VT, VF, Asystole, or PEA. This can be corrected with calcium chloride, sodium bicarbonate, insulin and glucose. Hypothermia can make the myocardium irritable and produce arrhythmias.

4. **D,** Page 37.
Some systems (e.g., the renal, gastrointestinal, musculoskeletal, and integumentary systems) are much more resistant to ischemia than the heart and brain are and rarely sustain irreversible primary damage after a duration of cardiac arrest compatible with successful resuscitation. CPR generates about 30% of the pre-arrest blood flow and can be associated with survival. The endocardium is more sensitive than the epicardium to the effects of ischemia.

5. **C,** Pages 36, 43.
Once ventricular fibrillation has been established repeated defibrillation attempts should be performed immediately, taking precedence over CPR, intubation, and the establishment of an intravenous line. Cardioversion is the synchronized mode of defibrillation and has no value in a patient with ventricular fibrillation.

6. **A,** Page 43.
Precordial thumps carry a risk of converting ventricular tachycardia (VT) into a more malignant rhythm like ventricular fibrillation (VF), asystole, or pulseless electrical activity. Too much current can result in myocardial damage. Transthoracic impedance is decreased by pressing firmly with 25 pounds of force and allows for lower current with initial shocks. Cardioversion differs from defibrillation and has no role in VF or pulseless VT.

7. **D,** Page 44.

The femoral vein, although very safe to cannulate, is not as effective as the internal jugular or the subclavian vein. When dosing medicines via the endotracheal tube, the doses of medicines should be increased 2 to 2.5 times the standard dose. Intracardiac epinephrine is recommended only when other routes are not readily available or when the chest cavity is opened and the heart is directly visualized.

8. **C,** Pages 45-46.

Atropine blocks the depressant effects of vagally released acetylcholine (ACH) at the sinus and atrioventricular nodes. Bretylium is a class III antidysrhythmic; lidocaine is class IB. The correct dose of procaine for VF arrest is 30 mg/min to a maximum of 17 mg/kg. Sodium bicarbonate may help to provide an additional buffer once adequate ventilation, oxygenation, and tissue perfusion have been restored.

9. **C,** Page 52.

Although ABCs are crucial in anyone presenting in extremis, this patient needs immediate defibrillation before any other intervention.

10. **E,** Pages 47-51.

End tidal carbon dioxide has been shown to be useful during CPR and in confirming proper positioning of the endotracheal tube. Tube placement must be constantly re-evaluated for position as well as possible complications such as a pneumothorax. Historical information via pre-hospital providers and the family can help guide therapy as well as define the etiology and prognosis for the patient. Return to sinus rhythm on the monitor does not always mean a pulse is present. Physical examination of the patient is essential to ensure adequate airway maintenance and ventilation, confirm the diagnosis of cardiac arrest, find evidence for the etiology of the cardiac arrest, and monitor for complications of the therapeutic interventions. Constant reassessment of therapies is suggested. Restoration of adequate cardiac function and return of spontaneous circulation with restoration of normal brain function is the definition of successful resuscitation. The likelihood of achieving both of these goals decreases with every minute the patient remains in cardiac arrest.

# 4 Neonatal Resuscitation

*Dale J. Ray*

1. **B,** Page 61.

Bradycardia with a heart rate of less than 100 almost always reflects inadequate ventilation and oxygenation. Congenital third-degree block, which is rare, is the only cardiac cause of bradycardia. The other choices all have multiple reasons to be abnormal.

2. **A,** Page 61.

Hypoglycemia, metabolic acidosis, and increased oxygen consumption may also develop.

3. **D,** Page 64.

Neonatal hypoglycemia is treated with 2-4 ml/kg of D10W. Higher concentrations should be avoided because they are hyperosmolar.

4. **D,** Page 65.

Complications from meconium aspiration can be avoided with aggressive intervention. As soon as the head is delivered, the mouth and nose are suctioned. Immediately after delivery, suctioning of the trachea is performed using an endotracheal tube and meconium aspirator. Reintubation and suction should be repeated until meconium clears.

5. **B,** Pages 63-64.

Ventilate at 40 breaths per minute. No current evidence supports the use of atropine. Epinephrine is used for asystole and heart rate less than 80 if ventilation with 100% oxygen and chest compression are not effective. Chest compressions are begun if the heart rate is 60 to 80 beats per minute and not increasing after 15 to 30 seconds of positive-pressure ventilations. To intubate, the head should be in neutral to slightly extended position. Further extension may actually occlude the airway.

6. **C,** Pages 64-65.

Atropine is not used in neonatal resuscitation. Hypoglycemia with glucose <40 mg/dl should be treated with D10W to avoid hyperosmolality and rebound hypoglycemia. Sodium bicarbonate 4.2% solution at 2 mg/kg is given only after documentation of significant metabolic acidosis. The use of high-dose epinephrine (0.1 mg/kg or 0.1 ml/kg of 1:1000 solution) is controversial and cannot be recommended. Whole blood at 10 ml/kg is given only with evidence of acute bleeding with signs of hypovolemia (pallor despite oxygenation, weak pulses with a good heart rate, poor response to resuscitation).

# 5 Pediatric Resuscitation

*Dale J. Ray*

1. **E,** Page 66.

In the pediatric population, cardiac arrest is most often the end result of a long period of hypoxemia due to inadequate oxygenation, ventilation, or circulation. Pediatric cardiac arrest has a wide range of etiologies. Once cardiac arrest occurs, the outcome of resuscitation is quite poor due to the prolonged period of hypoxemia, hypercapnia, or ischemia, which causes severe organ damage.

2. **B,** Page 68; Figure 5-1.

The treatment of choice in asystole is epinephrine. This may be administered via the intravenous, intraosseous, or endotracheal routes. Choices A, C, D, and E are incorrect because of the time delay associated with their placement. After the first dose of epinephrine through the endotracheal tube, an intravenous or intraosseous line may be placed and used for additional medications and volume replacement.

3. **C,** Page 68.

Rapid delivery of medication to the central circulation is an essential aspect of resuscitation. The most effective means of achieving this is by intravenous or intraosseous cannulation. Although certain medications (lidocaine, epinephrine, atropine, and naloxone) can be given by the endotracheal route, the kinetics of drug distribution do not favor this route. However, when the intravenous and intraosseous routes are not immediately available, the first dose may be given through the endotracheal tube. The intracardiac and subcutaneous routes have prohibitively high complication rates. Oral administration in an arrest setting is obviously contraindicated.

4. **C,** Pages 68-69.

Although epinephrine has both alpha- and beta-adrenergic effects, at the doses used in cardiac arrest, epinephrine's alpha-adrenergic effects predominate. It is used in all cardiac arrest situations including asystole, electromechanical dissociation, and ventricular fibrillation, as well as bradycardia due to cardiac ischemia. The initial cardiac arrest dose of epinephrine is 0.1 ml/kg of 1:10,000 solution IV and 0.1 ml/kg of 1:1000 solution endotracheal. Clinical data show that if there is no organized cardiac activity after two rounds of epinephrine, survival to leave the hospital does not occur.

5. **B,** Page 73.

Data suggest that hyperglycemia predisposes the brain to greater ischemic insult by causing increased lactate production. This produces a severe intracellular acidosis and thus cellular injury. Severe hyperglycemia can mimic hypoxemia by causing poor perfusion, diaphoresis, tachycardia, and hypotension.

6. **C,** Pages 70, 73.

Airway and ventilation problems are the usual cause of bradycardia in the pediatric population. However, if bradycardia persists in spite of adequate oxygenation, consideration of atropine is appropriate. The IV dose is 0.01-0.03 mg/kg, with a minimum dose of 0.10 mg to avoid paradoxical bradycardia.

7. **C,** Page 74.

Calcium is indicated only to treat the adverse cardiovascular effects of hyperkalemia and hypermagnesemia, to correct documented hypocalcemia, and to reverse the hypotension produced by calcium channel blocker toxicity. Calcium is not indicated for the treatment of cardiac arrest unless the above conditions are present.

8. **C,** Page 75.

The opening of the larynx assumes a superior and anterior position in infancy and descends with age. The narrowest portion of the trachea in the infant is at the cricoid ring, while it is at the vocal cords in the adult. The young child's tongue and head are proportionally larger than the adult's. The occiput is more prominent in the young child.

9. **E,** Page 76.

Endotracheal tube size in millimeters can be determined by the formula (age in years + 16) ÷ 4 for children greater than 1 year of age.

10. **A,** Page 76.

Clinical deterioration of an intubated patient occasionally occurs. Equipment failure, endotracheal tube malposition and blockage, and tension pneumothorax must initially be considered and ruled out.

11. **D,** Page 77.

The lower limit of systolic blood pressure can be approximated by the formula 70 + (2 × age in years).

12. **A,** Page 79.

Asystole is the most common pediatric arrest rhythm. Electromechanical dissociation, pulseless ventricular tachycardia, and fine and coarse ventricular fibrillation are significantly less common.

13. **E,** Pages 81-82.

Post-resuscitation patients are typically poorly perfused. This patient is hypotensive. The initial treatment would be a fluid bolus to treat the relative hypovolemia. Should the fluid treatment be unsuccessful, treatment with a vasoactive substance would be indicated. The initial treatment of choice in pediatric patients in this situation is epinephrine.

14. **E,** Page 82.

The rule of 6 is helpful in calculating administration of inotropic infusions. The rule states that 6 × body weight in kilograms is the number of milligrams of inotropic agent needed to be added to a final volume to make a 100-ml solution. Then 1 ml/hr delivers 1 mg/kg/min. This is useful for dopamine and dobutamine. For epinephrine, norepinephrine, and isoproterenol, the multiplier is 0.6 since these rates are run starting at 0.1 mg/kg/min.

# 6 Shock

*Chih Chen and Leo W. Burns*

1. **D,** Page 99.

The resuscitative fluid of choice for persistent hemorrhagic shock is packed red blood cells. Normal saline and Ringer's lactate are isotonic solutions used in the initial treatment of hemorrhagic shock, and shock unresponsive to fluid administration is a primary indication for blood transfusion. Neither 5% albumin nor 6% hydroxyethyl hetastarch is of proven benefit in the initial treatment of hemorrhagic shock.

2. **A,** Pages 100-101.

Colloid solutions have been suggested to decrease the incidence of post-resuscitative pulmonary edema and the severity of ARDS. Adequate blood concentrations will maximize oxygen delivery. However, supranormal concentrations would impair flow and decrease oxygen delivery due to increased blood viscosity. Broad-spectrum antibiotics are indicated when an infectious focus cannot be found. Directed monotherapy would be inappropriate.

3. **D,** Page 101.

Epinephrine given in small IV doses is the most effective treatment of severe hypotensive anaphylaxis because absorption of subcutaneous drugs is unreliable. Severe laryngeal edema and respiratory failure would also benefit from IV epinephrine administration.

4. **C,** Pages 95, 101.

In spinal cord lesions rostral to $T_1$, cardiac vagal influences dominate and bradycardia is prominent. Sympathetic efferent fibers are interrupted, which results in unopposed vagal stimulation. The heart receives sympathetic fibers from $T_1$ to $T_4$. Atropine should be given for hypotension to increase the heart rate and prevent sudden death. The vasoactive agent of choice should be an alpha-1-adrenergic-specific medication such as phenylephrine or ephedrine.

5. **E,** Page 96.

Tachypnea occurs early in shock because chemoreceptors sense a decrease in pH and increase ventilation to lower $PaCO_2$. Orthostatic vital signs are helpful in cases of >20% loss of blood volume.

6. **D,** Pages 95, 100.

Amrinone, a phosphodiesterase inhibitor, should be given for refractory hypotension and shock. Dobutamine and dopamine are the vasoactive agents of choice. Benzodiazepines and morphine should not be given routinely because in the shock state their negative inotropism is exaggerated. Fentanyl, etomidate, or ketamine should be considered. For the acute MI with cardiogenic shock, percutaneous transluminal coronary angioplasty is recommended, if it can be performed within 90 minutes. Intraaortic balloon pumps are contraindicated for patients with aortic insufficiency. Tachycardia is an early signal of cardiogenic shock in an anterior MI.

7. **E,** Page 94.

Intravascular volume depletion results in increasing sympathetic outflow to the heart, the blood vessels, the adrenal medulla, and the juxtaglomerular cells. Initially, a high peripheral resistance is reflected as an increased diastolic blood pressure. As hemorrhage progresses, the stroke volume decreases and the pulse pressure narrows. The degree of hemorrhage roughly predicts the heart rate. Heart rates greater than 150 beats/min may be seen in severe blood loss. The mortality for vascular decompensation, when vascular smooth muscle cells fail to respond to maximal alpha-adrenergic agonist, approaches 100%.

8. **C,** Pages 101-102.

Tris(hydroxymethyl)-aminomethane (THAM) is an organic buffer that accepts $H^+$ without increasing extracellular $CO_2$. Sodium bicarbonate, in contrast, combines with extracellular $H^+$ to form water and $CO_2$. The $CO_2$ freely diffuses into cells, combines with water intracellularly, and produces $H^+$. This is known as paradoxical acidosis and may potentially depress cell function. THAM has been shown to improve ventricular function and reduce post resuscitation edema.

9. **C,** Page 102.

Plasma concentrations of $Mg^{++}$ correlate poorly with intracellular stores. Cardiac irritability has been shown to be a better marker for magnesium deficiency. Replacement therapy is indicated for chronic alcoholics and malnourished patients who are likely to be depleted of total body stores and

for patients with low levels of plasma $Mg^{++}$ who show signs of cardiac irritability such as multiple extrasystolic beats. $Mg^{++}$ antagonizes $Ca^{++}$ channels and is primarily excreted by the kidneys.

10. **A,** Page 96.

During shock, the brain has the most highly preserved blood flow of all organs. The cerebrovasculature has remarkable autoregulatory ability. In fact, cerebral blood flow does not decrease until the mean arterial pressure falls below 50 mm Hg. Cerebral damage results only after prolonged and profound hypotension.

11. **A,** Pages 98-99.

In acute respiratory failure, adequate PEEP of 5 cm $H_2O$ or greater can prevent alveolar collapse. Ketamine and etomidate are preferable to the benzodiazepines, barbiturates, and morphine for induction or sedation because they depress cardiac function only minimally. A supranormal CVP of 10-15 cm $H_2O$ is often needed during shock to produce adequate filling volumes against stiff ventricles. The $FiO_2$ should be reduced to less than 0.8 as soon as possible to reduce oxygen toxicity.

12. **A,** Pages 97-98.

End-tidal $CO_2$ monitoring can provide a noninvasive estimate of cardiac output. When hypoperfusion occurs, $CO_2$ generated by cells cannot be transported the lungs. A patient in shock who is adequately resuscitated will have an end-tidal $CO_2$ value that rises as blood flow to the tissue and to the lungs increases. A decrease in bicarbonate level or an increase in lactate concentration will represent worsening acidosis. A drop in the mixed venous oxygen saturation would indicate increased oxygen extraction and worsening shock.

13. **D,** Page 98.

There are several reasons for early elective intubation of a patient. Strenuous use of accessory muscles can increase oxygen consumption by 50%-100%. Relieving the patient's work of breathing will decrease the total body oxygen requirement, decrease cardiac strain, and increase cerebral blood flow. Hyperventilation can reduce acidemia and cerebral edema. Intubation does not affect the relaxation of the bronchial smooth muscles. It can produce barotrauma and predispose the patient to have a spontaneous pneumothorax and should be avoided.

# 7  Brain Resuscitation

*Carol L. Henderson and Leo W. Burns*

1. **C,** Pages 107-108.
Cerebral blood flow (CBF) greater than 50% of normal has no detrimental effects due to autoregulation. When the cerebral blood flow falls below 35% of normal, transmembrane ion pumping becomes compromised. At this point the electroencephalogram becomes silent. At less than 35% of normal cerebral blood flow the neurons are still viable but nonfunctional. At cerebral blood flow less than 20% of normal, cell death occurs.

2. **C,** Pages 110-112.
The goal of optimizing neuronal recovery is many-fold. ABCs are paramount. Intubation, oxygenation with 100% oxygen, low PEEP, and adequate sedation and paralysis are necessary. Hyperventilating the patient to a $PaCO_2$ between 30 and 35 will prevent worsening of neurologic status. Hyperventilation is effective for only 4 hours and should be used judiciously. The kidneys and cerebral spinal fluid compensate for the alkalosis after 4 hours. Mean arterial pressures must be maintained between 90 and 100 mm Hg. Nothing has been shown to prevent anoxic seizures. If seizures occur, benzodiazepines are the first-line agents. Maintaining euglycemia or mild hypoglycemia is important because hyperglycemia has detrimental effects on cerebral blood flow, cerebral metabolism, edema formation, and neurologic outcome.

3. **B,** Pages 110.
Success in resuscitation is inversely proportional to the arrest time. If CPR is started 10 minutes after arrest, 0% cerebral blood flow (CBF) occurs. If started within 5 minutes of arrest, CBF is 28% of normal. Standard CPR can achieve 20%-30% of cardiac output. If CPR is started within 2 minutes of arrest, 50% of CBF can be attained.

4. **A,** Page 107.
ATP falls 90% within 1 minute of total ischemia. Anaerobic metabolism then takes over and the brain "shuts off," resulting in coma.

5. **A,** Page 107.
When the $PaO_2$ is less than 25 mm Hg, coma ensues. The stores of ATP are depleted. Short-term memory loss, difficulty with coordination, and changes in intellect and personality are all common occurrences following survival of cardiac arrest. The arterial boundary zones affect several vulnerable areas within the brain to cause such varied neurologic sequelae. The viability threshold is reached at a $PaO_2$ of approximately 12 mm Hg, compromising the potential survival of cardiac and brain cells.

6. **D,** Pages 109, 113.
Calcium accumulates within the red cell membrane, resulting in decreased deformability. It enters into smooth muscle, causing vasospasm. Calcium uncouples oxidative phosphory-

lation, which consumes ATP and significantly reduces its production. Calcium also releases aspartate and the neurotransmitter glutamate in addition to prostaglandins, thromboxanes, leukotrienes, and free radicals.

7. **D,** Page 112.
Hyperglycemia is detrimental to neurorecovery and should be aggressively treated. A sliding-scale insulin regimen should be implemented. Glucose potentiates edema formation in the brain. Glucose also has deleterious effects on CBF and metabolism. Oral hypoglycemic agents cannot be titrated and should be avoided. Hydration alone is not adequate in the treatment of hyperglycemia in brain resuscitation.

8. **B,** Page 113.
Barbiturates have been shown in several studies to reduce cerebral metabolism, edema formation, intracranial pressure, and seizure activity. Other studies have shown that barbiturates improve cell energy charge and cyclic AMP and free-fatty acid accumulation. No human studies validate the hypothesis that barbiturates should be given to all arrest survivors.

9. **C,** Pages 112-113.
Only moderate hypothermia has shown consistent findings of cerebral protection in well-established laboratory models of global ischemia and brain injury. The clinical use of steroids lacks documented efficacy. Without PEEP, alveoli collapse, requiring increased pressures to oxygenate a patient, thus raising ICP. Ischemia compromises the autoregulation of cerebral blood flow so that hypotension can cause a severe compromise of blood flow and significant brain damage.

10. **D,** Page 108.
The ischemic penumbra is the area of the brain containing cells that have lost function but not viability following an ischemic insult. It is this area that cerebral resuscitative efforts attempt to save.

11. **A,** Page 111.
This patient has signs and symptoms of neurologic deterioration. The patient needs to be intubated using rapid-sequence intubation and in-line stabilization of his neck. Despite the patient's wheezing, ketamine is a poor drug for induction in this patient because it raises intracranial pressure. The patient needs to be hyperventilated to a $PaCO_2$ between 30 and 35. Decadron is controversial and is not advisable. Osmotic agents such as mannitol or glycerine can be used to reduce intracranial pressure. Maintaining the mean arterial pressure (MAP) between 90 and 100 mm Hg is important to maintain adequate cerebral blood flow. Vasopressors are indicated if hydration with crystalloid fails to achieve adequate MAP.

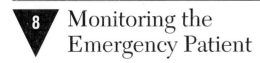

# 8 ▼ Monitoring the Emergency Patient

*David Hughes*

1. **C,** Page 120.
Intra-arterial catheters are the gold standard for blood pressure measurement followed by oscillometric devices which are more accurate, precise, and reliable than auscultation because the sensing devices are more sensitive than the human ear.

2. **C,** Page 121.
Pulse oximetry is based on light absorption at two different wavelengths, red and infrared, which are then canceled out and calculated. Carboxyhemoglobin is considered by the pulse oximeter to be mostly oxyhemoglobin and therefore will falsely elevate the pulse oximeter reading. Methemoglobin is absorbed at both wavelengths which forces the absorbance ratio toward unity, which corresponds to a pulse ox reading of 85%. This can artificially elevate or lower the pulse ox depending on the true oxyhemoglobin.

3. **E,** Page 123.
End tidal carbon dioxide detection can be falsely elevated when the metabolic production of carbon dioxide is high as in fever or hypothermia. Shock will cause errors secondary to decreased pulmonary perfusion. Abnormal respiratory patterns may affect readings due to sampling errors. If the gas sample is not at the end of an exhaled breath it may be falsely low. Obstructive airway disease may not allow an accurate assessment of the alveolar carbon dioxide.

4. **C,** Page 120.
The need for intraarterial BP monitoring solely due to Nitroprusside use is not supported in the literature.

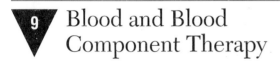

# 9 ▼ Blood and Blood Component Therapy

*Jack Horowitz and Denise J. Dunlap*

1. **A,** Page 124.
The majority of acute hemolytic reactions result from clerical error (mislabeling of blood product, misidentification of patient, etc.). Reactions to Rh, Kell, Kidd, and Duffy are usually delayed (5-7 days). Because the type O donor's antibody rich serum is removed prior to packed-cell transfusions, reactions are rare. Mild hemolytic reactions can occur with large amounts of fresh frozen plasma since the plasma retains the antibodies of the donor. Therefore it is preferable that the major blood groups be compatible.

2. **D,** Page 129.
An intravascular transfusion reaction may precipitate shock, renal cortical hypoperfusion, disseminated intravascular co-agulation, or death. If suspected, it necessitates immediate cessation of the transfusion and institution of vigorous fluid therapy to counteract shock. Furosemide (Lasix) or ethacrynic acid (Edecrin) will increase renal cortical flow as well as urine output, whereas mannitol does not increase renal perfusion and is therefore no longer the treatment of choice. Urine output should be maintained at 30 ml/hr.

3. **B,** Page 125.
The "type and screen" includes ABO grouping and Rh typing of the recipient's red cells. The additional "crossmatch" involves the mixing of donor cells with the recipient serum and serves as a check on ABO compatibility. If the patient actually needs the blood, the crossmatch can be done in 5 to 10 minutes after the type and screen has been completed. Since the "crossmatch" includes the "screen," it is both more costly and time consuming.

4. **B,** Page 128.
Factor VIII concentrate is the preferred treatment for a hemophilia A patient who is hemorrhaging. When refrigerated, it is stable for several months, making it useful for home administration. Also, heat-treated or solvent-detergent-treated factor VIII concentrates eliminate the hazard of HIV, hepatitis, and other viruses. Cryoprecipitate and fresh frozen plasma carry the risk of disease transmission. Factor IX concentrate is the treatment of choice for hemophilia B (Christmas disease).

5. **B,** Page 135.
Cryoprecipitate can be used to treat factor VIII and fibrinogen deficiencies. Other factors are present in insignificant amounts. The risk of hepatitis is about the same as with most other blood product transfusions. Patients who receive multiple packed red cell transfusions have enough residual donor serum to maintain some functional integrity of the coagulation system and do not require additional cryoprecipitate.

6. **C,** Page 125.
Intrathoracic blood is the only suitable blood for emergency reinfusion. Contraindications include abdominal blood or diaphragmatic rupture secondary to the possibility of enteric contamination, intrathoracic infections, and malignancies. Age and aspirin use are not contraindications.

7. **C,** Page 127.
Improvements continue to be made in storage techniques for blood products to extend their shelf life and improve posttransfusion survival. Current techniques include collection in citrate-phosphate-dextrose-adenine (CPDA-1) with or without additional additives.

8. **B,** Page 135.
Although concentrated factor VIII is the treatment of choice for bleeding with hemophilia A, cryoprecipitate contains 80-120 units of factor VIII:c and can be used if needed. Spontaneous bleeding is uncommon in patients with platelet counts above 20,000. The most common posttransfusion infection in the United States is hepatitis C. Although CMV and EBV can be transmitted by transfusion, they are not routinely screened for except for blood directed for neonates and infants.

9. **A,** Page 134.

Immune globulin is a form of passive antibody infusion that provides transient, acute protection against certain diseases such as tetanus, rabies, and hepatitis B. It should be given to all Rh-negative women with potential exposure to blood from an Rh-positive fetus to prevent hemolytic disease of the newborn. Patients with an up-to-date tetanus immunization status do not need hyperimmune globulin.

10. **D,** Page 132.

Multiple transfusions of stored blood at 4° C may result in a significant drop in body temperature. The preservative citrate can bind ionized calcium, resulting in a prolongation of the QT segment on an ECG. Citrate can also bind magnesium. Patients needing multiple transfusions may have injuries that can trigger disseminated intravascular coagulation. The consumptive coagulopathy plus the dilutional effect of the transfused blood can result in thrombocytopenia.

# 10 Approach to the Patient in the Emergency Department

*No questions*

# 11 Clinical Decision Making and "Best Practice" Systems

*No questions*

# 12 Geriatrics: Unique Concerns

*Norm Kalbfleisch*

1. **D,** Pages 162-163.

The elderly represent 13% of the U.S. population. Various studies have shown that the elderly utilize the ED at a rate proportional to or just slightly higher than this (13%-15%). All of the other statements are true.

2. **E,** Pages 163-165.

Very few ancillary tests change appreciably that would be attributable solely to the effects of old age. Q waves present in a regional pattern on an ECG suggest myocardial infarction and are never a consequence of normal aging.

3. **B,** Page 165.

As the elderly age, they are increasingly less likely to present with classic chest pain. For example, 60% of patients 65-74 years old will have chest pain with myocardial infarc-

tion (MI) or unstable angina. In the 75-84 age range, 50% will have classic pain. Only 40% of individuals in the mid-eighties or older have chest pain. The most common MI presentations for these oldest of the old are change in mental status or abrupt decline in activities of daily living (ADLs). Women are more likely than men to present atypically when matched for age throughout their adult lives.

4. **E,** Pages 166-168.

The physiologic changes of aging affect every organ system. Some estimate that physiologic reserve decreases roughly 1% per year after age 30 years. The elderly therefore have less reserve to handle *any* increased physiologic stress, including transient shock. This is particularly true in trauma. When comparing younger adults to the elderly and matching for severity of injury, the elderly are at least 4 to 6 times more likely to die of mild to moderate trauma than their younger counterparts. Nonfocal neurologic examinations with significant intracranial hemorrhage occur more frequently in the elderly than in the middle aged, in part due to the decrease in volume of the intracranial contents. The elderly may not manifest abnormal vital signs for a variety of reasons. For instance, an elder's typical blood pressure may be in the hypertensive range, and the individual may be receiving medications such as beta-blockers. On presentation after trauma, a heart rate in the 60s and a blood pressure of 130/60 may be falsely reassuring. Finally, as in the example of the elderly patient with multiple rib fractures, it may be prudent to admit or observe the patient rather than discharge him or her as would be likely for a younger patient.

# 13 Approach to the Immunocompromised Patient in the Emergency Department

*Lars Blomberg*

1. **A,** Pages 169, 170.

IgG and IgM activate the complement cascade through the classical pathway, whereas molecules with repeating chemical structure, such as bacterial cell walls, activate the alternative pathway.

2. **B,** Page 172.

Approximately 50% of bone marrow transplant patients acquire clinical cytomegalovirus disease (CMV). In all phases of transplantation, interstitial pneumonitis, most often tied to CMV, is a serious complication carrying a 15%-50% mortality.

3. **B,** Page 175.

Disseminated toxoplasmosis is a particular problem in heart transplant patients. Dormant toxoplasmosis can be reactivated during immunosuppression, resulting in myocarditis, encephalitis, or brain abscess. Myocardial toxoplasmosis has been mistaken for acute allograft rejection.

4. **D,** Page 173.

All drugs that inhibit cytochrome P-450 metabolism will produce elevated cyclosporin levels and enhance toxicity. In contrast, treatment with rifampin can increase cyclosporin metabolism and may lead to organ rejection.

5. **B,** Page 180.

Empiric treatment with the fluoroquinolones should be avoided in the febrile neutropenic cancer patient because of limited activity against streptococci and anaerobes. In addition, there has been a rapid emergence of resistance noted in gram-negative bacilli.

6. **C,** Page 183.

*S. aureus* infections are most common in hemodialysis patients. Up to 60% of patients on chronic hemodialysis are *S. aureus* carriers, and the carriage rate increases as time on dialysis increases.

7. **C,** Page 183.

Splenectomy or functional asplenia predisposes a patient to overwhelming infection from pneumococci and other encapsulated organisms. Young children, sickle cell anemia patients, and postsplenectomy patients for lymphoma or hematologic disorders are at highest risk.

 ## 14   Emergency Ultrasound

*Patrick Brunett*

1. **C,** Pages 188-189.

The amount of sound energy reflected back from a tissue interface depends on the density and compliance of the tissue. Dense, non-compliant, high impedance structures such as gallstones reflect most of the sound waves back to the transducer and appear bright. In contrast, low-density, high-compliance, fluid-filled structures such as the gall bladder reflect few sound waves and thus appear dark.

2. **A,** Page 188.

Lower transducer frequencies (2-3 MHz) are best suited for visualizing deep structures such as heart or abdominal organs. High-frequency transducers are used to visualize superficial structures such as neck vasculature, uterus, testes, and foreign bodies.

3. **D,** Page 189.

One study noted speech delay was twice as likely in children who had undergone prenatal ultrasound. No changes in school performance have been demonstrated. Childhood cancers are associated with prenatal radiographic studies, not with ultrasound. Tissue microcavitation is seen with acoustic intensities higher than those used in diagnostic ultrasound.

4. **C,** Pages 189-190.

With profound intravascular depletion and decreased filling pressures, physiologic responses including tachycardia and increased contractility result in a hyperdynamic myocardium despite absent pulses. All of the other choices (pulmonary embolism, hyperkalemia, hypothermia, and massive myocardial infarction) result in hypodynamic myocardial wall motion.

5. **D,** Pages 189-190.

The goal of emergency echocardiography in the hypotensive trauma patient is to identify pericardial fluid. If present, it is assumed to be hemopericardium with cardiac tamponade. All of the other choices are subtle findings of tamponade that are beyond the scope of emergency ultrasound in the unstable trauma patient.

6. **E,** Pages 190-191.

The sonographic appearance of fluid in Morison's pouch, as demonstrated here, does not distinguish between blood, ascites, or other fluid. Intraperitoneal fluid can be reliably detected at volumes >200 to 600 ml. The need for laparotomy is based both on sonographic findings and on the patient's hemodynamic instability. In the stable patient, a more specific test such as computed tomography may be indicated before laparotomy. Diagnostic peritoneal lavage is much more sensitive than either CT or ultrasound.

7. **A,** Pages 191-192.

In the patient with suspected biliary colic, the role of emergency ultrasound is to identify cholelithiasis. A sonographic Murphy's sign may also help distinguish cholecystitis from simple cholelithiasis. The identification of sludge, thickened gall bladder wall, and pericolic fluid are consistent with cholecystitis but less reliable in examinations not performed by a radiologist or sonographic technician. The same is true for common bile duct dilation as an indicator of biliary obstruction.

8. **E,** Page 193.

Subcutaneous fat and bowel gas may diminish sonographic resolution regardless of the study. Staghorn calculi may fill the entire renal pelvis and obscure dilation. In the dehydrated patient, urine production and thus the development of hydroureter may be delayed.

9. **C,** Pages 192-193.

The specificity of hydroureter as a criterion for diagnosis of renal calculus is near 100%. Ultrasound is accurate in visualizing actual calculi near the collecting system or the ureterovesical junction. It is less accurate in the middle third of the ureter, which may be obscured by bowel gas. If history and ancillary tests suggest renal colic and hydroureter is detected on the side of pain, computed tomography or intravenous pyelogram may not be necessary.

10. **D,** Pages 193-194.

The combination of abdominal pain and hemodynamic instability in patients with abdominal aortic aneurysm has been an accurate predictor of the need for surgical intervention. Elective repair is indicated in aneurysms greater than 5.4 cm, and spontaneous rupture rates rise significantly above this diameter. Murphy's sign is a test for cholecystitis.

11. **E,** Page 194.

Transvaginal sonography can reliably detect an intrauterine pregnancy (IUP) at β-hCG levels >1800, whereas transabdominal ultrasound can only detect an IUP with a serum β-hCG >6500.

12. **D,** Page 194.

Transvaginal ultrasound detects intrauterine pregnancy at an earlier gestational age. All of the other choices (wider, deeper view; use of 3.5 MHz probe; easier to learn; not reliable for cornual pregnancy) describe transabdominal ultrasound.

13. **B,** Pages 188, 194.

Emergency ultrasound is intended to answer simple clinical questions and thus expedite definitive treatment in the acute care setting. It does not replace (and in some cases may prompt) formal sonography, in order to provide definitive diagnoses. While ultrasound does indeed reduce patient exposure to ionizing radiation and contrast dye, these are not explicit goals.

# 15 Life and Death

*No questions*

# 16 Bioethics

*No questions*

# 17 Approach to Administration in the Emergency Department

*No questions*

# 18 Legal Issues in Emergency Medicine

*No questions*

# 19 Clinical Forensic Medicine

*No questions*

# 20 The Medical Literature: A Reader's Guide

*No questions*

# 21 Pain Management

*Ryan M. Kramer and Denise L. Dunlap*

1. **A,** Pages 284, 287.

The CNS toxicity of meperidine (Demerol) is caused by the metabolite normeperidine. Adverse CNS reactions include anxiety, disorientation, tremors, seizures, hallucinations, and psychosis. Both meperidine and morphine have a high abuse potential and a propensity for respiratory depression, especially when higher doses are given. Morphine produces hypotension as a result of peripheral venous and arterial dilation. Naloxone can be used, but usually is not effective in blocking this decreased peripheral vascular resistance because vasodilation is caused by histamine release. Treatment for hypotension is fluid administration.

2. **B,** Page 287.

Fentanyl is a synthetic opioid whose properties include a short half-life, lack of histamine release, and little effect on cardiac contractility. Since it is the only opioid analgesic that does not cause histamine release, it is ideal for the treatment of pain in patients with bronchospastic lung disease. Fentanyl given in high and repeated doses may produce muscle rigidity, which can be severe enough to interfere with ventilation, so that neuromuscular blockade may be required. Although a transmucosal (lollipop) preparation is available for children, this route is not ideal for this patient. Like all other opioid agonists, it can cause respiratory depression.

3. **D,** Page 287.

The most significant side effect of pentazocine is the psychotomimetic reaction that occurs in up to 7% of patients. Pentazocine is an opioid of the agonist-antagonists class. The advantages of the these drugs are minimal respiratory depression, decreased biliary tract spasm, and diminished abuse potential. It is thought that this class of drugs achieves analgesia by agonist action at the kappa receptors, while the reduced respiratory depression is due to antagonism of the mu receptors.

4. **B,** Pages 291-291.

The nitrous oxide/oxygen mixture is delivered to the patient through a demand valve activated when the patient inhales. The patient is in control of the system. However, because patient cooperation is necessary, this system is contraindicated in patients with an altered level of consciousness or head injury. At low temperatures, the mixture separates, with the lighter oxygen rising to the top and the heavier nitrous oxide settling on the bottom. Scavenger devices are required with nitrous oxide to prevent accumulation of the gas that could inadvertently affect health care workers or other patients.

5. **D,** Pages 293-294.

Lidocaine belongs to the amide class of local anesthetics. Other members include mepivacaine, bupivacaine, and etidocaine. Procaine belongs to the ester class, along with tetracaine. Since the two classes do not cross-react, a patient with an allergy to an agent in one class may be given an agent from the other class. True allergy to the amide class is rare. Allergy to the ester class has been reported and is believed to be caused by the preservative methylparaben and its breakdown products. Diphenhydramine (Benadryl) is another alternative for infiltration or nerve block.

6. **B,** Page 294.

Lidocaine is a safe and effective local anesthetic. However, toxicity may occur with inadvertent arterial injection or when the dose exceeds 3-5 mg/kg for lidocaine without epinephrine. Addition of epinephrine, which causes vasoconstriction and thus delayed systemic absorption, increases the maximum dose of lidocaine to 7 mg/kg. A 1% solution contains 10 mg per milliliter. Therefore, the maximum dose for this patient is 210 mg, equivalent to 21 ml of a 1% solution. Lidocaine toxicity includes CNS and cardiovascular effects. CNS toxicity includes altered mental status ranging from drowsiness, confusion, seizures, and coma and is initially manifest as light-headedness, headache, perioral paresthesias, tinnitus, slurred speech, and muscle twitches. Cardiovascular toxicity includes decreased cardiac contractility, impaired sinus and atrioventricular node function, and hypotension secondary to peripheral vasodilation. Hypotension should be treated with fluids and alpha-adrenergic agents.

 22 ## Sedation and Analgesia for Procedures

*Brian J. Levine and Angelo Grillo*

1. **B,** Page 304.

High-dose fentanyl may result in muscular and glottic rigidity, or "board chest." Rigidity, although often discussed, has never been reported with the use of fentanyl in the ED. This is most likely because of the much smaller doses associated with conscious sedation (2-3 μg/kg) when compared to the larger doses associated with general anesthesia used in the operating suite (50-100 μg/kg). The associated fall in chest compliance, glottic closure, or both may create difficulties in maintaining the airway. Studies have reported the onset of rigidity at an average dose of 9-17 μg/kg. Rigidity may also be associated with IV morphine and meperidine and is reversed with naloxone or succinylcholine. Fentanyl causes little or no histamine release compared to other commonly used opioids.

2. **B,** Page 304.

Proper monitoring is essential to ensure patient safety during conscious sedation. After completion of the procedure and removal of the pain stimulus, respiratory depression is increased. The half-life of fentanyl is 90 minutes; it is not affected by midazolam. Midazolam is water soluble and not stored in fat cells.

3. **D,** Page 306.

There is considerable experience with nitrous oxide in the ED. Some consider it the best agent for conscious sedation. Sedation and analgesia can occur in 1-2 minutes, and its duration of action is less than 5 minutes. Clinically, its sedative and anxiolytic effects are more evident than its analgesic properties. Higher concentrations are required at high altitudes (65%-70%). At least 30% oxygen needs to be administered along with the nitrous oxide to avoid hypoxia. The patient can control delivery of the nitrous oxide through demand valve opening with inhalation.

4. **C,** Page 306.

If a patient is overly sedated or experiences respiratory depression, partial reversal may be achieved by using small incremental doses of naloxone intravenously. At the same time it would be prudent to prepare for possible positive pressure ventilation should the need arise. Most authorities recommend doses of 0.1-0.2 mg initially to avoid withdrawal, although doses of 2 mg can be used at once to attempt complete reversal. Flumazenil antagonizes the effects of benzodiazepines.

5. **B,** Page 306.

Ketamine is a dissociative anesthetic that is structurally similar to phencyclidine. It produces a tonic state characterized by deep analgesia, maintenance of upper airway reflexes, and respiratory stability. On reawakening, emergent phenomena manifested by hallucinations and nightmares occur in up to 50% of adults and up to 10% of children. Ketamine also inhibits reuptake of catecholamines, resulting in mild increases in heart rate, blood pressure, cardiac output, and bronchodilation.

6. **C,** Page 307.

Flumazenil antagonizes the effects of benzodiazepines by competitively and reversibly binding to GABA-benzodiazepine receptors in the CNS. The peak effects occur 6-10 minutes after administration and elimination half-life is 41-79 minutes. Resedation may be a problem if flumazenil is used to reverse a long-acting benzodiazepine such as diazepam. Therefore, appropriate respiratory monitoring is important during the recovery phase despite the use of flumazenil. Due to the fear of precipitating withdrawal and seizures, flumazenil is currently not recommended as part of the "coma cocktail" for unknown polypharmacy ingestions. Seizures after flumazenil use have been associated with repeated doses of benzodiazepine administration, concurrent major sedative-hypnotic withdrawal, seizure activity before flumazenil use, and concurrent cyclic antidepressant poisoning.

7. **A,** Page 309.

A normal mental status and baseline cognitive and motor function are prerequisites to discharge. The patient should understand and follow directions, speak clearly, and ambulate unassisted (infants should sit unassisted). Children should be watched at home for at least 8 hours. Adults should not participate in potentially dangerous activities (drive, operate power tools, ride a bicycle) for the next 24 hours. Due to the short half-life of naloxone, patients who have been reversed from conscious sedation should be monitored for an additional 90 to 120 minutes.

8. **C,** Page 310.

Agents used for conscious sedation often have different pharmacokinetics in infants and children than in adults. Precise dosing according to weight and anticipation of their age-dependent responses to these medications are essential for their safe use. Midazolam has gained popularity for its effectiveness by many routes of administration (e.g., IV, IM, nasal, oral, rectal). Midazolam will not necessarily aid in making a child motionless, so additional medications may be needed for such studies as CT scans.

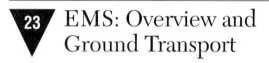

# 23 ▼ EMS: Overview and Ground Transport

*Daron P. Riley and Angelo Grillo*

1. **D,** Pages 317-318.

Although the 911 service has been promulgated by the national government since 1973, there are many communities who have not adopted it due to financial constraints. It is estimated that 30% of EMS calls are for nonemergent conditions and that 15%-20% actually constitute true emergencies. Provision of pre-arrival instructions in such medical emergencies as cardiopulmonary arrest, obstructed airways, hemorrhage control, and childbirth are an important part of emergency dispatching. Many studies have shown that dispatchers can identify those victims in need of CPR by bystanders and are skilled at providing such instructions. Priority-based systems of dispatching incorporate a defined list of common chief complaints, each having a subset of pre-determined prompts in order to gain more information about the seriousness of the call and therefore determine the level of response needed. Criteria-based dispatch recognizes one critical condition to determine the level of response, for example, chest pain selects for advanced life support crews regardless of the nature of the call. Systems status management refers to the matching of resources to demand during peak call times or in areas of high service volume by assigning ambulances to predetermined locations based on retrospective data. Obviously, the appropriateness of this management technique depends on EMS system size, population served, and resources available.

2. **B,** Page 319.

Deviations from specific protocols may indicate problems with the medical control physician, the individual EMT, or the protocol itself. Each incident needs to be analyzed individually by the medical director and continuing education and reassessment of all parties is essential. Pre-hospital providers are subjected to diverse emotional situations like domestic and child abuse, alcohol-related trauma, hostage situations, infant death, and hostile and abusive patients. Providing access to personnel counseling is an important function of the off-line medical director to ensure employee well-being. Off-line medical control includes prospective and retrospective patient care review. Retrospective call review using information from the run report and tapes assists the medical director in evaluating individual providers in protocol compliance and documentation skills. Communication and critique of medic performance between personnel in the ED after patient arrival is an important duty of the on-line physician if available. Pre-hospital protocols should include instructions for triaging patients for trauma center care. Standing orders allow a more streamlined approach in many medical emergencies; however, the use of standing orders for trauma has not significantly reduced scene times.

3. **D,** Pages 319-321.

Patents who are at a risk to themselves or others and refuse care are commonly encountered by pre-hospital providers. Competent, non-dangerous patients refusing care must be thoroughly assessed for injuries, and the attendant risks of refusal must be delineated. Usually a patient refusal form is filed in an attempt to prevent future litigation. Involuntary holds may be initiated in the pre-hospital setting by on-line physicians, safety officers, family members, or pre-hospital providers. The patient in this scenario needs to be evaluated by a physician for many reasons, including assessment of ongoing suicide risk and the potential for occult trauma with ongoing alcohol intoxication. When confronted with on-scene physicians, the medics should request proof of licensure and inform the physician that the on-line physician is accountable for all pre-hospital care. The medical control physician has authority to overrule any order given by on-scene physicians. Last, providers should not perform any procedure or function outside their level of education. The majority of lawsuits against EMS agencies deal with patient refusal-of-care issues. Scenario C deals with an adult patient who is clinically incompetent to decide for herself at the present time. This patient is at high risk for recurrent hypoglycemia due to the oral hypoglycemic. The on-line physician should ask to speak directly with the family to voice this concern and persuade them to allow transport. A hospital ED may go on diversion status when their maximal resources have been exceeded. Diversion prolongs pre-hospital times, delays definitive care, and puts logistic strains on the system and families. It is obvious that the patient presented here will need catheterization because of his contraindications to thrombolytic therapy and transport to the more distant hospital would only delay essential care. DNR orders are becoming more commonplace and EMS providers are frequently faced with decisions on resuscitation. Most states require that resuscitation attempts be performed regardless of the directive. When presented with DNR orders or advanced directives at the scene, the medic must decide if they are valid. If any doubt exists or the papers are not available, a reasonable alternative would be to transport to the closest hospital while instituting basic life support measures. Another important medicolegal point presented here is that the wife probably would have durable power of attorney for the patient.

4. **E,** Pages 315-316.
The Department of Transportation recognizes four common levels of EMS provider. The first responder (FR) provides quick scene response time, can assess the need for further resources, and can begin stabilization of the patient. The FR is skilled in basic life support and in some communities automatic external defibrillation (AED). They receive a set number of hours of didactic instruction but are not required to perform a clinical rotation. The EMT–B is the minimum level required to staff a BLS ambulance and is commonly used for convalescent transport services. The EMT–B can successfully deliver early defibrillation and thus increase out-of-hospital survival from cardiac arrest. The EMT–I has a variable scope of practice depending on the geographic region. Most systems allow EMT–Is to defibrillate, establish intravenous lines, and provide adjunctive airway procedures. They are best suited for areas where paramedics are unavailable or unaffordable such as in rural areas. The EMT–P is the most advanced pre-hospital provider, requiring a large number of hours of didactic and field instruction. The two most important procedures performed by paramedics are defibrillation and definitive airway control. Multiple medications are used by paramedics, many of which have yet to be clinically proven beneficial. Paramedic training requires on average 1000 hours of service and includes instruction in the invasive procedures.

5. **E,** Pages 314-315.
Basic life support crews are skilled in all of the procedures listed but do not have credentials in intravenous therapies. Hospital-based EMS systems are few in number but allow for better working relationships between pre-hospital and ED personnel because in less busy times the EMTs provide basic patient care services. Many public EMS systems were formed as their own entity of municipal third-service systems to avoid philosophic conflict between fire-based personnel and dedicated EMS providers. Third-service EMS systems are operated by county governments; a medical control committee usually oversees administration and basic operation. Multi-tiered systems and priority-based dispatch systems are optimally suited for large service areas with high volumes such as an inner city population. BLS transport of non-urgent patients allows a limited number of ALS ambulances to be available for potential critical patients. Most states incorporate an office of EMS or an EMS council to govern and oversee the provision of EMS activities to ensure the effective economic provision of optimal patient care. Their duties

include those stated in E as well as keeping all records and establishing examination guidelines for providers.

6. **B,** Page 321.
The Consolidated Omnibus Budget Reconciliation Act (COBRA) of 1986 governs the transfer of patients from Medicare-enrolled hospitals. The first statute stipulates that before transfer, an adequate screening examination must be performed to rule out an emergency condition, and if one is present, stabilization to prevent deterioration upon transfer must be completed. Patient transfer may then occur if no additional therapeutic measures are anticipated for at least 5 hours. In addition, the transfer must be communicated to and accepted by the receiving facility, performed by qualified and appropriately equipped personnel, and all records and test results must be transported with the patient. Cases in which diagnostic and therapeutic measures at the receiving hospital are of greater benefit may completely preclude stabilization of the patient.

## 24 Disaster Preparedness and Response

*Philip N. Salen and Anita H. Hodson*

1. **E,** Page 324.
In general terms, an event can be considered a disaster when it overwhelms response capabilities. It is the functional impact on the specific area that is the key concept in determining whether a disaster exists. Multiple-casualty incidents that take place in or near cities result in disaster scenarios when they overwhelm medical response capabilities in spite of multiple hospitals participating in a trauma system. Relatively small numbers of casualties in rural areas can overwhelm both the emergency medical service system and small rural community hospitals that do have the resources to treat multiple-casualty situations.

2. **E,** Page 326.
Rescue personnel often use a simple triage and rapid treatment (START) technique that depends on a quick assessment of respirations, perfusion, and mental status. Age, current injuries, ability to survive current injuries, and medical history are all important considerations but are not part of the initial triage criteria.

3. **C,** Page 326.
The goal of disaster triage is to do the most good for the most people. The only patient care interventions that should interfere with triage of patients into one of four categories (walking wounded, critically ill, ill but interventions can wait, and deceased) are opening an obstructed airway and placing direct pressure on obvious external hemorrhage. Under disaster conditions, cardiopulmonary resuscitation should not be performed. C-spine immobilization is important but should not be part of initial triage. Splinting of fractures should be done after triage has been completed and the critically ill patients have been cared for and transported.

4. **C,** Page 327.

The goals of disaster triage is to do the most good for the most people. Cardiopulmonary resuscitation should not be performed under disaster conditions. Therefore, CPR should not be initiated on the 8-year-old girl, and she should be last in the triage hierarchy. If after assessment and opening of airway, she does not regain pulse, she should be declared deceased. Because of his altered mental status and the extent of the burn wounds, the 40-year-old male should be first. The 70-year-old female should be next because in addition to the burn wounds, she has a potentially easily reversed medical condition, chest pain. The 20-year-old male is third because he is medically stable despite the burn wounds. The 25-year-old paramedic should be treated before other walking wounded because her medical conditions are easily treated and, once treated, she can assist in triage and care of wounded.

5. **A,** Page 328.

The incident commander has overall management responsibility for the incident. Physicians should understand that they are not in charge at the scene of a pre-hospital incident. In general, pre-hospital providers can handle the scene, and physicians should remain at the hospital to provide definitive care. The incident commander should appoint a command staff to handle public information, safety, and interagency liaisons. The incident commander, who most commonly does not have a medical background, leaves the responsibility of triage to the pre-hospital personnel.

6. **E,** Page 328.

An internal disaster is any event that disrupts daily routine hospital functions. This can be an infrastructure failure (e.g., the loss of electric power and water) or a threat to safety of patients and hospital personnel (e.g., a labor dispute). The geographic location of an event (internal or external to the facility) is not necessarily synonymous with its effect on the hospital's ability to provide patient care. The internal disaster plan directs the institutional response to such an event. An external disaster is an event occurring in the community that results in a sudden influx of patients requiring emergency care at hospitals.

7. **E,** Page 329.

Basic components of a hospital disaster plan must include an interdepartmental planning group, resource management plans, command structure plans, a designated committee to coordinate all media interactions, redundant communication systems, a roster of all critical personnel and a method for their mobilization, a systematic approach to patient management, and periodic disaster drills.

8. **C,** Page 330.

There are several important differences that occur in disasters involving hazardous materials. These include the need for effective decontamination of victims and the need for effective safety measures on the part of rescue personnel to prevent secondary contamination. Patients contaminated with hazardous chemicals should first be brought to the predesignated decontamination site containing a warm-water

shower with a container to hold drainage water. Rescuers and victims should remove all clothing, which is then bagged and discarded safely. Contaminated patients must never be brought into regular patient care areas because of the danger of contaminating other patients and hospital staff. The ED must close off the air intake vents in rooms to which contaminated patients are taken so toxic products do not enter the ventilation system and circulate to other parts of the hospital. The sooner individuals have been decontaminated, the sooner they can be treated as normal accident victims.

9. **D,** Page 331.

In responding to disasters, emergency health care providers frequently develop high levels of psychologic stress. If this excessive stress exceeds the capacity of normal coping mechanisms, it can potentially interfere with job performance or produce disturbing symptoms. Posttraumatic stress can result. In an attempt to reduce the psychologic impact of these events on medical responders, a technique known as critical incident stress debriefing (CISD) was introduced in 1983. The goal of CISD is to assist health care workers in regaining emotional control by facilitating ventilation of feelings and reactions through listening and support. Convened within 72 hours after the event, debriefings are coordinated by mental health and peer support staff and focus on education and ventilation of emotions; the sessions last about 3 hours.

10. **D,** Page 331.

FEMA is the primary federal agency for helping state and local organizations prepare for, respond to, and recover from emergencies, and it is a major source of funding for these endeavors. The National Disaster Medical System (NDMS) is the agency that is responsible for the duties listed in option A.

## 25 Aeromedical Transport and In-Flight Medical Emergencies

*Matthew P. Sullivan and Anita H. Hodson*

1. **C,** Pages 335-336.

Aeromedical missions may be described as primary, secondary, or tertiary. Primary responses, or scene flights, involve utilization of the aircraft as the sole means of patient transport to the receiving facility, whereas secondary responses involve inter-facility transport from an emergency department to another hospital. Tertiary responses occur when inpatients are transported to another facility for definitive care.

2. **C,** Page 338.

Boyle's law, as it applies to altitudes, states: As altitude increases and atmospheric pressure decreases, air expands and volume increases. Boyle's law, $P_1V_1 = P_2V_2$, means that, for any decrease in pressure (which occurs with an increase in altitude), there must be a proportional increase in volume (air expands).

3. **D,** Page 338.

At altitude, the molecules that compose air are farther apart and there are fewer oxygen molecules per unit area. The normal physiologic response to this situation is tachycardia and tachypnea. Subjects with a normal cardiopulmonary reserve will exhibit a compensatory tachycardia and tachypnea that restore adequate hemoglobin saturation and oxygen delivery to the body.

4. **A,** Page 339.

Charles' law, V1T2 = V2T1, indicates that the volume of a given unit of gas is directly proportional to its temperature. This relationship explains why temperature falls with altitude and why inadvertent hypothermia may be encountered at altitude.

5. **B,** Page 340.

Boyle's law predicts expansion of gases with increasing altitude. As such, the consequences of increased pressure exerted by endotracheal tube cuffs, air splints, and the pneumatic antishock garment may be predicted. In the case of air splints, this may lead to artificial compartment syndrome. Gaseous expansion within intravenous infusion bags not regulated by electronic pumps results in increased rate of infusion.

6. **D,** Pages 341-363.

Aeromedical transport is indicated for patients suffering from decompression sickness. These patients may be transported by air with an effort made to maintain as low an altitude as is safe. Patients in full cardiopulmonary arrest and those who are at risk for childbirth in flight are not suitable candidates for air transport, nor are patients who are potentially dangerous to the crew and themselves.

7. **B,** Page 344.

Pressurized commercial aircraft are unable to maintain a cabin altitude equivalent to sea level. Compressors aboard the aircraft require a safety valve to prevent structural damage. As a result, the internal air pressure generally approximates an altitude of 5000 to 8000 feet while at cruising altitude. Atmospheric pressure ranges between 632 and 565 mm Hg at these levels.

8. **B,** Page 345.

The present FAA regulations for onboard medical supplies date from 1986 and require syringes, needles, and basic medications such as dextrose and diphenhydramine injections and nitroglycerin tablets. Apart from epinephrine, no other ACLS medications are required. Oropharyngeal airways represent the only instruments for airway management, and defibrillators are not required by FAA regulation. Individual airlines, however, may carry more extensive supplies and medications.

9. **D,** Pages 346-347.

A pregnancy of less than 36 weeks' gestation is not a contraindication to commercial flight. Beyond 35 weeks' gestation, data suggest that birth weight is adversely affected by ascent to altitude, and there is an increased risk of delivery as the pregnancy approaches term. Therefore, flying during this period is contraindicated. Patients who are immobile are at risk because of logistic and safety considerations. Patients with contagious diseases pose a risk to their fellow passengers. Patients with severe anemia are at risk of complications when exposed to decreased oxygen at altitude.

# 26 ▼ Multiple Trauma

*Jeffery M. Tiongson and Neil B. Jasani*

1. **B,** Page 359.

This patient has vital signs consistent with Class II hemorrhage. Class III hemorrhage includes decreased BP and delayed capillary refill.

2. **A,** Page 353.

Duodenal hematoma is most commonly associated with handlebar injuries. Splenic rupture and pericardial tamponade are unlikely in a patient with minimal signs of shock.

3. **D,** Pages 355-357.

Trauma systems reduce the incidence of preventable death from trauma. They include all aspects of care for the patient, including all pre-hospital interventions.

4. **D,** Page 353.

This patient most likely has injuries involving the lower extremities and areas of transmitted force and therefore needs radiologic examination of the spine and pelvis.

5. **A,** Page 354.

Ejection from the vehicle is associated with injuries benefiting from treatment at a trauma center. The other injuries do not by themselves indicate need for a trauma team.

6. **B,** Page 356.

The trauma leader should not be distracted from the overall care of the patient while performing procedures. These should be delegated to other team members.

7. **E,** Pages 356-358.

This patient is likely to be experiencing upper airway occlusion caused by a mandible fracture. Stabilization of the airway is always the highest priority. IV access is also a high priority and may be required to facilitate intubation of this combative patient. Administration of a saline bolus is secondary to securing the airway.

8. **C,** Page 360.

This patient likely has a significant spinal cord injury. High dose methylprednisolone at 30 mg/kg has been shown to improve neurologic recovery when administered within 8 hours of injury. This treatment should not be delayed while obtaining other testing. Psychiatric consultation is important but may be deferred since initial resuscitation assumes priority.

9. **C,** Page 361.

This patient is not stable enough to wait 20 minutes for an abdominal CT. Diagnostic peritoneal lavage can be performed quickly and safely after the decompression of bowel and bladder with a Foley catheter and a nasogastric tube.

10. **C,** Page 362.

Victims of blunt trauma without signs of life before arrival at the hospital have no chance of survival. The other scenarios may benefit from an emergent thoracotomy.

11. **C,** Pages 362-363.

The indication for head CT scan should be more liberal in the elderly. Altered mental status should always be initially assumed due to a reversible cause and not attributed to senility.

12. **D,** Page 364.

Spinal cord injury without radiographic abnormality (SCIWORA) has been well described in children under age 8. A towel may be needed under the patient's shoulder to compensate for the relatively larger head size in children. Also due to the larger head size, injuries at the fulcrum point high in the cervical spine are more common.

 27 Trauma in Pregnancy

*Stephanie L. Ciccarelli and Neil B. Jasani*

1. **A,** Pages 372-373.

It takes only 1 cc of fetal blood exposure to Rh sensitize 70% of Rh negative mothers. 50 μg of RhoGAM will provide prophylaxis for up to 50 cc of fetal blood exposure and 300 μg for up to 30 cc (these are the two standard doses that are available). At 12 weeks' gestation, total fetal blood volume is only 4.2 cc. At 16 weeks' gestation, total fetal blood volume is 30 cc. Therefore, if dates are accurate and consistent with clinical evaluation, Kleihauer-Betke tests should be done for >16 weeks' gestation to determine if more than one dose of 300 μg of RhoGAM should be administered. The Kleihauer-Betke test is done on a maternal blood sample to measure the fetal-to-maternal blood ratio (fetal hemoglobin stains with this test and maternal does not). RhoGAM is effective when administered within 72 hours of exposure. The Kleihauer-Betke test may be falsely positive if maternal circulation contains persistent fetal hemoglobin (as seen in sickle cell trait and thalassemias). The persistent maternal hemoglobin F can be detected by noting incomplete staining and by hemoglobin electrophoresis.

2. **B,** Page 373.

Obstetric patients have reduced oxygen reserve and an increase in oxygen consumption, and the fetus is particularly vulnerable to hypoxia. Therefore all maternal trauma patients should be given supplemental oxygen until any significant injuries to both the fetus and the mother have been ruled out. Because of the increase in maternal blood volume (>50% by term), there is significant maternal reserve despite fetal compromise. Hence, maternal vital signs are not reliable predictors of fetal well-being. Risk of aspiration is increased in pregnancy because of decreased gastroesophageal sphincter integrity as well as the cephalad migration of diaphragm and intraabdominal organs. Also, the stomach contents during pregnancy are more acidic, making aspiration

more ominous. Therefore, a secure airway is critical, and if intubation is necessary, rapid-sequence intubation should be performed. For mechanical ventilation, it should be remembered that the pregnant woman has a chronic respiratory alkalosis (increased tidal volume and respiratory rate) with a $PCO_2 = 30$.

3. **B,** Page 374.

In blunt abdominal trauma during pregnancy, the mother may lose up to 35% of her blood volume before showing signs of hypotension, because of the increased blood volume. Diagnostic peritoneal lavage by open technique can be done safely in all three trimesters. Reduced maternal blood pressure is associated with fetal blood flow reductions of 10%-20%. The two most common causes of fetal death are maternal death and maternal shock.

4. **C,** Pages 33, 378.

Uterine contractions are the most common obstetric problem caused by trauma; 90% of cases are self-limiting. Persistent uterine contractions are an indication of an underlying pathologic process. During fetal monitoring, if more than three contractions are seen per hour, then the patient should be admitted for extended monitoring for 24 hours. Other signs of more serious injuries necessitating admission include persistent uterine tenderness, vaginal bleeding, and abnormal fetal strips (if fetal gestation is appropriate). Uterine rupture is a very rare event, usually occurring in the case of pelvic fractures and indicated by shock out of proportion to vaginal bleeding.

5. **A,** Page 376.

Tetanus toxoid and immunoglobulin are safe in pregnancy and should be given. The immunoglobulin does cross the placenta and, rather than causing any harm, is helpful in preventing neonatal tetanus.

6. **D,** Pages 376-377.

Maternal cardioversion can be performed safely in all three trimesters and in an elective as well as emergent situation. The energy delivered to the fetus is small and no adverse affects were reported in one study that used up to 200J of energy. However, fetal monitoring is still recommended.

7. **B,** Pages 372, 377-378.

Maternal stability and survival does not ensure fetal well-being, so trivial maternal injury should not be quickly dismissed. Although less likely to cause fetal injury than direct trauma, even minor indirect trauma may result in adverse fetal outcome, typically in the form of placental abruption. If normal, reactive strips are recorded for 4 hours, the patient may be discharged safely with close follow-up. Although controversial, fetal age between 20 and 24 weeks frequently merits monitoring (although the fetus often is not considered viable) because supportive intervention may allow enough fetal maturation for survival. All fetuses at 25 weeks' gestation or greater are considered viable.

8. **A,** Page 378.

Maternal survival does not guarantee fetal survival. Fetal death rates are three to nine times higher than maternal death rates. For a stable obstetric trauma patient, the focus of care is on the fetus. However, if the mother is unstable, maternal resuscitation is of first priority. If there are no signs of maternal life within several minutes of emergency department resuscitation, open cardiac massage and emergency C-section should be immediately considered. Since the time from cessation of maternal circulation is the critical factor in fetal outcome, no time should be wasted including time to obtain consent. A dead fetus is usually spontaneously aborted within 1 week of the demise and should not be an absolute indication for a C-section.

9. **E,** Page 1036.

In maternal carbon monoxide (CO) exposure, the fetus is more sensitive to CO since fetal hemoglobin binds CO more vigorously than does maternal hemoglobin. Fetal carboxyhemoglobin concentrates are 10%-15% greater than maternal levels and require 36 to 48 hours to plateau. Fetal CO elimination half-life is approximately 3.5 times longer than maternal half-life, and oxygen therapy is recommended for 5 times as long as is needed to reach acceptable maternal CO levels. Hyperbaric oxygen is not contraindicated in pregnancy.

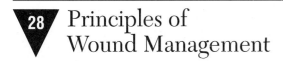

# 28 ▼ Principles of Wound Management

### *Michael E. Silverman and Scott P. Krall*

1. **D,** Page 383.
The static forces are demonstrated by the gaping of wounds following incision. Static forces of skin vary based on the area of the body but remain constant in any area of skin. Epithelialization bridges the defect by 48 hours in a surgically repaired laceration. Meticulous re-approximation of a jagged wound to a linear laceration may cause too much tissue loss and produce a wider, more visible scar. Lacerations parallel to skin folds, lines of expression, and joints do not impair function or cause unappealing scars.

2. **C,** Page 383.
Risk factors for wound morbidity and infection include prolonged time since injury; crush mechanism, deep penetrating wounds, high-velocity missiles, and contamination with saliva, feces, soil, or foreign matter. Bacterial proliferation leading to a level that may result in infection can occur in as little as 3 hours. Soil fractions render host defenses less able to perform normal duties. Lacerations produced by fine cutting forces resist infection better than crush injuries do.

3. **B,** Page 385.
Radiographs should visualize glass >1 mm thick if appropriate views are done. Most organic substances such as wood usually are not visible on plain films. A radiolucent shadow may be seen on close inspection because of displacement of tissue.

4. **C,** Page 385.
Lidocaine with epinephrine should be avoided in wounds with higher risks of infection and when tissue viability is a concern. Onset of action for direct infiltration occurs within seconds and lasts 20-60 minutes. Regional use of lidocaine for nerve blocks allows for an onset of action in 4-6 minutes. When epinephrine is added for vasoconstriction, there may be a delay in wound healing and a lower resistance to infection. Lacerations of the face, hands, fingers, feet, and toes are often well suited for regional anesthesia. Digital artery vasospasm may be successfully reversed with a local injection of 0.5 mg of phentolamine.

5. **B,** Page 385-386.
Tetracaine, adrenaline, cocaine combination (TAC) is more effective for anesthesia to the face and scalp but can be used on other parts of the body; however, mucus membranes must be avoided. TAC needs to be applied for 10-20 minutes to allow for effective anesthesia. Lidocaine injection is less painful if a smaller lumen needle is used and if it is injected slowly. When buffering, lidocaine-bicarbonate mixture should be 1:10. Bicarbonate-lidocaine buffering mixture will last 1 week at room temperature and 2 weeks if refrigerated.

6. **E,** Page 386.
Local anesthetics are divided into two different groups: amides and esters. Lidocaine and bupivacaine belong to the amide group, whereas tetracaine belongs to the ester group. The two allergen groups do not cross-react. One should consider allergy to the multidose vial preservative. Before attempting, a subcutaneous test dose can be given and the patient observed for 30 minutes. Normal saline potentially decreases pain via disruption for neuron function but is a less suitable alternative and is not an anesthetic. Another option may be aqueous diphenhydramine (1%) for local anesthesia.

7. **D,** Page 385-388.
The eyebrow is one of the exceptions to hair removal, because it is an important landmark for reapproximation and it grows back inconsistently. Disinfection and removal of devitalized tissue is important to decrease the incidence of infection. Irrigating the wound with normal saline using a 19-gauge needle and 30-ml syringe will provide the necessary pressure flow to clean the wound.

8. **E,** Page 389-390.
Vicryl is considered an absorbable suture, as are gut, chromic, polyglycolide, and polydioxanone. Nylon, silk, polypropylene, and stainless steel wire are nonabsorbable, as is mersilene.

9. **E,** Page 391.
The time necessary for closure is significantly lessened with staples compared with sutures. The monofilament stainless steel staples offer less risk of infection then even the least reactive suture. Acceptable wounds must be linear and subjected to weak skin forces. Staples are uncomfortable while in situ and when removed. Stapled wounds gain tensile strength sooner, and the staples can be removed 1-3 days earlier than sutures. Following their removal, staples should be replaced with wound closure tape for continued reinforcement.

10. **E,** Pages 394-395.

Up to 40% of all cases of tetanus occur in individuals who have either minor wounds or no recollection of any injury. The majority of patients who get tetanus are over 50 years old. The incubation period for tetanus is 7-12 days but ranges from 3-56 days. Immunization should be given as soon as possible but can be given days to weeks after injury. Tetanus immune globulin and tetanus toxoid may be administered in the same visit but should be given with a different syringe at separate sites. Tetanus toxoid, tetanus immune globulin, and diphtheria vaccination are safe and effective in pregnancy.

---

 ## 29 Injury Control

### Christine Milosis and Scott P. Krall

1. **D,** Page 398.

Central to the injury-control model is that injury is a disease rather than the consequence of random occurrence. The injury triangle consists of host, agent, and environment. Injury is the result of the host interacting with an agent in a dangerous environment. Environmental alterations are very effective and more easily instituted because they require no cooperation on the part of the host. The following is an example of factor modification to reduce motor vehicle crashes:

Agent: vehicle safety improvements
Environment: improved street lighting
Host: improved driving skills

2. **H,** Page 399.
3. **B,** Page 399.
4. **F,** Page 399.
5. **I,** Page 399.
6. **H,** Page 399.
7. **D,** Page 399.
8. **E,** Page 399.
9. **A,** Page 399.
10. **G,** Page 399.

A phase factor analysis of injury uses a nine-celled matrix that views each variable (host, agent, environment) in terms of pre-event, event, and post-event. This systematic approach is the mainstay of the injury model.

11. **C,** Pages 402-404.

Approximately 40,000 motor vehicle–related fatalities occur annually in the United States. Motor vehicle crashes are the greatest source of injury fatalities in the United States. Teenage drivers have the highest crash rate of all age-groups, and motor vehicle crashes are the leading cause of death and disability in this age-group. The elderly are another high-risk group with a high ratio of deaths to injuries because of pre-existing medical conditions. Persons older than age 70 are least likely to drive while intoxicated; however, visual and cognitive impairment lead to dangerous driving factors such

as misjudging distances and speed. Elderly persons are nine times more likely to be struck while turning left in front of an oncoming vehicle.

12. **E,** Page 403.

Injury occurs as energy is delivered to the vehicle occupant. To minimize energy transfer to the body, one must maximize stopping distance in a crash. The seat belt allows the occupant to decelerate when the vehicle begins decelerating rather than when the occupant strikes the interior of the vehicle after the car has slowed down or has struck an object. Air bags enable the occupant to decelerate over the distance of the inflated air bag. Collapsible steering wheels and deformable metals absorb crash energy and increase stopping distance.

13. **A,** Pages 404-405.

A firearm discharges a bullet from a cartridge case that has both gunpowder and primer. The cartridge is detonated by the firing pin of the firearm, hence the name. Not all guns are firearms because some guns (BB guns, air guns) discharge a projectile by the release of gas without burning gunpowder.

14. **B,** Pages 397-399.

For those 1 to 44 years of age, injury is the leading cause of death. Motor vehicle collisions are the leading cause of death and disability from unintentional injuries. One third of injuries are intentional.

15. **E,** Page 399.

The Haddon matrix is a "phase factor" definition of injury events. The emergency practitioner needs to understand the dynamics of this approach to manage the medical complications of the injury and help in injury prevention.

16. **C,** Page 399.

Using the three-phase Haddon matrix, an injury, like any other disease process, can be analyzed in terms of the host, the causative agent, and the environment in which the host and agent interact. Such analysis will encompass all other listed components.

17. **E,** Pages 403-404.

Lap and shoulder belts and air bags have been determined to be from 45% to 55% effective in preventing fatalities. The most common misuse of seat belts is wearing them under the arm, too loose, or too high, leading to injuries to the head, thorax, or abdomen. Injuries to the chest and abdomen may be seen even if seat belts are worn correctly.

18. **C,** Pages 404-405.

Homicide is the leading cause of death for African-American males ages 15 to 24, six times the rate for young white males. Firearms are used in approximately 60% of both homicides and suicides. Homicides occur at markedly varying rates in different metropolitan areas, but they are generally more an urban than suburban or rural problem, and they are most often associated with lower socioeconomic status. Victims and perpetrators tend to know each other. Women are most likely to be killed at home by a spouse or a lover as part of a pattern of battering.

# 30 Youth and Gang Violence

*No questions*

# 31 Head Trauma

### *Usamah Mossallam and Andrew Langsam*

1. **D,** Page 425; Table 31-1.
This patient receives 2 points for eye opening to painful stimuli, 2 points for moaning, and 4 points for flexion withdrawal from painful stimuli. The GCS score is thus 8.

2. **C,** Page 439.
Subdural hematomas are blood clots that form between the dura and the brain,. These are usually caused by the movement of the brain relative to the skull. These hematomas are common in patients with brain atrophy, such as alcoholic or elderly patients. In these patients the superficial bridging vessels traverse greater distances than in patients with no atrophy. As a result, the vessels are more prone to tearing with rapid movement of the head.

3. **B,** Page 440.
Death is more likely in patients who suffer from a subdural hematoma who are elderly, comatose, and present with a GCS of less than 8. The prognosis does not depend on the size of the hematoma but rather on the degree of brain injury caused by the pressure of the expanding hematoma. Survival is 35% to 50% in all such patients.

4. **D,** Page 426; Box 31-4.
Although nasal fractures may be associated with basilar skull fractures, they are not in and of themselves indicative of that more serious injury.

5. **A,** Pages 427-428; Table 31-5.
If hypotension is detected at any time in the course of the emergent management of a head-injured patient, a cause should be sought other than the head injury. Hypotension is rarely caused by head injury except as a terminal event. Important exceptions include profound blood loss from scalp lacerations and pediatric patients because they have relatively small circulating blood volume. Steroids have been shown to decrease vasogenic edema surrounding brain tumors but have no effect on the cytotoxic cerebral edema that develops and predominates after head injury as a result of secondary brain injury. High dose steroids cause detrimental infections and other complications. Seizure prophylaxis is indicated for intubation and paralysis, in addition to the other indications listed in Table 31-5. Barbiturates should not be administered early to patients with severe head injury, especially in the setting of multiple trauma because of the risk of profound hypotension. Mannitol is neuroprotective but is not indicated unless acute neurologic deterioration occurs.

6. **E,** Page 431; Box 31-6.
About 3% of all patients with minor head injury will deteriorate unexpectedly. A CT scan is recommended for high-risk patients. The presence of a skull fracture substantially increases the risk of an intracranial injury; therefore these patients should undergo CT scan evaluation.

7. **A,** Page 438.
The history given is the classic description of epidural hematoma. This occurs in only about 30% of all epidural hematomas. The lucid interval does not necessarily have to be a return to normal mentation but can represent an improvement in mental status.

8. **C,** Page 422.
Acute intracranial injury rarely causes hypotension or shock. The Cushing's reflex reflects a life-threatening increase in ICP. The triad of Cushing's reflex is hypertension, bradycardia, and respiratory irregularity and is seen in only one third of severe increases in ICP.

9. **B,** Page 426.
Blood behind the tympanic membrane or in the canal is presumptive of a basilar skull fracture. If the cribriform plate is fractured, the nasogastric tube may be passed into the cranial vault.

10. **B,** Page 428.
Hyperventilation decreases the $P_{CO_2}$, causing a constriction of the cerebrovascular bed and thereby lowering the ICP. This is usually accomplished within 30 seconds. Mannitol works as an osmotic diuretic to decrease ICP within 60 minutes. Steroids are no longer recommended and have no effect of decreasing ICP. Lasix and phenobarbital may be useful adjuncts to decreasing ICP, but they work far too slowly to have an immediate impact.

11. **A,** Page 429.
CT is rapid and noninvasive. Fresh or recent hemorrhage is readily visualized on CT. Bone windows are useful for locating skull fractures. MRI is slow and is often not available; in addition, it cannot always detect skull fractures. LP and ultrasound have no place in acute head trauma evaluation, and plain skull radiographs may miss significant intracranial findings.

12. **D,** Page 441.
Traumatic subarachnoid hemorrhage is defined as blood within the CSF and meningeal intima, probably due to tears of small subarachnoid vessels. It is detected on the first CT scan in up to 33% of patients with severe closed head injury and has an incidence of 44% in all cases of severe head injury. Traumatic subarachnoid hemorrhage is associated with a worse prognosis in these patients.

# 32 ▼ Facial Trauma

*Joseph B. Dore and Andrew Langsam*

1. **D,** Page 448.

In some series, as many as 50% of cases of facial trauma are caused by motor vehicle crashes. The severity of these injuries has decreased since the introduction of safety glass.

2. **E,** Page 449.

The Waters' projection is the single best view for the initial evaluation of these structures. This view is usually combined with posteroanterior and lateral views of the facial bones for improved visualization of bony structures. Computed tomography scans are very helpful in patients with complex facial trauma or with altered mental status following trauma but are generally not the initial study.

3. **A,** Page 458.

The patient described has sustained a right-sided orbital blowout fracture. Spontaneous resolution of the clinical problem may occur, but the orbital floor defect may need to be repaired surgically. For this reason, careful follow-up with a consultant is required. Many consultants will delay the decision to repair 10 to 14 days and base it on persistent diplopia or enophthalmos.

4. **A,** Page 450.

The most important aspect of facial trauma is airway control. Many patients with massive facial trauma will have sustained cervical spine injury, so the head-tilt/chin-lift method is contraindicated. Nasotracheal intubation is an alternative in the patient with a cervical spine injury but is contraindicated if there is a suspicion of cribriform plate fracture or laryngeal trauma. With the LeFort II fracture described, this patient is at high risk for a cribriform plate injury. Orotracheal intubation or surgical cricothyrotomy is indicated in this case. Radiographic studies and an operative tracheostomy would be an unnecessary delay for this patient.

5. **D,** Page 451.

Beveled lacerations on the face should be debrided perpendicular to the skin with the exception of lacerations through the eyebrow, which should be debrided parallel to the follicle. Animal bites should be considered dirty, and primary closure is not attempted. Traumatic abrasions with embedded debris should be scrubbed vigorously and all embedded material carefully removed. Delay in treatment may lead to permanent discoloration (traumatic tattooing).

6. **C,** Pages 454-456.

Injuries in the area of the parotid duct or submandibular duct require an evaluation of the patency of the duct, which includes observing the flow of saliva from the duct while milking the gland. A bloody discharge implies a ductal injury. If patency is in question, the patient should be referred for exploration and repair. Lid lacerations not involving the lid margin, loss of lid tissue, or damage to the lacrimal system may be repaired by the emergency physician. Through-and-through lacerations of the mouth may be repaired in a lay-

ered fashion, beginning with a watertight closure of the mucosa, irrigation, and then a layered closure of the muscle, subcutaneous tissue, and skin from the outside. Foreign bodies should be removed if present. Repair of the lacerated ear may be accomplished by the emergency physician by approximation of the cartilage with fine absorbable sutures followed by skin closure and supportive splinting.

7. **A,** Pages 451-452.

Facial wounds should be aggressively debrided, with removal of any debris to avoid traumatic tattooing. Tetanus prophylaxis should be an initial concern in all soft-tissue injuries. Wound age is an important consideration when deciding whether to close a wound. Uncontaminated facial wounds can be closed up to 24 hours after the injury. These wounds should be carefully explored to identify any involved structures that would need special consideration (e.g., nerves, salivary glands) and to rule out any retained foreign body. The resulting scar will usually be approximately the width of the wound before the sutures are placed.

8. **B,** Pages 452-453.

The choice of suture material in closing a wound is important. The deep layers should be approximated with absorbable sutures of 4-0 to 5-0 size. The absorbable synthetic sutures such as Dexon or Vicryl are probably better because they are stronger, last longer, and cause less tissue reaction as they are absorbed. This deep-layer closure is important because it obliterates potential dead space where exudate might collect. It is this closure which provides support to the wound because the skin does not regain adequate tensile strength for 5 to 6 weeks. Deep layers are best closed using a simple vertical stitch with a deeply buried knot.

9. **B,** Pages 458-459.

Orbital emphysema associated with orbital fractures is usually a benign, self-limited condition. This patient however, is complaining of a sudden decrease in visual acuity in the traumatized eye. The emergency physician must consider that air may have built up under pressure in the orbit, causing cessation of blood flow in the central retinal artery. The air must be released immediately or the patient may lose her vision. This may be done by performing a lateral canthotomy with cantholysis or intraorbital needle aspiration of the trapped air. Ballottement of the globe will not benefit this patient because the etiology of her visual loss is not embolic occlusion of the retinal artery. Iridocyclitis following trauma is painful but should not be associated with loss of visual acuity.

10. **C,** Page 455.

The lesion described is typical of septal hematoma. Prompt treatment is important to prevent necrosis of underlying nasal cartilage and should include incision, drainage, anterior packing, oral antibiotics, and referral for close follow-up with a plastic surgeon or otorhinolaryngologist. Management of the septal hematoma takes precedence over the treatment of most nasal fractures. Treatment within 1 week is inadequate. Clinical presentation argues against nasal polyps. Although a coagulopathy may exist, this would not preclude incision and drainage.

# 33 ▼ Spinal Injuries

*Robert T. Maroko and John F. Madden*

1. **B,** Pages 465, 498.

Although various types of vertebral injuries are associated with spinal cord injuries, it is important to note that bony injury need not be present in order for there to be a spinal cord injury. All patients with a history of significant injury, evidence of neurologic impairment, or radiographic abnormalities should be considered and treated in the emergency department on the assumption that they have mechanically and neurologically unstable injuries until proven otherwise. Emergency physicians should have a high index of suspicion for spinal cord injury. A spinal injury should be suspected in any trauma victim with the following:

• Impaired consciousness, including even mild alcohol intoxication with suspected trauma

• Complaints of neck or back pain

• Evidence of significant head or facial trauma

• Signs of focal neurologic deficit

• Unexplained hypotension

• A suggestive mechanism of injury associated with other painful injuries or distracting injuries

• A minor mechanism of injury but with patient discomfort or tenderness out of proportion to the mechanism

In addition to this, patients with severe osteoporosis, arthritis, metastatic disease, and other disorders of the spine may develop spinal injuries as the result of relatively minor trauma. Patients with cord injury may have a normal neurologic exam, at least initially. Central cord syndrome is not commonly seen in children.

2. **A,** Page 466.

This injury is associated with a high incidence of spinal cord injuries. The cause of this injury is secondary to flexion. The annulus fibrosis of the intervertebral disc and the anterior longitudinal ligament are disrupted. This leads to an extremely unstable condition. The inferior articulated facets of the upper vertebrae pass upward and over the superior facets of the lower vertebrae, causing anterior displacement of the spine. On x-ray this is demonstrated by the displacement of more than half of the diameter of the lower vertebral body.

3. **B,** Page 466.

The hangman's fracture occurs when the skull, atlas, and axis function as a unit that is put into extreme hyperextension as a result of abrupt deceleration. The pedicles of the axis are fractured bilaterally. This may occur with or without dislocation and is considered an unstable fracture. Despite this, spinal cord damage is usually minimal secondary to the diameter of the neural canal being at its greatest at the level of C2, and further because the bilateral pedicular fractures permit the spinal canal to decompress itself. Despite the name, death from hanging commonly results from strangulation rather than cord damage.

4. **D,** Page 473.

The Jefferson fracture of C1 is quite rare. It is caused by vertical compression forces transmitted through the occipital condyles to the superior pedicular surfaces of the lateral masses of the atlas. This force drives the lateral masses laterally, resulting in fractures of the anterior and posterior arches of the atlas and a disruption of the transverse ligament. On x-ray, a predental space in excess of 3 mm in adults or 5 mm in children is considered abnormal. There may be associated retropharyngeal swelling resulting from an associated prevertebral hemorrhage. This injury is considered extremely unstable.

5. **D,** Page 475.

The fractures of the odontoid process are classified into three types. Type one fractures involves the tip of the odontoid process, type 2 fractures occur at the base of the odontoid process, and type 3 fractures occur through the body of C2. All require surgical consultation. These fractures may be difficult to see on x-ray films because of problems with technique as well as normal anatomic variation.

6. **B,** Page 477.

Maximal deficit following blunt injury is often not seen immediately but progresses over the following hours. Although there are animal models for this as well as many theories for the mechanism of continuing injury including free radical damage, treatments have not been uniformly effective. Currently, steroids in blunt trauma have been shown to have improved neurologic outcome (this benefit is approximately one spinal level on average).

7. **A,** Page 498.

Other injuries may hint at the possibility of an associated spinal injury. Contusions about the scapula may suggest a rotation or flexion rotation injury of the thoracic spine. Injury to the gluteal region or feet and ankles as occurs with falls from considerable heights may suggest a compression type of spinal injury. Vertical compression injuries occur in any area of the spine that is capable of straightening at the time of impact. This is common in the cervical and lumbar regions.

8. **C,** Page 477.

The diaphragm is innervated by the phrenic nerve, which originates from the spinal cord at the levels of C3, C4, and C5. The intercostal muscles of the rib cage are supplied by nerves that originate in the thoracic spine. Thus diaphragmatic or abdominal breathing in the absence of thoracic breathing would indicate a lower cervical injury. Despite this, there may be delayed phrenic involvement as edema spreads upward from a cervical injury to the cord.

9. **C,** Page 477.

Neck pain and paralysis are not the only symptoms of cervical injury. Less obvious symptoms include occipital pain, which may indicate a C2 lesion, as well as burning and tingling in the hands, which may indicate a C6 to C7 injury. Painful dysesthesia ("burning hands") typically occurs in young football players who have sustained extension injuries to the cervical spine at the C6-C7 level and may be the only initial complaint in patients with significant spinal cord injury.

10. **A,** Page 481.

The likelihood of functional recovery in patients with neurologic deficits persisting longer than 24 hours is nil. A caveat to this is that any evidence of minimal cord function such as sacral sparing excludes the patient from this group. Further, this condition can be perfectly mimicked by a condition known as spinal shock, which usually lasts less than 24 hours.

11. **A,** Page 481.

The central cord syndrome is characterized by greater upper extremity involvement vs. lower extremity involvement and is the most common incomplete spinal cord lesion. It may present as almost complete quadriplegia with only sacral sparing. The injury is often seen in patients with degenerative arthritis of the cervical vertebrae who have hyperextension as the mechanism of injury. The ligamentum flavum encroaches into the cord, resulting in a concussion or contusion of the central portion of the cord.

12. **E,** Page 482.

Brown-Séquard syndrome is also known as hemisection of the spinal cord. The usual cause for this lesion is a penetrating lesion such as a gunshot or knife wound. However, it may also be seen following lateral mass fractures of the cervical spine. The typical findings include ipsilateral motor paralysis and contralateral sensory loss distal to the level of injury. Most patients have control of bowel and bladder function and have intact contralateral motor power.

13. **C,** Page 499.

Maintaining an airway, especially in cardiopulmonary arrest, is critical. During the intubation, in-line spinal immobilization should be maintained. This immobilization should not involve placing axial traction on the head or neck since it has been shown to cause both distraction and subluxation of unstable cervical spine injuries. Nasotracheal intubation does cause less spinal movement than orotracheal intubation but is often technically difficult to perform and time consuming and may result in injury to the nasopharynx and vocal cords. Orotracheal intubation causes greater movement of the cervical spine but is technically easier to perform, and retrospective reviews have not found it to cause or worsen neurologic injury in victims of spinal trauma. Cricothyroidotomy theoretically causes the least spinal movement but has not been studied adequately.

14. **A,** Page 503.

A neurosurgical consultation should be sought by the emergency physician in all cases of spinal injury. There are, however, three instances in which risk of cord injury is low:

• Musculoskeletal injuries of the spine involving only mild to moderate discomfort and no impairment with normal neurologic findings and no other injuries requiring hospitalization

• Patients with isolated spinous process fractures that result from direct blows or are secondary to flexion or extension injuries and that are not associated with neurologic deficit or with instability on flexion and extension x-ray films

• Simple wedge fractures of the cervical spine that involve only mild to moderate discomfort and that are not associated with neurologic impairment

Wedge fractures of the thoracic or lumbar spine, on the other hand, are unstable and are best managed in the hospital.

# 34 Neck Trauma

### M. Greg Amaya and John F. Madden

1. **A,** Pages 506, 508.

The neck is divided into three anatomical zones. Zone I is the base of the neck and upper mediastinum. Damage to the major thoracic structures in this zone makes this the most lethal site of injury in the neck. For this reason, symptomatic and asymptomatic injuries within this zone require emergent angiography to evaluate the great vessels. The boundary between zone I and zone II varies in the literature, but the cricoid cartilage is a commonly accepted dividing line. Zone II extends to the angle of the mandible, and zone III is above this to the base of the occiput. There is no zone IV.

2. **D,** Page 507.

In the past, paralytic agents and large doses of sedatives were contraindicated in controlling the airway in penetrating neck trauma because they take away voluntary muscle control of a potentially difficult airway. Although awake intubation with local anesthetic is an option, in the hemodynamically stable, non-distressed patient, rapid-sequence intubation is still the procedure of choice; studies show these patients do not lose airway patency. Blind nasotracheal intubation is contraindicated in the presence of facial or airway trauma. A cricothyrotomy or tracheostomy would be indicated only if attempted oral intubation was not successful.

3. **D,** Page 508.

Air embolism is a potentially fatal complication of neck trauma with vascular injury. In addition to tachypnea, tachycardia, and hypotension, a "machinery murmur" may be noted on auscultation of the chest. The left lateral decubitus position in Trendelenburg should prevent an air embolus from traveling through the heart to the brain. Pericardiocentesis of the right ventricle is indicated only if the patient's condition does not improve with proper positioning. The other positions are contraindicated because the likelihood of cerebral embolus is increased.

4. **E,** Pages 506, 507.

With penetrating neck trauma as with all trauma, the ABCs should be followed. This patient's airway is still intact, and other factors need to be considered before intubation such as the degree of respiratory distress, level of consciousness, bleeding into the airway, and extent of distortion or disruption of the airway. While intubation should be delayed, the patient must be vigilantly observed for signs of impending respiratory failure. Furthermore, wounds should never be blindly probed, especially in a poorly lit, moving ambulance. On the other hand, this patient may respond to direct pressure and fluid resuscitation as a temporizing measure prior to further evaluation. OR management may not be necessary at this point, although it still must be considered. Finally, MAST trousers have no role with neck injury and are playing a decreasing role in the pre-hospital setting overall.

5. **B,** Page 508.

Before any transport, it is important to optimally stabilize the patient while limiting delays in necessary treatment not available at the current medical location. Thus transferring a patient without any assessment or without securing an airway would most likely prove disastrous. Furthermore, delaying transfer for an ideal workup may prove deleterious. An orogastric tube should not be inserted because of the risk of encountering a pharyngeal hematoma, furthering airway trauma or causing retching that could reinitiate bleeding. Assessing platysmal violation by blind probing a wound outside of an operating room is not recommended. With bleeding into the oropharynx, once the airway is secured, packing with heavy gauze may provide internal compression and tamponade as a temporizing procedure before definitive management in the OR.

6. **C,** Pages 509-510.

Carotid artery injury usually results in thrombosis and delayed neurologic deficits, with a slower than expected evolution of symptoms. This injury can occur with blows to the side of the head or face that result in rotation and hyperextension of the neck that stretch the carotid artery across the vertebral bodies. In addition to Horner's syndrome and decreased level of consciousness with limb paresis, expanding hematomas and transient ischemic attacks are also characteristic. None of the other choices involves interruption of the sympathetic innervation and cortical blood supply.

7. **E,** Pages 509-511.

It is important to remember that aphonia or any alteration of voice quality is not necessarily present in laryngeal injury. It is, however, highly suggestive of such an injury, including recurrent laryngeal nerve injury, fracture of thyroid cartilage, hematoma of the vocal cords, or subluxation of the arytenoids. In addition, the edema and bleeding resulting from thyroid cartilage fractures results in loss of landmark definition. Furthermore, most authors recommend orotracheal intubation as the first option, given its user familiarity and high success rate. In terms of diagnostic imaging, CT and bronchoscopy are recommended with laryngeal injuries, but the flexible method is now preferred to the rigid by most.

8. **C,** Page 512.

For the respiratory complications of strangulation injuries, PEEP and fluid restriction have been the most useful in managing cerebral edema and centroneurogenic ARDS. Furthermore, hyperventilation, mannitol, and furosemide have proven helpful, hence the usefulness of intubation. Neither steroids, antibiotics, nor barbiturate coma have been very successful as treatment. Phenytoin helps to prevent ischemic cerebral damage by suppressing seizure activity and causing the reuptake of catecholamines in the CNS, decreasing the severity of centroneurogenic ARDS. Finally, calcium channel blockers may prove beneficial because calcium may contribute to poor postanoxic cerebral perfusion.

# 35 ▼ Thoracic Trauma

### *Sharon C. Amaya and Bonnie B. Matthaeus*

1. **B,** Page 515.

Previously, it was believed that a fracture of the first or second rib was associated with greater morbidity and mortality because of damage to important underlying structures. More recent studies have shown that routine aortography is not indicated unless there are signs of vascular injury. Furthermore, isolated first rib fractures have a mortality of only 1.5%. It is when this injury is associated with other rib fractures that there is a tenfold increase in mortality. Surgical intervention is not necessary for adequate bone union. The fracture is often more easily visualized on the AP cervical spine view.

2. **D,** Page 515.

Sternal fracture is of concern because of the possibility of myocardial contusion or rupture, cardiac tamponade, or pulmonary injury. The associated mortality is reported as 25%-45%. Diagnosis is frequently missed because lateral radiograph views are not usually obtained initially. Evaluation for cardiac injury is necessary in all of these cases. Admission, as well as further evaluation, should be considered in nearly all cases. Flail chest rarely occurs with sternal fracture. Endotracheal intubation may be needed if there is an associated flail chest, but it is not uniformly necessary.

3. **A,** Page 518.

All of the choices can be seen with a flail chest, but underlying pulmonary contusion is now thought to be the most significant factor in respiratory insufficiency. The pendelluft effect is the back-and-forth movement of a portion of the tidal volume between the flail side and the uninjured side with each respiration.

4. **E,** Page 518.

The mere presence of a flail segment is not an indication for intubation. Intubation should be strongly considered if the patient is in shock, has three or more associated injuries, has previous pulmonary disease, has fractures of eight or more ribs, is older than 65 years, or has an oxygen saturation of less than 92% on a non-rebreather mask. Chest tube thoracostomy is indicated if there is an associated hemopneumothorax. Severe pain should be adequately controlled. In the awake and cooperative patient, CPAP may obviate the need for intubation. External fixation is no longer advocated.

5. **B,** Page 519.

Traumatic asphyxia is caused by a severe compression of the thorax and retrograde flow of blood into the great veins of the head and neck, causing the characteristic appearance. The condition is usually benign and self-limiting, but may be associated with intrathoracic injury. Chest wall and pulmonary injuries may occur from the transmission of violent force involved. Retinal edema may occur but causes only transient visual disturbance, whereas retinal hemorrhage can cause permanent visual loss. Intracranial hemorrhages are rare. Venous thrombosis and tympanic membrane ruptures are not known complications.

6. **C,** Page 519.

Pneumomediastinum occurs when extrapleural tears allow air to leak into the mediastinum and soft tissues of the anterior neck. This typically causes subcutaneous emphysema over the supraclavicular area and anterior neck, whereas the presence of localized chest wall emphysema is an indication of a traumatic pneumothorax. A pneumomediastinum may be caused by an esophageal tear resulting from a Boerhaave's syndrome or penetrating injury, and has also been reported with asthma, emesis, Valsalva maneuvers, various respiratory tract infections, and breath-holding in cocaine and marijuana abusers. Only rarely does this progress into a tension pneumomomediastinum, usually in patients receiving positive pressure ventilation. If tension pneumomediastinum is suspected, immediate pericardiocentesis with aspiration of air is required, otherwise a benign pneumomediastinum may be treated with conservative measures. Beck's triad is typically indicative of a pericardial effusion.

7. **D,** Page 520.

Pulmonary contusions usually manifest within minutes of the initial injury and are thus usually apparent on the initial chest radiograph. Contusions are always present within 4 to 6 hours and tend to last 48 to 72 hours. Many of the worst contusions occur in patients without rib fractures, although rib fractures are commonly associated. Pulmonary contusion is the most significant chest injury in children, who tend to have more elastic chest walls. There are no specific signs for pulmonary contusion, but hemoptysis may be present in up to 50% of patients.

8. **D,** Page 521.

Arterial blood gases may be helpful in making the diagnosis of pulmonary contusion because most patients have hypoxemia. The earliest and most accurate means of assessing these patients is a widening alveolar-arterial oxygen difference, which indicates a decreasing pulmonary diffusion capacity of the contused lung. Although CT scan has been found to be sensitive for contusion, it is a static measurement and would be a difficult and expensive way to follow the progression of a pulmonary contusion. Serial chest radiographs are not the most accurate means of assessing the patient's status. Pulmonary artery pressures and pulmonary function tests are not commonly used to assess this injury.

9. **C,** Page 521.

The treatment for pulmonary contusion has changed dramatically over the last 40 years and now conservative therapy is the standard unless criteria for intubation and ventilation are met. These include a $PaO_2$ <60 mm Hg on room air or <80 mm Hg on supplemental oxygen. A trial of continuous positive airway pressure can be attempted, but if this does not correct hypoxemia, the patient requires intubation. It has been suggested that large volumes of crystalloid increase interstitial edema and intrapulmonary shunting in the injured lung; therefore restriction of fluids is suggested if the patient is hemodynamically stable. Steroids and diuretics have yet to be shown to be effective in the treatment of pulmonary contusion.

10. **D,** Page 522.

All of the choices are indications for chest tube placement except for multiple rib fractures, unless associated with a pneumothorax or hemothorax. Respiratory symptoms, regardless of the size of the pneumothorax, increasing size after initial conservative therapy, hemopneumothorax and bilateral pneumothorax regardless of size are all indications for chest tube thoracostomy.

11. **A,** Page 524.

A patient with a tension pneumothorax can become acutely ill within minutes. The cardinal signs of a tension pneumothorax are tachycardia, jugular venous distention, and absent breath sounds on the affected side. Hypotension will not occur as early as hypoxia and may represent a preterminal event. Diagnosis and treatment should not be delayed because the patient is normotensive. Ideally, diagnosis and treatment should be completed without a chest radiograph, but one may be required when the diagnosis is obscure. A needle thoracostomy should be done immediately once the diagnosis is suspected. Although this patient will eventually require a chest tube, it should follow the life-saving therapy of needle decompression. Intubation delays definitive treatment, and with positive pressure ventilation it could potentially worsen the situation.

12. **D,** Page 524.

As pressure outside the visceral pleura increases, it will become increasingly more difficult to deliver a breath to the patient. This will be apparent to the person bagging the patient or will trigger pressure monitors if the patient is attached to a ventilator. Distended neck veins, hypotension, and tracheal deviation can occur but are later signs of a tension pneumothorax. Cyanosis is unlikely to be seen.

13. **E,** Page 525.

Thoracotomy for hemothorax is indicated if the size of the hemothorax is increasing on chest radiograph, if the initial chest tube drainage is greater than 20 ml/kg of blood, if there is persistent bleeding at a rate greater than 7 ml/kg/hr, if the patient remains hypotensive despite adequate blood replacement (and other sources of blood loss have been ruled out), or if the patient decompensates after an initial positive response to resuscitation.

14. **E,** Page 525.

Patients with tracheobronchial disruption have a wound that opens into the pleural space, causing a large pneumothorax. A chest tube fails to re-expand the lung, and there is continuous bubbling of air in the underwater seal device. These patients typically have hemoptysis, dyspnea, subcutaneous and mediastinal emphysema, and cyanosis. A communicating pneumothorax should be detected on physical examination. Both a communicating pneumothorax and a pneumothorax associated with a flail chest should be adequately treated with chest tube placement. Diaphragmatic rupture and laryngeal fracture typically do not present in this manner.

# 36 Cardiovascular Trauma

### Shobhit Arora and Bonnie B. Matthaeus

1. **E,** Pages 527-530.
Sinus tachycardia is the most sensitive sign of myocardial contusion. However, it is nonspecific and should be interpreted in the context of the clinical setting. Other factors that may be responsible for tachycardia that must be considered are pain, hemorrhage, and pneumothorax. Chest contusion and associated tenderness are common signs, but they are not sensitive. CPK-MB lacks both sensitivity and specificity.

2. **E,** Page 529.
Biopsy and autopsy are the only ways to make a definitive diagnosis of myocardial contusion. The other studies and laboratory tests can assist in making a diagnosis when combined with clinical interpretation, but they are not diagnostic.

3. **B,** Page 528.
Pericardial effusions complicate approximately 50% of myocardial contusions. Most occur during the second week after contusion. They are usually small but occasionally do become symptomatic. The delayed presentation favors the diagnosis of effusion.

4. **E,** Pages 527-542.
Blunt and penetrating trauma to the chest can cause any of a number of life-threatening injuries that the emergency physician must be prepared to diagnose and treat. Myocardial contusion, myocardial rupture, pericardial tamponade, tension pneumothorax, massive hemothorax, and aortic rupture can all result from the injuries described in this patient.

5. **C,** Page 531.
Penetrating trauma to the chest and upper abdomen is the most common cause of traumatic pericardial tamponade, with a reported incidence of 2% in patients with these injuries. Blunt trauma and penetrating trauma to the lower abdomen are rarely implicated.

6. **D,** Pages 531-532.
Elevated CVP (>15 cm $H_2O$), tachycardia, and hypotension are the most reliable signs of pericardial tamponade. Beck's triad—distant heart sounds, distended neck veins, and hypotension—is often difficult to demonstrate clinically, especially in the setting of hypovolemia. An elevated pulsus paradoxus is nonspecific and can be caused by numerous other conditions such as pneumothorax, COPD, asthma, and pulmonary edema.

7. **B,** Pages 532-533.
Electrical alternans is a highly specific sign of pericardial tamponade, but it usually occurs with chronic pericardial effusion and is rare in the acute setting. Very small volumes of fluid in the pericardial space can cause tamponade when the accumulation is acute. Hence a normal cardiac silhouette on chest x-ray does not rule out acute pericardial tamponade.

8. **C,** Pages 533-534.
A patient with acute pericardial tamponade who sustains cardiac arrest is most effectively resuscitated with a left lateral thoracotomy, which allows direct access to the pericardium for pericardiotomy. Blind pericardiocentesis is not as effective as pericardiotomy in the arrested patient. It is, however, very useful for both diagnostic and therapeutic reasons in the pre-arrest setting. Closed-chest CPR is ineffective in the presence of tamponade. Bilateral needle decompression would not be useful in this patient.

9. **D,** Pages 535-536.
Myocardial rupture with hemopericardium can cause an enlarged cardiac silhouette in the acute setting. More often, an enlarged heart on x-ray represents preexisting cardiac or valvular disease. Aortic rupture should not produce an isolated enlargement of the cardiac silhouette but of the superior mediastinum.

10. **E,** Page 538.
Interscapular pain is the most common symptom present with traumatic aortic disruption, but it occurs in only 25% of these patients. Hypertension is present in more than 70% of patients with an aortic tear. Other less common clinical findings include dyspnea, stridor or hoarseness from laryngeal nerve compression, and extremity pain from ischemia.

11. **A,** Pages 538-541.
Aortography is the gold standard for diagnosing aortic disruption. It allows determination of the precise location of the sites of rupture, which are multiple in up to 15% of cases. Chest CT scans are neither sensitive nor specific. Transthoracic echocardiography is far less sensitive than the transesophageal approach that is being utilized by many centers.

12. **D,** Page 541.
Elevated blood pressure in a patient with an aortic disruption requires emergent regulation because this theoretically reduces the shear forces on the intact adventitia surrounding the area of rupture. Short-acting beta-blockers and nitroprusside are particularly useful because of their titrateability. Reducing heart rate and providing oxygen, while likely useful, are not essential in the management of these patients.

# 37 Esophageal and Diaphragmatic Trauma

### Suzanne F. Beavers and Ross E. Megargel

1. **E,** Pages 546-548.
Esophageal perforation due to foreign body usually occurs at the cricopharyngeal muscle, the level at which the esophagus crosses the left mainstem bronchus and aortic arch, or the gastroesophageal junction. NG tubes and nasotracheal intubation have both been associated with esophageal tears, most commonly at the pyriform sinus. The most common cause of esophageal perforation is iatrogenic. Liquefaction necrosis does lead to more esophageal injuries than does coagulation necrosis, but it is more commonly associated with alkali burns.

2. **B,** Pages 547-548.

Boerhaave's syndrome is classically associated with vomiting, but it can also be seen with blunt trauma, seizures, childbirth, laughing, straining at stool, and heavy lifting. The pressure leading to this syndrome is usually 3-6 psi. The diagnosis of Boerhaave's syndrome is often subtle, and the history and physical must be accompanied by radiologic and laboratory studies. The tear is longitudinal and occurs at the left posterolateral aspect of the esophagus.

3. **C,** Page 548.

Most experts agree that Gastrografin should be used before barium; it does not obscure visualization on subsequent endoscopy. Barium is better than Gastrografin for mucosal detail. Endoscopy depends on the size of the tear, and the operator and is not infallible.

4. **A,** Pages 548-550.

Herniation of abdominal contents after a diaphragmatic tear may occur many years after the initial injury. The defects caused by blunt injury average between 5 and 15 cm, whereas those caused by penetrating injury are usually less than 2 cm long. The most common organ to herniate through a right-sided diaphragmatic defect is the liver. Diaphragmatic tears occur in a 4:1 male to female ratio, according to one comprehensive review of the English literature.

5. **C,** Page 551.

When using diagnostic peritoneal lavage to evaluate for isolated diaphragmatic injury, a level of 5000 RBC/mm³ should be used. Using a standard of 100,000 RBC/mm³ can lead to a false negative rate of up to 25%. CT and ultrasound are not sensitive for diaphragmatic injury in the absence of herniation. Contrast instilled through a diagnostic peritoneal lavage catheter may be helpful in diagnosing a diaphragmatic tear, but its sensitivity in evaluating for injury is unknown. Liver-spleen scans are not helpful in the absence of liver or splenic herniation through the diaphragmatic tear.

6. **E,** Pages 548-550.

Penetrating trauma is a more common cause of diaphragmatic injury than blunt trauma. A patient with a penetrating wound to the lower chest or flank is at high risk for diaphragmatic hernia. Defects in the diaphragm do not heal spontaneously regardless of size.

Diaphragmatic trauma caused by penetrating trauma is more commonly due to knives than guns.

7. **E,** Pages 548-550.

A nasogastric tube is useful for diagnosis and therapy in a diaphragmatic hernia. Chest x-ray is a valuable screening tool and yields radiographic abnormalities in 50%-100% of patients. Performing contrast studies in patients with suspected diaphragmatic hernia can often be helpful in diagnosis, as can repeating the chest x-ray, since the herniation is often intermittent.

8. **E,** Pages 551-552.

As with tension pneumothorax, chest tubes are used to treat a tension viscerothorax. A NG tube can be both diagnostic and therapeutic in a diaphragmatic hernia. Surgery is ultimately required to repair the defect in all patients with di-

aphragmatic tears. Trocars should not be used in placing chest tubes in patients with diaphragmatic hernias, and careful palpation of internal chest structures should be performed before tube placement is initiated.

## 38 ▼ Abdominal Trauma

*Gregory P. Cuculino and Ross E. Megargel*

1. **A,** Page 555.

Injuries to the liver and spleen often refer pain to the right and left shoulders respectively because of diaphragmatic irritation. This is increased if the patient is in the supine position. Injuries to retroperitoneal organs, especially the duodenum and parts of the GU tract, refer pain to the testicles. Although renal colic often radiates to the testicle, in the setting of trauma, a missed duodenal injury poses a much higher morbidity. In addition, renal colic often causes one-sided testicular pain. The fact that this patient is older and the pain is bilateral favors against torsion. Physical examination would also aid in the decision process.

2. **E,** Page 556.

Although plain abdominal films have a limited role in the evaluation of a trauma patient, at times they are useful. Free air indicates rupture of a hollow viscus. Loss of renal and psoas shadows may represent a retroperitoneal injury. Shifting of the gastric bubble may indicate an expanding splenic hematoma.

3. **B,** Page 557.

After trauma the WBC can be elevated to as high as 20,000. This may be accompanied by a bandemia and last for several days. Without abdominal trauma and complaints of abdominal pain, an abscess is highly unlikely. Empirically treating with antibiotics is unwarranted. Evaluating for other possible sources of infection should have been done on initial examination. The elevated white blood cell count should prompt an extensive work-up.

4. **B,** Page 557.

An elevated amylase level is a nonspecific indicator of intraabdominal injury, especially on initial evaluation. The blood alcohol level has no clinical significance except to lead to questioning of the validity of the physical examination. Initial measurements of hemoglobin and hematocrit are nonspecific when taken alone. These may appear relatively normal because the patient has not had time to hemodilute to maintain blood volume. Also the patient may have a baseline anemia. Therefore, finding a trend in the hemoglobin and hematocrit levels is more helpful. The one concerning laboratory value is the patient's base deficit. A base deficit >6 without other explanation raises the concern of an intraabdominal injury.

5. **A,** Page 569.

Following penetrating trauma to the abdomen, there are seven indications for urgent laparotomy: hemodynamic instability, peritoneal signs, evisceration, diaphragmatic injury, gastrointestinal hemorrhage, implement in situ, and intraperitoneal air.

6. **D,** Pages 563-564.

A retroperitoneal injury, by virtue of its anatomy, will give a falsely negative DPL. The other injuries may falsely elevate the red blood cell count in the lavage fluid.

7. **D,** Page 565.

Emergency department thoracotomy is a last-ditch effort. Its primary purpose is to shunt available blood into the coronary and cerebral circulation. It also allows for proximal bleeding control and provides direct atrial access for fluid administration. If vital signs are reestablished, the next step is the operating room. Survival following an ED thoracotomy is more likely following penetrating rather than blunt trauma. Survival is also increased in thoracic versus abdominal trauma and if vital signs were present immediately before the procedure.

8. **A,** Page 568.

Penetrating trauma to the abdomen can be managed in a stepwise fashion. If no clinical indicators for celiotomy exist (i.e., hemodynamic instability, evisceration, peritoneal signs, diaphragmatic injury, gastrointestinal hemorrhage, implement-in-situ, or intraperitoneal air), then evaluation for peritoneal entry must be done. The first step is local wound exploration. If that definitively demonstrates no peritoneal entry, the patient can be safely discharged from the emergency department. If local wound exploration is positive or there is a question of peritoneal entry, a further workup is mandated.

9. **C,** Pages 569-570.

Clinical examination and chest x-ray are rarely diagnostic in diaphragmatic injuries. Ultrasound is accurate in detecting hemoperitoneum but very inaccurate in detecting diaphragmatic injuries. Blunt trauma to the diaphragm may cause small tears; the red blood cell count criteria is lowered to 5000 to increase the sensitivity of DPL to pick these up. In this case a DPL with a red blood cell count of 300 most strongly argues against a diaphragmatic injury.

10. **C,** Page 570.

Medium- and high-velocity missiles have an explosive effect and create a temporary passage in the tissue. This displaces nearby organs and vascular structures, which may cause injury. In several cases, high-velocity missiles have caused intraperitoneal injury without entering the peritoneum.

11. **A,** Page 560.

This picture demonstrates the presence of a hemoperitoneum. The picture is of Morrison's pouch. It is a potential space between the liver and kidney. Fluid is represented as the black (anechoic) stripe between the kidney and liver. In the setting of trauma this represents blood; the next step is celiotomy.

12. **E,** Pages 560-561.

Ultrasound is a quick, portable method for detecting the presence of fluid in the abdomen. Sensitivities for detecting 100 ml of fluid in the abdomen range from 60%-95% in current studies. As experience is gained, sensitivities increase. However, ultrasound is very insensitive for detecting solid viscera injury and bowel injury.

13. **E,** Pages 562-563.

In cases of blunt abdominal trauma, a DPL with a red blood cell count in the lavage fluid greater than 100,000/mm³ is considered positive and highly specific for intraabdominal injury. RBC counts ranging from 20,000 to 100,000 are considered equivocal and warrant further investigation.

14. **C,** Page 568.

An indeterminate local wound exploration mandates further investigation for the possibility of intraabdominal injury. This may include a DPL and serial abdominal examinations. Significant GI bleeding, evisceration, peritoneal irritation, hemodynamic instability, and evidence of diaphragmatic injury require urgent laparotomy.

15. **C,** Page 568.

When wound exploration reveals peritoneal penetration, further studies are mandated. In completing the wound exploration, wounds should be anesthetized and may be extended carefully to obtain adequate visualization. Blind probing with anything is inaccurate and hazardous.

# ▼ 39 Genitourinary Trauma

*Eric Gallagher and Christopher J. Murphy*

1. **B,** Page 586.

If a partial tear is identified on retrograde urethrography, one careful attempt can be made to pass a catheter coudé and if any resistance is met, a urologic consult must be obtained for suprapubic drainage of the bladder. The treatment for a partial tear is stenting with a Foley catheter, or suprapubic drainage if a Foley cannot be passed. Most tears will heal without operative management.

2. **D,** Page 596.

In penetrating trauma the presence or absence of hematuria is of no consequence in predicting the likelihood of upper urinary tract injury. Rather, the location of the wound in relationship to the urinary tract is the most important factor in determining the need for further imaging.

3. **B,** Page 596.

The guidelines for evaluating hematuria in adults do not apply to children. Children may have undiscovered congenital malformations and do not have the muscle or skeletal mass of adults. Children also have the ability to compensate for moderate blood loss without becoming hypotensive. For these reasons, children are more likely to sustain significant injury than adults given the same mechanism of injury and must undergo complete urologic evaluation for any degree of hematuria.

4. **D,** Page 595.

Single-shot IVP is to be discouraged due to the unacceptable rate of both false-negative and false-positive results. When life-saving surgery is needed for non-urologic emergencies, an intraoperative bolus IVP should be performed to ensure the integrity of both kidneys before clamping a vascular pedicle to control retroperitoneal bleeding. A retrograde urethrogram can be performed in the operating room before attempting to pass a Foley catheter. This procedure will also allow the evaluation of the bladder, and if a suprapubic catheter is needed it can be placed in the operating room.

5. **A,** Page 588.

The literature clearly defines gross hematuria alone or in conjunction with a pelvic fracture as a hallmark of significant bladder injury. Grossly clear bladder urine in a trauma patient virtually eliminates bladder rupture in all but 2% of patients. That 2% of patients with clear urine and only microhematuria often have an associated pelvic fracture, and clinical judgment must be used in deciding which patients require a retrograde cystogram.

6. **A,** Page 600.

In cases of testicular trauma often the only sign of injury is a small hematoma. Therefore color Doppler ultrasound is the procedure of choice to evaluate the structural integrity of the testis. If the testis is dislocated, it will be found under the abdominal wall in 80% of cases. Most penile fractures require drainage of the hematoma and repair of the tunica albuginea. Bleeding from an amputated penis can usually be controlled via direct pressure. If this fails, a Penrose drain can be used as a short-term tourniquet.

7. **C,** Page 583.

Unlike with male urethral injuries, urethrography is not helpful in the female trauma patient because of the urethra's short length. The inability to pass a Foley catheter in a premenopausal female with a pelvic fracture mandates suprapubic drainage of the bladder because of the high likelihood of urethral injury.

8. **A,** Page 586.

Although a pelvic fracture is commonly associated with urethral injury, by itself it does not mandate evaluation of the urethra. Gross blood at the meatus, a high riding or absent prostate or perineal hematoma all mandate evaluation of the urethra via retrograde urethrography.

# 40 ▼ Orthopedic Injuries: Management Principles

### *Leonardo Huertas and Christopher J. Murphy*

1. **B,** Page 613.

The man is complaining of increased severe pain and edema, as well as the hallmark sign of compartment syndrome: pain out of proportion to injury or physical finding. An immediate fasciotomy should be considered. Occult fractures are gen-

erally not visible for 7-10 days, so another x-ray examination on the arm this soon would most likely not show the fracture. Doppler ultrasound showing good blood flow does not rule out compartment syndrome. Splinting and giving pain relief would not be adequate for this presentation without first ruling out compartment syndrome.

2. **C,** Page 610.

The ulnar nerve and the medial nerve are the most commonly injured structures in elbow dislocation. Musculocutaneous nerve injury is most commonly seen with forearm injuries, whereas axillary nerve injuries are seen with shoulder dislocations. A proximal radial head fracture can be seen with an elbow fracture but distal radial head fracture is not a common occurrence.

3. **B,** Pages 602-604.

Fragments are described relative to their normal position. Any deviation from normal is termed displacement. In Figure 40-1, the portion of the distal fragment is described in relation to the proximal one. Thus there is volar displacement of the fractured radius in relation to the proximal portion of the bone.

4. **A,** Page 610.

Intravascular fat droplets appear in nearly one of five patients admitted with major trauma although not all would be systemic or require treatment. The fat embolism syndrome most commonly follows long bone fracture in a young adult, usually the tibia and fibula. Other associated signs would be jaundice, retinal changes, and renal involvement, with fat globules seen in the blood in approximately 50% of patients with long bone fractures within 3 days of the injury. To treat the patient with heparin would not help since this is not a blood clot embolism. Treating this as either a viral or bacterial infection would be inadequate in the face of dyspnea after a long bone fracture without first ruling out fat emboli.

# 41 ▼ The Hand

### *Bret M. Levy and Sunanda Nabha*

1. **A,** Pages 636-637.

Although occurring at times in the forearm, injury to the median nerve occurs most commonly in the wrist. This is usually due to laceration or compression via the carpal tunnel. Opposition of the thumb to the second finger indicates an intact distal median nerve.

2. **D,** Pages 636-638.

Extension and radial deviation of the wrist and pointing of the finger, as well as sensation over the anatomic snuff box, are functions of the radial nerve. Pronation is a function of the median nerve and is lost with damage to the median nerve above the elbow. With ulnar nerve damage there is loss of finger abduction and abduction against resistance because the interosseus muscles are innervated by the ulnar nerve. The patient would not be able to tightly pinch a piece of paper.

3. **E,** Pages 658-659.
Trephination of the hematoma should be performed to provide symptomatic relief. Antibiotics, if indicated in this scenario, should cover such gram-positive organisms as staphylococcus and streptococcus. A first-generation cephalosporin would be appropriate. Kirschner wire fixation is indicated only in the event of displaced fracture, despite manipulation. Protective splinting is rarely needed for more than 2-4 weeks unless the fracture is intraarticular. Nail removal would not likely be indicated since a 25% subungual hematoma only has about a 20%-25% risk of nail bed laceration and repair would be of questionable benefit.

4. **C,** Pages 643-645.
As little as 10 degrees of malrotation may lead to improper hand function. On flexion, all the fingers should point to the scaphoid region. Any variance should cause suspicion of malrotation.

5. **E,** Pages 647-648.
Metacarpal neck fractures are usually dorsally angulated due to flexion of the interosseous muscles. Metacarpals of the second and third fingers are rigidly fixed to the distal carpal row. The carpometacarpal joint does not allow for flexion or extension; therefore all angulated fractures must be reduced. This is best accomplished with percutaneous pinning.

6. **D,** Pages 650-651.
Swelling and bony joint tenderness following hand trauma warrants x-ray evaluation. DIP joint dislocations are quite rare; the DIP joint is supported by two collateral ligaments as well as a volar plate. All planes should be assessed to check ligamentous stability. For lateral PIP dislocation, at least two supporting structures must be damaged, including the volar plate. Pain on ligamentous testing associated with a stable joint is likely due to a partial ligamentous tear and is treated with 2-5 weeks of buddy taping.

7. **A,** Page 653.
Ulnar collateral ligament sprain, otherwise known as gamekeeper's thumb, is usually due to forced radial deviation or abduction at the metacarpal-phalangeal joint. Volar base avulsion fractures may be associated, but ligamentous disruption alone is more common. This injury is commonly missed in the emergency department. Diagnosis is made by checking the thumb in extension; if >20 degrees of ulnar ligament instability is present compared to the other hand, injury should be suspected. Complete rupture should be surgically repaired to prevent chronic pain and instability.

8. **C,** Page 655.
Zone III injuries include the common extensor tendon on the dorsum of the hand. This injury is zone I (DIP joint and distal). Inadequate treatment may result in mallet finger deformity. Boutonniere deformity results from injury to the PIP joint (zone II). Interarticular fractures involving more than one third of the joint are optimally treated with K-wire fixation.

9. **E,** Pages 640-658.
Fracture caused by a foreign body that penetrates the skin should be considered an open fracture. A specialist trained to handle these injuries should be consulted while the patient remains in the emergency department since operative debridement may be indicated. This is especially true when there is suspicion of wound contamination.

10. **B,** Pages 658-659.
Treatment of this injury clearly mandates symptomatic relief as well as thorough evaluation of the injury. Digit block should provide analgesia as well as allow a thorough wound exploration. Epinephrine should be avoided because of the risk of ischemia and necrosis. Treatment is controversial, and no guidelines are established. Exposed bone lends to poor healing and generally requires skin grafting or bone shortening to allow primary or secondary closure. This is the most common extremity injury. Successful reimplantation distal to the nail has been described but is not usually indicated in adults. Treatment often depends on the digit involved and age of the patient. Injuries with less than 1 cm of skin loss have been shown to heal best by secondary intention.

11. **C,** Pages 658-659.
Nail substance is made at the nail matrix. Matrix, if avulsed, should be replaced with horizontal mattress suture. Nail bed lacerations require precise repair to prevent nail deformity. The nail body provides support for volar fingertip during "pinching." Zone I line injury may be closed by secondary intention.

12. **B,** Pages 662-663.
All human bite wounds should be scrubbed, irrigated, and left open. Antibiotics should include both penicillin (for aerobes) and agents that cover beta-lactamase producing staphylococci. Diabetic patients often have polymicrobial infections, and broad-spectrum antibiotics should be used. Paronychia usually results from nail biting or aggressive manicures and early signs of inflammation without purulence may be treated with warm soaks, immobilization, and a first-generation cephalosporin. Treatment of an eponychia may require bilateral paronychia incisions as well as elevation of the eponychium with proximal nail bed removal. Regardless of the choice, frank pus usually requires incision and drainage of abscess.

13. **C,** Pages 663-664.
The infection described would be diagnosed a felon. Initial treatment should be within the realm of the emergency department physician. Choice B describes traditional management of a felon. Incision through the fibrous septa is needed to provide adequate drainage. Incisions should be made on the ulnar aspects of the second, third, and fourth digits, with radial incisions of the first and fifth fingers. Closure of the skin edges is contraindicated. Complications, although relatively uncommon, include soft tissue and bony necrosis lymphangitis and osteomyelitis.

# 42 Forearm and Wrist

### R. Alan Shubert and Sunanda Nabha

1. **C,** Pages 672-674.

The scaphoid is the most commonly fractured of the carpal bones, composing nearly 60% of all carpal fractures. These fracture are typically seen in young adults between the ages of 15 and 30 years of age and result from a fall onto an outstretched hand. Fractures of the hamate, lunate, and trapezium are rare, together accounting for less than 10% of all carpal bone fractures.

2. **C,** Page 673.

Fractures may be extremely subtle on plain film radiography, which may fail to detect up to 15% of scaphoid fractures. The associated risk of nonunion is much higher if the diagnosis is delayed. For this reason, patients in whom there is clinical suspicion of scaphoid fracture should be treated with immobilization and have a repeat x-ray in 10-14 days.

3. **D,** Page 673.

If the 10-14 day follow-up x-rays remain negative, but the clinical examination indicates a possible fracture, then a technetium bone scan or CT scan of the scaphoid should be obtained to confirm the diagnosis of a fracture. The other modalities listed are of little use in evaluating the scaphoid for fracture.

4. **D,** Page 675.

According to the Mayfield and Yeager classification, carpal dislocations are staged according to the progressive degree of intercarpal injury. Lunate dislocation is by definition a stage IV injury. Stage I injury involves widening of the scapholunate joint, stage II is perilunate dislocation, and stage III is identical to stage II with the addition of dislocation of the triquetrum.

5. **A,** Page 676.

By definition, a Colles' fracture involves the distal radius. This is the most common fracture seen in adults. The fracture is a transverse fracture of the distal radial metaphysis with dorsal displacement and angulation. The fracture usually occurs within 2 cm of the distal radial articular surface and may extend into the joint.

6. **B,** Page 683.

Sustained wrist flexion (Phalen's test), is the most sensitive (76%) test on physical examination for carpal tunnel syndrome. It carries an associated specificity of approximately 80%.

7. **C,** Page 685.

Monteggia's fracture involves the junction of the proximal and middle thirds of the ulna associated with dislocation of the radial head. The site of the ulnar fracture and degree of radial head dislocation determine the type of Monteggia fracture.

8. **A,** Pages 681-682.

The patient in question displays some classic symptoms of carpal tunnel syndrome, including: wrist pain with tingling in the fingers and worsening pain at night. She also has a positive Phalen's test on physical examination.

9. **D,** Page 673.

The patient depicts the classic presentation of a scaphoid (navicular) fracture. Well-localized tenderness in the anatomic snuffbox is diagnostic. Treatment is with a short arm thumb spica cast with re-examination in 10 to 14 days.

10. **A,** Page 675.

The "piece of pie" configuration of the lunate on PA views of the wrist is pathognomonic of a true lunate dislocation, not a perilunate dislocation.

# 43 Humerus and Elbow

### Paul R. Sierzenski and Leonard A. Nitowski

1. **D,** Pages 690-691.

The posterior compartment of the upper arm contains two structures; the radial nerve and the triceps brachii. The anterior compartment contains three muscles; the biceps brachii, the brachialis, and the chorachobrachialis. The brachial artery, median nerve, musculocutaneous nerve, and the ulnar nerve are also found in the anterior compartment. The radial nerve exits the axilla and winds posteriorly behind the humerus between the heads of the triceps in the "radial groove," then crosses the elbow anterior to the lateral epicondyle. It is this posterior position that makes the radial nerve susceptible to injury from fractures of the humerus.

2. **D,** Page 692.

When examining the elbow of a child, it is helpful to determine the carrying angle. The "carrying angle" is formed by the intersection of lines drawn parallel to the long axis of the humerus and ulna (Rosen Fig 43-5). The mean measurement in children is 15 degrees. A carrying angle difference of greater than 12 degrees between the injured and uninjured arms is often associated with fractures. In children this is frequently a supracondylar fracture. The carrying angle has no diagnostic relevance to early compartment syndrome. Anterior elbow dislocations present with the arm fully extended with the forearm supinated; often the olecranon fossa is palpable posteriorly. Axillary nerve injury would be evident by severe sensory and muscular deficits including radial, ulnar, and possible median nerve deficits.

3. **A,** Pages 692, 611.

Compartment syndrome is an acute emergency due to increased pressure in an enclosed osseofascial space; it is a potential complication of long bone fractures. Pain is the only dependable early sign of this condition. Passive extension of the fingers produces extreme pain in the forearm if flexor (volar) compartment syndrome is present. The remaining signs of compartment syndrome (the five Ps) are pain, paresthesia, pallor, pulselessness, and paralysis. This condition requires measurement of compartment pressures and emergent orthopedic consultation.

4. **D,** Page 693.

Occult intraarticular fracture is often diagnosed by the "fat pad sign" (also known as "sail sign") on x-ray. Fat around the proximal elbow is usually hidden by the olecranon and coronoid processes. Often a thin anterior strip of lucency can be normal. If intraarticular hemorrhage is present, the joint capsule bulges, displacing the fat pad. Although anterior, posterior, or both fat pad signs may be present with a fracture, in the setting of trauma, more than 90% of patients with posterior fat pad sign have an intraarticular skeletal injury. In adults an occult radial head fracture is often implicated, whereas children often have a supracondylar fracture. Superficial soft tissue swelling is not itself diagnostic and is present in multiple disease processes including trauma, infection, and cancer. Periosteal elevation is classically associated with osteomyelitis but can also be noted in callus formation of bone and suppurative arthritis.

5. **C,** Pages 693-694.

Evaluation of x-rays for supracondylar fractures in children should included measurement of Bowman's angle (Rosen Fig. 43-9). This angle usually measures 75 degrees and is often equal in both arms. It is helpful in assessing accuracy of supracondylar fracture reduction. An increase in Bowman's angle indicates medial tilting and can predict the final carrying angle. Comparison x-rays are helpful for assessing Bowman's angle.

6. **D,** Pages 694-695.

15% to 20% of humerus fractures result in radial nerve injury. The radial nerve courses posteriorly to the humerus and is fixed in position by the intramuscular septum of the triceps muscle. This places the radial nerve at risk of entrapment between fracture fragments, especially when reduction is attempted. The radial nerve innervates the extensor muscles of the wrist and fingers; evidence of radial nerve injury requires emergent orthopedic evaluation. Injury to the radial nerve from midshaft humerus fractures often results in a benign neuropraxia that resolves spontaneously 80% of the time. The ulnar nerve courses under the medial epicondyle and can be injured with fractures of this structure.

7. **B,** Pages 695-696.

Supracondylar fracture results from extension/hyperextension injuries 98% of the time, most often because of falling on an outstretched hand with the elbow locked in extension. This is primarily a childhood injury. In children the tensile strength of the collateral ligaments is greater than the immature bone strength. During the injury, the ulna levers against the distal humerus and causes the humerus to fracture. Direct blows to the elbow often result in olecranon fracture, anterior elbow dislocation, and to a lesser extent, supracondylar fractures. A spiral injury, commonly a result of arm torsion, necessitates a thorough evaluation to exclude child abuse. It is essential to remember that bones in children are softer than adults, and a great deal of force is needed cause a fracture.

8. **E,** Pages 691-692.

Ulnar nerve injury is characterized by weakness of the interosseous muscles (inability to abduct the fingers against resistance), and loss of sensation over the palmar aspect of the fifth digit and hypothenar eminence. Radial nerve function is best evaluated by wrist extension and abduction of the thumb and sensation over the lateral aspect of the thumb. Median nerve function is tested by finger flexion and sensation over the tip of the index finger.

9. **D,** Pages 705-706.

Posterior elbow dislocation occurs after a fall on an outstretched hand or wrist, with the elbow either extended or hyperextended. Patients present with the elbow in flexion at about 45 degrees with marked prominence of the olecranon. Fractures of the distal humerus, radial head, and coronoid process are often associated with posterior elbow dislocation. Posterior elbow dislocations are reduced emergently when neurovascular compromise is evident. Reduction is accomplished by elbow flexion and posterior pressure applied on the distal humerus while an assistant immobilizes the humerus.

10. **A,** Page 706.

Complications of posterior elbow dislocations include median nerve injury and brachial artery injury. Brachial artery injury is a serious complication that, when suspected, requires emergent angiography and immediate orthopedic consultation. Signs of brachial artery injury can include presence of a bruit/thrill, loss of distal pulses, or signs consistent with ischemia (pain, pallor, paresthesia). Severe joint disruption results in brachial artery injury 8% of the time. The presence of distal pulses does not rule out brachial artery injury. Ulnar and radial nerve injuries are less common with posterior elbow dislocations.

11. **A,** Page 707.

"Little leaguer's elbow" results in a constellation of injuries to the adolescent elbow, including compression fracture of the radial head and capitellum (lateral elbow tenderness), but more commonly an avulsion fracture of the medial epicondyle. The adolescent athlete who presents with this injury should rest the elbow if throwing causes pain and should be referred for orthopedic consultation. Olecranon bursitis is often related to repetitive injury with the elbow in flexion (e.g., plumbing or gardening); symptoms are pain, swelling, and tenderness over the olecranon. Infectious causes for septic bursitis must be considered, and if doubt exists, bursa aspiration should be performed.

12. **D,** Pages 706-707.

Radial head subluxation represents 20% of upper extremity injuries in children. This injury results from a sudden longitudinal pull on the forearm in pronation and a displacement of the annular ligament between the capitellum and the radial head. The child presents with the arm in slight flexion at the elbow and with resistance to attempted supination. X-rays are not needed for this clinical diagnosis, unless there is suspicion of child abuse or the child refuses to use the arm after reduction. Reduction is by supination of the forearm, putting pressure over the radial head, followed by elbow flexion (this is performed in one continuous motion). Ninety percent of patients regain use of the arm within 30 minutes.

# 44 Shoulder

*Greg Ledbetter*

1. **D,** Pages 713-714.
The transthoracic is the least preferred orthogonal view (two films viewed at right angle to each other) because of image overlap. The axillary or transscapular (Y view) views are the preferred orthogonal projections.

2. **A,** Pages 718-719.
The majority of scapular fractures, including those that are severely comminuted, can be managed conservatively. Selected fractures, especially those involving the articular surface, may benefit from surgical correction.

3. **B,** Pages 719-721.
Epiphyseal fractures are uncommon fractures that have a high potential for growth disturbance. All epiphyseal fractures in the proximal humerus should have early orthopedic consultation.

4. **B,** Pages 720-723.
This injury is usually seen in young males between 11 and 17 years of age in whom the joint capsule is stronger than the epiphyseal plate.

5. **A,** Page 723.
The costoclavicular ligament remains intact with grade II injuries of the sternoclavicular joint.

6. **B,** Pages 726-731.
This is the classic clinical presentation of a posterior shoulder dislocation. Similarly, limited adduction and internal rotation are the clinical hallmarks of an anterior shoulder dislocation.

7. **C,** Pages 727-729.
An impaction fracture of the posterolateral humeral head is responsible for the Hill-Sachs deformity.

8. **B,** Page 729.
The incidence of axillary nerve injury with anterior dislocations is between 2.8% and 4%. The axillary nerve supplies sensation to the lateral aspect of the shoulder (regiment's band), and its motor branches innervate the teres minor and deltoid muscles.

9. **C,** Pages 730-731.
Radiographs can be deceptively normal in posterior shoulder dislocations. An impaction fracture of the anteromedial humeral head or reverse Hill-Sachs deformity is another radiographic clue to a posterior shoulder dislocation.

10. **C,** Page 735.
The tendon of the supraspinatus is the most commonly torn tendon.

11. **D,** Pages 734-735.
A rotator cuff tear is usually associated with chronic overuse of the dominant extremity. Patients will have problems with pain in the shoulder and decreased flexion and abduction. Radiographs can be normal but classically show superior displacement of the humeral head with complete tears. Only 10% of rotator cuff tears are associated with a specific traumatic event.

12. **A,** Pages 735-737.
This clinical presentation is classic for adhesive capsulitis. Calcific and bicipital tendinitis are associated with more localized pain.

# 45 Pelvis and Hip

*Greg Ledbetter*

1. **D,** Page 740.
The AP view demonstrates most fractures and dislocations but often does not show the degree of bony displacement. The CT scan of the pelvis and inlet/outlet views are usually needed to further delineate the injury. The normal width of the pubic symphysis is less than 5 mm wide, and the SI joint is 2-4 mm wide on AP view.

2. **B,** Page 742.
Turner's sign is ecchymosis on the abdomen or flanks from a retroperitoneal hemorrhage. Maisonneuve's fracture is a fracture of the proximal fibula with an associated ankle fracture.

3. **C,** Pages 749-750.
To assess for the possibility of occult acetabular fractures, internal and external oblique (Judet) views should be obtained next. If these are not positive and concern still exists, then tomography, CT scan, or radionuclide bone scans can be ordered.

4. **C,** Page 758.
Avascular necrosis occurs most commonly after fractures of the neck of the femur. Tears of the posterior capsule such as those that occur during dislocations of the hip account for a significant number of cases as well.

5. **A,** Page 761.
The most important late complication following traumatic hip dislocation is femoral head ischemia leading to avascular necrosis.

6. **C,** Pages 757-758.
Transient synovitis of the hip is a common, short-lived, nonspecific inflammation of the synovium of the hip. This is often attributed to a mild traumatic episode or a low-grade febrile illness such as tonsillitis or otitis media.

7. **C,** Pages 757-758.
Transient synovitis of the hip occurs most often in boys between the ages of 5 and 6. The onset of the condition is usually insidious, with the child complaining of hip pain that radiates down into the thigh and the knee. The temperature is usually normal to slightly elevated and is rarely high.

8. **B,** Page 759.
Posterior dislocations are 10 to 20 times more common than anterior dislocations. They are suggested by a shortened, flexed, adducted, and internally rotated leg. The femoral head comes to rest posterior to the acetabulum, just anterior to the sciatic nerve, and may cause compression or traction injuries. Slipped capital femoral epiphysis occurs in children. To prevent complications and late sequelae of hip disloca-

tion, reduction should be performed as soon as possible, and certainly within 12 hours.

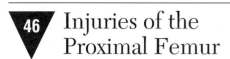

# 46 Injuries of the Proximal Femur

*Greg Ledbetter*

1. **D,** Page 766.
An open fracture that occurs in a highly contaminated environment such as a farm needs coverage for gram-positive and gram-negative bacteria, and specifically for clostridia.

2. **D,** Pages 767-771.
Avascular necrosis of the femoral head is a common and very serious complication of proximal femur fractures. Early diagnosis and early orthopedic consultation are imperative in decreasing the incidence of this devastating complication.

3. **B,** Pages 776-778.
Premature muscle loading can lead to re-traumatization and delayed healing. Pain is the usual guideline for increasing mobilization.

4. **A,** Page 767.
Femoral head fractures usually occur in young patients and are associated with either anterior or posterior hip dislocations (most commonly anterior dislocations). Elderly patients usually sustain a femoral neck fracture with a similar mechanism. Seventy-five percent of femoral head fractures are the result of automobile accidents. The patient has moderate to severe pain and is unable to bear weight.

5. **E,** Pages 767-769.
All of the statements are true. Femoral neck fractures occur most frequently in elderly women. These fractures may occur with only minor trauma, and often the patient may not recall any incidence of trauma. Garden I and II femoral neck fractures are nondisplaced, and the patient may be able to ambulate. In contrast, Garden III and IV fractures are displaced and are unstable, the patient is unable to walk.

6. **C,** Pages 769-771.
The most common femur fracture is an intertrochanteric fracture. Open reduction and internal fixation of an intertrochanteric fracture is the most commonly performed orthopedic operation in the United States.

7. **D,** Page 773.
Femoral shaft fractures are usually the result of high-energy trauma and, as a consequence, commonly produce associated hip, knee, and patellar injuries. In addition, vascular injury is common and may produce large-volume hemorrhage. In contrast, nerve injuries are relatively rare because the muscles of the thigh cushion the nerve from the fracture.

8. **E,** Page 775.
The patient described has classic findings of a slipped capital femoral epiphysis (SCFE). SCFE most frequently occurs in males between 10 and 17 years old. SCFE is more common in obese patients with underdeveloped genitalia or in long, slender, rapidly growing adolescents. The pain is usually grad-

ual in onset over days to months and often starts as groin pain that radiates to the anterior medial thigh. Acute exacerbation may occur after only minimal trauma. Radiographic findings are often subtle, and abnormalities are best seen on lateral views of the hip. Hip dislocations require significant trauma, and Legg-Calvé-Perthes disease usually occurs in younger children (3 to 12 years old). While the signs and symptoms described are similar to those associated with femoral stress fractures, stress fractures tend to occur in vigorous patients involved in extensive athletic or military training.

9. **E,** Page 766.
Sciatic nerve injury and an open femur fracture are both contraindications to application of traction with a Hare splint. Application of traction may worsen the deficit caused by a stretched or partially torn sciatic nerve. In open fractures with exposed bone ends, traction should be applied only after the contaminated wound is débrided in the operating room. Internal bleeding from a femur fracture is often controlled only after application of traction.

10. **D,** Pages 773-775.
Selected stress fractures and isolated greater and lesser trochanteric fractures may initially be treated on an outpatient basis. Internal fixation is recommended for a slipped capital femoral epiphysis.

11. **E,** Page 773.
All of the statements are true. Greater and lesser trochanter fractures do not usually require any treatment other than conservative management. In reliable patients, treatment can easily be done on an outpatient basis. Some fractures may, however, require surgery. Avulsed fragments displaced more than 1 cm in greater trochanter fractures or more than 2 cm in lesser trochanter fractures may require open reduction and internal fixation, especially in younger patients.

12. **E,** Page 774.
Early diagnosis of femoral stress fractures is extremely important because they may progress to displaced fractures if treated inappropriately. In reliable patients, treatment may be done on an outpatient basis and consists of 6 weeks of no weight bearing followed by 6 more weeks of partial weight bearing. Elderly patients with superior neck stress fractures or patients with a complete fracture line may require internal fixation. Orthopedic consultation is required.

13. **D,** Pages 779-780.
Distal pulses are usually present in femoral venous injuries and may be present in 25% of patients with major arterial injuries.

14. **D,** Pages 779-780.
Initial treatment should consist of direct pressure over the injury in order to control bleeding. In addition, fluid resuscitation via large-bore IV catheters should be initiated in patients with either arterial or venous injuries.

15. **C,** Pages 779-780.
While major hemorrhage via arterial injuries is more common, patients with venous injuries require an average of six units of blood in addition to crystalloid infusion. Ligation or clamping of venous or arterial injuries is not recommended in most cases.

# 47 Knee and Lower Leg

*Greg Ledbetter*

1. **A,** Page 802.

Evaluation of traumatic dislocation of the knee may not reveal an obvious gross deformity because of the high incidence of spontaneous relocation. The most common mechanisms include motor vehicle accidents, industrial falls, and athletic injuries. Arterial injury may exist even in the face of intact pedal pulses, if a nonocclusive intimal tear is present. To rule out subclinical arterial injuries, arteriography is recommended in all cases of suspected knee dislocation.

2. **A,** Pages 798-799.

Partial disruption of the quadriceps mechanism is treated by placing the patient in a knee immobilizer with the knee in full extension. Complete tears are treated with surgical repair.

3. **C,** Page 807.

Overuse syndromes are often seen in the ED. Iliotibial band or tract tendinitis is an overuse injury seen commonly in long-distance runners. The patient may complain of increasing pain when running hills or climbing stairs. On physical examination the patient has superficial localized tenderness of the lateral epicondyle of the femur.

4. **C,** Page 812.

Osgood-Schlatter disease occurs in children, particularly active 10- to 15-year-old boys, and symptoms have an insidious onset. The disease may be confused with superficial infrapatellar bursitis.

5. **C,** Page 810.

The clinical situation described is that of a Baker's cyst, which is inflammation of the gastrocnemius-semimembranous bursa.

6. **A,** Page 792.

The Segund fracture results from excessive internal rotation and varus stress. It is uniformly associated with a detachment of a portion of the lateral collateral ligament and tears of the anterior cruciate ligament. In the majority of cases, there are associated injuries of the menisci and other supporting ligamentous structures.

7. **A,** Page 809.

Prepatellar bursitis secondary to trauma commonly becomes infected as in this case. Fluid should be aspirated and Gram stain, culture, and white blood cell count should be done.

8. **B,** Page 816.

The vast majority (95%) of stress fractures in athletes occur in the lower extremities. Sites of injury include the tibia (50%), metatarsals (18%), fibula (12%), and femur (6%), with other sites accounting for <1%. Most of these occur in runners and make up 6% to 15% of all running injuries.

9. **C,** Page 801.

Chondromalacia patella is a disorder most commonly seen in the young active female. The pain is poorly localized in the knee without effusion or any history of trauma.

10. **C,** Page 789.

The Lachman's test is 99% sensitive for diagnosing anterior cruciate ligament injury. Anterior drawer test is 70% sensitive and is less reliable in acute injuries. A knee x-ray will show a probable joint effusion with an anterior cruciate injury but is neither specific nor sensitive.

11. **D,** Page 792.

Tibial plateau fractures produce a high percentage of vascular complications. A thorough neurovascular examination should be done on all of these injuries.

12. **C,** Page 800.

The quadriceps angle is formed by lines that are drawn from the tibial tubercle to the center of the patella and from the center of the patella to the anterior iliac spine. The Q angle should be less than 10 degrees in men and 15 degrees in women. A Q angle larger than that should suggest patellofemoral problems.

13. **C,** Pages 804-805.

The Lachman's test is for diagnosing damage to the anterior cruciate ligament. Valgus laxity is caused by damage to the medial collateral ligament. The lateral meniscus is commonly injured in this setting of combined ligament injuries.

# 48 Ankle and Foot

*Greg Ledbetter*

1. **B,** Pages 824-827.

The Maissonneuve fracture is a sequela of external rotation of the foot with resultant rupture of the anterior tibiofibular ligament and fracture of the proximal third of the fibula. The fibula fracture would be missed on routine ankle views.

2. **A,** Pages 830-831.

A patient with a grade II (second-degree) sprain will have immediate pain, whereas first- and third-degree sprains may be painless initially.

3. **D,** Page 834.

When the diagnosis of retinaculum injury is suspected, immediate orthopedic surgical consultation is appropriate. The patient should be splinted in midplantar flexion to remove tension from the retinaculum.

4. **C,** Pages 852-853.

This is the classic description of tarsal tunnel syndrome, caused by compression of the abductor digiti quinti or the posterior tibial nerve.

5. **B,** Pages 849-850.

Nondisplaced fractures are treated with padding and taping to an adjacent uninjured toe, "dynamic splinting," also known as buddy taping. Unstable displaced fractures often require open reduction and internal fixation.

6. **D,** Page 824.

Although it is associated with many ankle fractures, soft tissue swelling is not by itself a reason to order ankle films according to the Ottawa Ankle Rules.

7. **D,** Page 827.

Lateral malleolar fractures distal to the tibiotalar joint line without associated injuries are very unlikely to affect the congruity of the ankle joint. Casting and non–weight bearing status is an acceptable conservative option for these injuries. The patient should have close orthopedic follow-up to ensure proper healing. All potentially unstable ankle fractures require orthopedic consultation.

8. **D,** Page 833.

The Thompson test is performed with the patient prone and the knee flexed at 90 degrees. Squeezing the calf muscle should cause passive plantar flexion of the foot.

9. **C,** Pages 843-844.

Significant calcaneal fractures commonly have complications. All but minor extraarticular calcaneus fractures should have orthopedic consultation, and all fractures need close orthopedic follow-up.

 **49** Foreign Bodies

*Greg Ledbetter*

1. **D,** Page 862.

Patching the opposite eye to prevent consensual movement is appropriate. Once a perforated globe is confirmed, procedures on the affected eye beyond a brief examination are inappropriate, including slit-lamp exam and instillation of any drops. Immediate referral is mandatory and should not be delayed to the next day.

2. **B,** Pages 863-864.

The auditory canal is an elliptical cylinder. Therefore, directing irrigation at the periphery of the foreign body (i.e., past the object, against the tympanic membrane, and against the posterior of the object) facilitates removal. The pinna must be pulled posteriorly and superiorly to straighten the canal. The canal is very sensitive, and forceps are often helpful. Trendelenburg's position does not facilitate removal.

3. **B,** Page 864-865.

Nose picking is a nonspecific sign for nasal foreign body. The common history is of the patient being observed placing the object in the nose or the classical clinical presentation of purulent, unilateral, malodorous nasal discharge. A nasal foreign body is less commonly discovered incidentally after routine dental radiograph studies. One report suggests that bad body odor may be the presenting complaint in up to 25% of cases.

4. **B,** Page 867.

Foreign bodies of the upper esophagus are usually oriented in the coronal plane, whereas tracheal objects are in the sagittal (i.e., anteroposterior) plane.

5. **D,** Page 867.

The films show an essentially normal inspiratory film. On forced expiration, the left lung remains expanded with relative hyperlucency, diaphragm is fixed, and there is a shift of the mediastinum to the right. These findings are consistent with the "one-way valve" effect of a partial obstruction of the left mainstem bronchus. The findings would be exactly reversed for the right mainstem. Early findings for complete mainstem bronchus obstruction are atelectasis on the involved side, with mediastinal shift toward the involved side on inspiration and toward the uninvolved side on expiration. In late complete obstruction, the findings are atelectasis of the involved side, with mediastinal shift toward the involved side during both inspiration and expiration.

6. **A,** Pages 867-868.

This situation represents complete obstruction of the larynx or trachea. The Heimlich maneuver and finger sweep have already been performed and have failed to relieve the obstruction, and the patient is unconscious. Therefore an immediate cricothyrotomy should be undertaken to open the airway. Choices C, D, and E would not facilitate opening the airway, and tracheostomy (B) is a more complicated, time-consuming procedure.

7. **A,** Page 870.

Subcutaneous emphysema found on palpation of the neck indicates probable esophageal perforation. Only if perforation is not a concern should barium be used, because it is inert in tissues and is not reabsorbed. Water-soluble contrast could be considered, although its use is controversial. The other choices are all acceptable approaches for attempting visualization and removal of the bone.

8. **B,** Pages 870-871.

Foley catheter technique can be effective, but it is contraindicated in complete obstruction. Glucagon is also effective, but if given too rapidly may produce nausea and vomiting, which can lead to rupture of the obstructed esophagus. This patient's chest pain suggests perforation, so gas-forming agents are contraindicated. In addition, the impaction has been present for 10 hours, and gas-forming agents are much less likely to succeed after 6 hours. Suspected esophageal perforation also contraindicates use of papain, because continued proteolytic action in the mediastinum creates a medical disaster. Thus the only appropriate approach in this case is endoscopic.

9. **E,** Page 872.

If the disk battery has passed into the stomach, the patient can be observed expectantly for spontaneous passage, and induced emesis is not indicated. Immediate endoscopic removal is indicated if the disk battery is lodged in the esophagus. Lack of formal follow-up is inappropriate, because follow-up radiography may be needed to rule out disintegration of the battery. Only then might chelation therapy based on heavy metal levels be indicated.

10. **D,** Page 874.

The radiograph indicates a rectosigmoid foreign body. The free air on the upright film is diagnostic for bowel perforation. Therefore surgical intervention is indicated. If perforation was not suspected, all of the other techniques for removal could be attempted.

11. **A,** Page 875.

The history and physical findings are consistent with a missile wound passing near the popliteal artery. Missile wounds near major vessels, with or without obvious clinical involvement, require arteriography to rule out a vascular injury. The other imaging studies listed all have utility in the diagnosis of foreign bodies, but are not mandatory for management of this patient.

12. **C,** Page 875.

In cases of impaled foreign objects, no attempt should be made in the field to remove the object. Impaled foreign bodies should be left in place and stabilized as well as possible. If the impaled object is too long to allow for easy transportation, it should be cut off close to the patient and the patient then moved. Impaled foreign bodies often compress or tamponade potentially life-threatening bleeding points and therefore should be left until they can be removed in the operating room. Otherwise, normal trauma protocol should be followed, and transport should not be delayed when a solution is possible.

13. **D,** Pages 875-876.

High-pressure injection injuries involving chemical foreign material (e.g., paint, grease, turpentine) should generally be considered surgical emergencies requiring decompression and debridement. Failure to recognize the seriousness of what externally appears to be a minor wound can lead to extensive tissue necrosis and ultimately amputation. The other choices are all important in general wound management, but are not as important as prompt surgical care.

14. **C,** Pages 872-873.

The physician should perform those procedures and interventions that can be medically justified as reasonable steps to protect the patient from injury resulting from the ingested object or substance. Use of ipecac to induce vomiting following ingestion of cocaine-filled condoms is medically justified because of the risk to the patient should a condom burst. Hospital or infirmary observation is equally justified to watch for passage of the condoms or for signs of overdosage. Gut decontamination is medically indicated for drug intoxication and thus appropriate. Requesting clarification is always acceptable but should not interfere with appropriate care. However, the patient in question shows no sign of intestinal obstruction or intoxication. Emergent laparotomy is not medically indicated and is thus inappropriate.

## 50 Soft-Tissue Spine Injuries and Back Pain

*Barbara N. Wynn*

1. **D,** Page 879.

The only radiographic abnormality seen with torticollis would be a rotational curvature of the cervical spine. If a cervical spine fracture is possible, a minimum of lateral AP and odontoid views are required. A radiograph cannot prove cer-

vical strain; it will demonstrate only the presence or absence of bony abnormalities and ligamentous instability. MRI is the modality of choice for investigating cervical disk disease, and it is also safer in pregnant women than CT.

2. **E,** Pages 881-884.

Most patients do not notice or complain of neck discomfort immediately after an injury but will develop symptoms minutes to hours later. Variation in the presenting symptom is marked. Neurologic complaints can occur, with the most common involving numbness or paresthesias down one or both arms. The use of motor vehicle headrests at the proper height was expected to drastically reduce the incidence of cervical hyperextension injuries, but head restraints have made either little or no difference in the incidence of injury. Patients should be advised to expect fairly rapid recovery from the injury (between 2 and 12 weeks), and several studies find better results with early motion compared with use of the collar; in general neck collars for soft tissue injury cannot be recommended.

3. **D,** Page 885.

Plain radiographs of the thoracic spine are felt to be important in the initial investigation of suspected thoracic disk herniation. In addition to helping rule out potentially dangerous lesions, plain radiographs can actually suggest the presence of disk herniation in up to 80% of cases. Calcification within the thoracic disk space is most suggestive. In suspected cases, further imaging studies such as MRI need to be done.

4. **B,** Page 887.

Back problems are not unique to the industrialized world; however, the attitude toward the pain is different in developing countries. Reliable predictors of who will have low back pain are limited to those with previous back problems or back surgery; the patient's attitude toward and degree of satisfaction with his or her job is also a factor. Disk herniation is most common in the 30- to 40-year-old age-group, and despite the fact that between 48% and 76% of pregnant women have back pain, there is no increased incidence of disk herniation in pregnancy.

5. **A,** Page 889.

Suggested criteria for lumbar radiographs in the emergency department include extremes of age (<18 or >50 years old), trauma other than simple lifting, unresolved back pain for 4-6 weeks, prior referral, and patients in whom something other than simple diskogenic or musculoskeletal pain is suspected. See Rosen Box 50-1.

6. **B,** Page 892.

Scheurmann's disease, which causes kyphosis, vertebral wedging, and endplate irregularities, seems to be associated with premature disk disease. Spondylosis refers to degenerative changes of the vertebrae and can include osteophyte formation at the disk spaces. It has not been found to have any correlation with symptoms. Spondylolysis refers to a defect in the pars interarticularis (the isthmus of bone between the superior and inferior facets). Stress fractures of the pars interarticularis are thought to be responsible for some instances of low back pain in young athletes. Spondylolisthesis refers to frank slippage of the anterior portion of the superior vertebral body forward on the inferior vertebral body. Spondylolysis in itself is not a clinical problem but may contribute to spondylolisthesis, which seems to predispose to sciatica. The slippage is most often at the L5 to S1 level and is graded from stage 1 to stage 4 depending on percentage of slippage. Transitional vertebrae, a congenital anomaly, may also cause back pain. The only type that may do this is the one involving contact between the transverse process of L5 and the sacrum or ileum.

7. **B,** Pages 895-896.
A positive straight leg test occurs if the pain radiates down the back and below the knee. Dorsiflexion tests L5. The L5 dermatome involves the medial foot web space and the web space of the great toe. The S1 dermatome involves the posterior calf and lateral foot. S1 motor function is tested by having the patient walk on toes.

8. **A,** Page 896.
Back pain greater than leg pain is indicative of nondisk pain. True disk pain should have leg pain greater than back pain. The other answers are all seen with disk pain. See Rosen Box 50-3.

9. **B,** Page 898.
Cauda equina syndrome, severe neurologic deficit, and progressive neurologic deficit are consistent with a severe disk problem. Severe unremitting pain is of no real diagnostic value. Multiple nerve root involvement may be suggestive of a spinal tumor requiring operative intervention.

10. **D,** Pages 898-900.
In approximately 80%-90% of cases, patients with mechanical back pain have improvement within 2 months regardless of therapy. Absence of saddle area sensation and anal sphincter tone indicates acute cauda equina syndrome, and emergency neurosurgical consultation is mandatory. Recovery from back injury is aided by early motion rather than prolonged immobilization and it is clear that bed rest should not be strict nor should it exceed 2 days for most patients.

# 51 ▼ Animal Bites and Rabies

*Barbara N. Wynn*

1. **E,** Pages 906, 909, 911, 912.
Pig bites are the fourth most common bite reported among veterinarians after horses, cats, and dogs. The wounds are often deep, although they may be small on the surface, and they have a high risk of infection. With dog bites to the scalp, children under 2 years old may suffer perforation of the skull. Primate bites must be scrubbed immediately with a concentrated soap solution to prevent possible *Herpesvirus semiae* (also known as B virus) infection. Suturing should not be done. Cat wounds to the face are the only ones that should be sutured. Cefuroxime, amoxicillin/clavulanate, and doxycycline plus penicillin are all drugs of choice for cat bites; cephalexin is a drug of choice for dog bites.

2. **E,** Pages 909-910.
For dog bites, the infection rate of hand wounds is as high as 30%, whereas the infection rate of wounds elsewhere averages 9%. Hand wounds from cat bites have an infection rate of 19%; those on the lower extremity 20%; and wounds on the arms, neck, or trunk have an infection rate of 5% or less. Also contributing to risk for infection are the wound type (puncture, extensive crush, contaminated, old) and the patient (elderly, diabetic, asplenic, alcoholic, steroid dependent). See Rosen Table 51-2.

3. **A,** Page 910.
*C. canimorsus* is a gram-negative rod that occurs in patients most commonly after dog bites, but the illness has also followed nonbite contact with dogs and cats, including scratches. In a number of cases there is no report of any animal exposure. Onset of illness is within a few days of contact. Purpura, particularly on the face, and petechiae are common findings. Cutaneous gangrene at the site of the bite strongly suggests the presence of this organism.

4. **A,** Pages 912-913.
Human bites are tetanus-prone wounds; therefore the patient's immunization status would need to be boosted. Human bite locations other than the hand do not have a particularly high rate of infection, nor does the CDC consider human bites to carry a high risk of transmission for HIV. Studies of bacteriology of human bites to the hand showed a polymicrobial picture with an average of five organisms per wound.

5. **B,** Pages 912-913.
Involvement of the deeper structures of the hand requires hospitalization and parenteral antibiotics. Lacerations of the face may be closed primarily within 24 hours of injury. Because *Staphylococcus* species are common in wound infections, penicillinase-resistant antibiotics should be added if penicillin is used. Local wound care is more important than antibiotic prophylaxis. Prophylactic antibiotics do not reduce the incidence of infection in mucosal bites. Through-and-through lacerations require a layered closure, and prophylactic antibiotics appear to reduce the risk of infection in these wounds.

6. **A,** Pages 914-916.
High-risk animals are raccoons, skunks, fox, and bats. Rodents such as squirrels, rats, chipmunks, gophers, and guinea pigs are very unlikely to carry rabies and thus are considered low risk. Domestic animals, particularly dogs and cats, are generally low risk. Petting a rabid animal and contact with its blood, urine, or feces are not considered exposures because the virus is transmitted in the saliva.

7. **E,** Pages 915-916.

The incubation period for rabies is 30 to 90 days; however, bites on the head and neck have a much shorter incubation period (as short as 15 days), whereas those on the trunk or lower extremity have a longer incubation period. The initial symptoms of rabies are nonspecific, and paresthesias or pain at the bite site may be the first neurologic symptom. Difficulty in swallowing is a much later symptom and is seen when rabies has become full blown. No specific, effective treatment exists for rabies. Only three patients are known to have survived clinical rabies, and all had received some form of preexposure or postexposure prophylaxis. The cost of postexposure prophylaxis is about $1000.00 per series.

8. **D,** Pages 915-917.

Most cases of rabies are transmitted by bites, which are considered the most infectious form of exposure. Risk of transmission by a bite is about 50 times that of a scratch. Cats are the domestic animal most commonly reported rabid, representing 48% of all domestic animal bites. Animals are capable of transmitting rabies once they start secreting the virus in their saliva; they may not become ill until several days after secretion begins, and then they usually die within 3 to 9 days. Initial symptoms may be ataxia, anorexia, and lethargy or excessive salivation. In a wild animal there may be a change in instinctive behavior. The only U.S. state that remains rabies free is Hawaii.

---

 ## 52 Venomous Animal Injuries

*Gwen L. Hoffman*

1. **A,** Page 925.

In the United States (1950-1969) insects were responsible for 52% of the fatalities, snakes 30%, and spiders 13%. More specifically, bees are responsible for the most fatalities, followed by rattlesnakes, wasps, and spiders.

2. **C,** Page 927.

Venomous snakes have a triangular head, elliptical pupils, pits, fangs, and a single row of subcaudal plates. The pit, a heat-sensitive organ that enables the snake to locate warm-blooded prey, is found midway between the eye and the nostril on both sides of the head.

3. **A,** Pages 927-928, 931.

Venom spread can be retarded by keeping the patient calm and preventing movement of the extremity. Suction is helpful if done within the first 15 minutes after the bite occurs. The wound should not be incised. An ice bag wrapped in a towel and applied to the area may reduce the pain but will not slow the spread of venom. Packing the extremity in ice is dangerous and only adds to tissue destruction. A constricting band may be applied proximal to the wound only tightly enough to impede lymph flow but not arterial flow.

4. **E,** Page 930.

It is important to appreciate the degree of envenomation to determine whether and how much antivenin should be ad-

ministered. Grade I is described in choice B; grade II is choice E; grade III is choice C, and grade IV is answers A and D.

5. **C,** Page 931.

The smaller the body of the patient, the larger the initial dose required. A bitten child usually receives more venom in proportion to body weight and thus requires more antivenin to neutralize it. Pregnancy is not a contraindication to antivenin therapy. A skin test should be performed in every patient before each administration of a foreign antiserum, regardless of the patient's clinical history. Antivenin should never be injected around the wound or into a finger or toe. Serum sickness usually develops about 1 week after administration of 10 or more vials. It can be treated with diphenhydramine 50 mg and cimetidine 300 mg every 6 hours. If serum sickness is severe, steroids can be initiated; this is the only indication of steroid use in connection with snakebite.

6. **C,** Page 933.

For a urticarial reaction epinephrine 0.3 ml SQ and diphenhydramine 50 mg IM is appropriate treatment. If symptom free after 1 hour, the patient may be discharged and given antihistamines every 6 hours for 24 hours. An emergency insect sting kit should be prescribed and referral made for desensitization. With a severe reaction, 5 ml of epinephrine in a 1:10,000 dilution slowly IV and oxygen by mask may be needed, and a beta-agonist is given for wheezing. Close monitoring is necessary, and 100 mg of methylprednisolone, 50 mg of diphenhydramine, and 150 mg of cimetidine are given intravenously in addition to normal saline IV. Hospitalization and referral for desensitization are required.

7. **A,** Pages 934-935.

Antivenin is suggested for patients (1) younger than 16 years of age and older than 65, (2) with severe envenomations, (3) who are pregnant, or (4) who are not able to stand the stress of envenomation. An ice pack should be applied to the area for relief of pain. Hypertension usually occurs and can be treated with nitroprusside if the diastolic pressure is >130 mm Hg. Dapsone is used for brown recluse spider bites. Severe muscle cramps are present and are treated with calcium gluconate. Methocarbamol and diazepam may also be used.

8. **D,** Page 935.

Antivenin is not currently available in the United States. Excision of the lesion has not been shown to aid healing and may be detrimental. After 6 hours of observation with no evidence of envenomation, discharge with follow-up may be appropriate. Systemic symptoms include fever, chills, rash, petechiae, nausea, vomiting, malaise, and weakness. Hemolysis, thrombocytopenia, shock, jaundice, renal failure, hemorrhage, and pulmonary edema are evidence of severe envenomation. Fatalities are more common in children, most often the result of severe intravascular hemolysis.

9. **D,** Pages 937-938.

Antivenin is available only for stone fish (scorpion fish) envenomation. At least as many deaths are caused by drowning after envenomation as by toxic effects of the venom. With stingray wounds, the area should be put in water as hot as can be tolerated for 30-40 minutes because the venom is heat labile; the heat will help neutralize the venom. Tetanus prophylaxis is indicated for all marine bites as indicated. Nematocysts should be treated as described.

---

 # Thermal Burns

## 53

*Dale J. Ray*

1. **A,** Page 944.
Nonaccidental burns often have clear-cut edges and "stocking" distribution, and they tend to occur on the back of the hands and feet, the buttocks, perineum, and legs. Accidental burns, such as those which occur with spills, often have fuzzy, uneven edges and are located on the head, trunk, and palmar surface of the hands and plantar aspects of the feet.

2. **D,** Page 945.
If a fourth-degree burn is present, charring of the skin and destruction of the subcutaneous tissues is observed. Blistering may be present with full-thickness burns and is not solely characteristic of partial-thickness burns.

3. **B,** Page 945.
Many physiologic changes seen after burns are a response to diminished circulating blood volume. The immediate cardiovascular response is a reduction in cardiac output accompanied by an elevation in peripheral vascular resistance. In the absence of heart disease, the ventricular ejection fraction and velocity of myocardial fiber shortening are actually increased during thermal injury. With replacement of plasma volume, cardiac output increases to levels that are above normal.

4. **E,** Page 947.
Placement of ice directly on the burn may worsen the injury by potential freezing. The use of ice may also lead to hypothermia. The burn wound should be immersed in cold water (1° to 5° C) for approximately 30 minutes if immediate transport is impossible; this must be done in the first 30 minutes to be beneficial. Cold inhibits lactate production and acidosis, thus promoting catecholamine function and cardiovascular homeostasis. Cold also inhibits burn wound histamine release, and it suppresses the production of thromboxane. Intravenous fluids are needed if the transport time is >30 minutes and burns >20% of BSA or evidence of burn shock.

5. **C,** Pages 946-947.
According to the rule of nines, the right arm burn would be 9% of his body surface area and the front of his chest and abdomen would be 18%, leading to a total of 27%.

6. **D,** Pages 947-949.
This patient has an estimated burn, according to the rule of nines of 36% BSA. The Parkland formula for fluid resuscitation is 4 ml/kg/% BSA burned of lactated Ringer's solution to be administered over the first 24 hours, with the first half over the first 8 hours. The fluid loss is calculated from the time of injury. Any formula is only a guideline, and clinical parameters must be closely followed. The calculation in this case is 36 × 4 × 70 kg = 10,080 ml over first 24 hours. One half of this is 5040 ml/first 8 hours or 630 ml/hr.

7. **A,** Pages 948-949.
Because of accompanying ileus, burns >20% BSA preclude the use of oral fluid hydration. Burned children frequently have greater evaporative water loss and therefore have greater fluid resuscitation needs because of their larger BSA relative to weight. The most common error during resuscitation is overhydration. Hypertonic saline resuscitation has not led to the anticipated benefits of fewer escharotomies and limited ileus. Fluid replacement is calculated from the time of injury.

8. **C,** Page 952.
All patients with major burns require hospitalization. Major burns include in adults, second degree with >10%-20% TBSA and in children, second-degree with >5%-10% TBSA. Other indications are significant chemical or electrical burns; significant burns to the airway, face, hands, feet, or perineum; and significant preexisting medical disorders or special psychosocial needs.

9. **D,** Page 952.
The ointment vehicle, rather than the Neosporin, is the removal factor. The ointment contains polyoxyethylene sorbitan, which will dissolve the tar and, because it is water soluble, will facilitate washing off of the residue. Alternative agents are Tween 80, Neosporin cream, or De-Solv-It.

---

 # Frostbite

## 54

*Scott A. Carlson*

1. **C,** Page 954.
Thyroid stimulation and shivering thermogenesis, along with catecholamine release and peripheral vasoconstriction, are processes orchestrated by the preoptic anterior hypothalamus, meant to prevent hypothermia, not frostbite. Acral skin structure's arteriovenous anastomoses facilitate drastic reductions in blood flow. The "hunting response" of recurrent cycles of vasodilation occurs at 10° C and below. Cold stress can trigger marked reductions in cutaneous blood flow.

2. **E,** Pages 954-955.
Because of extracellular fluid ice-crystal formation, the osmotic gradient causes fluid shifts out of the cell into the extracellular space, resulting in intracellular dehydration, cell shrinkage, and ultimately collapse. Blister fluid contains tissue-damaging substances like thromboxane. Early tissue edema resolves after a few days, leading to necrosis, with ultimate mummification and sloughing. Microvasculature injury, with stasis and sludging, is the ultimate determinant of progressive tissue damage.

3. **A,** Page 956.
Trench foot (immersion foot) and chilblains (pernio) are both nonfreezing injuries. Trench foot results from exposure to wet cold. Chilblains is a mild form of dry-cold injury often following repeated exposure. Plaques, blue nodules, and ulcerations can develop as a result of persistent vasospasm and vasculitis. Most patients with trench foot have numbness. Its hallmark after rewarming is very painful erythematous, dry skin.

4. **A,** Pages 960-961.

The common sequelae of frostbite are thought to occur as a result of direct neuronal damage and sympathetic tone residual abnormalities.

5. **B,** Page 956.

Numbness is present in more than 75% of patients.

6. **A,** Page 958.

Rewarming of frostbitten extremities should never be initiated in the field if there is any potential for interrupted or incomplete thawing. Tissue refreezing is disastrous.

7. **D,** Page 958.

Frozen or partially thawed tissue should be rapidly and actively rewarmed by immersion in gently circulating water maintained at 40°-42° C. Frozen parts should be kept away from dry heat sources to prevent a gradual, partial thaw. Direct tissue massage is not efficacious and will increase tissue loss.

8. **D,** Pages 958-959.

Tissue massage can increase tissue loss and should be avoided. Digital exercises should be encouraged after thawing to prevent venous stasis. Edema formation is common; therefore splints and casts should be avoided and elevation encouraged. Silvadene does not have a role in frostbite, although topical aloe vera may be helpful as a thromboxane inhibitor (limiting arachidonic acid breakdown products). Ibuprofen also inhibits thromboxane and should be part of the treatment protocol.

9. **E,** Page 955.

Final demarcation between viable and nonviable tissue often requires more than 60 to 90 days; thus the surgical aphorism "Frostbite in January, amputate in July."

10. **A,** Pages 958-959.

For hemorrhagic blisters, aspiration is preferable to debridement because the latter can cause injury extension from secondary desiccation of deep dermal layers. Splints and compressive dressings should be avoided. Aloe vera is recommended for *direct* application to frostbitten areas, which intact blisters preclude.

---

 ## 55 Accidental Hypothermia

*Scott A. Carlson*

1. **B,** Pages 963-964.

Conductive heat loss is increased 25 times with immersion in cold water. Insensible heat loss is responsible for 20%-27% of total heat loss. Radiant heat loss is dependent on the temperature gradient between the environment and the exposed body surface area. Greater heat losses occur in a cool, dry, windy environment (wind-chill index). Convective losses increase with shivering.

2. **A,** Pages 964-965.

In hypothermia, the PR, QRS, and QT intervals may be prolonged, with QT prolongation being most characteristic. Spontaneous ventricular fibrillation and asystole are findings associated with profound hypothermia. A large, multicenter

hypothermia study did not find ventricular fibrillation to be iatrogenic. The J wave, while associated with hypothermia, may be present in other conditions, especially central nervous system lesions. Atrial fibrillation typically converts spontaneously as the patient is rewarmed. Reentrant dysrhythmia is common because of decreased conduction rates.

3. **C,** Pages 964-965.

Shivering ceases at approximately 32° C. The other associations are correct.

4. **E,** Pages 966-967.

Hyperthyroidism is not associated with hypothermia. The other choices may be.

5. **D,** Pages 968-969.

Dopamine infusions should be reserved for disproportionately hypotensive patients who do not respond to crystalloids or rewarming. The value of prophylactic heparin administration is unknown. The optimal dosage of bretylium tosylate is unknown in the hypothermic patient. Empiric treatment with thyroxine should be reserved for patients thought to have myxedema. Although cold exposure induces adrenal unresponsiveness to ACTH, steroids are not thought to be beneficial.

6. **C,** Pages 968-969.

Most dysrhythmias associated with hypothermia spontaneously convert during rewarming. Contrary to dysrhythmias in normothermic patients, asystole is not more ominous than ventricular fibrillation in hypothermic patients. Atrial fibrillation is a common and usually innocent rhythm. Because of delays in conduction, it is usually associated with a slow ventricular response. Lidocaine has not been useful in facilitating defibrillation in hypothermic patients. Although the optimal dose is unknown, canine studies and human case reports confirm the choice of bretylium in patients with ventricular fibrillation.

7. **D,** Pages 966, 969-970.

The knee jerk is the last of the peripheral reflexes to disappear, at about 26° C. The corneal reflex persists until approximately 23° C.

8. **E,** Page 970.

Blood gas analyzers typically warm blood to 37° C, giving an uncorrected result. "Correction" of this result for the patient's temperature should not be used to guide therapy, and maintenance of corrected ABG neutrality depresses coronary blood flow and cardiac output while increasing the incidence of ventricular fibrillation. The neutral pH of water rises with cooling, as does blood pH, leading to a relative alkalinity that offers some myocardial protection.

9. **E,** Pages 970-971.

Hyperkalemia may be seen in association with renal failure, rhabdomyolysis, or metabolic acidosis. Hypokalemia is less common and results from intracellular flux caused by an increased pH. Hyperglycemia caused by catecholamine-induced glycogenolysis is seen in early hypothermia. Cold-induced diuresis decreases plasma volume, and an increase in the hematocrit of 2% per 1° C drop in temperature is expected with hypothermia. Hematocrit and BUN levels are both poor indicators of a patient's actual fluid status.

10. **B,** Page 971.
Laboratory tests of coagulation are performed at 37° C, accounting for the disparity between normal values and a clinically evident coagulopathy. The only effective treatment is rewarming, as the enzymatic nature of activated clotting factors is temperature dependent. Thrombocytopenia is common in hypothermia.

11. **D,** Page 972.
Attendants should handle the patient gently, allowing no exertion. Heat loss, particularly by conduction in this circumstance, should be minimized. No stimulants or heated oral fluids should be given. Skin rubbing suppresses shivering thermogenesis and promotes cutaneous vasodilation and should be avoided. This patient is alert and therefore not a candidate for intubation.

12. **C,** Pages 976-977.
Sinus tachycardia is not indicative of cardiovascular instability. Uncontrolled shivering in an otherwise stable patient indicates a temperature greater than 32° C with the ability to generate heat. Frostbite is not an indication for active rewarming. Moderate or severe hypothermia is defined as core temperature less than 32.2° C. Patients with pharmacologically induced peripheral vasodilation are incapable of sufficient thermogenesis and will require active rewarming.

13. **C,** Pages 976-979.
Airway rewarming is indicated in all cases of moderate or severe hypothermia. Complete humidification is necessary for heat delivery. Heat transfer from irrigation fluids is usually very limited because of minimal surface area. Truncal active external rewarming is preferred, as cardiovascular collapse can occur by increasing metabolic demands with vasodilation of the extremities if they are heated.

14. **D,** Pages 973-974.
Studies have found that intubation is safe, with induced dysrhythmias rare. It is always necessary unless the patient is alert with intact protective airway reflexes. Secretory bronchorrhea accumulation from depressed ciliary activity produces a frothy sputum and chest congestion, often mistaken for pulmonary edema. Blind nasotracheal intubation is often required when trismus is present. A nasogastric tube is indicated in moderate and severe hypothermia after endotracheal intubation.

 **56** Heat Illness

*Dale E. McNinch*

1. **D,** Pages 987-988.
Evaporation of sweat from the skin is the most important mechanism of heat dissipation. Cooling is achieved by evaporation from the body surface; sweat that drips from the skin does not cool the body. In humans, respiratory mechanisms are minimal sources of heat loss. A 70-kg man's average basal metabolic rate is 100 Kcal/hour. Eccrine glands produce

"thermal" sweat. Individuals exercising in hot environments commonly lose 1-2 L of sweat per kg per hour.

2. **B,** Page 988.
Acclimatization usually results in a lower baseline heart rate and a higher stroke volume, with generally no change in cardiac output. There is an earlier onset of sweating (at a lower core temperature), increased sweat volume, and lowered sweat electrolyte concentration.

3. **B,** Pages 989-990.
Neurologic malignant syndrome is clinically similar to malignant hyperthermia but differs in that it is induced by antipsychotic medications, usually haloperidol (Haldol). It is characterized by muscular rigidity, severe dyskinesia or akinesia, hyperthermia, tachycardia, dyspnea, dysphagia, and urinary incontinence. Malignant hyperthermia is seen in certain patients undergoing general anesthesia and is also treated with dantrolene.

4. **D,** Pages 991-993.
Heat stroke is diagnosed only in the presence of severe CNS dysfunction (delirium, seizures, coma) and severe hyperthermia (core temperature usually 40° C or greater). Heat exhaustion, if left untreated, may progress to heat stroke. Heat edema is defined as swollen feet and ankles in an nonacclimatized individual, especially the elderly. Heat syncope is seen in individuals who stand for protracted periods, which allows pooling of blood in the lower extremities. This, combined with volume loss and peripheral vasodilation, results in inadequate central venous return, a drop in cardiac output, and a cerebral perfusion inadequate to maintain consciousness. Lying down cures the condition.

5. **A,** Pages 994-995.
Although anhidrosis is a dramatic finding in some patients with heat stroke, persistent sweating may be present in up to 50% of cases. In 80% of cases, heat stroke has a sudden onset. Hepatic injury is evidenced by markedly elevated levels of hepatic enzymes. Coma, seizures, and delirium are seen. Core temperature is usually 41° C or more but may be lower.

6. **E,** Page 995.
Although described, pancreatitis in heat stroke is rare. Liver damage is such a consistent feature of heat stroke that its absence should cast doubt on the diagnosis. CNS dysfunction is an invariable feature of heat stroke. Myoglobinuria with resultant renal failure is common. Myocardial injury, particularly right-sided cardiac failure, is also common.

7. **D,** Page 995.
Classic heat stroke (CHS) is usually the result of poor environmental heat dissipation, whereas exertional heat stroke (EHS) results from excessive endogenous heat production. EHS typically occurs in healthy young men and has much more pronounced laboratory value abnormalities than CHS; in CHS abnormalities are generally mild and a respiratory alkalosis is usually seen.

8. **D,** Pages 995-996.

Respiratory alkalosis is a physiologic response to active or passive heating and may be severe enough to produce tetany in patients with heat stroke. Most patients with classic heat stroke have respiratory alkalosis, whereas those with exertional heat stroke usually have a relatively pure lactic acidosis. All the other choices are seen.

9. **C,** Page 997.

Ice water immersion (and subsequent loss of body heat through conduction) is 20-30 times more rapid for dissipating heat than evaporation or convection. Cooling is the cornerstone of treatment in heat stroke and should precede any time-consuming search for the cause. Mortality increases significantly when cooling is delayed.

10. **D,** Pages 997-998.

Heat loss into a cool liquid occurs 20-30 times more rapidly via conduction than in air. Therefore, if the patient is stable enough, immersion is the modality of choice. If highly unstable (intubated), evaporative cooling using large circulating fans and skin wetting may be the best choice. In most instances this method is the easier to accomplish. The other modalities may be used as adjuncts.

11. **B,** Pages 998-999.

Malignant arrhythmias are not a common feature of heat stroke. Chlorpromazine is used only if cooling is not adequate because of vigorous shivering. Seizures may be treated with diazepam or phenobarbital. Myoglobinuria can be treated with mannitol. The urine can be alkalinized with bicarbonate as well. If hypokalemia is present, the potassium deficits must be replaced cautiously.

12. **E,** Page 999.

Through alkalization and diuresis, mannitol and bicarbonate are useful adjuncts to prevent the development of acute renal failure secondary to rhabdomyolysis. See Rosen Box 56-7.

# 57 Chemical Injuries

*Warren F. Lanphear*

1. **B,** Page 1003.

Although some chemicals produce considerable heat as the result of an exothermic reaction when they come in contact with water, their ability to produce direct chemical changes in the skin accounts for the most significant injury. After skin contact, the absorption of some agents may cause toxicity.

2. **A,** Page 1004.

Ideally, the patient should be thoroughly decontaminated *before* arrival in the emergency department. The command post for a large incident should be established away from the exposure site. The hazardous material needs to be identified before initiation of the site plan. Dry chemicals are removed from victims by being brushed off, then copious water irrigation is delivered under low pressures.

3. **B,** Page 1004.

Because contact time is a critical determinant of the severity of injury, hydrotherapy of skin exposed to a toxic chemical must be initiated immediately by the victim or witness to the injury. When clothes are soaked with such agents, valuable time is lost if clothing is removed before copious washing is commenced. Gentle irrigation with a large volume of water under low pressure is recommended.

4. **C,** Pages 1004-1008.

Elemental metals (sodium and potassium) are harmless unless activated by water, which causes a highly exothermic reaction and tremendous heat production. The result is significant chemical and thermal burns. Copious water irrigation is recommended for acids, alkalis, phosphorous, and hydrofluoric acid.

5. **E,** Page 1005.

Acid (not alkali) is rapidly neutralized and typically causes only epithelial and basement membrane damage. Acid burns of the periphery often heal uneventfully. Acid burns of the central cornea may lead to corneal ulcers, neovascularization, and scarring. Alkali can destroy the anterior segment, leading to perforation, endophthalmitis, and eye loss.

6. **A,** Page 1006.

Infiltrative therapy with calcium gluconate is necessary to adequately treat deep and painful hydrofluoric acid burns. Immediate irrigation for hydrofluoric acid skin exposure is done with copious amounts of water. Intraarterial infusion of calcium gluconate is effective and has less disadvantages than infiltration. All blisters should first be removed because necrotic tissue may potentially harbor fluoride ions. Topical gel is effective only for mild, superficial burns.

7. **E,** Pages 1007-1008.

White phosphorous ignites spontaneously in air at temperatures greater than 34° C. Tissue injury appears to be caused primarily by heat production. Exposures are treated with immersion in cool water, then washing with 5% sodium bicarbonate and 3% copper sulfate. The elemental metals potassium, sodium, and lithium are activated by water.

8. **D,** Page 1007.

A quick swipe of the skin with PEG 300 or 400 reduces burn severity. The exposed area should be irrigated with large volumes of water delivered under low pressures until PEG is available. Gentle swabbing of exposed skin with water-soaked sponges causes more rapid absorption because of dilution. Resorcinol is a phenol derivative and it is not indicated for treatment in these cases.

**Electrical and Lightning Injuries**

*Scott A. Carlson*

1. **B,** Pages 1011-1012.
Nerves are designed to carry electrical impulses, while muscle and blood have a high electrolyte and water content making them good conductors. Bone, tendon, and fat, which contain a lot of inert matrix, tend to heat up and coagulate, rather than transmit current.

2. **B,** Pages 1011-1012.
At 1-4 mA, a tingling sensation is felt. The let-go current is 4 mA in children and from 6-9 mA in adults. At 10-21 mA, freezing to the circuit occurs. Respiratory arrest from thoracic muscle tetany occurs at 20-50 mA, and ventricular fibrillation occurs at 50-100 mA.

3. **B,** Pages 1011-1012.
Moisture, increased vascularity, skin breakdown from prolonged contact, and blistering all decrease skin's resistance, thus potentially allowing more current to enter the body. Areas of skin thickening, like callousing, have increased resistance.

4. **C,** Page 1013.
In addition to falls, blunt injury can be caused by violent muscle spasms associated with AC injuries. Signs of neural damage may develop immediately or may be delayed by hours to days. An arc burn can cause deep thermal burns at the point at which it contacts the skin. Furthermore, the arc may also ignite clothing and cause secondary burns, thereby making it difficult to determine the exact mechanism of the patient's burns. Small vessel intimal damage can result in delayed thrombosis and "progressive" tissue necrosis. Muscle damage can be spotty, with periosteal muscle damage occurring with normal-appearing overlying muscle.

5. **D,** Pages 1013-1014.
There are five mechanisms of lightning injury. Side splash is described, and direct strike is obvious. Contact results from the individual's touching an object that is directly struck. Step voltage occurs as current spreads radially through the ground, potentially into a victim's legs. Blunt trauma can occur either from the victim's being thrown or from a massive explosive/implosive force (rapid superheating of body tissues with air expansion followed quickly by reversal).

6. **E,** Pages 1015-1016.
Cataracts develop in about 6% of cases of high-voltage injuries. Blunt abdominal injuries are rare in lightning injuries. Shoulder dislocations have been reported but do not seem to be as common as most texts would stress. The most common areas of ground are the heels. Tympanic membrane rupture is commonly found in lightning victims and may be secondary to the shock waves, direct burn, or basilar skull fracture.

7. **C,** Page 1015.
Oral commissure injuries often involve children under the age of 4 years sucking on electrical extension cords that carry household current. They may involve the orbicularis oris muscle, damage developing dentition, and cause significant cosmetic deformity. "Kissing burns" are arc burns seen at moist flexor creases.

8. **E,** Page 1014.
Unlike most mass casualty triage situations, in lightning injuries priority of care should be given to those that appear to be in arrest. Initial arrest is from the lightning acting as a massive DC countershock, causing asystole. Intrinsic cardiac automaticity can restart the heart, but secondary hypoxic arrest from CNS injury can be avoided with oxygenation and ventilation. The safest approach to high-voltage incidents is to have the local power company turn the power source off. EMS groups have condemned the use of insulated electrical gloves. Victims of electrical incidents may have sustained significant blunt trauma and injury; therefore they should be approached like any other trauma victim (i.e., evaluation and possible immobilization before ambulation).

9. **B,** Pages 1015-1018.
Acute myocardial infarction appears to be rare. An elevated CK level by itself is not indicative of myocardial damage in the presence of an electrical injury because of the large amount of skeletal myonecrosis that may result. Furthermore, skeletal muscle damaged by electrical current may produce an inordinate rise in the CK-MB fraction. The other statements are accurate.

10. **E,** Pages 1018-1019.
The use of burn formulas to calculate fluid requirements in electrical injuries is unreliable because of the large amount of tissue damage that may exist under normal skin. A urine output of at least 0.5 to 1.0 ml/kg/hr in the absence of heme pigment is a good clinical indicator of adequate tissue perfusion.

11. **A,** Pages 1016-1019.
Feathering burns are not true burns and show no damage to the skin itself. Most lightning victims do not sustain the deep-tissue damage seen with electrical injuries, and rhabdomyolysis is rare. Fluid restriction is often advisable to avoid cerebral or pulmonary edema. Peripheral nerve damage is common, and recovery is usually poor. Most victims behave as though they have had electroconvulsive therapy and are confused with antegrade amnesia for several days. If further neurologic deterioration occurs, a CT is indicated. Poorly colored extremities usually return to normal quickly as vasospasm resolves.

12. **C,** Pages 1016-1018.
The most common cause of renal injury following electrical injury is from the massive amount of myoglobulin that may be released from destruction of skeletal muscle. The damage can be reduced or prevented by alkalinization of the urine, aggressive rehydration, and osmotic diuresis. Urine output should be maintained at 1.0-1.5 ml/kg/hr.

13. **E,** Page 1020.
An obstetric consultation should be obtained for all patients in their second or third trimester because of the increased risk of stillbirth. Electronic fetal monitoring should be performed and the patient followed as a high-risk patient for the remainder of her pregnancy. Patients in the first trimester may have an increased risk of spontaneous abortions and may be discharged with close obstetric follow-up if no other indications for admission exist.

# 59 ▼ Diving Injuries

*Dale E. McNinch*

1. **D,** Page 1022.
DAN is a membership association with a mission to enhance diving safety, avoid injury, and provide assistance when injury occurs. DAN provides a 24-hour medical emergency hotline (919-684-8111) and training courses for physicians and nonphysicians.

2. **D,** Page 1023.
Middle ear barotrauma, also known as barotitis or "ear squeeze," is the most common complaint of scuba divers. It occurs when a negative differential pressure is created within the middle ear because the diver could not equilibrate to ambient pressure. The others are not as common but do occur.

3. **C,** Page 1023.
Water is more dense than air. Each foot of sea water exerts an additional pressure of 23 mm Hg or 0.445 psi on the diver.

4. **B,** Pages 1023-1024.
If equilibration of the middle ear pressure does not occur at a depth of only 4 feet, a 90 mm Hg pressure differential exists and the eustachian tube collapses shut, making further attempts at equilibration futile. Tympanic membrane rupture occurs when the pressure differential is between 100 and 500 mm Hg corresponding to a depth of 4.3 to 17 feet.

5. **A,** Pages 1024-1025.
Prophylactic use of pseudoephedrine, 60 mg, 30 minutes before diving may reduce the incidence and severity of middle ear barotrauma in healthy divers, but use of this or nasal decongestants or antihistamines to facilitate diving with a URI is not recommended. Diving should be avoided for 2 weeks after resolution of a URI. URI increases the likelihood of suffering barotitis because it causes edema and obstruction of the eustachian tubes.

6. **A,** Page 1027.
Because of its high lipid content, the CNS is particularly susceptible to DCS. The spinal cord, particularly the upper lumbar area, is more often involved than cerebral tissue. Limb weakness, paralysis, paresthesias, numbness, and back pain are common complaints. Bladder symptoms, fecal incontinence, and priapism may occur. Spinal DCS can occur alone or in combination with cerebral, inner ear, or pulmonary symptoms.

7. **B,** Pages 1027, 1029.
The slow release of nitrogen that has been dissolved in tissues during the dive ("off-gassing") continues after the diver has surfaced. It takes 12 hours at the surface for nitrogen stores to return to normal sea level values. Repetitive dives within several hours result in increased accumulation of nitrogen in tissues, and thus longer time is needed to return to normal.

8. **D,** Page 1028.
Recompression is the only definitive treatment for DCS and AGE; no drugs can be given prophylactically to prevent or lessen symptoms. Cardiac arrhythmias may be refractory to standard treatments until after recompression. If air transport to a hyperbaric chamber is required, cabin pressure must be maintained at 1000 feet (most commercial aircraft typically pressurize to 5000 to 8000 feet). Most of these aircraft are capable of near-sea-level cabin pressures if flying no higher than 20,000 to 25,000 feet. Intravenous fluid administration should ensure a urine output of 2 ml/kg/hr to facilitate tissue perfusion and washout of inert gases.

9. **E,** Page 1028.
Almost all cases of AGE present within the first 10 minutes of surfacing, whereas DCS presents more typically after 10 minutes, and up to 24 hours, after surfacing. AGE is precipitated by rapid ascent ("out of air") and has life-threatening complications. DCS is precipitated by fatigue, dehydration, obesity, overexertion, or hypothermia, and has milder, more vague neurologic symptoms.

10. **D,** Page 1028.
Panic or inexperience ("out of air") increases the likelihood of rapid, uncontrolled ascent, which may precipitate AGE. Dehydration, fatigue (overexertion), cold ambient water (hypothermia), fever, diving at high altitude (flying after diving), patent foramen ovale, obesity, and tobacco or alcohol use increase susceptibility to DCS.

11. **A,** Pages 1028, 1030.
This patient has decompression sickness. The only definitive treatment for DCS or AGE is treatment in a hyperbaric chamber.

12. **B,** Page 1029.
The safe interval recommendations between diving and flying range from 2 to 48 hours. Most authorities recommend that flying be delayed for at least 12 hours after diving if less than 2 hours of total dive time was accumulated in the preceding 48 hours (for longer total dive time, delay should be 24 hours).

13. **A,** Page 1029.
Drowning is the most common cause of death in sports divers. AGE accounts for approximately 30% of diving-related deaths.

# 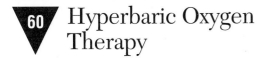 Hyperbaric Oxygen Therapy

*Warren F. Lanphear*

1. **E,** Page 1034.
A pneumothorax may progress to a tension pneumothorax, particularly during decompression. HBO therapy is relatively contraindicated in COPD and otitis media. COPD with air trapping, especially bullae, increases the risk of barotrauma which can be prevented by maximal bronchodilator therapy and slow ascent. Otitis media may cause inability to equalize pressure in the ears but may be pretreated with a decongestant. HBO therapy is not detrimental to the fetus when performed appropriately. Oxygen-induced seizures are unpredictable and rare. They have no known permanent neurologic sequelae and do not contraindicate continuation of therapy.

2. **B,** Pages 1034-1035.
Middle ear barotrauma or "ear squeeze" is the most common side effect caused by inadequate equalization of pressure in the middle ear. Claustrophobia has an incidence of approximately 1 in 2000 patients. The incidence of oxygen-mediated seizures from HBO therapy is about 1 in 10,000 patients treated at 2.4 ATA. Sinus "squeeze" or barotrauma is the second most common complication. Changes in refraction caused by a progressive myopia are reported only in some patients undergoing daily HBO therapy multiple times.

3. **A,** Pages 1034, 1036.
In CO poisoning during pregnancy, the fetus is more susceptible to the toxic effects of CO than the mother is. Fetal CO levels at equilibrium are higher and elimination time is longer than for maternal CO levels. The fetal oxyhemoglobin dissociation curve is shifted to the left and the fetal $Po_2$ is normally low; thus a small decrease in maternal and fetal oxygen tension and a relatively low level of fetal carboxyhemoglobin can result in significant fetal tissue hypoxia or anoxia. HBO treatment should be used more liberally in the pregnant patient because of enhanced fetal vulnerability to CO and hypoxia.

4. **B,** Page 1036.
HBO therapy for CO poisoning is 2.4-3 ATA for 60-90 minutes. 1.5-2.0 ATA for 60-75 minutes is too little pressure for too short a duration. Retreatment is controversial but is used if symptoms persist after treatment. Multiplace chambers are compressed with air, and the oxygen is delivered by face mask or a head tent. Most chambers in the United States are monoplace, which are usually compressed with 100% oxygen. Oxygen therapy is not recommended after HBO therapy.

5. **D,** Pages 1036-1037, 2678.
HBO therapy at oxygen tensions of 250 mm Hg will inhibit alpha toxin production. HBO has a bacteriostatic effect on clostridia; it does not kill them. HBO improves polymorphonuclear leukocyte function. The combined approach of aggressive surgical debridement, antibiotics, and HBO ther-

apy has been well studied and is recommended. Late presentations have very high mortality regardless of any therapy. HBO therapy may be effective very early in this disease.

6. **C,** Pages 1033, 1038.
Although it is still investigational, it is believed that HBO therapy can affect the anaerobic flora and potentially reduce edema in cases of perifocal brain swelling or elevated intracranial pressure. All others are approved for HBO by the Undersea and Hyperbaric Medical Society (UHMS). A full listing is provided in Rosen Box 60-1.

#  High-Altitude Illness

*Dale E. McNinch*

1. **D,** Page 1043.
High-altitude illness depends on many variables, including the rate of ascent, final altitude reached, and duration of stay at the altitude. Young age may be a factor slightly favoring the development of AMS, but gender does not affect the incidence of AMS.

2. **B,** Page 1045.
With arrival at high altitude, the peripheral chemosensors in the carotid bodies respond to a decrease in a $PaO_2$ and signal the respiratory control center in the medulla to increase ventilation. This is known as the hypoxic ventilatory response (HVR) and may be inhibited or stimulated by alcohol, sleep medications, caffeine, cocoa, prochlorperazine, and progesterone. Respiratory alkalosis occurs and the kidneys begin to excrete bicarbonate to compensate; as the pH normalizes, ventilation rises slowly, maximizing after 6 to 8 days. The ability to achieve an adequate HVR varies among individuals and is closely related to the ability to acclimatize.

3. **C,** Pages 1045-1046.
Hypoxia is a potent pulmonary vasoconstrictor but causes vasodilation in the cerebral circulation. Hypoxemia results in an increase in 2-3 DPG, causing a rightward shift of the oxyhemoglobin dissociation curve that favors release of oxygen from the blood to the tissues. With early exposure to hypoxic conditions there is an increase in hemoglobin concentration of up to 15% principally caused by a fluid shift into the extravascular space. Longer term acclimatization leads to an erythropoietin-induced production of red blood cells. Red blood cell mass increases in proportion to the degree of hypoxemia. Within 24 to 48 hours of ascent the kidneys begin to excrete bicarbonate in an effort to compensate for the respiratory alkalosis.

4. **E,** Pages 1045, 1049-1050.
Acclimatization may be enhanced by allowing for gradual ascent (sometimes over several weeks). Medications and foods such as sleep aids, alcohol, antihistamines, caffeine, cocoa, and a low-carbohydrate diet may hinder acclimatization. Slowly ascending (less than 1000 feet per day when above 10,000 feet), and sleeping at an altitude lower than the maximal elevation achieved for the day will aid in adaptation.

**5. E,** Page 1049.

An isolated mild bitemporal headache occurring at over 8000 feet of elevation probably represents acute mountain sickness. Further ascent to a higher sleeping altitude is contraindicated. If the symptoms do not progress or worsen, the affected hiker may remain at this elevation, but exercise should be avoided. Further treatment is not necessarily indicated at this point. Aspirin and acetaminophen are useful for the treatment of headache, but narcotic analgesics should be avoided because they may depress the HVR and the respiratory drive during sleep.

**6. A,** Page 1049.

Acute mountain sickness may be manifested by a bitemporal throbbing headache, nausea with or without vomiting, general fatigue, increased dyspnea on exertion, periodic breathing, and decreased urine output. The presence on examination of ataxia or confusion, crackles, dyspnea at rest, or cyanosis indicates a more serious condition and mandates immediate descent.

**7. C,** Page 1049.

AMS-associated headache may be treated with aspirin or acetaminophen. All symptoms of AMS may be addressed with the administration of supplemental oxygen. AMS may respond to acetazolamide, which is a carbonic anhydrase inhibitor, resulting in a renal bicarbonate diuresis. The resulting metabolic acidosis increases ventilatory rate and arterial oxygenation. The diuretic effects may be of benefit for the fluid retention common in AMS. Prochlorperazine, unlike other emetics, may stimulate the HVR and can be effective in the treatment of nausea and vomiting. The use of benzodiazepines and other sedative hypnotics should be avoided because of their tendency to decrease ventilation during sleep. Dexamethasone may reduce symptoms secondary to its euphoric effects.

**8. D,** Page 1049.

Acetazolamide is a carbonic anhydrase inhibitor and a sulfa drug. In addition to options A, B, C, and E, less common adverse reactions are transient myopia, crystalluria, and renal calculus.

**9. A,** Pages 1050, 1053.

HAPE and HACE typically develop days (usually 1 to 4 days) after arrival at high altitude. AMS often develops within hours after arrival at altitude. The other answers are typical of both HAPE and HACE.

**10. A,** Pages 1051, 1052.

Dyspnea at rest is a serious symptom and must be considered to be an indication of high altitude pulmonary edema (HAPE). The patient may have an associated cough productive of clear, watery, or blood-tinged sputum. Chest x-ray will reveal fluffy alveolar and patchy infiltrates, but since HAPE is noncardiogenic, cardiomegaly and Kerley B lines will not be seen. The ECG may reveal tachycardia and rarely will show right heart strain. It is unlikely, however, that a previously healthy 40-year-old skier will show ischemic ECG changes. Mild pulmonary edema can be treated at altitude with 1 or 2 days of bed rest. However, if the dyspnea progresses and the patient's condition deteriorates, immediate

descent is mandated. Descents of 1500 to 3000 feet should be adequate.

**11. E,** Pages 1053-1054.

High-altitude cerebral edema (HACE) may be manifested by severe headache, ataxia, altered mentation, confusion, stupor, seizures, and coma. The only treatment of proven value for HACE is descent. Other therapies, including steroids, intubation, and diuretics, are of secondary importance.

**12. E,** Page 1054.

High-altitude retinal hemorrhages are commonly seen at elevations above 17,000 feet. Because generally no symptoms are associated with these hemorrhages, they are noted only if retinoscopy is performed. Generally, they are benign and self-limited unless the macular region is involved, in which case return to high altitude would be contraindicated. High-altitude retinal hemorrhages are not generally related to the presence of mild AMS but do seem to be related to strenuous exercise at high altitudes.

**13. A,** Page 1056.

Patients with sickle cell disease are affected by the hypoxemia occurring at low to moderate altitude (5000 to 7000 feet). Patients at higher elevations are at risk for vasoocclusive crisis, particularly splenic ischemic or infarction. This patient should be advised not to consider an ascent of such magnitude.

 **62** ▼ Near-Drowning

*Michael D. Brown*

**1. E,** Page 1061.

Secondary drowning refers to death occurring from a complication minutes to days following a near-drowning. Drowning refers to death from suffocation by submersion in a liquid, usually water. Immersion syndrome is sudden death after submersion in very cold water, probably resulting from dysrhythmias induced by vagal stimulation.

**2. C,** Page 1062.

Lysis of red cells may occur from the effects of hypotonic fresh water. Pulmonary edema may occur with salt water secondary to the created osmotic gradient across the alveolar membrane. Serum electrolytes are not often significantly altered with either fresh or salt water since most victims do not aspirate a large amount of fluid. Pulmonary injury can occur though with little as 2 mg/kg of fluid. Injury to pulmonary surfactant may result in hypoxia, infection, pulmonary edema, and ARDS.

**3. A,** Pages 1063, 1064.

Initial evaluation at the scene involves assessment of airway, breathing, and circulation. Treatment of hypoxia is next, followed by protection of the cervical spine. Procedures to drain fluid from the lungs are not effective and are potentially dangerous. Wet clothing should be removed after the initial priorities are addressed.

4. **E,** Pages 1063-1064.

Shock is uncommon, but when it is present, a determination should be made as to whether it is related to hypoxia, spinal cord injury, or hypovolemia.

5. **A,** Page 1065.

Caution is advised in discharging near-drowning victims. The absence of radiographic abnormalities does not necessarily indicate normal pulmonary status. Asymptomatic near-drowning patients who have a normal physical examination, chest x-ray, and ABG can be discharged from the ED after 4 hours of observation. Attempts to drain fluid from the lungs are useless and potentially dangerous. Prophylactic usage of antibiotics or steroids is generally not indicated.

6. **E,** Pages 1064-1065.

Prophylactic antibiotics have not been shown to improve survival and should be reserved for those with clinical signs of infection. The use of steroids for treatment of pulmonary aspiration is controversial, and several outcome studies do not support their routine use. Chest x-ray and ABGs are done but initial management is providing oxygen. Initial chest x-ray may be normal.

7. **A,** Page 1062.

The mammalian diving reflex is present in infants and children but is diminished in adults. This may account for the higher salvage rates in children. The resulting hypothermia may have both beneficial and disastrous effects. In addition to initiating the diving reflex, hypothermia decreases metabolic demands and prevents or delays severe cerebral hypoxia. Hypothermia may, however, induce ventricular fibrillation and death (immersion syndrome). Successful resuscitation with neurologic recovery following submersion for up to 40 minutes has been reported. It is important to remember that a severe hypothermic state may be indistinguishable from death.

# 63 Radiation Injuries

### Dale J. Ray

1. **B,** Page 1069.

Alpha particles are emitted by elemental decay, as with plutonium or uranium. They have the lowest penetration capabilities of all ionizing particles; it is limited to the thickness of epithelium.

2. **D,** Page 1069.

Neutrons are able to make a stable atom radioactive by being "captured" and thus induce radioactivity in previously non radioactive material.

3. **D,** Page 1070.

A Gray (Gy) is equal to 100 radiation absorbed doses (rad).

4. **C,** Pages 1070, 1073.

The patient is displaying central nervous system effects soon after an exposure. He definitely has received at least 2000 rads or 20 Grays (1 Gy = 100 rads). In a mass casualty situation this person would be placed in the impending or expec-

tant death category and further resuscitation measures withheld.

5. **D,** Pages 1070, 1073.

The median lethal dose ($LD_{50}$) is estimated to be between 3 and 5 Gy (300-500 rads). In mass casualty situations where intensive care resources are limited, the $LD_{50}$ is in the range of 3.5 Gy; in other situations, it is probably 4.5 Gy.

6. **D,** Page 1070.

Those systems with the most rapid cellular division will be most affected. Death is usually caused by infection secondary to leukopenia.

7. **E,** Page 1071.

Significant ongoing radiation exposure is possible if skin and clothing are not fully decontaminated. This is a potential risk not only to the patient but to ED personnel as well.

8. **A,** Pages 1070, 1073.

The most accurate early prognostic indictor is the absolute lymphocyte count 48 hours after exposure. If it is greater than 1200, the chances of a lethal exposure are small. With massive exposures the peripheral granulocyte count may be more accurate. However, the nadir of the granulocyte count does not occur until 8 to 30 days after exposure.

# 64 The Pediatric Patient: General Approach And Unique Concerns

### Sandra K. Dettmann and Gwen L. Hoffman

1. **A,** Page 1076.

All vital signs, except for temperature, change with age. The resilience of a child's chest wall results in a lower occurrence of rib fractures, sternal fractures, and flail chests. In a 1-month-old infant, meningitis is more likely to be caused by group B streptococci or *Escherichia coli* than *Haemophilus influenzae*. Most pediatric cardiac arrests are the result of respiratory failure. A child's diaphragm is oriented in a more horizontal plane than an adult's, which causes the liver and spleen to be more anterior and caudal and at greater risk of injury.

2. **D,** Page 1077.

SCIWORA is a cervical spinal cord injury without radiographic abnormality. The pediatric spine is more elastic, so momentary intersegmental displacements may endanger the spinal cord without disrupting bone or ligaments. Transient paresthesias, clumsiness, tingling, or "total body paralysis" after flexion, extension, distraction, or compression forces put children at risk for SCIWORA. A neurosurgical consultation should be obtained despite normal x-rays and neurologic examination.

3. **B,** Page 1079.

Incomplete ossification makes interpretation of alignment difficult and can mimic fracture lines. Increased preodontoid spaces can be seen in 20% of normal children. Widened prevertebral spaces can be caused by neck positioning, increased retropharyngeal lymph nodes, crying, and expiration. Pseudosubluxation of C2 on C3 (3 mm) can be seen in 40% of children less than 7 years old. Flatter and more horizontal facet joints can be seen and can be a factor when evaluating for SCIWORA.

4. **E,** Page 1079.

Frequencies are trauma, 55%; CNS, 17%; metabolic/toxicologic, 10%; cardiorespiratory, 9%; medical arrest, 1%; and other, 8%.

5. **C,** Page 1081.

A, B, D, and E signify moderate impairment. Severe impairment would be cyanotic, mottled or ashen color, no smile, inconsolable, and weak, moaning, or high-pitched cry. Factors evaluated are quality of cry, reaction to parent stimulation, state variation, color, hydration, and response to social overtures. See Rosen Table 64-3.

6. **E,** Page 1082.

Parental consent is not needed in an emergency, and care should not be delayed because of consent issues. As time permits, efforts to obtain parental consent over the telephone should be made and documented. Most states have case law or legislation allowing physicians to render care without parental consent in cases in which "prompt" treatment it required.

7. **B,** Page 1082.

All states allow minors to consent to diagnosis and treatment of sexually transmitted diseases and drug abuse without parental consent. In such cases, billing should be done in such a way as to protect the minor's confidentiality.

8. **E,** Page 1084.

A 2 month old holds head in midline, lifts chest off table, no longer clenches fists tightly, smiles socially, and recognizes parents. A 3 month old supports self on forearms, holds head up steadily, holds hands at rest, coos, and reaches for familiar people or objects. A 4 month old rolls front to back, reaches with arms in unison, laughs, and enjoys looking around the environment. A 5 month old rolls back to front, sits supported, transfers objects, and says "ah-goo."

# 65   Fever in Children

*Sandra K. Dettmann*

1. **D,** Pages 1088-1089.

Children 24 to 36 months of age are less likely than those under 24 months of age to be bacteremic. Children under 36 months of age with a rectal temperature of 39° C and no obvious source of fever have an incidence of bacteremia of 3% to 5%. Each degree of temperature elevation above 39° C increases the risk of bacteremia. The most common pathogen is *Streptococcus pneumoniae,* accounting for more than 85% of the positive cultures. The presence or absence of a drop in temperature after administration of acetaminophen does not influence the risk of bacteremia. With pneumococcal bacteremia, most children become afebrile in 3 to 4 days with or without antibiotic coverage; however, in the cases of *H. influenzae* and *N. meningitidis,* complications such as persistent bacteremia, pneumonia, meningitis, and sepsis commonly occur.

2. **C,** Page 1089.

Febrile seizures affect approximately 2% to 5% of all children. The greatest risk for meningitis is in patients younger than 18 months of age. The peak incidence of seizure is between 8 and 20 months, and it usually occurs during the upslope of the fever curve. Brief, generalized seizure in a 12 to 18 month old who is playful and nontoxic after the postictal period can be treated without lumbar puncture.

3. **E,** Pages 1098-1099.

Kawasaki syndrome is a vasculitis that causes a prolonged fever (more than 5 days), which usually exceeds 39.5° C to 40° C. Major diagnostic criteria are fever in addition to at least four of the following:

• Changes in extremities, including edema, erythema, desquamation

  • Polymorphous exanthem

  • Bilateral conjunctival injection

  • Changes in the lips and oral cavity including an injected pharynx, cracked lips, and strawberry tongue

  • Cervical lymphadenopathy with nodes greater than 1.5 cm in diameter, usually unilateral.

   Treatment consists of gamma globulin and aspirin.

4. **D,** Page 1091.

In addition to its being the most accurate method of temperature determination, rectal temperature is the basis for most algorithms for risk of serious illness. The tympanic and axillary methods can yield a falsely low temperature. In older children and adolescents the temperature may be taken by the oral route if the patient has not recently been eating, drinking, or smoking; these factors as well as hyperventilating can falsely raise or lower the oral temperature. Forehead strips are unreliable in a sick child.

5. **B,** Page 1094.

After 4 weeks of age, ampicillin and cefotaxime are the drugs of choice, because they cover both the neonatal and the community-acquired pathogens. Ampicillin is needed in addition to a cephalosporin until at least 6 to 12 weeks of age to treat for *Listeria monocytogenes* and enterococci. Empiric treatment for the infant under four weeks of age traditionally consists of ampicillin plus an aminoglycoside. This combination provides excellent coverage for the typical pathogens in neonates (group B streptococci, *E. coli, L. monocytogenes,* and enterococci). The combination of ampicillin and a third-generation cephalosporin is also acceptable. Advantages to using a cephalosporin rather than an aminoglycoside include no need for time-consuming, and expensive aminoglycoside levels; little or no associated otic or nephrotoxicity; excellent penetration into the meninges; and superior coverage against *H. influenzae.*

6. **E,** Page 1095.

When the fever source is known and the child does not appear toxic, oral antibiotics alone are sufficient in the 3 to 24 month old. If no source is found and the temperature is below 39° C, fever instructions with follow-up the next day are appropriate.

7. **B,** Page 1095.

If the temperature is 39° C or greater, a CBC should be obtained. If the WBC is less than 15,000/mm³, the patient should be discharged with fever instructions and next-day follow-up. If the WBC is 15,000 mm³ or greater, a blood culture should be obtained and the patient treated with a single dose of ceftriaxone, 50 mg/kg IV or IM. For patients receiving antibiotics, a blood culture and a urinalysis and urine culture by bladder catheterization should be obtained before the first dose. The urinalysis and culture may be omitted if the patient is a boy older than 6 months of age or a girl older than 2 years of age. Urinalysis and culture should also be obtained if the fever has persisted for 3 days or the temperature is 40° C or greater. Next-day follow-up is needed.

8. **D,** Page 1096.

Central and peripheral blood cultures should be obtained. Chest films, urine evaluation, and lumbar puncture may also be indicated. Neutropenic patients should not have the temperature taken rectally. They also need IV antibiotics as soon as the blood cultures are obtained. Flushing of the Broviac should be avoided until well after initial antibiotics have been given via a peripheral IV and after consultation with the child's oncologist.

9. **A,** Page 1097.

When the possibility of osteomyelitis is present, coverage must include *Salmonella.* Ceftriaxone, a third-generation cephalosporin, will provide this whereas the others do not.

10. **D,** Pages 1097-1098.

Patients with ventriculoperitoneal shunts and fever must be evaluated for shunt infection. Especially in cases in which the patient displays headache, stiff neck, vomiting, or irritability, the shunt reservoir should be aspirated under sterile conditions and the fluid examined for pleocytosis and bacteria. The most common bacterial pathogen is *Staphylococcus epidermidis.* A CT scan of the head is also warranted.

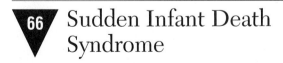

## 66 ▼ Sudden Infant Death Syndrome

*Scott A. Carlson*

1. **D,** Pages 1101-1102.

Maternal cigarette smoking and mother's age less than 20 years at first pregnancy are factors with the highest relative risk. The other options do not increase the risk.

2. **A,** Page 1101.

SIDS rarely occurs in children younger than 1 month (1%) or older than 12 months (2%). Peak occurrence is between 2 and 4 months, with 88% younger than 5½ months of age.

3. **C,** Page 1102.

Educating parents to place their children to sleep on the back or side has led to a 50% decline in the incidence of SIDS in several countries. Avoidance of the other factors may be important but have yet to be proved.

4. **A,** Page 1103.

An infant in the appropriate age-group for SIDS (as this one) with an ALTE should be admitted for evaluation.

5. **B,** Page 1104.

Theophylline also reduces periodic breathing in infants at risk for SIDS, but its usefulness in preventing SIDS has not been established. Theophylline normalizes a pneumogram in 94% of users and improves the pneumogram in 100%. It acts as a respiratory stimulant. Therapeutic levels of 10-15 µg/ml are effective.

6. **D,** Pages 1104-1105.

The NIH Consensus Development Conference on Infantile Apnea and Home Monitoring has identified the following groups that may benefit from home monitors: symptomatic premature infants with continued apnea, infants with tracheostomies or severe BPD, and infants with a history of ALTE who required vigorous stimulations.

7. **D,** Page 1105.

Providing an explanation for the cause of death and allowing the family to vocalize their feelings are among several interventions that have been found useful. The words "dead" and "died" should be used to avoid confusion, and the message should not be delayed with explanations of the details of the resuscitation. Emotional responses are extremely varied and may include being detached or unemotional.

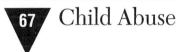

## 67 ▼ Child Abuse

*Sandra K. Dettmann*

1. **A,** Pages 1108-1111.

Subdural hematomas are common with shaken baby syndrome, with an incidence of 38%-100%, with 80% being bilateral. Homicide is the leading cause of death in infants from 6 to 12 months of age. Failure to thrive is partially or totally caused by neglect in more than 50% of cases, particularly in those with impaired weight gain only. The younger the child, the higher the potential is for abuse. The age distribution can be broken down into thirds: One third of cases occurs before 6 months of age, one third in children from 6 months to 3 years of age, and one third in those older than 3 years of age. Up to 50% of fractures in children less than 1 year old are caused by abuse.

2. **C,** Pages 1108-1109.

The families of abuse are often socially isolated, have inadequate support systems, and find it difficult to reach out and ask for help. Although poisoning accounts for only a small number of abuse cases, it carries a high mortality rate of 17%. Ninety-five percent of abuse cases involve the parents. Women are more often involved than men because the mother is usually the primary caretaker. Most abused children are younger than 4 years of age. This is probably because of the large discrepancy between the young child's limited developmental capacity and the parent's mistaken expectation and perception of what it should be. Infants, usually those less than 15 months of age, may be violently shaken by a frustrated parent.

3. **B,** Pages 1109-1110.

The caretaker in Polle's syndrome can have a hysterical personality disorder and often has previous medical experience or education. He or she does not seem as concerned about the child's illness as is the medical staff, and is overly attentive with prolonged visiting or living in with the child in the hospital. Another characteristic is a caretaker who has had symptoms similar to the victim's within the last 5 years.

4. **C,** Page 1113.

Common sites for inflicted bruises include buttocks and lower back from beatings; genitals and lower thighs from toilet training or sexual abuse; cheeks from slapping; earlobes from pinching; neck from choking; and upper lip, frenulum, and floor of mouth from forced feeding. Accidental bruising usually occurs over bony prominences such as the knees, anterior tibia, chin, elbows, and forehead, and tends to produce bruises on only a single body plane.

5. **B,** Pages 1114-1115.

Although epiphyseal, metaphyseal, and periosteal injuries are the most pathognomonic skeletal lesions of abuse, they are not the most common. Diaphyseal transverse and spiral fractures of the long bones are more common, followed by skull fractures. Fewer than 20% of abused children exhibit skeletal injuries. Joint dislocations, other than nursemaid's elbow, require a fair degree of force and are uncommon in small children. Nuclear scanning is now being used as an adjunctive diagnostic technique because it can pick up changes as early as 24 to 48 hours after injury. The radiographic changes in child abuse are subtle, and usually only the healing phase of fractures is recognized.

6. **E,** Page 1115.

Shaken baby syndrome may result in increased intracranial pressure caused by diffuse cerebral edema or subdural hematomas. With increasing intracranial pressure, the infant may be irritable or lethargic or have nuchal rigidity, decreased muscle tone, a full fontanelle, increasing head circumference, focal signs of an intracranial mass, coma, seizures, bradycardia, bradypnea, apnea, or cardiopulmonary arrest. Retinal hemorrhages are present in 50%-80% of these cases and are the most important physical sign of shaken baby syndrome.

7. **A,** Pages 1118-1119.

Gonorrhea is the most commonly encountered infection in sexual abuse, with an incidence of 2.3% to 11.2%. Incest is common and involves a parent or guardian in 46%-75% of cases. Offenders are known to the child or family in 75%-80% of cases. False accusations by a child do occur but are rare, and all accusations must be investigated. Violence is seldom a factor, but coercion and threats are common.

8. **E,** Pages 1120-1121.

Anal dilation in children is abnormal and suspicious and requires further investigation but is not in itself proof of anal abuse because it may also be caused by chronic constipation or other pathologic conditions. Greater variation exists in the appearance of the normal hymen—annulate, septate, cribriform, fimbriated, imperforate. Labial fusion can be caused by chronic trauma and vulvovaginitis and as such is much more common in sexually abused than non-abused children. It may also be caused by congenital failure of separation, dermatitis, and fecal soiling. A vaginal opening of 4 mm, especially in children less than 5 years of age, is suggestive of penetration; others suggest that an opening of greater than 1 mm/year is suggestive. An opening of greater than 8 mm is definitely indicative.

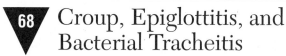

# 68 ▼ Croup, Epiglottitis, and Bacterial Tracheitis

*Jeffrey S. Jones*

1. **C,** Pages 1123-1124.

Croup is most common between 6 months and 3 years. Boys are at a higher risk than girls by 1.73 times. It is most common in fall and winter between the hours of 6 PM and 6 AM, and on days with lower temperatures.

2. **A,** Pages 1124-1125.

In the majority of cases, no certain pathogen is identified, either by blood culture or by throat culture. All of the organisms listed have been recovered, but *H. influenzae* is the most common.

3. **B,** Pages 1125-1127.

Croup is characterized by a barky cough, low-grade fever, and upper respiratory infection symptoms for a couple of days. Spasmodic croup is similar to viral croup (laryngotracheobronchitis) except that attacks tend to be recurrent and occur suddenly without warning or prodrome. They usually improve with exposure to cold outside air or misted saline. Bacterial tracheitis has features of both croup and epiglottitis, which can include URI symptoms for several days, barky cough, and then toxic appearance and high fever. Epiglottitis presents rapidly with high fever, toxic appearance, drooling, severe respiratory distress and a preference for sitting and learning forward. Since the introduction of the *H. influenzae* vaccine, it is now rarely seen.

4. **E,** Page 1126.

In comparison, croup is most commonly seen between 6 months and 3 years.

5. **D,** Page 1127.

The most common complication other than airway obstruction of bacterial tracheitis is pneumonia or pulmonary infiltrates. As in other types of staphylococcal infection, toxic shock has also been reported. Airway obstruction may also occur after intubation because of the thick tracheal secretions. Cervical adenitis, meningitis, and otitis media may all be seen as complications of epiglottitis.

6. **C**, Page 1129.

The possibility of foreign body should be considered in every child who has acute airway symptoms. This is especially true without other symptoms such as fever. Foreign bodies are most common in children younger than age 5. Signs and symptoms may vary from complete obstruction and respiratory arrest to minor stridor or distress. Expiratory stridor generally indicates an obstruction below the carina.

7. **D**, Page 1130.

No attempt should be made to draw blood until a secure airway has been established. The other steps can be done without upsetting the child. The child must be kept as calm as possible while awaiting transport to the operating room for definitive airway management.

8. **E**, Pages 1130-1131.

In bacterial tracheitis fuzziness of the normally sharply defined borders of the tracheal air column is visible on x-ray. Thickened aryepiglottic folds are specific for epiglottitis. The other choices may be seen in croup as well as epiglottitis.

9. **A**, Page 1132.

Croup is viral (usually caused by the parainfluenza virus, especially type 1) and does not require antibiotics. All of the other answers are important aspects of management.

10. **A**, Page 1133.

Often a child can be temporarily ventilated using positive-pressure bag-mask ventilation. If not, orotracheal intubation should be attempted, followed by cricothyrotomy or tracheostomy if necessary. Optimally this should be done in the operating room. Racemic epinephrine can worsen the epiglottitis.

11. **B**, Page 1134.

Steroids and racemic epinephrine have no proven benefit in bacterial tracheitis. Intubation in the operating room or tracheostomy is needed for suctioning of secretions. This must be done quickly and efficiently as with epiglottitis. Intravenous antibiotics should be a penicillinase-resistant penicillin to cover *S. aureus*, the most common pathogen, and will need to be started after an airway is established. Adequate hydration is also important.

 **69** Asthma and Bronchiolitis

*Jeffrey S. Jones*

1. **E**, Page 1138.

Asthma associated with inhaled allergens interacting with airway tissues (atopy) is the second most common cause. The other choices are also common triggers.

2. **E**, Pages 1138-1139.

Use of accessory muscles correlates best with the degree of obstruction and oxygen saturation. Tachycardia occurs with respiratory distress. Agitation may signal hypoxia. Dyspnea can be assessed by asking the patient to count to 10 or to speak a sentence. Wheezing is one of the most unreliable signs in evaluating the degree of distress. Its absence may represent severe obstruction and with improvement of the condition, wheezing may become more prominent.

3. **B**, Page 1144.

It is estimated that 1 mg/kg of IV aminophylline will increase serum theophylline concentration approximately 2 μg/kg.

4. **D**, Pages 1140-1144.

Arterial blood gases are most useful when the ventilatory status is uncertain. Peak expiratory flow is noninvasive and will suffice, unless there is a real concern for $CO_2$ retention or developing respiratory failure. Chest x-ray should not be ordered routinely. It is helpful if pneumothorax, pneumonia, or pneumomediastinum is suspected. In the acute setting, theophylline has not been proven to be helpful. Corticosteroids act by altering various components of the inflammatory response. Because home albuterol administration is not working for this child and he has a borderline pulse oximetry, adding a corticosteroid for a short time should help him. It is best to give it early in the ED because up to 6 hours may pass before improvement is seen.

5. **D**, Pages 1145-1147.

Bronchiolitis is a lower airway disease of infancy, with 11.4% of cases occurring in the first year of life. The principal etiologic agents are respiratory syncytial virus (RSV) and parainfluenza virus. Steroids are not recommended as routine therapy, but supplemental oxygen is routine and bronchodilator therapy may be helpful. Very young infants are at risk for apnea, and hypoxia is common.

6. **D**, Page 1146.

Supplemental oxygen should be routine and is the mainstay of therapy. Most infants with bronchiolitis are hypoxemic. Bronchodilator therapy is controversial. Steroids are not routinely recommended, and theophylline is not beneficial. Because bronchiolitis is secondary to a virus, antibiotics are not helpful. Ribavirin should be used in high-risk infants with proven RSV.

7. **C**, Page 1144.

Ipratropium has been shown to be effective during acute exacerbations when used together with adrenergic nebulizer agents. It does not cause the dry mouth, blurred vision, tachycardia, and urinary retention that are commonly seen with atropine.

8. **E**, Page 1144.

Cromolyn also decreases the migration of eosinophils during the late phase of allergic asthma. It is used in the chronic management of asthma, often in conjunction with beta-agonists.

9. **B**, Page 1144.

Nedocromil inhibits acute and late allergen-induced asthmatic responses. More experience is needed to determine its therapeutic role.

10. **A,** Page 1141.

Terbutaline acts to relax smooth muscle and may decrease mediator release from mast cells and basophils. Albuterol is the most commonly used.

11. **D,** Page 1143.

Theophylline is a methylxanthine with bronchodilator properties but is not as potent as beta-agonists. It may also promote mucociliary clearance and inhibits the late-phase inflammatory response of asthma.

# 70 Pneumonia

### Gwen L. Hoffman

1. **E,** Pages 1150-1152.

The other choices are seen but are not as common. Since the introduction of HIB immunization, the evidence of *H. influenzae* type B disease has decreased by 90%.

2. **D,** Page 1151.

The other choices may all be present, but tachypnea is the best (and may be the only) indicator present. Auscultatory findings may be helpful in the older child but are much less consistent in the younger child. Rales, for example, may be masked by poor inspiratory effort or noisy upper airway sounds.

3. **A,** Page 1151.

Dehydration results from decreased intake secondary to malaise and excessive respiratory effort. Fluid loss is also increased because of vomiting, fever, and tachypnea. The other complications can develop as infectious foci secondary to bacteremia.

4. **A,** Page 1154.

All children younger than 6 months of age with presumed pertussis should be observed in the hospital for monitoring and supportive care and should be treated with erythromycin. Disease begins with mild URI symptoms and cough (catarrhal stage). It progresses to severe paroxysms of a staccato cough. This is followed by post-tussive emesis and may be accompanied by the characteristic inspiratory "whoop." Apnea is common in children under 6 months of age, and fever is usually absent. Immunization is only 80% effective in providing immunity after three doses.

5. **C,** Pages 1154-1156.

Bacterial pneumonia is abrupt in onset, with fever, cough, and a toxic appearance. Chlamydia is most often seen in the 4-16 weeks age-group, with nasal congestion and often conjunctivitis, followed by a staccato cough. The infant can be afebrile. Pertussis is usually seen in infants younger than 6 months of age. It consists of a catarrhal stage and paroxysms of a staccato cough, followed by a convalescent stage. Viral pneumonia has a gradual onset often associated with cough, coryza, and low-grade fever. Tachypnea may be the only physical finding.

6. **D,** Page 1155.

Erythromycin is preferred, although tetracycline is an alternative for the child older than 10 years of age. Choices A through C could be used for the treatment of bacterial pneumonia. Clarithromycin may also be an appropriate single agent. It has proven efficacious in adults with fewer gastrointestinal effects than erythromycin.

7. **C,** Page 1156.

With viral pneumonia, no specific antibiotic therapy is warranted. Care should include fever control and ensuring adequate hydration with close follow-up.

8. **B,** Page 1156, Rosen Table 70-1.

Pertussis does not have related conjunctivitis, which is seen in up to 50% of those with chlamydia. The cough in pertussis is staccato but it occurs in paroxysms. Wheezing is more common with RSV. Mycoplasma pneumonia is most common in the 5- to 18-year-old age-group and is characterized by a hacking cough. With bacterial pneumonia there is usually a high fever, productive cough, and confined rales.

# 71 Cardiac Disorders

### Gwen L. Hoffman

1. **D,** Pages 1162, 1165-1166.

Still's murmur, a short ejection systolic murmur, is the most common of all innocent murmurs. Innocent flow murmurs are (1) located in early systole, (2) of short duration, (3) of low intensity (grade 1 or 2), (4) well localized and nonradiating, and (5) not associated with other cardiovascular abnormalities.

2. **E,** Page 1163.

Increased pulmonary vasculature may be seen in cases of pulmonary artery hypertension, which may be the result of high flow from a left-to-right shunt as with ventricular septal defect. The other conditions have either decreased or normal pulmonary flow.

3. **A,** Page 1164.

The hyperoxia test is a clinically useful bedside test. If the PaO$_2$ does not exceed 100 mm Hg after breathing 100% oxygen for at least 10 minutes, a significant right-to-left shunt is present. When alveolar hypoventilation is the cause of cyanosis, the PaO$_2$ usually rises above 150 mm Hg. Diaphragmatic hernia, as well as the other options, can result in this.

4. **D,** Pages 1164-1166.

Central cyanosis occurs when oxygenated and deoxygenated blood mix before arterial circulation. Transposition of the great vessels is the most common cyanotic defect that appears in the first week of life. With surgery, the prognosis is excellent. All of the other answers are acyanotic conditions.

5. **B,** Page 1165.

Cyanosis is the outstanding clinical feature that develops as the ductus arteriosus closes. Exertional dyspnea and hemoptysis are also present. Clubbing of the fingers and toes appears in long-standing cyanosis.

6. **B,** Page 1167.

Jugular venous distention is seldom obvious, and more generalized edema involving the eyelids, sacrum, and legs is seen.

Splenomegaly is not a feature of uncomplicated congestive heart failure. Marked tachycardia is present, and a gallop rhythm is often heard. Hepatomegaly is usually present.

7. **B,** Page 1168.

All of the choices are used, but digoxin is the most frequently used preparation and remains the mainstay in medical therapy. Infants can be placed in a semi-reclining position in an infant seat. Sedation with morphine may also be needed, and diuretics can relieve edema and pulmonary congestion. Feeding should be IV fluids only to prevent aspiration. Oximetry is useful to follow oxygenation.

8. **D,** Pages 1168-1172.

Myocarditis affects children of all ages and is the leading cause of end-stage dilated cardiomyopathy. The hallmark presentation is CHF. In children, endocarditis is most often associated with congenital heart disease. Acute rheumatic fever and Kawasaki syndrome have specific diagnostic criteria. (See Rosen Boxes 71-6 and 71-7) Pleuritic or positional chest pain is a common symptom of pericarditis.

9. **D,** Pages 1172-1176.

Supraventricular tachycardia is by far the most common dysrhythmia seen in pediatric patients, but it is most common in infancy. All of the other dysrhythmias are seen but with much less frequency.

10. **B,** Pages 1173-1174.

Vagal manipulation can be attempted in the stable patient by the application of an ice bag to the facial area. Ocular pressure and other Valsalva techniques are useless. Medical management with adenosine or electrical cardioversion may be needed.

11. **E,** Page 1174.

Verapamil should never be given to children younger than 1 year of age because of its association with severe hypotension and sudden death. All the others may be tried. Adenosine is effective in terminating nearly all forms of supraventricular tachycardia, including Wolff-Parkinson-White syndrome.

# 72 Gastrointestinal Disorders

*Sandra K. Dettmann*

1. **A,** Pages 1179-1182.

The neonate with suspected upper GI bleeding should have gastric aspirate or vomitus examined by the Apt test to determine the presence of maternal blood. To perform this test, a specimen is placed on a filter paper, and 1% NaOH is added. Fetal hemoglobin is more resistant to reduction and remains pink or bright red. Adult hemoglobin reduces more readily and turns the specimen yellow or rusty brown. Most often, GI bleeding is painless. Significant pain in the presence of lower GI bleeding suggests an obstructive or vascular occlusive process. For melena to exist, a blood loss >50-100 ml/24 hr is present. Hematochezia is the hallmark of lower GI bleeding; however, massive upper GI bleeding may produce red or maroon stool as a result of the cathartic effect

of fresh blood. Meckel's diverticulum may cause bleeding in a child older than 1 month of age. This occurs in 2% of the population, but only a small percentage of the children become symptomatic.

2. **A,** Pages 1182-1183.

In the school-age child, the most common symptom associated with constipation is recurrent abdominal pain. The pain is spasmodic, intermittent, and usually periumbilical. The pain is usually of mild to moderate intensity but occasionally can be severe, suggesting an acute surgical condition. If other systemic symptoms such as fever or vomiting are present, surgical consultation should be obtained. A fecal mass can sometimes be palpated in the left lower quadrant and suprapubic region. Mild tenderness over the mass is common, but abdominal rigidity and guarding are generally absent. Radiographic studies may be necessary for diagnosis in complicated cases. The objective of initial disimpaction is emptying the rectal vault. This is generally accomplished with enemas.

3. **E,** Page 1184.

Esophageal impactions caused by food boluses are uncommon in children with a normal esophagus. All other objects are commonly ingested.

4. **C,** Pages 1184-1186.

In the past, routine removal of disc batteries was advocated, but recent experience indicates that they pose little risk if they are smaller than 20 mm in diameter. Foreign bodies that do not pass the pylorus within 3-7 days, as well as those in patients who develop symptoms, should be endoscopically removed.

5. **B,** Pages 1186-1188.

Plain abdominal radiographs are seldom helpful and should not be obtained to prove or disprove appendicitis. C-reactive protein level is elevated in acute appendicitis, but it can also be elevated with other illnesses. Total leukocyte count and neutrophil percentage should be interpreted only in conjunction with physical findings, given that the tests have false-positive and false-negative results. Ultrasonography is gaining popularity, and some studies show an overall sensitivity of 98%, with a specificity of 100%. At this time, clinical judgment remains the best predictor of appendicitis.

6. **B,** Pages 1187-1188.

Triple antibiotic therapy is recommended once the patient is considered to have a perforated appendix and is continued for 7-14 days postoperatively.

7. **A,** Pages 1188-1189.

Children receiving ceftriaxone, a third-generation cephalosporin that is largely excreted in bile, are reported to develop gallbladder sludge. Ultrasound is the most sensitive and safest method for identifying gallstones. The stone discovery rate can be as high as 98% with this method. Acute noninflammatory distension of the gallbladder without bacterial infection or congenital anomaly of the gallbladder is defined as hydrops of the gallbladder. It is a rare condition and has a good prognosis. Gallstones in younger children are usually the result of a hemolytic disease. Many children with gallstones are asymptomatic.

8. **C,** Pages 1189-1191.

Rectal examination reveals a small, compact ampulla empty of feces. The disease occurs four to five times more often in males. Hirschsprung's disease accounts for 15%-25% of cases of intestinal obstruction in early infancy. Small volumes of stool (usually of ribbon- or pellet-like consistency) may be passed. Definitive therapy for Hirschsprung's disease is corrective surgery.

9. **B,** Page 1191.

Intussusception (the telescoping of one segment of intestine into another segment) occurs when one part of the intestine prolapses into the lumen of an immediately adjoining part. The central invaginated bowel is termed the intussusception, and the surrounding bowel is termed the intussuscipiens. Four types occur: ileocolic, ileoileocolic, ileoileal, and colocolic. The vast majority of intussusceptions are ileocolic.

10. **B,** Pages 1191-1193.

In a typical presentation, a healthy infant who recently had a mild viral upper respiratory infection appears to have a brief episode of sudden, severe abdominal pain, manifested by screaming and drawing the legs up against the abdomen. These episodes recur at 15- to 20-minute intervals. Between episodes, the infant is quiet or may become progressively lethargic, with marked alteration in mental status. There may be recurrent vomiting and diarrhea. The patient ultimately passes typical currant-jelly stools. This classic picture is easily recognized as intussusception. The cardinal features include intermittent severe abdominal pain, vomiting, rectal bleeding, right upper quadrant sausage-shaped abdominal mass, lethargy, and hypotension.

11. **A,** Page 1194.

With pyloric stenosis, there is non-bilious vomiting and a 4:1 male to female ratio. There is no clear relationship to maternal age, season of birth, or ABO and Rh factors. A positive family history may be present.

12. **D,** Page 1194.

Ultrasonography and radiographic studies are sometimes required to confirm the diagnosis. Ultrasonography is the procedure of choice because it is reliable and noninvasive. If the ultrasound is non-diagnostic or not available, a barium swallow may be used, looking for a "string" or "beak" sign. Vomiting and aspiration may occur with a barium swallow.

13. **D,** Pages 1194-1195.

The persistent vomiting causes loss of chloride, potassium, and hydrochloric acid, resulting in hypochloremic, hypokalemic alkalosis.

14. **C,** Page 1196.

In addition to hypoglycemia, elevated levels of LDH, bilirubin, and alkaline phosphatase, as well as increased prothrombin time, are usually present. BUN is often elevated.

15. **E,** Page 1196.

A midgut volvulus is usually seen in the neonate or during the first year of life. The infant commonly has bilious vomiting, abdominal distension, and a palpable abdominal mass. Appendicitis, Meckel's diverticulum, and Reye's syndrome do not typically present with an abdominal mass. Pyloric stenosis classically presents with non-bilious vomiting.

# 73 Acute Infectious Diarrhea Disease and Dehydration

*Sandra K. Dettmann*

1. **C,** Page 1201.

The most common bacterial organisms causing acute diarrhea in the United States are, in order of frequency, *Shigella* species, *Salmonella* species, *Campylobacter jejuni*, and *Yersinia enterocolitica. Clostridium perfringens, Staphylococcus aureus, Vibrio cholerae,* and *Vibrio parahaemolyticus* each make up less than 1% of cases.

2. **E,** Page 1201.

Rotavirus causes acute febrile illness with vomiting and diarrhea. Severity may vary, but the diarrhea has a watery consistency, and the volume is large enough to cause significant and rapid intravascular volume depletion. Rotavirus may also involve symptoms of upper respiratory tract infection. The incubation period is 1-3 days. No specific therapy is available, although a vaccine may be available in the future.

3. **E,** Pages 1201-1202.

Infection with *Giardia* may be asymptomatic or may cause nausea, flatulence, bloating, epigastric pain, abdominal cramping, and watery diarrhea. Norwalk agent usually causes odoriferous, nonbloody diarrhea. There is often vomiting but not usually a fever. Rotavirus causes acute febrile illness with vomiting and diarrhea. With *Salmonella,* vomiting is common, and fever may or may not be present. The stool is loose and foul-smelling but rarely bloody.

4. **B,** Pages 1201-1202.

Older children and adults have more nonenteric symptoms, presenting with an appendicitis-like illness as a result of mesenteric adenitis. Others have generalized abdominal cramping. Stools may be green with *Salmonella, Shigella,* and *Yersenia,* and with *Shigella* they may be bloody as well. Fever is seen with *Yersinia, Shigella,* and *Campylobacter* infection, and vomiting may be present in any type of bacterial gastroenteritis. *Yersinia* is the only type of gastroenteritis with pain that locates in the right lower quadrant.

5. **B,** Page 1202.

Signs and symptoms of pseudomembranous colitis are diarrhea, abdominal cramps, and fever. Pseudomembranes, friable rectal mucosa, and the presence of C. *difficile* toxin in the stool are diagnostic. Stopping intake of the offending agent and therapy with vancomycin, 40 mg/kg/24 hr, is indicated.

6. **C,** Pages 1203, 1206.

15% dehydration constitutes severe dehydration. Rapid re-expansion of the intravascular space is the goal of immediate resuscitation and can be achieved with an isotonic crystalloid solution. Administration of 20 ml/kg of 0.9% saline (or other appropriate isotonic crystalloid solution) IV at a rapid rate should result in reversal of signs of shock within 5 to 15 minutes. Oral rehydration is usually adequate in the child who is less than 5% dehydrated and who will tolerate oral fluids.

7. **C,** Pages 1205-1206.

Oral rehydration therapy has been reported as a safe and effective treatment for fluid repletion in infants and children with acute gastroenteritis and volume depletion. Oral rehydration therapy may be instituted even if the patient continues to vomit or has diarrhea. Children with severe volume loss or significant sodium derangement should be identified by a thorough physical examination and should not receive oral rehydration therapy. The desired volume of oral rehydration solution is 60 ml/kg for mild and 80 ml/kg for moderate volume depletion. This technique requires that the emergency department have the facilities and personnel to observe and monitor the patient for the 4 to 8 hours required to determine whether oral rehydration therapy is going to succeed or fail.

8. **C,** Page 1208.

If the serum glucose is low (<50 mg/dL), administration of dextrose D25 at 2 ml/kg IV (in neonates younger than 3 months of age use D10 at 2 to 4 ml/kg) should correct the deficit. Glucose should be monitored (every 30-60 minutes until stable) to ensure improvement and to identify future needs.

9. **B,** Page 1208.

The fluid requirement for a child weighing 10 kg or less is 100 ml/kg/24 hr. For a child 11-20 kg, it is 1000 ml plus 50 ml/kg/24 hr for each kg over 10 kg. For a child weighing more than 20 kg, the formula is 1500 ml plus 20 ml/kg/24 hr for each kg over 20 kg.

---

# 74 Neurologic Disorders

*Dale J. Ray*

1. **A,** Page 1213.

Group B streptococcus accounts for half of the cases of neonatal meningitis, and coliforms account for one fourth. The other organisms can occur, but are much less frequent in neonates.

2. **B,** Page 1215.

Children older than the age of 1 year usually have a headache along with symptoms of fever, chills, vomiting, and photophobia. Only a small percentage will present in septic shock or with coma on admission; most cases in this age-group have insidious findings. The most frequent cranial neuropathy is of the abducens (cranial nerve VI) nerve.

3. **E,** Page 1216.

Focal neurologic signs may be present in brain abscess patients but are rare in viral meningitis. In a patient with focal neurologic signs, especially if at risk for brain abscess because of prior history of head trauma, meningitis, chronic otitis media and sinusitis, or congenital heart disease, a CT of the brain should be performed before lumbar puncture. The CSF glucose, cell count, and Gram stain are not likely to be helpful, and the India ink stain is used to diagnose cryptococcal meningitis.

4. **C,** Pages 1216-1217.

This patient most likely has bacterial meningitis and developing uncal herniation related to increased ICP. A lumbar puncture is contraindicated and a brain CT is indicated. However, before this, immediate antibiotics should be administered (usually following obtaining a blood culture which should not delay therapy). In addition, emergent treatment of elevated ICP should be carried out.

5. **B,** Pages 1218-1219.

Polymorphonuclear leukocytes may be the predominant white blood cell type in early viral meningitis, but it is best to assume these represent a bacterial cause. The CSF glucose level must be interpreted relative to the serum glucose. The normal ratio of CSF/serum glucose is about 0.6, with a lower level down to 0.4. CIE is most useful in patients with prior antibiotic treatment. The most common bacterial agents in meningitis in the older infant and child age-group are *N. meningitidis*, *S. pneumoniae*, and *H. influenzae*. Blood cultures in this group are positive in 80%-90% of cases. C-reactive protein is insensitive and has little value in the evaluation of meningitis in the emergency department.

6. **B,** Pages 1220-1221.

The preferred third-generation cephalosporins are ceftriaxone and cefotaxime. Because of susceptibility of the most common etiologic agents, ampicillin is recommended in children up to the age of 3 months. Rifampin chemoprophylaxis is recommended for medical personnel with intimate exposure such as administering mouth-to-mouth resuscitation, intubation, and suctioning.

7. **C,** Page 1224.

Infantile spasms are characterized by bilateral symmetric clustered spasms. Most affected children have an underlying CNS disorder. The syndrome usually presents in the first year of life with a peak onset between 4 and 7 months of age. It has a poor outcome and typically does not respond to anticonvulsant medications.

8. **B,** Page 1224.

Febrile seizures are benign when they are tonic or tonic-clonic without focal features, last less than 15 minutes, have a source of fever outside the CNS, the age of the child is between 6 months and 5 years, there has been normal growth and development, and there is no family history of epilepsy. Most febrile seizures have an associated viral illness (including roseola) and have also been associated with *Shigella* gastroenteritis.

9. **D,** Page 1225.

The overall risk of a second febrile seizure is about 33%, and this increases if the child is younger than 1 year of age or there is a family history of febrile seizures.

10. **A,** Pages 1228-1229.

Although it may be clinically difficult to distinguish a seizure from another type of attack, most seizures are followed by some period of lethargy and confusion. Syncope is characterized by loss of motor tone and may have associated light-headedness, pale appearance, and diaphoresis. Vasovagal syncope is secondary to loss of postural tone and is often secondary to fright or pain. Pseudoseizures are often exacerbated by stress without postictal episodes and may be characterized by quivering, pelvic thrusts, opisthotonic posturing, side-to-side movements, and other atypical behavior and movements.

11. **C,** Pages 1230-1231.

Lorazepam is the drug of choice to treat status epilepticus, and the dose is 0.05 to 0.10 mg/kg IV. Diazepam IV dose is 0.2 mg/kg and rectal dose is in the range of 0.5 mg/kg. Phenytoin and phenobarbital both have initial loading doses of 18-20 mg/kg IV.

12. **B,** Page 1232.

The current general recommendation is to withhold anti-convulsants after a first seizure; however, each patient needs to be considered individually. Factors that increase risk include abnormal EEG and neurologic lesions. In addition, a patient who has the first unprovoked seizure while sleeping has twice the recurrence rate of those who have the first seizure while awake. Environmental circumstances (e.g., swimming) must be considered when evaluating risk.

13. **C,** Pages 1235-1237.

Headaches that are maximal at onset, especially if associated with strenuous activity, are suspicious for a subarachnoid hemorrhage. If scanning results are negative, lumbar puncture must be done to completely rule out bleeding (see Rosen Box 74-8).

14. **A,** Page 1238.

Breath-holding spells typically occur by age 1, and virtually all children have had their first spell by age 2. The attacks are commonly triggered by an emotional episode that causes crying. In a complex spell, cyanosis or pallor occur, leading to loss of consciousness. The child experiences loss of motor tone and may occasionally have anoxic seizures with body jerking and incontinence. This may be difficult to differentiate from other disorders. However, breath-holding spells are characterized by cyanosis preceding loss of muscle tone and lack a postictal period. Orthostatic hypotension is not usually preceded by crying and resolves once a patient is horizontal.

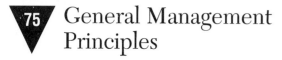

## 75 General Management Principles

*Greg Ledbetter*

1. **D,** Pages 1245-1247.

Toxidromes are a distinct set of signs and symptoms associated with characteristic classes of agents. There are several classic toxidromes that, when recognized, enable rapid diagnosis and guide therapy. SLUDGE is a useful mnemonic for the cholinergic toxidromes. Sedative-hypnotics will classically present with flaccidity and areflexic coma but occasionally with hyperreflexia, rigidity and clonus. The classic triad for opiate poisoning is coma, respiratory depression, and miosis, not mydriasis.

2. **B,** Page 1244.

Naloxone and Thiamine can be safely administered to unconscious patients with respiratory depression. Recent studies have shown that glucose administered to unconscious patients who are not hypoglycemic may have deleterious side effects. Flumazenil should rarely if ever be given in this scenario.

3. **A,** Page 1247.

Although few agents produce microscopic changes in the urine, ingestion of ethylene glycol has been shown to produce oxalate crystalluria. An initial CBC should always be documented as a reference to help identify developing marrow toxicity, hemolytic anemia, or idiopathic thrombocytopenic purpura. Serum and urine toxicologic screens may not provide the answer in many cases and most often do not influence treatment. Acidosis may develop late in methanol and ethylene glycol ingestions and therefore may not be reflected in the arterial blood gas, especially if drawn early.

4. **B,** Page 1247.

Many substances not routinely screened for are causes of serious overdoses. In addition, substances such as cocaine and marijuana have metabolites still traceable in the urine long after ingestion. Positive or negative toxicologic screens are not definitive, although they can be helpful when combined with a thorough history and physical examination.

5. **A,** Pages 1247-1249.

The current recommendation is to administer activated charcoal to all patients who have orally ingested adsorbable toxins or poisons. The efficacy of ipecac or lavage has been found to be inferior to that of activated charcoal alone. Both ipecac and lavage have been shown to move drugs from the stomach into the intestine, where absorption is enhanced.

6. **B,** Page 1245.

Specific odors can provide diagnostic information. Arsenic leaves a garlic-like odor.

7. **B,** Page 1246.

These are all typical symptoms of the toxidrome associated with anticholinergic poisoning.

8. **C,** Page 1247.

Serotonin syndrome is caused by the drug interaction between and among selective serotonin reuptake inhibitors, monoamine oxidase inhibitors, and other antidepressants, meperidine, dextromethorphan (found in decongestants), and lithium.

9. **D,** Page 1248.

Deferoxamine is the antidote for iron, not lead.

# 76 Aspirin, Acetaminophen, and Nonsteroidal Agents

*Greg Ledbetter*

1. **B,** Page 1251.
Salicylates are rapidly absorbed from the gastrointestinal tract. Two thirds of an ingested dose is absorbed within 1 hour, and, in most preparations, peak levels are reached 2 to 4 hours after ingestion. Because of the large surface area, most of the ingested dose is absorbed in the small intestine, regardless of whether the tablet is enteric coated. With enteric-coated tablets, peak serum concentrations may occur 6 to 9 hours after ingestion.

2. **B,** Page 1251.
Salicylate intoxication results in uncoupling of oxidative phosphorylation, producing a hypermetabolic state and increased glucose demand. Gluconeogenesis and lipid metabolism begin, producing hyperglycemia, glucosuria, and ketonuria. In addition, the hypermetabolic state produces hyperthermia and diaphoresis. Direct stimulation of the medullary respiratory center produces hyperventilation and respiratory alkalosis. Lactic and pyruvic acids are generated, producing an anion gap metabolic acidosis. The tendency to generate organic acids, however, decreases with age, and metabolic acidosis is often absent in older children and adults.

3. **A,** Page 1251.
Children younger than 2 years old have a predominant metabolic acidosis as compared with older children and adults, in whom respiratory alkalosis predominates.

4. **E,** Page 1252.
All of the signs and symptoms listed may be seen with salicylate intoxication. In addition, other signs and symptoms include hyperventilation, hyperthermia, acute renal failure, hemorrhage, and a deficit of ionized calcium.

5. **D,** Page 1253.
A toxic dose of aspirin is 200 to 300 mg/kg, and more than 500 mg/kg is potentially lethal.

6. **A,** Page 1253.
The Done nomogram is useful only after a single acute ingestion of salicylates. It is not useful in patients taking aspirin chronically, in ingestions that occurred over several hours, or when other salicylates (such as Pepto Bismol or Alka-Seltzer) have been ingested within the last 24 hours. In addition, the Done nomogram will not work if the aspirin is enteric coated, even if the ingestion is acute. When using the nomogram, the first blood level should be established 6 hours after the ingestion.

7. **C,** Page 1254.
All of the treatment modalities listed are appropriate except forced diuresis, which has the potential for exacerbating cerebral and pulmonary edema. To enhance excretion of sa-

licylates, the urine should be alkalinized to a pH of 7.5 to 8.0 using 1 to 2 mEq/kg sodium bicarbonate over 1 to 2 hours. When bicarbonate is excreted into the urine, serum potassium must be sufficient to supply a counter cation for excretion. If the serum potassium is low, hydrogen ions will be preferentially excreted, thereby preventing urine alkalinization. Activated charcoal with a cathartic is a useful modality for decontamination, especially since aspirin may inhibit gastric emptying. In order to treat dehydration and prevent hypoglycemia, intravenous fluids should contain a minimum of 5 g/dl glucose and be infused at a rate to maintain urine output at 2 to 3 ml/kg/hr.

8. **E,** Pages 1251-1253.
All of the statements are true. The mortality of chronic salicylate intoxication is 25%, whereas it is only 1% in acute ingestions. The difference usually relates to the fact that the diagnosis of salicylate intoxication is frequently delayed in chronic ingestions. Many patients are admitted to the hospital with pulmonary edema, coma, hyperthermia, or dyspnea without the proper diagnosis of salicylate intoxication.

9. **E,** Page 1255.
Patients with toxic ingestions of APAP may progress through four stages. Stage one is between 7 and 24 hours after ingestion; symptoms include nausea, vomiting, anorexia, and diaphoresis. Some patients, however, remain asymptomatic throughout stage one. CNS depression does not occur unless there was a co-ingestion of a narcotic or other CNS depressant. In stage two (24 to 48 hours), symptoms, if initially present, tend to decrease, but the patient develops right upper quadrant pain, and AST, SGPT, and LDH levels increase dramatically. In stage three (72 to 96 hours), patients develop hepatic necrosis with jaundice, hypoglycemia, and coagulation defects. Death may occur from hepatic failure. If the patient survives to stage four, the recovery phase, hepatic regeneration and normalization of liver function tests occurs rapidly over 1 to 3 weeks.

10. **B,** Pages 1256-1257.
The initial dose of NAC is 140 mg/kg PO, followed by 70 mg/kg every 4 hours for 72 hours (17 doses). If the time or amount of ingestion is unknown or if serum APAP levels are not available, NAC should be administered until levels are available.

11. **B,** Page 1257.
Because there is continued absorption from the gastrointestinal tract, serum APAP levels are not useful until 4 hours after ingestion. After 4 hours, a serum APAP level should be obtained and the value plotted on the Rumack-Matthew nomogram to ascertain the need for treatment. NAC will prevent hepatotoxicity if it is given within 8 to 10 hours after ingestion of APAP, so therapy can be withheld until the 4-hour level is obtained. The patient should not be discharged or transferred to a psychiatric facility until the 4-hour level is confirmed to be in the nontoxic range. Gastric lavage and charcoal are usually ineffective if initiated beyond 1 hour after ingestion. Forced diuresis is not effective in removing APAP.

12. **C,** Pages 1255, 1258.

For unknown reasons, hepatotoxicity rarely occurs in young children with toxic serum APAP levels. This difference in toxicity may be due to metabolic differences between children and adults. In spite of this difference, all children with toxic APAP levels should receive N-acetylcysteine. Barbiturates induce the microsomal P-450 system and thereby increase the rate of conversion of APAP to its toxic metabolite. Acute alcohol ingestion inhibits the P-450 system and is hepatoprotective. In alcoholic patients, however, APAP toxicity usually produces fatal hepatic necrosis.

13. **A,** Page 1259.

The incidence of NSAID toxicity is low. Patients usually follow a benign course even if a large amount of NSAID was ingested. Drug levels are not useful in acute or chronic ingestions.

14. **D,** Page 1257.

N-acetylcysteine provides hepatoprotection for the first 8 hours after ingestion. Although there is a decrease in efficacy after 8 hours, studies have shown N-acetylcysteine to be efficacious up to 24 hours after ingestion.

15. **E,** Page 1254.

Hemodialysis should be considered for patients with salicylate levels >100 mg/dl, coma, renal or hepatic failure, pulmonary edema, severe acid-base imbalance, rising serum salicylate levels, severe toxicity, or failure of more conservative treatment.

# 77 Alcohol-Related Disease

### *Greg Ledbetter*

1. **B,** Page 1264.

Alcoholism is the leading cause of morbidity and mortality in the United States.

2. **A,** Page 1265.

The oxidation of alcohol is a complex process involving three enzyme systems. The primary pathway is alcohol dehydrogenase, which is located in the liver and gastric mucosa. The gastric metabolism of alcohol is decreased in women. Alcohol is eliminated at a rate of 15 to 20 mg/dl per hour in the nonalcoholic. Its elimination may be increased to greater than 30 mg/dl per hour in the chronic drinker.

3. **C,** Page 1265.

The physiologic effects of different blood alcohol levels are outlined in Rosen Table 115-1.

4. **B,** Page 1265.

In most states, the acceptable legal level of intoxication is 80-100 mg/dl (0.08%-0.1%). An easy approximation to remember is that 1 mg/kg of 100% ethanol produces a level of 100 mg/dl 2 hours after ingestion.

5. **C,** Page 1267.

Minor alcohol withdrawal occurs within 24 hours after a significant decrease in alcohol ingestion. It is characterized by mild autonomic hyperactivity, including nausea, vomiting, anxiety, insomnia, tachycardia, hypertension, hyperreflexia, and tremor.

6. **C,** Page 1268.

Benzodiazepines are currently the mainstay of treatment for alcohol withdrawal.

7. **D,** Page 1266.

Opioid withdrawal, not intoxication, will appear similar to the autonomic hyperactivity of alcohol withdrawal.

8. **C,** Pages 1273-1274.

As with viral hepatitis, the severity of alcoholic hepatitis can be easily assessed in the ED by prothrombin time.

9. **E,** Pages 1274-1275.

Both the cardiovascular and neurologic signs of thiamine deficiency can become abruptly evident following the administration of glucose to thiamine-depleted, asymptomatic patients. Thiamine should be administered with glucose to any patient in whom subclinical thiamine deficiency is suspected.

10. **D,** Page 1276.

Although there are a variety of causes of bacterial pneumonia in alcoholics, *Streptococcus pneumoniae* is, as in the general population, still the most common.

11. **A,** Page 1279.

Iron deficiency in alcoholics is usually secondary to gastrointestinal blood loss. The serum ferritin level is the best screening test for iron deficiency anemia in this population.

12. **B,** Page 1278.

Elevated urine glucose and ketones are a sign of diabetic ketoacidosis.

13. **A,** Page 1278.

Ketonuria without glucosuria is indicative of alcoholic ketoacidosis.

14. **C,** Page 1278.

The presence of oxalate crystals in the urine signifies ethylene glycol poisoning.

15. **D,** Page 1278.

Proteinuria, cellular casts, and low specific gravity are indicative of renal failure and uremia.

16. **D,** Page 1267.

Delirium tremens is a rare manifestation of alcohol withdrawal. It represents the extreme end of the spectrum, with symptoms including gross tremor, profound confusion, fever, incontinence, visual hallucinations, and mydriasis. With aggressive ICU care, the mortality rate from delirium tremens is much lower than 15%. Other causes for delirium should also be considered. The differential diagnosis for delirium in an alcoholic patient should include sepsis, meningitis, hypoxia, hypoglycemia, hepatic failure, and intracranial bleeding.

17. **C,** Pages 1268-1269.

Phenothiazines are contraindicated for patients with alcohol withdrawal syndrome because they lower the seizure threshold, interfere with thermoregulation, and may cause hypotension. Hydration, thiamine, multivitamins, folic acid, and magnesium sulfate are acceptable treatment considerations. Dextrose and naloxone should be considered if the patient is obtunded. Benzodiazepines are indicated in virtually all cases of alcohol withdrawal syndrome.

18. **D,** Page 1271.

An alcoholic patient with a documented history of alcohol withdrawal seizures who has a seizure but is now alert with normal vital signs and physical examination findings requires treatment only for alcohol withdrawal. New onset seizures or focal seizures require a full seizure work-up including head CT and lumbar puncture. Beginning anticonvulsants in alcohol withdrawal seizures is controversial and should be done only in consultation with a neurologist or the primary care physician.

19. **A,** Pages 1274-1275.

The classic triad of Wernicke's encephalopathy is oculomotor disturbances, ataxia, and global confusion. The oculomotor disturbances include nystagmus (usually horizontal) and ophthalmoplegia, which most often involves both lateral rectus muscles. Untreated Wernicke's encephalopathy will develop into Korsakoff's psychosis, which involves anterograde and retrograde amnesia. Treatment is parenteral thiamine 50-100 mg daily.

# 78 Other Alcohols

*Greg Ledbetter*

1. **C,** Page 1293.

A distinguishing feature of isopropyl alcohol ingestion is ketosis from acetone formation without acidosis. Isopropyl alcohol is broken down by alcohol dehydrogenase into acetone, which is cleared by the liver and the kidneys. The serum osmolal gap increases 0.17 mOsm/kg for every 1 mg/dl rise in blood isopropyl alcohol concentration. Ingestion of isopropyl alcohol causes hypotension, which is an indication for dialysis.

2. **D,** Pages 1297-1298.

Because the alcohols are rapidly absorbed, gastric lavage is indicated if the patient arrives in the ED within only 1 to 2 hours after ingestion. Activated charcoal is not useful unless co-ingestion of other substances is suspected. Forced diuresis with fluids, furosemide, and mannitol will help clear toxic metabolites, but dialysis is a better means of removing these compounds. Unlike lactic acid, the acids produced by the breakdown of methanol and ethylene glycol are not metabolized to bicarbonate; therefore large amounts of bicarbonate may be necessary to correct acidosis. Ethanol IV can prevent further production of the toxic metabolites by competing for the enzyme alcohol dehydrogenase. IV folate is recommended for methanol poisoning because it is a cofactor in the degradation of formic acid (the toxic acid byproduct of methanol metabolism).

3. **C,** Pages 1293-1294.

Methanol ingestion has serious sequelae, including permanent blindness, neurologic dysfunction, and death. The lethal dose of methanol can be as low as 0.4 ml/kg of 40% methanol. Methanol is converted to formic acid by alcohol dehydrogenase. Formic acid is responsible for the serious toxicity of methanol. Formic acid is degraded to carbon dioxide by a folate dependent pathway, so folate-deficiency can prolong the half-life of formic acid.

4. **C,** Page 1294.

For unknown reasons, patients with methanol ingestion have ocular toxicity with as little as 4 ml of 40% methanol. Ocular symptoms include cloudy, blurred, indistinct, or misty vision. Patients may see yellow spots, central scotomata, or in rare cases have photophobia. Patients may describe their ocular symptoms as the feeling of "stepping out into a snowstorm." Visual symptoms are an indication for hemodialysis.

5. **A,** Page 1294.

Patients will typically have an increased anion gap metabolic acidosis primarily due to the increased levels of formic acid in methanol ingestion and glycolic and glyoxylic acid in ethylene glycol ingestion. Patients will also have an elevated osmolal gap because of the presence of these low-molecular-weight solutes in the blood.

6. **D,** Page 1296.

The hallmark of ethylene glycol poisoning is calcium oxalate crystalluria. Also, because antifreeze commonly has fluorescein added to detect radiator leaks, another useful test is the examination of freshly voided urine for fluorescence with a Wood's lamp. However, the absence of calcium oxalate crystals or of fluorescence does not rule out ethylene glycol ingestion. Blood can be tested for ethylene glycol, but it takes a long time and is not commonly available. Head CT and lumbar puncture are useful to rule out other diagnoses.

# 79 Anticholinergics

*David Hughes*

1. **E,** Page 1301.

In addition to the usual anticholinergic drugs such as atropine, scopolamine, and ipratropium, many other drugs possess anticholinergic properties. These include the $H_1$ receptor blockers (antihistamines, such as diphenhydramine, meclizine, hydroxyzine), antiparkinsonian agents related to antihistamines (such as benztropine, trihexyphenidyl), phenothiazines, tricyclic antidepressants, carbamazepine, cyclobenzaprine, and many over-the-counter preparations (e.g., Dristan, Excedrin PM, Nytol, Pamprin, Sominex).

2. **A,** Page 1303.

The typical signs and symptoms of anticholinergic poisoning are the result of muscarinic receptor blockade and include mydriasis, dry mucous membranes, absent sweating, flushed skin, fever, tachycardia, decreased gastric motility, and urinary retention. In addition, blockage of central muscarinic receptors initially produces stimulation; the patient is usually alert but may be silly, agitated, violent, or incoherent. Massive overdoses may produce coma and cardiovascular collapse.

3. **D,** Page 1303.

It is often very difficult to differentiate between anticholinergic, cholinergic, and adrenergic toxicity on physical examination. Determination of increased or decreased bowel sounds, mydriasis or miosis, dry skin versus diaphoresis, and tachycardia versus bradycardia is often helpful. Adrenergic stimulation results in mydriasis, tachycardia, diaphoresis, and increased bowel sounds.

4. **D,** Page 1303.

EKG changes from anticholinergic toxicity are exceedingly rare. Their presence should suggest either a massive exposure or the presence of a more cardiotoxic agent with antimuscarinic side effects, such as tricyclic antidepressants, carbamazepine, or a phenothiazine.

5. **E,** Page 1304.

The patient's most significant problem at this time is his agitation and hyperthermia. In this setting, hyperthermia may produce hepatic necrosis, myoglobinuric renal failure, cerebral edema, or disseminated intravascular coagulation. Therefore the morbidity and mortality from the hyperthermia far outweigh the morbidity of the drug overdose itself. Appropriate initial treatment is to decrease the patient's agitation, initiate cooling measures, and begin rehydration. After management of the patient's immediate life-threatening condition, the toxicologic issues should be addressed.

6. **D,** Page 1304.

Aggressive treatment of agitation in the presence of an anticholinergic overdose is necessary to prevent exacerbation of hyperthermia and the development of myoglobinuric renal failure, as well as to prevent harm to the staff or patient. Benzodiazepines are ideal drugs for this purpose because they produce minimal hypotension, decrease the chance of the patient's developing seizures, and lack intrinsic anticholinergic properties. Phenothiazines (chlorpromazine) have anticholinergic side effects and may exacerbate the signs and symptoms of the overdose. Butyrophenones (droperidol and haloperidol), although lacking anticholinergic properties, do not protect against seizures and may exacerbate hypotension.

7. **B,** Page 1305.

Physostigmine antagonizes the effects of anticholinergic medications by inhibiting acetylcholinesterase and thereby increasing the concentration of acetylcholine in the synaptic space. In the absence of a significant anticholinergic overdose, however, physostigmine may exacerbate asthma and may produce seizures, bradycardia, salivation, diarrhea, and bronchorrhea. It should therefore be used with caution and never as a first-line drug. The proper dose is 1 to 2 mg slow IV push in adults and 0.5 mg slow IV push in children. Doses may be repeated as needed. Rapid infusion, even with significant anticholinergic toxicity, may produce seizures.

8. **D,** Page 1305.

See answer to Question 10.

9. **C,** Page 1305.

See answer to Question 10.

10. **A,** Page 1305.

Any patient with a significant anticholinergic ingestion within the last 1 to 2 hours should have gastric lavage. In addition, any comatose and intubated patient should be lavaged. In patients with small ingestions and minimal symptoms, multidose activated charcoal with a cathartic is usually sufficient without gastric emptying. A cathartic should not be utilized in patients with absent bowel sounds. The patient in Question 10 needs immediate intubation and gastric decontamination. Physostigmine is never a first-line drug; it is usually used only in pure anticholinergic overdoses, and its use is contraindicated in tricyclic antidepressant overdoses. Patients with moderate to severe anticholinergic ingestions should be admitted to the intensive care unit for treatment and observation. Patients with small ingestions may be observed 4 to 8 hours in the ED and discharged if they have only mild or no symptoms. Psychiatric assessment or an assessment of a pediatric patient's home situation should be made before discharge.

11. **C,** Page 1305.

Initial decontamination in a patient with suspected anticholinergic toxicity and slowed GI motility indicated by decreased bowel sounds should be with charcoal and water via nasogastric tube. A cathartic, such as sorbitol, is contraindicated in the presence of decreased GI motility. Lavage performed more than 2 hours after ingestion in an agitated patient has the inherent risk of aspiration. Charcoal with water enemas is the safest method for repeated dosing of the decontaminant.

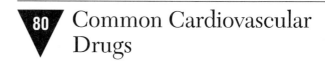

# 80 ▼ Common Cardiovascular Drugs

### *David Hughes*

1. **E,** Page 1308, Box 80-2.

Many drugs and disease states may alter absorption, volume of distribution, and protein binding and elimination and render the heart more susceptible to digoxin toxicity.

2. **C,** Pages 1308-1309.

Chronic digitalis intoxication has been found to have an $LD_{50}$ at a level of 6 ng/ml. The $LD_{50}$ for acute intoxication is not known but is much higher, especially in children. Most patients with chronic toxicity have comorbidity such as heart disease. The treatment of chronic versus acute intoxication differs in that in chronic toxicity the total body potassium may be low and treatment with supplemental potassium may be needed. In acute intoxication, life-threatening hyperkalemia may develop and empiric potassium therapy is contraindicated.

3. **A,** Page 1311, Box 80-4.

Studies before the availability of Digibind revealed a mortality of 23% for digitalis toxicity. This has been reduced to less than 10% with Digibind. Indications for treatment include instability of hemodynamics as well as a serum potassium above 5 mEq/L. One study showed no survivors of those who presented with a serum potassium >5.5 mEq/L. Supportive measures should also be undertaken including treating hyperkalemia without using calcium, which is contraindicated.

4. **D,** Pages 1314-1315.
Ventricular dysrhythmias are uncharacteristic of beta-blocker overdoses and should be addressed using ACLS protocols.

5. **C,** Page 1316.
Verapamil has the deadliest profile for the reasons listed. Diltiazem has only one third of the myocardial depressant effects. Nifedipine acts primarily on vascular smooth muscle, causing peripheral vasodilation.

6. **B,** Pages 1312, 1315, 1318.
Patients who have taken regular release beta blockers and calcium channel blockers and who remain asymptomatic may be discharged if psychiatric treatment is not necessary. The half-life of digoxin is 30 hours, so it may cause rhythm disturbances and toxicity remote to its ingestion.

7. **A,** Pages 1310, 1314.
This patient has severe and sudden cardiovascular collapse, which is most consistent with acute overdose of propranolol. One must also consider the possibility of digoxin toxicity, and for that reason calcium would be contraindicated because it may increase the effect of digitalis. One of the most important features of beta-blocker overdose is the early and often abrupt onset of life-threatening toxicity, which can include cardiovascular collapse, apnea, and seizures even within the first hour after overdose. High-dose IV glucagon is the most effective treatment; it can be administered through continuous infusion if an initial result is obtained. Atropine should be administered for symptomatic bradycardia. Decontamination after beta-blocker overdose has not been well studied, but ipecac is contraindicated because of the possibility of sudden deterioration and aspiration. Gastric lavage is useful only within 2 hours of ingestion, and it may increase bradycardia by increasing vagal tone. Activated charcoal should be used.

# 81 Corrosives

### David Hughes

1. **D,** Pages 1321-1322.
Acid ingestions produce coagulative necrosis with a protective eschar from thermal and dehydrating factors. The eschar causes acid ingestions to accumulate in the stomach, causing gastric injury. Alkalis produce a liquefactive necrosis that rapidly penetrates the oropharynx and esophagus. Early complications of both acid and alkali ingestions are perforation and infection. A late complication of alkali ingestion is esophageal stricture. Late complications of acid ingestions are gastric outlet obstruction and achlorhydria.

2. **D,** Page 1323.
An ingested alkaline battery needs to be removed immediately if lodged in the esophagus because the alkali can rapidly penetrate and damage tissue by liquefactive necrosis. The use of emetics like ipecac may reexpose the esophagus to additional corrosive contact. Disk batteries usually pass without serious results once they reach the stomach.

3. **D,** Pages 1323-1324.
As opposed to alkali ingestions, for strong acid ingestions aggressive gastric aspiration should be performed immediately. Acid corrosive ingestions have a tendency to accumulate and create more damage in the stomach than in the esophagus, and perforation is unlikely. Ice water lavage should only follow continuous aspiration, because dilution of a strong acid with water can result in a large amount of heat production (increase of approximately 80° C). Water added to a concentrated acid may cause boiling and explosive steam formation. The use of corticosteroids and antibiotics is not recommended for acid corrosive ingestion. Emetics, absorbants, and cathartics are not indicated in cases of corrosive ingestions.

4. **B,** Pages 1321-1322.
Alkalis typically produce more severe injury due to the rapidly penetrating liquefactive necrosis that occurs. Acids tend to produce a coagulative necrosis which forms an eschar that will delay its caustic effects. Oxidants have an associated morbidity and mortality but they are not as great as those of alkalis.

# 82 Antidepressants and Monoamine Oxidase Inhibitors

### David Hughes

1. **D,** Page 1330 (Rosen Table 82-2).
Classic electrocardiographic changes of cyclic antidepressant toxicity include QRS and QT prolongation and bundle branch blocks, usually right. In an obtunded patient with a rightward terminal QRS vector or a QRS duration of >0.10 seconds, the diagnosis cyclic antidepressant overdose should be entertained. PR prolongation rather than shortening is a common finding.

2. **B,** Page 1331.
Some patients may be discharged after 6 hours of observation if they never develop evidence of significant ingestion ventilatory insufficiency, desaturation on pulse oximetry, QRS >100 msec, sinus tachycardia >119, dysrhythmias, hypotension, decreased level of consciousness, seizures, abnormal or inactive bowel sounds. The presence of normal bowel sounds indicates that charcoal and cathartic are passing through the digestive tract and the CA is being eliminated.

3. **A,** Page 1331.
Treatment of brief seizures is of questionable benefit, but protracted seizures must be treated. Lorazepam or diazepam is the first-line treatment of protracted seizures followed by continuous IV midazolam or phenobarbital. Physostigmine can cause seizures. Sodium bicarbonate alkalinization is not a treatment for seizures but should be carried out to minimize cardiovascular toxicity.

4. **A,** Pages 1329-1330 and Rosen Table 82-2.

Maintaining pH around 7.5-7.55 seems most beneficial. Hyperventilation alone is often effective, but use of bicarbonate may be indicated. Sodium loading also may be helpful. Phenytoin, lidocaine, and bretylium may be used with caution in cases of life-threatening tachyarrhythmias. Physostigmine has been shown to have detrimental effects.

5. **B,** Pages 1336-1339.

Patients taking an overdose of MAOIs may have a long latency period before onset of symptoms, and most patients require observation for 24 hours. Tachycardias are usually the sinus type and do not require treatment. Beta blockers are contraindicated. Bradycardias are usually reflex secondary to stretch receptors and are protective and should not be treated. Phase I is a latent period. Hypertension should be treated with short-acting titratable drugs that can be stopped if hypotension occurs.

6. **B,** Pages 1136-1139 and Rosen Table 82-8.

Wines, aged cheeses and fava beans all can precipitate MAOI interactions. Activated charcoal is indicated and ipecac contraindicated. Symptoms of interaction usually occur in minutes, whereas with overdose the symptoms are delayed. Overdose manifests as a CNS sympathomimetic storm, with interaction evident as both CNS and PNS sympathomimetic storm.

7. **C,** Page 1325.

The therapeutic effects of cyclic antidepressants are thought to be secondary to the inhibition of serotonin and norepinephrine reuptake. Anticholinergic effects, especially muscarinic, are responsible for the toxidrome often seen with cyclic antidepressant overdose as well as some of the cardiovascular effects. Alpha blockade can result in hypotension with reflex tachycardia. Sodium channel blockade is similar to that of quinidine and prolongs QRS duration through inhibiting conductance through the fast sodium channels. Calcium channel blockade is not associated with CA overdose.

8. **D,** Page 1329.

Phenytoin has been found to have no reliable therapeutic effects and may even increase the frequency and duration of ventricular tachycardia. Procainamide, which is a class Ia antiarrhythmic, exerts similar effects on the fast sodium channels as do the cyclic antidepressants. Lidocaine has been found to be only transiently effective in treating PVCs and has a negative effect on blood pressure. Sodium bicarbonate has been shown to be effective in terminating ventricular tachycardia.

9. **C,** Pages 1329-1331 (Table 82-2).

Hyperventilation, sodium bicarbonate, and hypertonic saline all act to increase serum pH. It is thought that alkalinization of serum increases conductance of sodium through sodium channels in the myocardium and thereby partially corrects conduction abnormalities. Physostigmine is contraindicated in cyclic antidepressant overdoses despite the significant anticholinergic signs and symptoms. It has been associated with seizures, cardiac arrest, and death when used in cyclic antidepressant overdoses.

10. **E,** Page 1333 (Rosen Box 82-4).

Sternbach (1991) suggested diagnostic criteria for diagnosing serotonin syndrome that include the following:
- Adding a serotonergic agent to a regimen or increasing the dose of such an agent
- Adding or changing the dose of a neuroleptic to a regimen
- Ruling out other etiologies.

The patient must have at least three of a list of signs and symptoms that includes the following:
- Agitation
- Ataxia
- Diaphoresis
- Diarrhea
- Hyperreflexia
- Hyperthermia
- Mental status changes
- Myoclonus
- Shivering
- Tremor

Nausea and vomiting are not among the signs and symptoms.

# 83 ▼ Hallucinogens

### *David Hughes*

1. **B,** Page 1349.

Buspirone is an antidepressant that does not cause agitation in overdoses. Each of the other choices must be considered. The acute psychosis of either cocaine or LSD intoxication may be indistinguishable from psychiatric disease. Mixed-drug intoxications must always be considered, because coingestions may require specific treatments (such as cyclic antidepressants and phencyclidine).

2. **E,** Page 1348.

*A. muscaria* requires supportive care only. Mistreatment has been common because the name implies cholinergic effects from muscarine, yet it contains only a very small amount. Atropine worsens the anticholinergic effects already present. Diazepam may worsen the deep sleep associated with this ingestion. Admission to the ICU is unnecessary unless anticholinergic effects, seizures, or mixed ingestion are present. Intubation and lavage are not indicated.

3. **B,** Pages 1352-1353.

Most patients recover uneventfully from intravenous marijuana use but may exhibit cyanosis, fever, bleeding diatheses, and renal insufficiency. "Toxic psychosis" is rare and does not occur with inhalation. Schizophrenics commonly do not like the effects of marijuana; it can turn borderline schizophrenics into overt schizophrenics. The most common presenting complaint among marijuana users is panic, particularly among novice users.

4. **E,** Pages 1358-1359.

Phencyclidine (PCP) is excreted mainly by the liver. Acidification of the urine will cause or exacerbate myoglobinuric renal failure. Supportive care is indicated, as is gastric suction after lavage, because there is ion trapping of PCP in gastric juice. Because PCP production laboratories use many toxic chemicals (such as cyanide), the avoidance of skin absorption of these and of the PCP is crucial.

5. **A,** Pages 1357-1359.

Hyperthermia can be treated with cooling blankets, ice, fans, or sponging. Temperature greater than 40.5° C may be treated with dantrolene, 1 to 1.5 mg IV, as well. Hypertension may resolve or may require treatment with diazoxide or sodium nitroprusside. Bronchospasm, rhabdomyolysis, and myoglobinuric renal failure are treated in the traditional manner. Tachycardia, rather than bradycardia, is common and typically does not require treatment. Beta blockade, if necessary, should be used with caution because of the risk of bronchospasm.

6. **D,** Pages 1357-1359.

Among the drugs classified in the hallucinogenic category, PCP has the most unpredictable and physiologically dangerous side effect profile. Ingestion can result in myoglobinuric renal failure secondary to rhabdomyolysis, hyperthermia, coma, seizures, and cardiac arrest. The side effect profile of the remaining hallucinogens is mainly related to psychologic problems such as panic and paranoia.

7. **A,** Page 1344.

LSD is the most potent psychoactive drug, with doses as low as 1.0 μg/kg causing psychedelic effects. Despite its high potency there has never been a reported death, disregarding behavioral toxicity, due to LSD, even with doses of thousands of micrograms.

8. **B,** Page 1356 (Rosen Table 83-4).

A good prognostic indicator of PCP intoxication is the clinical classification of intoxication developed by McCarron (1985). The minor patterns include lethargy or stupor, bizarre behavior, violent behavior, agitation, euphoria, and asymptomatic patterns. If the patient's worst clinical state exhibits only a minor pattern, the patient may be safely discharged after several hours of observation. Cardiac arrest, respiratory depression, hyperthermia, status epilepticus, and rhabdomyolysis have all been associated with clinically major patterns.

sure control are relatively contraindicated. Pulmonary edema is a real threat, so fluid administration should be titrated judiciously. This patient needs a chest radiograph on arrival to establish his baseline before his respiratory status declines.

2. **A,** Page 1366.

Two questions must be answered before discharge of a patient exposed to hydrocarbons: "Was the ingestion intentional?" and "Are there any symptoms suggestive of toxicity?" Intentional ingestions are often underreported by the patient. Formal psychiatric clearance must be obtained before discharge. Patients symptomatic on arrival should be admitted expeditiously, as should those who develop symptoms. A patient who remains asymptomatic may be discharged with definite follow-up arranged.

3. **B,** Page 1362.

Hydrocarbons usually enter the body through the lungs although skin and GI tract are also routes of exposure. The primary organ of toxicity is the lung, usually as a result of aspiration. There are several mechanisms of toxicity, including bronchospasm and inflammatory response, displacement of oxygen, and direct alveolar and capillary injury. CNS toxicity over the short term is related to its narcotic-like effects. Long-term exposure may lead to peripheral neuropathy, cerebellar degeneration, neuropsychiatric disorders, and chronic encephalopathy. Cardiac toxicity is related to ventricular dysrhythmia because of its sensitizing effect on the myocardium to catecholamines.

4. **E,** Pages 1362-1363.

Despite the many different types of hydrocarbons, these four characteristics will dictate their potential toxicity. Lower viscosity is considered more toxic because it will spread faster. Higher volatility allows gasses to displace oxygen. Low surface tension allows a substance to disperse easily. Chemical side chains such as heavy metals can increase toxicity.

5. **B,** Pages 1365-1366.

The aphorism "the safest place in the body for hydrocarbons is in the duodenum" holds true for most hydrocarbon ingestions regardless of the volume ingested. This is due to the high pulmonary toxicity if aspirated and the relatively low GI toxicity. There are specific cases in which aggressive GI decontamination is indicated; these can be remembered by the mnemonic CHAMP, which stands for camphor, halogenated, aromatic, metals, and pesticides.

# 84 Hydrocarbons

### David Hughes

1. **E,** Pages 1363-1366.

A key element of hydrocarbon exposure management is to remove any possible source of further exposure. Gastric emptying would be indicated if the exposure had been oral. Adrenergic medications for dysrhythmia and blood pres-

# 85 Acute Iron and Lead Poisoning

### David Hughes

1. **A,** Page 1367.

Maternal prenatal vitamins, as well as children's vitamins, are a common source of iron poisoning.

2. **B,** Pages 1367-1369.

Patients who ingest more than 60 mg/kg of elemental iron may experience severe symptoms. The primary determinant of shock may be the action of free iron as a direct cardiac toxin. The TIBC may be measured inaccurately in iron poisoning and is not as useful in assessing toxicity as previously thought. Ingestion of toxic amounts of iron produces hyperglycemia and an increased white blood cell count. However, these conditions do not correlate well with the degree of toxicity.

3. **C,** Pages 1369-1370.

Either ipecac or gastric lavage could be indicated in this child; however, the use of bicarbonate in the lavage fluid has not been shown to be of benefit and has significant potential complications. Because iron forms bezoars, the abdominal film is needed. Whole-bowel irrigation may be beneficial. Serum iron is the laboratory test most useful in estimating the seriousness of the ingestion, and the TIBC, although less useful, is still recommended. The deferoxamine challenge will determine if free iron is present in the serum.

4. **B,** Page 1369.

Peak serum iron levels, which should be obtained at 3 to 5 hours and again at 6 to 8 hours if sustained-release forms are suspected, can be helpful for prognostic purposes. Levels less than 350 µg/dl indicate minimal toxicity, levels 350-500 µg/dl may cause moderate toxicity, and levels greater than 500 µg/dl are potentially lethal. TIBC is not accurate in the face of acute iron poisoning. A leukocytosis has been found to correlate with elevated serum iron levels, but this has poor predictive values. A radiograph will demonstrate radiopaque iron tablets, but dissolved tablets may not be radiopaque.

5. **A,** Pages 1369-1370.

Iron salts bind very weakly to activated charcoal, and unless there is a co-ingestant, activated charcoal is not indicated. Induced emesis or gastric lavage is useful in acute poisoning although may be difficult because of the clumping of pills with resultant embedded fragments in the mucosal wall. Deferoxamine, whether given orally or intravenously, will chelate ferric iron, which can then be renally excreted.

6. **B,** Pages 1375-1376.

The ingestion of a single foreign body is unlikely to produce lead toxicity unless it is retained for longer than 2 weeks. If it does not pass, invasive procedures should be undertaken to reduce the risk of toxicity. Lead levels should be drawn initially to rule out chronic exposure. Chelation therapy is indicated in levels greater than 25 µg/dl.

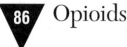

# 86 Opioids

### *David Hughes*

1. **A,** Pages 1380, 1381 (Table 86-1).

Although time to onset of both toxic and therapeutic effects will vary by agent, in general the effects are reached within 10 minutes by IV, 30 minutes with IM injection, and 90 minutes with subcutaneous injection or oral administration.

With this in mind, an observation period of 2 to 3 hours after ingestion in an asymptomatic patient is sufficient to discern the nontoxic nature of the ingestion. An important exception to this is diphenoxylate (Lomotil), which has a slower onset of action than other opioids.

2. **D,** Page 1380.

Narcotics are widely distributed throughout the body, resulting in low blood levels; this renders hemodialysis ineffective as a detoxifying method. Generally speaking, narcotics are not fat soluble. Important exceptions include propoxyphene (Darvon) and fentanyl, which therefore have a prolonged duration of action. Narcotics undergo a significant first-pass effect resulting in the dosing difference between orally and parenterally administered agents. Hepatic metabolism is fairly rapid (less than 8 hours), but certain agents such as methadone and diphenoxylate (Lomotil) are metabolized more slowly. Prolonged metabolism is also seen with hepatic disease and delayed gastric emptying.

3. **D,** Pages 1380-1382.

Despite its agonist effects, nalorphine enjoyed immense popularity until naloxone was developed. Nalorphine was capable of causing respiratory depression, miosis, and sedation through its agonist activities. Naloxone (Narcan) more closely resembles a pure antagonist by blocking the mu, kappa, and sigma receptors. Naltrexone is a new agent that may be administered orally and provides antagonist effects lasting up to 72 hours.

4. **E,** Pages 1382-1384.

Tolerance is common among addicts, resulting in the need to use higher doses. Certain exceptions to tolerance occur, including miosis and GI spasmogenic effects. Opioids cause analgesia and respiratory depression before a decrease in level of consciousness occurs; thus if the patient is truly unconscious, other causes should be sought. A patient experiencing narcotic overdose has slow, deep respirations with little change in tidal volume. The mechanism is a decrease in responsiveness of the respiratory center to rising arterial $CO_2$, while maintaining sensitivity to hypoxic stimuli. Opioids produce orthostatic hypotension with no effect on heart rate, heart rhythm, or blood pressure in the supine patient. The anticholinergic effects of meperidine may cause pupillary dilation.

5. **C,** Page 1383.

Noncardiogenic pulmonary edema never occurs after a therapeutic dose. The mechanism is unknown, but hypoxia-induced pulmonary edema is suspected. Even with treatment, the mortality rate approaches 20%.

6. **A,** Pages 1384, 1386-1388.

Nausea and vomiting are produced by central stimulation of the chemoreceptor trigger zone. Following stimulation the zone is depressed, making induction of emesis difficult. Convulsions are routine in children, but in adults indicate the use of specific agents such as meperidine or propoxyphene. Fentanyl and meperidine are known to cause twitching, increased tendon reflexes, and rigidity from increased neuromuscular tone. Opioids decrease GI transit, especially from the stomach as a result of increased duodenal tone. The ingested drug may therefore be accessible in the stomach by lavage or emesis for hours after ingestion.

7. **E,** Pages 1385-1386.

All the statements are true.

8. **D,** Page 1386.

Because of the delay in gastric emptying, activated charcoal should be given regardless of when the ingestion occurred. Naloxone is useful in oral narcotic overdoses even when signs and symptoms are absent, because it acts to decrease gastric emptying. Most ingestions involve combination agents, and an acetaminophen level as well as an acetylsalicylic acid level should also be obtained. All oral and parenteral overdoses should be observed for 12 to 24 hours.

9. **D,** Pages 1386-1388.

All may require high doses of naloxone because of a demonstrated resistance to reversal.

10. **C,** Pages 1386-1388 (Table 86-4).

Methadone is a long-acting agent. Overdoses may require a naloxone drip for up to 48 hours.

11. **D,** Page 1389.

Withdrawal from opioids differs from alcohol and barbiturate withdrawal in that the syndrome is very unpleasant but in the absence of severe underlying disease has no associated mortality. Very rarely is it necessary to administer opioids to an addict. Twenty to 30 days of sustained use are required before a patient is likely to show signs of withdrawal.

12. **D,** Page 1386.

The treatment of opioid overdose complicated by significant pulmonary edema should include a naloxone bolus followed by an infusion at two thirds the original bolus per hour. Oxygen via face mask in mild cases or via endotracheal tube in severe cases will be required. PEEP is rarely needed. Steroids and digitalis have not been found to have therapeutic use. Diuretic administration may cause severe hypotension and should be avoided.

13. **D,** Page 1386.

Toxic symptoms of propoxyphene ingestion can be seen at five times the therapeutic dose, and death is common in overdoses of 15 times the therapeutic dose. Collapse and death can occur within 15 minutes of ingestion and significant sequelae almost always occur within 2 hours. Large and repeated doses of naloxone are often required to treat respiratory depression and hypoxia. Naloxone does not have predictable effects on seizures or cardiovascular problems, and standard supportive treatment is recommended.

 **87** Lithium Intoxication

*David Hughes*

1. **E,** Pages 1392-1393.

Weakness, difficulty with attention and memory, and gastrointestinal distress may occur as side effects of lithium therapy and do not necessarily indicate toxicity. Lithium crosses cell membranes with difficulty and, as a result, the time to initial therapeutic effects and the half-life in the serum are prolonged.

2. **B,** Pages 1392-1393.

Dialysis rapidly clears the serum, but as lithium enters the serum from the cells, levels once again rise. Therefore, prolonged dialysis is needed. Activated charcoal is ineffective, and the value of forced saline diuresis appears limited. Patients with very high lithium levels (3.5-4 mEq/L), even without symptoms, are at grave risk and should be considered for dialysis. The patient with lithium toxicity often has mild hyperkalemia, with an ECG suggestive of hypokalemia.

3. **C,** Page 1392.

Lithium is entirely renally excreted and depends on the glomerular filtration rate and the rate of sodium reabsorption in the proximal tubules. Any situation that leads to decreased GFR or sodium depletion such as hypovolemia secondary to gastroenteritis will lead to reabsorption of lithium in the proximal tubules along with sodium. This may create toxic levels of lithium despite unchanged dosing.

4. **D,** Page 1392.

Lithium intoxication mimics hypokalemia on ECG, with flattened T-waves and nonspecific ST-T changes.

5. **E,** Page 1393.

All of these common medications have been found to increase lithium levels, mainly by increased renal reabsorption, especially the diuretics.

6. **A,** Page 1393.

Activated charcoal does not effectively bond lithium. Gastric lavage is indicated in patients with suspected large ingestions who arrive shortly after ingestion. Cation exchange resins such as Kayexalate have been found to reduce absorption of orally administered lithium. Whole-bowel irrigation may be useful, especially in situations in which slow-release lithium was ingested.

 **88** Neuroleptics

*David Hughes*

1. **B,** Pages 1395-1396.

Life-threatening dysrhythmias, including slow ventricular tachycardia, occasionally occur during routine therapy. Although phenothiazines lower the seizure threshold, they rarely produce seizures. Tardive dyskinesia occurs most commonly with the least potent neuroleptics and those with the greatest anticholinergic activity. The potential to produce acute dystonia is a result of the balance between cholinergic and dopaminergic input to the central neurons.

2. **C,** Pages 1395-1396.

Despite the predominance of anticholinergic effects in overdose, paradoxical miosis is common. Phenothiazines act as class 1A antidysrhythmics; therefore other class 1A agents are contraindicated. Phenytoin and lidocaine are effective, and magnesium should be used for torsades de pointes. Neuroleptic malignant syndrome is extremely rare but may occur following a single exposure to almost any neuroleptic. Respiratory depression is very unusual.

240

3. **D,** Page 1397 (Table 88-2).

Tardive dyskinesia results from prolonged neuroleptic use and may occur after cessation of long-term therapy as a result of the increased sensitivity of dopamine receptors. Akathisias (sometimes referred to as "motor restlessness"), dystonia (which can mimic tardive dyskinesia), and NMS all occur early in the course of neuroleptic use.

4. **D,** Page 1396.

The most serious adverse extrapyramidal side effect of neuroleptic use is NMS. The diagnosis is one of exclusion. NMS presents as hyperthermia, muscle rigidity, altered mental status and autonomic nervous system instability. There are multiple predisposing factors. Therapy consists of drug withdrawal, active cooling, and possibly neuroparalytic therapy for muscle rigidity.

5. **D,** Page 1399.

Patients with life-threatening adverse or overdose effects of neuroleptic agents, such as CNS or respiratory depression, hypotension, ventricular dysrhythmias, and NMS should be admitted to the ICU. Extrapyramidal side effects other than NMS and laryngeal dystonia rarely require hospitalization. It is recommended that anticholinergics be given by IV initially, because higher serum concentrations may thus be obtained; discharge and oral anticholinergics for 48 hours follow if symptoms improve.

# 89 Pesticides

### Lars Blomberg

1. **B,** Page 1402.

Because of their high lipid solubility, organophosphates are readily absorbed through the skin, GI tract, and respiratory tract and are also stored in fatty tissues. The organophosphates act as competitive inhibitors of acetylcholinesterase and cause build-up of acetylcholine at both muscarinic and nicotinic receptor sites. The build-up of acetylcholine causes general hypersecretion and a classic cholinergic syndrome. Morbidity and mortality are related to hypersecretion and bronchorrhea early, while hyperstimulation of skeletal muscles with fatigue and respiratory insufficiency occur later in the course.

2. **D,** Page 1404.

Cholinesterase levels should be obtained in both serum and red blood cells, because serum levels tend to fall first, with later decreases noted in the RBCs. Atropine, the definitive treatment agent, should be given early to reverse hypersecretion and prevent patients from "drowning in their own secretions." Two to 5 mg should be given IV every 5 minutes until the secretions are controlled. This may require 200 mg or more by IV in the first hour, followed by 50 mg/hr for several days. Pralidoxime chloride will break up the organophosphate-acetylcholinesterase complex and is usually given

in 1- to 2-mg IV doses dictated by serial cholinesterase levels. It may be necessary to treat for days or weeks because the pesticide continues to leach out of the adipose tissue.

3. **B,** Page 1405.

The carbamate insecticides are another class of acetylcholinesterase inhibitors that are differentiated from the organophosphates by their short duration of action. Treatment usually requires lower doses of atropine than in organophosphate poisoning, and pralidoxime is not indicated.

4. **E,** Pages 1405-1406.

Both DDT and lindane (Kwell) are well-known agents in this class. DDT was a popular insecticide until its ban in 1972. The chlorinated hydrocarbons act to irritate and excite neuronal membranes. Common signs and symptoms are seizures, which are generally the initial complaint, and myocardial irritability. Because of the high lipid solubility, chlorinated hydrocarbons are readily stored in adipose tissue.

5. **D,** Page 1406.

The diagnosis of chlorinated hydrocarbon poisoning relies heavily on clinical suspicion because laboratory results are not readily available and are unreliable. Treatment is mainly symptomatic for seizures and cardiac dysrhythmias. The cardiac instability is related to catecholamine hypersensitivity and should be treated with beta blockers, not antiarrhythmic agents. Because of high lipid solubility and wide distribution, hemodialysis should not be considered.

6. **B,** Page 1406.

Following seizure control and cardiac stabilization, treatment of chlorinated hydrocarbon poisonings is directed toward potential complications. Rhabdomyolysis and associated myoglobinuria, known to occur after seizures, could lead to renal dysfunction. Pralidoxime is used to treat organophosphate poisoning, not chlorinated hydrocarbon poisonings.

7. **A,** Pages 1406-1408.

The substituted phenols have found widespread popularity in many over-the-counter insecticides. In addition, they have been used for weight reduction, although they are no longer legal for this purpose. They act by uncoupling oxidative phosphorylation, which leads to hyperthermia, hypermetabolic states, ATP deficiency, and neurologic changes. They produce a yellow discoloration on contact with skin and organ surfaces. Those agents that substitute nitrogen may lead to methemoglobinemia.

8. **D,** Pages 1408-1409.

The best known chlorophenoxy compound is "agent orange." Other agents are relatively commonplace in over-the-counter herbicides. Skeletal muscle is the primary organ involved, with symptoms ranging from muscle weakness to acute rhabdomyolysis. High doses can cause uncoupling of oxidative phosphorylation similar to the substituted phenol pesticides. Symptoms develop quickly, and if the patient is asymptomatic after 6 to 8 hours, discharge is reasonable. Laboratory evaluation is not very helpful in diagnosing chlorophenoxy compound poisonings.

9. **D,** Pages 1409-1410.

Paraquat is a very corrosive agent that commonly causes chemical burns of the oropharynx. Although pulmonary injury is quite striking, its progression is generally slow, developing over 1 to 3 weeks. Mediastinitis following esophageal perforation is a frequent cause of death with ingestion. Treatment is geared toward decontamination using cleansing of contaminated skin surfaces, activated charcoal, and catharsis for oral ingestions, and rapid initiation of charcoal hemoperfusion to decrease serum levels.

10. **B,** Pages 1402, 1405-1408.

Many pesticides, including organophosphates, chlorinated hydrocarbons, and phenols, have very high lipid solubilities resulting in drug deposition in body fat. Over time, toxic systemic levels may accumulate with repeated exposures. In contrast, chlorophenoxy compounds have a very low lipid solubility, and cumulative toxicity does not occur.

11. **D,** Page 1406.

Ventricular dysrhythmias following chlorinated hydrocarbon exposure are most commonly due to high levels of catecholamines and should be treated with beta-antagonists. (e.g., propranolol, esmolol).

12. **D,** Pages 1410-1411.

Pyrethrins and pyrethroids are most commonly used as aerosols; therefore inhalation is the most common exposure. Only the natural pyrethrin-based aerosols are likely to cause allergic reactions; however, this severe asthma-like picture is the most serious possible complication. Cumulative toxicity is not found.

 # 90 Sedative-Hypnotics

*Lars Blomberg*

1. **C,** Pages 1413-1414.

Barbiturates induce hepatic microsomal enzymes, increasing the metabolism of such drugs as oral anticoagulants, digitoxin, doxycycline, tricyclic antidepressants, quinidine, theophylline, acetaminophen, and oral contraceptives. Barbiturates are active at the GABA receptor by opening the chloride channel, making excitatory depolarization more difficult. The reticular activating system in the brain stem, the cerebellum, and the cerebral cortex are the most sensitive areas in the CNS. The lower the lipid solubility, the longer the duration of action and the longer the onset of action.

2. **A,** Pages 1416-1417.

Forced alkaline diuresis will only enhance the renal clearance of long-acting barbiturates such as phenobarbital. Late gastric lavage (after 4-6 hours) may be beneficial, because barbiturates slow gastric emptying. Maximal extraction is accomplished by gastric lavage within 4 hours. Oral activated charcoal effectively absorbs barbiturates in the GI tract. Hemodialysis is most efficient for long-acting barbiturates but can be effective for short-acting agents. Indications for hemodialysis include a severe overdose, unstable vital signs regardless of resuscitative efforts, organ failure, potentially fatal doses, and prolonged coma.

3. **B,** Pages 1422-1423.

Unlike barbiturate ingestion, methaqualone use can create pyramidal tract signs such as myoclonus, hyperreflexia, and hypertonicity, which can progress to seizures. Diazepam will treat both the hypertonicity and the seizures. Barbiturate anticonvulsants are contraindicated. Methaqualone ingestion causes a less severe respiratory depression than barbiturates. Abstinence syndrome occurs in both types of ingestions, and the presentation and the treatment are almost identical. Forced alkaline diuresis is ineffective in methaqualone and short-acting barbiturate ingestions, because the drugs are metabolized primarily in the liver with very little renal clearance.

4. **B,** Pages 1420-1421

All of the listed sedative-hypnotic drugs were popularized in the 1950s-1960s as safe, nonaddicting medications. Methaqualone, glutethimide, methyprylon, and ethchlorvynol all had early recognizable abuse potential. The glutethimide-codeine combination is used as an oral substitute for heroin, because it produces a cheap, long-lasting euphoria. Glutethimide has anticholinergic effects that produce dilated, unreactive pupils and grand mal seizures; otherwise its clinical occurrence and management are similar to the barbiturates.

5. **C,** Pages 1418-1419.

Chloral hydrate has prominent side effects, which include GI irritation such as nausea and vomiting, gastritis, and cases of transmural gastric necrosis and esophageal stricture. Chloral hydrate is similar to other halogenated hydrocarbons and appears to sensitize the myocardium to circulating catecholamines, producing dysrhythmias. Supraventricular and ventricular tachyarrhythmias are the most common. Chloral hydrate is rapidly metabolized in the liver by alcohol dehydrogenase, which produces the active metabolite trichloroethanol. Trichloroethanol inhibits the breakdown of ethanol, while ethanol aids the production of trichloroethanol, producing a synergistic reaction. The popular combination of the two drugs alcohol and chloral hydrate is referred to as a "Mickey Finn" or as "knockout drops."

6. **A,** Pages 1423-1424.

Over-the-counter nighttime sleep aids (OTC-NSAs) usually contain the antihistamines diphenhydramine and doxylamine with hypnotic, antihistaminic, anticholinergic, and local anesthetic properties. The patient described has symptoms indicating anticholinergic toxicity, especially the dry skin and absent bowel sounds. Hyperthermia is treated with ice water bath or evaporative cooling. Dantrolene, used for malignant hyperthermia, has no support for its use in anticholinergic toxicity. Physostigmine is a controversial agent in the management of anticholinergic overdoses, mainly because it has potent side effects such as bradycardia. If it is used, physostigmine should be infused slowly in repeated doses and never as a continuous infusion. Cardiopulmonary arrest has been reported in children, who are more likely to arrive at the ED with CNS excitation, usually delirium or confusion.

7. **A,** Page 1425.

Unique characteristics of a bromide toxic ingestion are pseudohyperchloremia and a low anion gap. The falsely elevated level of chloride is due to the laboratory's inability to differentiate the positive interference of other halides.

8. **A,** Page 1418.

Symptoms of phenobarbital withdrawal usually begin 10-14 days after birth. This late onset of symptoms is thought to be due the poorly developed renal and hepatic function in neonates. The other symptoms listed are all common with neonatal withdrawal syndrome.

9. **C,** Page 1424.

Cardiac toxicity secondary to antihistamine toxicity is rare. When it occurs, QT prolongation and QRS widening are most likely due to quinidine-like effects. Following antihistamine poisoning, children usually present with CNS agitation or delirium.

10. **C,** Pages 1413-1414.

Barbiturate duration of action depends on several factors including lipid solubility, protein binding, and pKa. In general, short acting and intermediate acting barbiturates are more lipid soluble than long acting. Rosen Box 90-1 lists some barbiturates based on duration of action.

# 91 Cocaine, Amphetamines, and Other Sympathomimetics

*Lars Blomberg*

1. **A,** Page 1438.

Forced acid diuresis is no longer recommended because the risk of acute tubular necrosis from rhabdomyolysis is thought to outweigh any benefit from increased renal excretion. All of the other answers are recommended in the appropriate setting.

2. **A,** Page 1432.

The most common complaint is altered mental status, usually intoxication with euphoria. In one series, 40 of 137 patients had altered mental status alone whereas another 17 had altered mental status and some other complaint. Other complaints were chest pain in 17, syncope in 15, suicide attempt in 13, palpitations in 12, and seizures in 3.

3. **D,** Pages 1435-1436.

Although most cocaine users will have a normal urine drug screen in 1 to 3 days after use, a large dose can take 10 to 20 days before a negative test result is obtained. Although serum cocaine level can confirm the presence of cocaine, it does not help with management, which is symptomatic. Cocaine can cause virtually any tachyarrhythmia but none is pathognomonic. Urine should be checked for blood, which can indicate myoglobinuria and the accompanying risk of renal failure. Ninety percent of body packers will have positive plain films locating the cocaine-filled condoms, which should be removed in the operating room.

4. **D,** Pages 1431-1433.

Although 80% of chest pain in cocaine users is noncardiac, there is a real risk of infarct even in a patient known to have normal coronary arteries. An elevated CPK is not definitive, because only 5 of 19 cocaine patients with chest pain and an elevated CPK proved to have an infarction. Thrombolytics must be used with caution because of the increased risk of intracerebral bleeds from mycotic aneurysms. Besides myocardial ischemia there are many important causes of chest pain that must be considered, including pulmonary infarction, endocarditis, and pneumothorax.

5. **D,** Pages 1429-1430.

Of the drugs listed, MDMA (ecstasy) is not conducive to regular or frequent use because tolerance develops quickly to the positive effects and the negative effects increase with use.

6. **A,** Page 1433.

Although nausea, vomiting, and abdominal pain have all been reported, in general gastrointestinal symptoms are uncommon with sympathomimetic ingestions. Caffeine is an important exception; it can cause significant abdominal symptoms. Symptomatology often results after ingestions of 0.5 to 1.0 gm.

7. **C,** Page 1436.

Because of the short half-life of cocaine, patients presenting to the emergency department with immediate hypertension or tachycardia may be observed or treated with benzodiazepines. Atrial and ventricular tachycardias unresponsive to sedation should be treated with beta-blockers. Initially, lidocaine may increase toxicity because of its similarity to cocaine; however, ventricular dysrhythmias presenting several hours after cocaine use are thought to more likely represent cardiac ischemia, and lidocaine is believed to be appropriate.

# 92 Toxic Inhalations

*Lars Blomberg*

1. **B,** Page 1447.

The half-life of carboxyhemoglobin is 4 to 6 hours when breathing room air, 90 minutes at an $FiO_2$ of 21% at 1 atm, and 30 minutes at the typical hyperbaric level of 100% at 3 atm.

2. **A,** Pages 1447-1448.

Carboxyhemoglobin shifts the oxygen dissociation curve to the left. Because of the effects on oxygen delivery, patients with dyshemoglobinemias are far more symptomatic than patients whose oxygen delivery capacity is decreased secondary to blood loss. $Po_2$ is unaffected by CO poisoning, and carboxyhemoglobin is misinterpreted as oxyhemoglobin by pulse oximetry. Serum carboxyhemoglobin levels do not correlate well with toxicity.

3. **A,** Page 1448.

Because fetal hemoglobin has a higher affinity for carboxyhemoglobin, the fetus is exposed to hypoxia after the mother's carboxyhemoglobin has returned to normal. Fetal carbon monoxide poisoning has been associated with demise, and hyperbaric therapy is relatively safe in pregnancy. Therefore some authors recommend dropping the standard for hyperbaric therapy in pregnancy.

4. **D,** Page 1450.

This patient may be suffering from carbon monoxide and/or cyanide poisoning. Treatment with the nitrite components of the antidote kit will produce methemoglobin, which could be disastrous in the non-cyanide-poisoned patient with high carboxyhemoglobin levels. However, failure to treat the cyanide-poisoned patient may be fatal. Treatment with sodium thiosulfate may be sufficient to stabilize a cyanide-poisoned patient while the carboxyhemoglobin level reading is pending. Once the carboxyhemoglobin level is known, the remainder of the cyanide antidote kit may be given. It should be given after hyperbaric therapy is started if the carboxyhemoglobin level is high.

5. **A,** Page 1450.

Laryngeal edema and cardiac arrest are both associated with a high incidence of noncardiogenic pulmonary edema (NCPE). Ozone, phosgene, and ammonia are pulmonary irritants, but of the three, only ammonia is rarely associated with NCPE. Sulfur dioxide and chloramine are also pulmonary irritants rarely associated with NCPE.

6. **B,** Pages 1445, 1447-1448.

Although rare, red skin may be found with carbon monoxide or cyanide poisoning. Bullae may be found with carbon monoxide poisoning. Amyl nitrate causes methemoglobin, which typically causes "chocolate cyanosis." Cyanide and hydrogen sulfide may be associated with bright red venous blood as the oxygen extraction falls. Phosgene is a pulmonary irritant that is associated with delayed noncardiogenic pulmonary edema.

7. **B,** Page 1444.

Exposure to carbon tetrachloride, a respiratory depressant, results in hypoventilation, retention of carbon dioxide, and respiratory acidosis. The A-a gradient, however, is unaffected. Because carbon tetrachloride sensitizes the myocardium to catecholamines, administration of epinephrine or norepinephrine may exaggerate dysrhythmias. Complications are usually related to hypoxia, and treatment is supportive.

8. **D,** Pages 1445-1446.

Hydrogen chloride is a highly water soluble pulmonary irritant. Exposure generally results in immediate irritation of mucous membranes and upper airways. Nebulized sodium bicarbonate may be helpful through neutralization of the hydrochloric acid produced in the alveoli, although beta-agonists are the treatment of choice for patients with bronchospasm. NCPE is unlikely, but if present, corticosteroids are generally not indicated.

9. **B,** Pages 1443, 1449.

ABG, CXR, and EKG are all essential diagnostic tests to be performed on a patient with a presumed toxic inhalation. Because amyl nitrite inhalers are relatively inefficient, if IV access has already been established the physician can move im-

mediately to administration of sodium nitrite in cases of cyanide poisoning.

 **93** Benzodiazepines

*Lars Blomberg*

1. **D,** Page 1453.

All benzodiazepines are highly bound to plasma albumin. Diazepam is a benzodiazepine that is rapidly distributed from the blood to fatty tissues, causing the prompt termination of drug effect. Cimetidine and ethanol (each inhibits the cytochrome P-450 enzyme system) alter the metabolism of benzodiazepines. Several benzodiazepines are metabolized to active metabolites that produce pharmacologic effects.

2. **D,** Page 1454.

Tachycardia is typical, but hypotension is rare. Profound coma suggests a concomitant depressant ingestion. Hyperreflexia is commonly seen.

3. **A,** Pages 1454-1455.

Flumazenil is effective in mixed benzodiazepine and ethanol overdoses. Hypotension, marked respiratory depression, and profound coma would be consistent with an overdose of a benzodiazepine and a large quantity of ethanol.

4. **B,** Page 1455.

Flumazenil may precipitate a severe withdrawal reaction in chronic benzodiazepine users. It may precipitate seizures. Recovery is rapid, usually within 5 minutes, when flumazenil is given to reverse benzodiazepine sedation and coma. The recommended dosage is 0.1-0.2 mg intravenously initially with incremental additional doses of 0.1 mg to a total of 2 mg.

5. **D,** Page 1456.

Benzodiazepine withdrawal is difficult to distinguish from the original anxiety disorder. Withdrawal can result in rebound, which is an exacerbation of the original symptoms being treated. Withdrawal symptoms are seen 1 to 11 days (average 3 to 4 days) after drug discontinuation. Gradual discontinuation prevents severe withdrawal symptoms.

6. **C,** Page 1456.

Buspirone lacks the muscle relaxant and anticonvulsant properties of benzodiazepines. It has minimal interaction with ethanol. There is no evidence for development of tolerance or a withdrawal syndrome.

7. **C,** Page 1453.

Benzodiazepines metabolized primarily by oxidation are affected by changes in the hepatic cytochrome P-450 pathway. These include all of the answers listed except lorazepam.

8. **C,** Page 1453.

Drugs with short half-lives do not sustain high tissue concentrations and therefore do not produce physical dependence. Long-acting benzodiazepines are eliminated slowly and cause only mild withdrawal symptoms. In contrast, drugs with intermediate half-lives can produce severe and rapid withdrawal symptoms.

9. **D,** Pages 1454-1455.

Rosen Table 93-3 lists the contraindications for flumazenil. Flumazenil administration is particularly helpful in co-ingestions with alcohol.

# 94 Dyspnea

### Michael S. Buchsbaum and Leonard A. Nitowski

1. **D,** Page 1461.

The vagus nerve transmits sensory information from the airways. Motor control of respiration involves the diaphragm (phrenic nerve), intercostal muscles (T1 to T12), scalene muscles (C4 to C8), and sternocleidomastoid muscles (spinal accessory nerve). Damage to any component of this system may impair respirations.

2. **B,** Page 1463.

Generally, a pleural effusion large enough to impair respirations will take several days to develop. The other conditions may occur suddenly, including a COPD exacerbation after exposure to allergens. The exception is a pleural effusion after a traumatic event (hemothorax), which requires chest tube drainage.

3. **C,** Pages 1465-1466.

This patient has several significant findings of acute CHF, including dyspnea, orthopnea, high blood pressure, and a paradoxical split second heart sound. Wheezing is not specific to asthma and can be seen in COPD and CHF (i.e. "cardiac asthma").

4. **B,** Page 1466.

Patients with COPD often have cor pulmonale.

5. **A,** Page 1447.

Headache is a prominent symptom of carbon monoxide poisoning.

6. **D,** Page 1466.

Perioral tingling is seen often in hyperventilation syndromes.

7. **C,** Page 1466.

An $S_3$ gallop is characteristic of an overloaded ventricle in congestive heart failure.

8. **E,** Pages 1463 to 1468.

Although the most common findings of pulmonary embolus are chest pain (88%), tachypnea (82%), and dyspnea (84%), it is an important cause of syncope that always needs consideration.

9. **A,** Page 1465.

High-altitude pulmonary edema occurs with rapid ascent to elevations above 3000 meters. Signs and symptoms include dyspnea, fatigue, dry cough, cyanosis, tachypnea, and tachycardia. The most effective treatment is oxygen therapy and immediate descent.

10. **C,** Page 1466.

This individual has signs of significant cor pulmonale (right-sided heart failure) with jugular venous distention and pretibial edema. The symptoms are consistent with both congestive heart failure secondary to cardiomyopathy and exacerbation of COPD; however, clear lungs would be an unlikely finding in CHF. Further evaluation of this patient should include a chest radiograph to differentiate the two conditions. With COPD, the causes of acute exacerbation must be evaluated.

# 95 Adult Acute Asthma

### Kenneth D. Katz and Gordon D. Reed

1. **E,** Page 1470.

Increases in asthma morbidity and mortality have been reported in the United States as well as other countries since the early 1970s. For example, in 1977, 1674 deaths were caused by asthma in all ages in the U.S.; deaths rose to 3564 in 1984 and then 5106 in 1991. Increases in mortality due to asthma were also seen in the late 70s and 80s in New Zealand, Australia, England, and France. The death rate is also higher in certain populations; African-Americans and urban dwellers are among those at highest risk. In addition, the factors mentioned in responses A through D have also contributed to the increased asthma mortality. For a variety of reasons, including some of those cited above, low socioeconomic status is believed to predispose to higher rates of asthma deaths.

2. **A,** Pages 1472-1473.

Extrinsic (allergic) asthma is characterized by a well-defined sensitivity to specific allergens, a family history of allergic disease, increased IgE levels, and positive skin tests. The immunologic response in allergic asthma may be divided into early and late responses. The early response has been shown to be mast cell dependent and is best treated with beta-agonist therapy. The late response is mainly inflammatory, with an influx of neutrophils, eosinophils, and mononuclear cells into the bronchoalveolar tissue. Consequently, therapy directed against the inflammatory reaction in the form of steroids may alleviate the late phase of asthma.

3. **C,** Page 1475.

Aspirin-induced bronchospasm has been described since the early 1900s. The typical patient is female in the third to fourth decade of life, who develops intense vasomotor rhinitis and, later, chronic nasal congestion. The physical examination reveals nasal polyps. Subsequently, the patient develops asthma and aspirin sensitivity. Acute attacks usually begin shortly after aspirin ingestion (minutes to hours) and are characterized by rhinorrhea, conjunctival infection, and flushing of the head and neck. Shock may occur with as little as 300 mg of aspirin ingestion. There is cross-reactivity with many NSAIDs, and, recently, acetaminophen has been demonstrated to induce bronchospasm in the poorly controlled aspirin-sensitive patient. The mechanism is thought to be related to inhibition of cyclooxygenase rather than IgE mediated.

4. **A,** Page 1477.

Most patients with asthma have cough, dyspnea, and wheezing. The cough is probably generated from subepithelial vagal stimulation; it starts early and can be associated with a sense of chest tightness. Dyspnea may represent the awareness of disproportionate inspiratory effort for a given ventilatory output. Wheezing depends on air movement velocity and turbulence. Severe obstruction results in the disappearance of wheezing and should alert the emergency physician to impending respiratory failure.

5. **E,** Page 1487.

Intubation of the asthmatic patient requires that certain principles be followed. Airway pressures should be kept low by providing low tidal volumes (<10 cc/kg) and low respiratory rates (<10 breaths/min) to prevent auto-PEEP and stacking of breaths, thus minimizing barotrauma. In addition, prolonged inspiratory to expiratory ratios may be implemented to allow the patient to exhale since the problem is one of airway obstruction. Muscle paralysis may be implemented to sedate the patient. Additional agents such as aminophylline, ketamine, and isoflurane may be given for bronchodilation.

6. **A,** Page 1482.

The correct dosage of subcutaneous epinephrine is 0.2-0.5 cc, 1:1000, given every 20-30 minutes as needed for a total of three doses. The intravenous dosing of epinephrine is 2-10 cc, 1:10,000, given over 5 minutes, which may be repeated for severe asthmatic attacks. Epinephrine, an endogenous catecholamine, possesses both alpha and beta effects and can generate tachycardia, hypertension, arrhythmias, and vasoconstriction; it can be used in an attempt to avert intubation of the severely asthmatic patient.

7. **C,** Pages 1478-1480.

There are clinical as well as objective parameters, that may be implemented to evaluate the severity of an asthma attack. Presence of wheezing indicates not only bronchoconstriction but also that there is enough airflow to generate sound. Thus absence of wheezing in the patient in extremis should alert the emergency physician that intubation may be needed. Initially, as the asthmatic experiences dyspnea and tachypnea, a respiratory alkalosis will be seen. However, as the attack progresses and further airway obstruction occurs, the patient may not be able to release $CO_2$, and normalization of the arterial blood gas occurs despite the patient's increased ventilatory efforts. This worsening clinical picture correlates to the $FEV_1$; normalization of the $PaCO_2$ occurs at the $FEV_1$ of 15%-25% predicted, and eventual respiratory acidosis occurs at a $FEV_1$ of <15% predicted.

8. **E,** Page 1480.

In patients with a good clinical response to initial therapy (PEFR, $FEV_1$ >70% predicted) disposition includes observation for 30-60 minutes and discharge with close follow-up and on appropriate outpatient medications. For patients with an incomplete response (PEFR, $FEV_1$ >40%-<70% predicted) continued beta-agonist therapy and subcutaneous epinephrine or terbutaline should be administered. Clinical and objective monitoring should occur every 30-60 minutes

with reassessment at 4 hours. At that point, a decision can be made regarding hospitalization. Magnesium sulfate is generally reserved for severe non-responding acute asthma attacks in an attempt to avoid intubation.

9. **C,** Page 1483.

Steroids are an integral part of asthma therapy and have been shown not only to reduce relapses after treatment of acute exacerbations of asthma, but also to reduce hospitalization rates. Methylprednisolone is the intravenous drug of choice and is five times more potent as an antiinflammatory agent than hydrocortisone. Hydrocortisone has marked mineralocorticoid activity, resulting in sodium retention. There has been no evidence that intravenous steroids are more effective than the oral forms, but the intravenous form can be used in patients who are extremely ill or cannot swallow. Oral steroid therapy includes prednisone and prednisolone; prednisone is converted to prednisolone via hepatic metabolism.

10. **D,** Page 1485.

Theophylline may be used as adjunct therapy in severe asthmatics, since it possesses bronchodilatory properties. The correct loading dose of aminophylline is 5-6 mg/kg actual body weight over 20 minutes IV, with each 1 mg/kg of aminophylline raising the serum level approximately 2 μg/ml. The optimal serum level is 10-20 μg/ml. Theophylline has a rather narrow therapeutic window, and many side effects, including nausea, vomiting, nervousness, headache, arrhythmias, CNS disturbances, and metabolic abnormalities may be seen. In addition, medications that affect hepatic metabolism can affect theophylline levels; the drugs listed in response E will decrease serum levels. Ciprofloxacin, erythromycin, clarithromycin, cimetidine, propranolol, allopurinol, and the influenza A vaccine may all increase serum levels. Recent studies reveal that the IV route shows no advantage over oral ingestion (aminophylline dose × 0.80 = theophylline dose) in mild to moderate asthma. A therapeutic serum concentration of theophylline can be achieved rapidly by the oral route using the alcohol-based elixir of theophylline.

11. **C,** Page 1487.

It is important for the emergency physician to understand how to use the metered dose inhaler (MDI) so that the patient can be instructed to take the inhaler correctly. The correct sequence to use the MDI includes assembling the MDI, shaking the canister, placing the mouth piece between the teeth, exhaling, actuating the inhaler at the beginning of a slow inhalation and then holding the breath for at least 10 seconds.

12. **D,** Pages 2395, 2404.

In pregnancy, one third of asthmatics will improve, one third will remain the same, and another third will become worse. Terbutaline can be used in pregnancy but can inhibit uterine contractions. Corticosteroids are safe in pregnant patients. Theophylline use may result in adverse fetal effects because it crosses the placenta, but it has not been linked to fetal abnormalities. Epinephrine, however, has been associated with an increased incidence of fetal malformations.

13. **B,** Page 1484.

Ipratropium bromide is an anticholinergic medication used in the treatment of asthma. The drug's effects are exerted by blocking the smooth muscle constrictor and secretory consequences of the parasympathetic nervous system. Ipratropium bromide's bronchodilatory effects are less potent and slower than those of a beta-agonist and, consequently, should not be used alone in treating a severe asthmatic. Nebulization with ipratropium and a beta-agonist alone. The correct dose of ipratropium is 0.25-0.5 mg via wet nebulization. Ipratropium bromide should be used as a first-line agent added to the beta-agonists (mixed together in the same nebulizer) for patients with severe bronchoconstriction.

14. **B,** Page 2396.

The Collaborative Perinatal Project demonstrated a significant rise in the incidence of congenital anomalies in mothers receiving epinephrine. As a result, this agent should be avoided in pregnant asthmatics. Steroids and anticholinergics have been shown to be safe in pregnancy. Beta-agonists should be used as first-line therapy, and supplemental oxygen should be implemented early to avoid hypoxemia.

15. **E,** Page 1482.

Terbutaline is a beta-2 specific, long-acting adrenergic agent with bronchodilatory effects equivalent to epinephrine in acute or stable asthma. Epinephrine is the agent of choice for suspected allergic asthma. Medication doses administered by inhalation are much lower when compared with equipotent oral or intravenous doses, and terbutaline provides much more specific delivery with rapid onset. Recent studies indicate that subcutaneous terbutaline is less effective than nebulized albuterol as initial therapy for asthma.

16. **C,** Pages 1483-1484.

Ipratropium bromide, which may be more effective in patients over 40 years of age, is effective in reversing bronchospasm secondary to beta-blocking agents and is particularly useful in patients with psychologic factors contributing to asthma. Anticholinergic therapy should not be used as first-line therapy but should be considered for its additive effect in someone who is on maximal beta-agonist therapy or who cannot tolerate adrenergic side effects. Theophylline therapy in acute asthma should be reserved for patients not responding to beta-agonist and steroid therapy. Hydrocortisone has marked mineralocorticoid properties that result in sodium retention. Magnesium sulfate should be used in patients with severe, nonresponding asthma.

17. **B,** Page 1485.

The loading dose for the listed conditions will be equivalent, but maintenance doses should be reduced for patients with liver dysfunction. Other conditions requiring lower theophylline maintenance doses include age over 50, congestive heart failure, and COPD.

18. **D,** Page 1485.

Theophylline possesses weak to medium bronchodilatory effects of an uncertain mechanism. Other pharmacologic properties of the methylxanthines include enhancing diuresis, cardiac output, mucociliary clearance, ventilatory drive, and contractility of the diaphragm. The methylxanthines also inhibit release of inflammatory mediators, reduce systemic and pulmonary resistance, and suppress microvascular permeability.

---

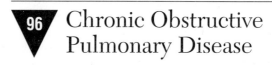

# 96 Chronic Obstructive Pulmonary Disease

### *Janice K. Balas and Gordon D. Reed*

1. **C,** Page 1498.

The ability to speak in only phrases or short sentences, diaphoresis, use of accessory muscles of respiration, visible retractions, and high-pitched wheezes on auscultation are all signs of worsening respiratory status. However, a silent chest on auscultation indicates that very little air exchange is taking place and is an extremely worrisome finding.

2. **B,** Pages 1501-1503.

In bronchitis, hypoxia, hypercapnia, and acidosis all produce pulmonary artery vasoconstriction. This combines with increased blood viscosity to produce chronic right-sided heart strain, termed cor pulmonale. The bronchitis patient's blood pressure is normal or even slightly elevated. Chronic ventilatory failure and cor pulmonale account for the prominent peripheral edema. Heat intolerance, along with anorexia and insomnia, become prominent symptoms in stage D emphysema.

3. **C,** Pages 1501, 1503.

In emphysema, there is gross lung overinflation, giving rise to a low, immobile diaphragm and increased anteroposterior (AP) diameter of the thorax. In bronchitis, the thorax AP diameter is normal, and the diaphragm is not abnormally low. There is normal lung volume, minimal or modest hyperaeration of upper lung fields, coarse reticulation of lower lung fields, and a slightly enlarged globular cardiac silhouette. Most importantly, impingement on the retrosternal airspace by the enlarged right ventricle can be seen on the lateral film. Neither emphysema nor bronchitis classically elevates the diaphragm.

4. **E,** Page 1507.

Acutely ill patients not previously taking aminophylline should receive approximately 5 mg/kg IV over 10-15 minutes to achieve the desired low therapeutic level of 10 mg/ml. Therefore a 70-kg patient should receive a loading dose of 5 mg/kg × 70 kg, or 350 mg.

5. **B,** Page 1507.

Administration of 1 mg/kg of aminophylline results in approximately a 2 mg/ml increment in blood level. The observed level is 6 mg/ml, and the desired level is approximately 10 mg/ml. The blood level must be increased by 4 mg/ml, which would be accomplished with a dose of 2 mg/kg, or 140 mg.

6. **B,** Page 1507.

The dose is 0.5 mg/hr in adults without impaired liver function. Reduced doses may be needed in patients who are also taking erythromycin, ciprofloxacin, or histamine blockers, or who have liver failure, alcoholism, or heart failure.

7. **C,** Page 1497.

The antibiotics neomycin and kanamycin can affect neuromuscular function by interfering with motor end-plate activity.

8. **B,** Page 1498.

Aspirin can induce bronchospasm.

9. **D,** Page 1498.

Alcohol is a cause of respiratory depression.

10. **B,** Page 1507.

Acetylcysteine can also induce bronchospasm.

11. **A,** Page 1507.

Ciprofloxacin may cause increased blood aminophylline levels.

12. **D,** Page 1508.

MAT can be seen in COPD patients and can be confused with atrial fibrillation. It should be treated (beyond initial measures to maximize pulmonary function and correct any possible electrolyte disturbances) if the patient is suffering from hemodynamic compromise, CHF, or ischemia. Two drug regimens are acceptable. A cardioselective beta-blocker such as metoprolol may be used in doses of 2 to 3 mg IV every 2 to 3 minutes to a total dose of 15 mg. As an alternative, verapamil may be used in doses of 2.5 to 5.0 mg every 2 to 4 minutes to a total dose of 15 mg. Pretreatment with calcium may help avoid hypotension. Propranolol is not cardioselective and may possibly cause worsening of bronchospasm.

13. **D,** Page 1508.

Cor pulmonale (right heart failure) occurs in COPD secondary to chronic lung disease. Theophylline is the only medication listed that has been found to be of possible benefit in pulmonary vasodilation. Calcium channel blockers, ACE inhibitors, and alpha-blockers have not been found to be effective.

14. **B,** Pages 1499-1503.

See answer to Question 25.

15. **A,** Pages 1499-1503.

See answer to Question 25.

16. **D,** Pages 1499-1503.

See answer to Question 25.

17. **C,** Pages 1499-1503.

See answer to Question 25.

18. **B,** Pages 1499-1503.

See answer to Question 25.

19. **A,** Pages 1499-1503.

See answer to Question 25.

20. **A,** Pages 1499-1503.

See answer to Question 25.

21. **A,** Pages 1499-1503.

See answer to Question 25.

22. **C,** Pages 1499-1503.

See answer to Question 25.

23. **A,** Pages 1499-1503.

See answer to Question 25.

24. **D,** Pages 1499-1503.

See answer to Question 25.

25. **A,** Pages 1499-1503.

Emphysema is irreversible. The patient hyperventilates and is typically thin, anxious, alert and oriented, dyspneic, and tachypneic. Dyspnea is the hallmark. The pathognomonic posture of pursed lips on expiration (puffing) increases intraluminal bronchial pressure and supports bronchial walls that have otherwise lost their elastic support. The patient assumes a sedentary existence. Supporting the torso with the elbows on the knees produces the subtle but characteristic signs of tanning and induration of the skin just proximal to the knees.

In chronic bronchitis, a cough is prominent and is the hallmark. The bronchitis patient has a normal or slightly elevated blood pressure and an increased cardiac output. The hypoxemia that develops will, over time, produce polycythemia, which increases blood viscosity. Hypoxia is seen in both the emphysema and bronchitic patients. Cor pulmonale may also develop in both; however, it is more commonly associated with bronchitis.

Wheezing is the hallmark of asthma. Electrocardiographic changes are not specific for COPD but can be suggestive. Right ventricular hypertrophy suggests established cor pulmonale. "P pulmonale" suggests COPD. However, the classic descriptions of low RS voltage, clockwise rotation, and poor R wave progression are interesting correlates of COPD, but both are insensitive and nonspecific findings.

 ## 97 Pleural Disease

### *Martin A. Bennett and Robert A. Rosenbaum*

1. **B,** Page 1513.

*Pneumocystis carinii* pneumonia is commonly associated with secondary pneumothorax. In patients taking pentamidine the incidence is 5%. The mechanism appears to involve rupture of necrotic lung tissue, which results from an inflammatory response to *Pneumocystis*. Bilateral pneumothoraces and delayed re-expansion are common complications. Treatment is therefore tube thoracostomy, not simple aspiration.

2. **C,** Page 1511.

The incidence of primary spontaneous pneumothorax is 2.5 to 18 per 100,000. After the first pneumothorax has occurred, the risk of another is 23%-30%.

3. **B,** Page 1511.

Secondary pneumothorax occurs most commonly in the 50 and older age-group, particularly in smokers with COPD. Acute bronchitis is not associated with pneumothorax. Tuberculosis, lung cancer, and pneumonia are all associated with increased risk but less so than COPD.

4. **E,** Page 1511

Primary pneumothorax occurs most commonly in young, tall, healthy men. 65% occur in the 20- to 40-year-old age-group. It should be noted that, overall, pneumothorax is more common during the neonatal period than any other time in life (occurring in up to 2% of neonates), but this is often secondary to barotrauma from positive pressure ventilation and resuscitation efforts required for mucous, meconium, or RDS in these neonates.

**248**

5. **B,** Page 1514.

Chest pain is the most common symptom associated with spontaneous pneumothorax, occurring in 90% of cases. Dyspnea is present in 80%, and cough in only 10%. Anxiety and weakness occur less frequently.

6. **B,** Page 1518.

The definitive diagnosis is by chest x-ray. A significant pneumothorax is a 20% loss in lung volume by chest x-ray. Beyond this point, shunting of arterial blood past non-ventilated lung occurs, causing a significant A-a gradient.

7. **C,** Page 1514.

In the COPD patient, pneumothorax often presents with dyspnea and anxiety out of proportion to the degree of collapse, often without significant chest pain. The classic physical signs of decreased breath sounds, hyperresonance to percussion, and decreased chest wall movement may be absent or simply attributed to the underlying lung disease. Mortality is up to 16%.

8. **B,** Page 1521.

The most common cause of pleural effusion is congestive heart failure, which usually causes a bilateral transudate. Features of a transudative effusion include (p. 1523) LDH <200 Units, fluid-to-blood LDH ratio <0.6, and fluid-to-blood protein ratio <0.5. A transudative pleural effusion is seen in 30%-50% of patients with pulmonary embolism.

9. **C,** Page 1525.

The parietal pleura is richly innervated by somatic sensory nerves, and inflammation leads to localized pain. With central diaphragmatic involvement, pain may be referred to the neck or shoulder via the phrenic nerve (C3-C5). Pulmonary embolism frequently presents with pleuritic chest pain and must always be considered in the differential diagnosis of pleuritis. Bornholm disease is caused by Coxsackie virus infection. Indomethacin or other nonsteroidal agents are the treatment of choice for idiopathic pleuritis. Opiates should be avoided because of associated decreased respirations, level of consciousness, and cough reflex.

10. **D,** Page 1526.

Three clinical features which help distinguish pulmonary embolus from viral pleuritis include pleural effusion on chest x-ray, risk factors or history of DVT or PE, and physical signs of phlebitis. Tachypnea, low grade fever, decreased $PO_2$, and abrupt onset of pleuritic chest pain may be present in either PE or viral pleuritis.

11. **B,** Page 1522.

The most common cause of exudative pleural effusion is bacterial pneumonia. Usual causative agents include *Streptococcus pneumoniae*, anaerobes, *Staphylococcus*, *Klebsiella*, and *Pseudomonas*. Less commonly, *Mycoplasma* and viral agents cause effusions, but these tend to be small and serous. *E. coli* is not a common causative agent in pleural effusions.

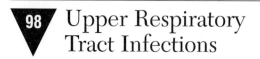

# 98 Upper Respiratory Tract Infections

*Dana A. Ger and Robert A. Rosenbaum*

1. **C,** Page 1529.

Epiglottitis has a bimodal age distribution of 1-4 and 20-40 years old. Older adults may also have epiglottitis; therefore age alone should not be used to exclude the diagnosis.

2. **A,** Page 1529.

*Haemophilus influenzae* is the most commonly isolated bacterial pathogen causing epiglottitis, however; in most cases no organisms can be cultured from the blood or supraglottic structures.

3. **B,** Page 1529.

The prodrome in epiglottitis resembles that of a benign upper respiratory tract infection, with fever and cervical lymphadenopathy. The prodrome usually lasts 1-2 days but may last from several hours to 7 days. Hoarseness is not found because inflammation does not extend below the vocal cords. Pharyngeal pain may be severe and out of proportion to clinical findings.

4. **C,** Page 1531.

Apart from airway management, initial treatment includes supplemental humidified oxygen, IV hydration, and monitoring. Antibiotics should include *Haemophilus influenzae* coverage with cefotaxime or ceftriaxone.

5. **D,** Page 1532.

In chronic pharyngitis, the tonsillar crypts rather than the tonsils themselves are involved.

6. **B,** Pages 1532-1533.

See answer to Question 12.

7. **D,** Pages 1532-1533.

See answer to Question 12.

8. **G,** Pages 1532-1533.

See answer to Question 12.

9. **E,** Pages 1532-1533.

See answer to Question 12.

10. **F,** Pages 1532-1533.

See answer to Question 12.

11. **A,** Pages 1532-1533.

See answer to Question 12.

12. **C,** Pages 1532-1533.

Viral pharyngitis is usually seen in conjunction with cough, rhinorrhea, myalgia, headache, and odynophagia. Influenza pharyngitis is usually seen in epidemics and is manifest by high fever, myalgia, and headache. Adenovirus pharyngitis is usually seen in conjunction with follicular lesions and often unilateral conjunctivitis. Mononucleosis pharyngitis is usually seen in conjunction with tonsillar exudate, generalized lymphadenopathy, and splenomegaly. Herpes pharyngitis usually presents with painful superficial vesicles on an erythematous base. Streptococcal pharyngitis is usually seen in conjunction with temperature greater than 38.3° C, tonsillar exudates, tender cervical lymphadenopathy, and an absence of cough or rhinorrhea. Diphtheria pharyngitis is usually characterized by pharyngeal erythema with gray-green adherent pseudomembrane.

13. **B,** Page 1533.

Rapid Strep tests will also be positive in patients in a carrier state who are at low risk for transmission and complications. This test also can be negative in the setting of low-bacterial-count pharyngitis; these patients actually do still require treatment.

14. **A,** Page 1534.

Waiting for culture results can delay treatment of streptococcal pharyngitis and therefore increase the risk of transmission, although rheumatic fever can be prevented with up to a 9-day delay in treatment. Interestingly, the incidence and course of poststreptococcal glomerulonephritis is unaffected by antibiotic therapy. The antibiotic of choice is penicillin, either via injection of 1.2 million units of benzathine penicillin or in penicillin V 250 mg orally 3 to 4 times a day for 10 days.

15. **B,** Page 1535.

Antitoxin should be started upon clinical suspicion of diphtheria. There is no need to wait for positive test results. The dose is variable depending on the severity of symptoms and the time elapsed since the onset of symptoms. The antitoxin is given over 60 minutes.

16. **C,** Page 1537.

Neuromuscular blockade causes muscular laxity, which may worsen the degree of airway obstruction. The surgical airway of choice is cricothyrotomy. See Figure 98-4.

17. **B,** Page 1537.

Peritonsillitis usually occurs in patients ages 20-40 years. Recurrence rates are 33%-50%.

18. **B,** Page 1538.

The diagnosis of peritonsillitis is a clinical diagnosis. Contrast-enhanced CT with ultrasound needle aspiration can be used.

19. **A,** Page 1538.

Dental disease is the cause of Ludwig's angina 70%-98% of the time. Deep space infection may occur as the disease progresses, but Ludwig's angina is a cellulitis by definition.

20. **D,** Pages 1536, 1538, 1540.

Hoarse voice is seen in all other listed conditions.

21. **D,** Page 1541.

Retropharyngeal abscess is usually seen in children younger than 6 years old because the retropharyngeal lymph nodes atrophy after age 4-6. The fluctuant mass should not be palpated because this can cause rupture of the abscess. The tracheal "rock" sign is often positive with retropharyngeal abscess and is evidenced by eliciting pain when moving the larynx and trachea side to side.

22. **D,** Page 1541.

This is most likely retropharyngeal abscess, but epiglottitis must be excluded.

23. **C,** Pages 1541-1542.

The mean retropharyngeal space is 3.5 mm in children and 3.4 mm in adults, with top normal being 7 mm in both adults and children. This question asked for the normal retrotracheal space dimensions.

24. **A,** Page 1544.

Lemierre syndrome usually occurs after pharyngitis that initially improves but is then followed by severe sepsis. It can involve metastatic infections in the lung, manifested by bilateral nodular infiltrates, pleural effusions, and pneumothoraces. This can present with leukocytosis and increased bilirubin and liver enzymes.

25. **B,** Pages 1545-1547.

CT scan is the gold standard of imaging for sinusitis. Usually sinusitis involves copious yellow-green discharge versus the clear discharge of rhinitis. Antihistamines should not be used because these impede sinus drainage.

---

 ## 99  Pneumonia

*Robert D. Hagan and Donnita M. Scott*

1. **E,** Page 1555.

The most common cause of community-acquired pneumonia among adults is *S. pneumoniae.* The other listed pathogens can cause community-acquired pneumonia but are less common.

2. **B,** Page 1556.

Fungal infections should be considered in anyone from an appropriate geographic location who is involved in activities that disturb the soil (e.g., mountain biking). This patient had traveled to the desert Southwest where *C. immitis* is endogenous. Clinically this infection is characterized by either acute or chronic pneumonia, or the patient may be asymptomatic with granulomas or hilar adenopathy as an incidental finding on chest radiograph.

3. **B,** Pages 1557-1558.

These findings are classic for patients with psittacosis. The exposure to birds is a critical piece of history necessary for this diagnosis.

4. **B,** Pages 1555, 1557.

*K. pneumoniae* rarely causes disease in a normal host but can cause disease in patients with alcoholism, diabetes, or other debilitating diseases. The pathogen results in severe pneumonia with a cough productive for currant-jelly–like sputum. The sputum takes on that character because of the necrotizing and hemorrhagic nature of the infection.

5. **C,** Page 1558.

Infection with *Legionella* presents as a severe systemic illness with dry cough, pleuritic chest pain, and high fever. In addition, these patients frequently have GI complaints that are often a predominant feature of their illness. The drug of choice for *Legionella* is erythromycin.

6. **C,** Pages 1559-1561.

When blood cultures are positive, they reflect the causative agent more accurately than sputum cultures. Cold hemagglutinins are present in 60% of patients with *Mycoplasma* species infection, but they can also be present with a number of viral illnesses and therefore are nonspecific. Although a chest radiograph is important for determining the presence of pneumonia, it does not point to a specific etiology and may in fact be normal in patients with clinically evident pneumonia.

7. **C,** Page 1561.

PCP is an uncommon finding in those patients whose CD4 count is >200. If the CD4 count and HIV status are unknown, the following findings can be used as a guide: a CD4 count of <200 is suggested by a total lymphocyte count of <1000 and physical findings of oral candidiasis, hairy leukoplakia, and weight loss.

8. **E,** Pages 1561, 1568.

The LDH level above 220 IU has been proven to have diagnostic significance in distinguishing patients with PCP from those patients with non–*Pneumocystis carinii* pneumonia. Factors that portend a poorer survival outcome for patients with PCP are prior episodes of PCP, tachypnea, abnormal chest radiograph, WBC count >10,300, elevated LDH, hypoxemia, and hypoalbuminemia.

9. **B,** Page 1561.

Each of these factors increases the likelihood of PCP except for the productive cough. Actually patients at risk for PCP typically present with a nonproductive cough, dyspnea, and weight loss.

10. **E,** Page 1563.

The "best" treatment for an aspiration pneumonitis remains somewhat controversial. It is recommended that antibiotics be initiated if the patient develops signs of bacterial pneumonia such as increased fever, expanding infiltrates on chest radiograph more than 36 hours after the aspiration, or a deterioration in the patient's condition that cannot be otherwise explained. Most experts agree that the use of steroids is not indicated. The "best" treatment for these patients is to protect the airway by intubating, thereby preventing further aspiration, and then providing supportive care.

11. **E,** Pages 1556, 1564.

Ribavirin is primarily used to treat respiratory syncytial virus but is thought to have activity against Hantavirus. Hantavirus is a rare cause of pneumonia in the United States and is spread by contaminated rodent feces. The prodrome consists of fever, myalgias, and malaise, and, in severe cases, is followed by hypoxia, ventilatory failure, and death.

12. **A,** Page 1566.

Because patients with cystic fibrosis are at increased risk for *P. aeruginosa* pneumonia, a combination of ceftazidime and an aminoglycoside is a good choice for empiric treatment.

13. **C,** Page 1566.

For patients younger than 60 years of age who are otherwise healthy, a macrolide or tetracycline is a good choice for empiric antibiotic therapy. These cover the atypical pneumonia agents (*M. pneumoniae, C. pneumoniae, Legionella* sp.) in addition to typical pathogens (*S. pneumoniae, M. catarrhalis*). Extended azalides such as azithromycin have the advantage of additional activity against *H. influenzae*.

14. **E,** Page 1566.

All of the antibiotics listed have activity against PCP; however, only trimethoprim-sulfamethoxazole has the benefit of being effective against the typical pneumonia pathogens as well.

15. **B,** Page 1567.

Peripheral neuropathy is a common side effect of isoniazid. Therefore, pyridoxine should be given to patients in which neuropathies are common including diabetics, alcoholics, and those who are malnourished.

# 100 Syncope

### Richard S. Hartoch

1. **E,** Page 1573.

A Prolonged QT interval indicates a prolonged duration of ventricular repolarization. This delay increases susceptibility to dysrhythmias brought on by discrepancies in local myocardial excitability. The medications most frequently cited as potentially causing prolonged QT interval syndrome include disopyramide phosphate, amiodarone, phenothiazines, tricyclic antidepressants, and terfenadine (Seldane) or astemizole (Hismanal), especially in combination with ketoconazole or erythromycin. Other conditions known to cause QT interval prolongation include hypothyroidism, hyperuricemia, myocarditis, CVA, pituitary tumors, and diffuse ischemic heart disease. The inherited form may be associated with hearing loss.

2. **B,** Page 1573.

Syncope in association with strenuous physical activity suggests the diagnosis of aortic stenosis. Exercise generally lowers systemic vascular resistance and therefore requires increased cardiac output. When cardiac output is limited by a fixed outflow obstruction such as aortic stenosis, syncope may result. The classic triad of symptoms associated with aortic stenosis are exertional dyspnea, angina pectoris, and syncope.

3. **B,** Page 1574.

Glossopharyngeal neuralgia is characterized by a tic-like pain emanating from an irritated ninth cranial nerve. It is paroxysmal and lancinating in nature. It may be felt in the oropharyngeal, cervical, and aural regions. The specific mechanism of syncope is not known, although it is generally believed that some degree of vagal stimulation precipitates the faint. Carbon monoxide toxicity can cause syncope, presumably secondary to hypoxemia and a leftward shift of the oxyhemoglobin dissociation curve. Massive pulmonary embolism causes syncope, presumably via an acute obstruction of blood flow. The subclavian steal syndrome involves a narrowing of the subclavian artery proximal to the origin of the vertebral artery, most commonly on the left side. Exercise of the arm creates a demand shunt, diverting blood into that arm from the vertebrobasilar system. Syncope can result from the reduction of cerebral blood flow.

4. **B,** Page 1574.

In one study, 47% of subjects who had cough syncope experienced some degree of clonic or repetitive motion during the unconscious period. Syncopal patients may exhibit 6-8 seconds of body movement that is not considered a true seizure. As opposed to patients with true underlying seizure disorders, patients with syncope generally demonstrate motion that is brief and less intense. They are usually not incontinent of urine and experience rapid return to premorbid cognitive function without the postical confusion characteristics of a true seizure. An EEG is generally not considered useful in determining the cause of syncope.

5. **C,** Page 1578.

Two thirds of patients with suspected cardiac syncope are 60 years of age or older. A syncopal episode in this age-group that cannot be explained as noncardiac in the ED should be managed as cardiogenic. This patient should be admitted to the hospital. Cardiac syncope has the highest 1-year mortality of all syncopal syndromes, about 30%.

6. **B,** Page 1579.

The enlarged uterus of pregnancy may compress the inferior vena cava and impede venous return. A pregnant patient experiencing syncope should be placed in left lateral decubitus position to remove mechanical obstruction.

7. **C,** Page 1579.

In the pediatric population, syncope is caused by vasovagal stimulation in up to 50% of cases. Pressure applied to the optic globe can be employed to make the diagnosis of vagal hypersensitivity. This procedure may be considered a pediatric version of carotid massage. One review of pediatric syncope indicated that in approximately 5% of patients it may be useful in detecting PR and QT interval abnormalities. Blue or cyanotic breath-holding syncope in children resolves spontaneously following loss of consciousness. White or pallid syncope is believed to result from reflex asystole from carotid sinus hypersensitivity. It may be treated with atropine if indicated.

8. **B,** Page 1580.

Specific situation syndromes, such as cough, micturition, or defecation syncope, can be managed on an outpatient basis without an extensive work-up.

9. **B,** Page 1575.

Cannon A waves result from atrial contraction against closed mitral valve, indicating A-V electrical block. They may be seen in third-degree heart block and ventricular tachycardia, but not PSVT. Adenosine would not be useful. Abdominal aortic aneurysm must be considered in an elderly patient with syncope and back pain. An abdominal ultrasound or CT scan may be of benefit.

10. **C,** Page 1573.

Carotid sinus hypersensitivity (CSH) occurs in about 10% of the adult population. It is most common in elderly males who have underlying ischemic heart disease, diabetes, or hypertension. CSH may result in a vasodepressor reaction in which pure hypotension without bradycardia occurs. More commonly, isolated heart rate slowing occurs, with ventricular asystole being a potential extreme consequence. Medications such as beta-blockers, digitalis and alpha-methyldopa potentiate CSH.

---

## ▼ 101  Dysrhythmias

*Richard J. Harper*

1. **C,** Page 1611-1613.

Multifocal atrial tachycardia (MAT) is most often seen in patients with chronic obstructive pulmonary disease and hypoxia. There is also a strong correlation to treatment with theophylline. Treatment is difficult at best and should in general be directed toward the underlying pulmonary problem. However, agents that are often used to treat COPD, specifically beta-agonists, can worsen the tachycardia. Procainamide, digitalis, and magnesium have all been advocated for use in the treatment of MAT.

2. **B,** Pages 1600-1605.

This is a classic demonstration of second-degree type I AV block, showing a gradually prolonging PR interval until finally there is a nonconducted beat. Note the grouping of beats into pairs of QRS complexes following the dropped beat. It is important to distinguish type I from type II AV block, which has a much more ominous prognosis.

3. **B,** Pages 1606-1609.

While all of the answers help to distinguish between PACs with aberrancy and PVCs, the only one that is absolutely specific for PVCs is the presence of fusion beats. Fusion beats are caused by depolarization of the ventricle from an atrial source simultaneous with that from a ventricular source.

4. **D,** Pages 1613-1617.

Cardioversion, either electrical or pharmacologic, is an increasingly accepted practice in the ED. However, it should not be attempted unless the atrial fibrillation is known to be of recent (<72 hours) onset because there is significant risk of embolization associated with cardioversion. Pharmacologic cardioversion can be attempted using several agents including procainamide, ibutilide, amiodarone, or quinidine. If the atrial fibrillation is not known to be of recent onset, the patient should be fully anticoagulated before cardioversion. In this case the job of the emergency physician is to provide rate control. Magnesium is a second-line agent for rate control but will not cause cardioversion.

5. **C,** Pages 1617-1621.

Although a patient with an accessory pathway (Wolff-Parkinson-White syndrome) will have a delta wave when in sinus rhythm, it completely disappears when he or she develops a reentrant tachyarrhythmia. In this situation, antegrade conduction occurs forward over the AV node, with retrograde conduction occurring backward over the accessory pathway. The surest sign of a reentrant tachycardia with an accessory pathway is the presence of an inverted P wave 0.07 seconds after QRS complex, which is seen in virtually 100% of these patients. This particular configuration is seen in only 4% of those with AV nodal reentry. Unstable patients with a narrow complex tachycardia should be electrically cardioverted. Stable patients with either accessory pathway or AVNRT can be treated with adenosine, calcium channel blockers, or beta blockers; procainamide may also be used.

6. **C,** Pages 1595-1596.

Adenosine can cause chest pressure that exactly mimics coronary artery disease. Patients with angina will be convinced that they are having an anginal attack. However, adenosine is a coronary artery dilator and does not precipitate ischemia. Palpitations, which are seen with almost all cardiac drugs, are not reported with adenosine. The action of adenosine is antagonized by aminophylline and other methylxanthines. Adenosine may be augmented by benzodiazepines, calcium channel blockers, and digitalis.

7. **C,** Pages 1583-1585.

The single most important factor in determining the negative intracellular charge in any given cell is the extreme difference in concentration of $K^+$ across the cell membrane. Eighty mV of the total electrical charge is generated by $K^+$ flowing down its concentration gradient. As each positively charged ion leaves the intracellular space, a net negative charge builds up.

8. **E,** Page 1585.

Pacemaker cells by definition exhibit phase 4 spontaneous depolarization. This means that a pacemaker cell will gradually depolarize while at rest (phase 4) until it reaches the threshold to generate a new action potential. Pacemaker cells also have a less negative resting membrane potential.

9. **E,** Page 1595.

Magnesium has been used as an antidysrhythmic for many years. It is useful as a second-line agent in many dysrhythmias, usually providing rate control. It is considered the drug of choice for polymorphic ventricular tachycardia. Torsade de pointes is associated with a low serum $Mg^{++}$ but has been effectively treated with $Mg^{++}$ even when serum levels are normal.

10. **D,** Pages 1611-1613.

This patient has multifocal atrial tachycardia, a common dysrhythmia in patients with chronic obstructive pulmonary disease. If the patient is unstable, cardioversion is the treatment of choice. If the patient is stable but symptomatic, particularly due to presumptive ischemia, treatment with a beta-blocker or calcium channel blocker may be instituted. Mag-

nesium is a second-line agent that may be used to provide rate control. In general, multifocal atrial tachycardia is very resistant to antidysrhythmic treatment. It is most likely to resolve spontaneously when hypoxia improves.

11. **E,** Pages 1603-1604.

This patient's blood pressure and heart rate are stable for now. The nature of Mobitz type II block is sudden deterioration to complete heart block, sometimes with a very slow rate. Pharmacologic treatment of type II second-degree block is not indicated. The preferred treatment, should the rate deteriorate, is a pacemaker. A transcutaneous pacemaker can provide adequate treatment without the need for an invasive procedure. Even though the patient is currently stable, pacemaker pads should be in place, ready for use as needed. If the pacer is enabled, the patient must be warned that the pacer may begin operation should the heart rate drop.

12. **E,** Pages 1600-1604.

The treatment for type II AV block is pacing. Pharmacologic agents should be used only if pacing is not available because they can worsen type II block by increasing the number of atrial impulses reaching the AV node without improving conduction. Carotid massage may improve conduction in type II block by decreasing the number of atrial impulses reaching the node.

13. **D,** Pages 1627-1628.

This ECG demonstrates a markedly prolonged QT interval of 0.48 sec. The normal QT interval is rate dependent, but any QT over 0.4 (two big boxes) should be considered abnormal. Causes of a prolonged QT interval are type I antidysrhythmics; psychotropic agents (phenothiazines and tricyclics); electrolyte disturbances such as hypocalcemia, hypokalemia, or hypomagnesemia; and certain congenital conditions. These patients are at particular risk for torsade de pointes. This ECG is from a patient with pancreatitis who has a calcium level of 4.8.

14. **D,** Page 1589.

Propafenone is a class 1C agent. This group of antidysrhythmics prolongs repolarization and action-potential duration. They also greatly slow depolarization and conduction. Lidocaine, phenytoin, and mexiletine are all class 1B agents. Quinidine is a class 1A agent.

 **102** # Heart failure

*J. Leibovitz*

1. **B,** Pages 1637-1638.

Heart failure patients are classified according to the underlying cause of their disease. The two leading causes of heart failure are ischemic heart disease and dilated cardiomyopathy. In the former, prolonged occlusion and stenosis in atherosclerotic coronary arteries leads to myocardial cell death resulting in scarring and fibrosis. In the latter, a number of specific etiologies (idiopathic, postviral, chronic alcoholism, cocaine, familial, metabolic, and connective tissue disorders) lead to heart dilation and decreased contractility. Valvular heart disease and hypertension, which were the leading causes of heart disease in the early 1900s, are less common today but still represent the third most common causes. Hypertension is present in up to 75% of heart failure patients; however, it is not considered the primary cause of heart failure in these patients. Endocarditis leads to heart failure through a valvular mechanism, while chronic alcohol use can lead to a dilated cardiomyopathy.

2. **E,** Pages 1642, 1643.

Epidemiologic studies have identified several risk factors for developing heart failure, including advanced age, heavy smoking, diabetes mellitus, obesity, heart disease of any type, and electrocardiographic rhythm abnormalities. Thyroid disease is not considered a risk factor for developing heart disease, although hyperthyroid states (thyrotoxicosis) can precipitate acute (high-output) heart failure.

3. **C,** Page 1631.

Epidemiologic studies have shown changes in trends, etiology, incidence, and prognosis of heart failure. The 5-year mortality due to heart failure is approximately 50%, and of the patients with severe disease, half die within the first year. Fatal ventricular dysrhythmias account for 40% of the deaths, while progressive hemodynamic deterioration leads to close to 50% of the mortality. Despite current advances in antidysrhythmic therapy, medical intervention has not decreased the frequency of dysrhythmic deaths in heart failure patients. ACE inhibitors have decreased the rate of hemodynamic deterioration in affected patients by improving pump function and have improved CHF functional class.

4. **B,** Pages 1633-1634.

Heart rate is of importance in determining cardiac output. Increases in heart rate will increase cardiac output. However, beyond heart rates of 150-160 beats per minute, cardiac filling is inefficient and cardiac output will decrease because of decreased diastolic filling time resulting in reduced stroke volume. In addition, myocardial perfusion is impaired because coronary blood flow occurs during diastole, which decreases with severe tachycardia and can even result in ischemia. Cardiac cell performance depends on fiber length (preload) as well as contractility of the cell. Preload is the stretching force that determines cardiac muscle length. Optimum preload is the filling pressure that achieves the greatest stroke volume. The Frank-Starling mechanism shows a relationship between force of contractility and muscle fiber length. Elastic tissue in the aorta and large arteries is responsible for transforming pulsatile flow from the heart into continuous flow through blood vessels. Poiseuille's law states that vascular resistance is directly related to the fourth power of the vessel's radius, with the highest resistance found at the peripheral arterioles.

5. **E,** Pages 1637-1640.

Heart failure can occur from primary disease of many tissues, including the coronary arteries, myocardium, cardiac valves, pericardium, lungs, and the peripheral vessels. Coronary artery disease leads to focal myocardial necrosis with scarring and fibrosis. Valvular dysfunction leads to impaired output or regurgitation. Pulmonary disease can cause hypoxia, which reduces the cardiac oxygen supply resulting in ischemia while at the same time increasing peripheral tissue demand. In addition, prolonged hypoxia leads to constriction of the pulmonary vasculature and results in increased afterload and right-sided heart failure (Cor pulmonale). The emergency physician must be familiar with these categories in order to determine if treatment of the underlying disease is possible and can improve or reverse heart failure. Disease of the peripheral blood vessels can lead to hypertension, which may precipitate failure.

6. **B,** Page 1638.

Dilated cardiomyopathy is the most common of the three types of cardiomyopathies. Common causes include idiopathic, postviral, rheumatologic, neuromuscular, metabolic, drug induced, nutritional deficiency, and postpartum status as in this patient.

7. **A,** Pages 1638-1639.

This 17 year old has symptoms of hypertrophic cardiomyopathy. Usually asymptomatic, it often presents with sudden death in a young adult. Other symptoms include dyspnea on exertion or syncope. Findings include left ventricular hypertrophy without chamber dilation. It is hereditary in half the cases commonly associated with mutations of the beta myosin protein. Diastolic dysfunction is the primary factor leading to heart failure.

8. **C,** Page 1639.

Restrictive cardiomyopathy is the least prevalent. It is found in disease states including amyloidosis, hemochromatosis, and sarcoidosis, in which the heart muscle is replaced with other substances such as protein, iron, or granulomas. The heart becomes noncompliant due to the infiltrated substances resulting in diastolic dysfunction. Restrictive disease can mimic restrictive pericarditis and often requires endocardial biopsy.

9. **D,** Page 1639.

Myocarditis is an inflammatory disease of the myocytes, interstitium, coronary vessels, or pericardium. There are numerous causes of myocarditis, including infectious agents, toxins, drugs, physical agents, or hypersensitivity reactions. Thyroid disease is not a cause of myocarditis. Viral agents are the most frequent causes of myocarditis in North America, and myocarditis is a well-known complication of Lyme disease. Several drugs and toxins, including cocaine, tricyclic antidepressants, lead, carbon monoxide, and others, are known to cause myocarditis. Autoimmune disorders and hypersensitivity reactions (e.g., transplant rejection) may also cause myocarditis.

10. **E,** Pages 1639-1640.

Valvular heart disease is the third leading cause of heart failure after ischemic heart disease and dilated cardiomyopathy. Involvement of the aortic and mitral valves is most common in adults and usually results in fulminant regurgitant lesions. Type A aortic dissections may involve the annulus, resulting in aortic regurgitation that can sometimes result in cardiac tamponade if the dissection continues through the pericardium. Complete rupture of the papillary muscle often occurs days after an acute myocardial infarction and leads to sudden valvular regurgitation and acute pulmonary edema. Although prosthetic valves become incompetent, the most common etiology leading to heart failure is acute stenosis secondary to thrombus formation, which can lead to symptoms of syncope or obstructive shock.

11. **E,** Page 1640.

High-output failure is a condition in which the patient has clinical signs of heart failure with increased cardiac output and abnormal pressure-volume relationships in the ventricles. Although these patients have elevated cardiac outputs, diastolic dysfunction and elevated central venous pressures result in pulmonary congestion. Patients are warm and flushed and have a widened pulse pressure. Conditions causing high-output failure include chronic anemia, hyperthyroid disease, hyperthermia, and beriberi.

12. **C,** Pages 1636-1637.

The onset of heart failure in a diseased heart leads to a series of compensatory responses including mechanical responses and neurohormonal responses. Sensory receptors in the heart and great vessels detect decreased blood flow, activating a reflex arc to stimulate the sympathetic nervous system. Increased levels of catecholamines increase the discharge rate and speed of conduction of cardiac pacemaker cells, leading to an increased heart rate in acute heart failure. Changes in preload provide an immediate compensatory response by raising stroke volume by increasing the number of cross-bridges between muscle fibers, resulting in greater output. This effect is limited, and beyond a certain level of stretch, cardiac output will start to decrease. The heart hypertrophies by increasing the number of myocardial cells and by increasing contractile proteins within the cell. Vasopressin levels are increased in heart failure, leading to mild vasoconstriction and renal water retention.

13. **E,** Page 1645 (Table 102-2).

There are several causes of acute cardiogenic pulmonary edema. In a study by Goldberger in 1986, worsening of heart failure was the most common precipitating cause of acute cardiogenic pulmonary edema. The emergency physician must be diligent in the search for the precipitating event that led to heart failure. Other causes exist, including acute ischemia, myocardial infarction, valvular rupture, dysrhythmia, hypoxia, medication noncompliance, and trauma.

14. **A,** Page 1645.

Patients can have varying degrees of pulmonary congestion. Most patients with acute pulmonary edema will have an elevated blood pressure with bounding pulses and cool, clammy skin. An $S_3$ gallop is present 25% of the time. Most patients have rales or wheezes. Half have jugular venous distention, and one third have pedal edema. The most common acid base abnormality is a metabolic acidosis with respiratory compensation. Lactic acidosis results from decreased systemic perfusion, hypoxia, and increased work of breathing. The majority of patients compensate by increasing their respiratory rate (respiratory alkalosis) in order to reduce the total $CO_2$ and increase the pH. The mortality for acute pulmonary congestion is approximately 17% per admission and 40% for the first year after admission. An elevated systolic blood pressure >160 mm Hg in the ED is a good prognostic sign revealing significant myocardial reserve, with more than twice the survival rate of patients with lower blood pressures on presentation.

15. **E,** Pages 1642-1643.

The emergency physician must always search for a precipitating event that led to decompensation in the heart failure patient. Causes include myocardial infarction, valvular rupture, cardiac dysrhythmia, acute hypoxia secondary to pulmonary embolism or pneumonia, blood loss, medication noncompliance, dietary noncompliance, hypertensive crisis, or trauma. A large proportion of cases of acute pulmonary edema will be attributed to transient ischemia or progression of the disease process.

16. **C,** Pages 1646,1648-1649.

The patient described is in heart failure with pulmonary edema and borderline hypotension. Appropriate management should be aimed at controlling pulmonary congestion and raising cardiac output. To attain this goal, the ED physician must decrease preload and afterload and maintain adequate blood pressure for perfusion. Dopamine, a dose-dependent catecholamine precursor, is an effective pressor agent, but it is not successful as a single agent to correct pulmonary edema. At higher doses it causes increased contractility by acting on beta-1 receptors, but at these doses it can also lead to significant elevation of systemic vascular resistance (afterload) and exacerbate pulmonary edema despite its positive inotropic effect. Its use in heart failure patients with pulmonary edema is recommended only in combination with a vasodilating agent.

17. **D,** Pages 1648-1649.

Dopamine is a dose dependent, naturally occurring catecholamine precursor of norepinephrine with direct inotropic and chronotropic effects on the heart. At low doses (2-5 $\mu g/kg/min$), it acts primarily on dopaminergic receptors found in the kidney, and results in increased renal perfusion and urinary output. At medium doses (5-15 $\mu g/kg/min$), dopamine acts on beta-1 and beta-2 receptors, resulting in increased contractility, faster heart rate, and peripheral vasodilation. At high doses (>15 $\mu g/kg/min$), it acts similar to norepinephrine, raising systemic vascular resistance by causing significant vasoconstriction.

18. **A,** Page 1649.

Dobutamine is a synthetic catecholamine with primarily beta-1 and slight beta-2 and alpha-agonist effects. Administration leads to increases in cardiac output and decreases in pulmonary capillary wedge pressures.

19. **C,** Page 1647.

Nitroprusside is a potent venous and arterial smooth muscle dilator resulting in significant reductions in both preload and afterload. It is the drug of choice in patients with heart failure due to malignant hypertension. The drug should be avoided in patients with coronary ischemia because of its ability to dilate less diseased vessels to a greater degree than diseased ones resulting in diverting blood flow away from ischemic regions (coronary steal).

20. **B,** Page 1646.

Morphine sulfate is a narcotic that reduces pulmonary congestion via a central sympatholytic effect, leading to vasodilation.

21. **D,** Pages 1641, 1646-1648.

This patient has an acute inferior myocardial infarct. About one third of patients with inferior infarct will have involvement of the right ventricle. Right ventricular infarct can cause acute isolated right-sided heart failure without pulmonary congestion. Patients usually have symptomatic hypotension that responds to administration of normal saline, which increases right ventricular output. Diagnosis of right ventricular infarct can be confirmed by observing ST elevation in a right-sided V4 ECG lead. An intraaortic balloon pump can be beneficial, but a fluid challenge and other therapeutic modalities should be initiated first. Nitroprusside and nitroglycerin should be avoided initially because they may drop peripheral vascular resistance, resulting in significant cardiogenic shock. In addition, nitroprusside should be avoided when there is coronary ischemia due to coronary steal syndrome. Dopamine may increase vascular resistance, leading to a rise in blood pressure, but it should not be used as first-line agent in acute right-sided myocardial infarctions because it may increase ischemia.

22. **C,** Page 1649.

Cardiac glycosides are plant derivatives with a long history of use for heart failure. The ED physician should consider digitalis therapy in heart failure associated with atrial fibrillation and left ventricular hypertrophy. Glycosides have a low toxic-to-therapeutic ratio and must be used with caution, especially in patients with systemic acidosis, hypokalemia, and hypoxia, all conditions that enhance toxicity. They work by inhibiting cell membrane Na-K ATPase, leading to increased inotropy. Variable clinical responses have been found. Patients with atrial fibrillation respond well to glycosides, whereas patients with right heart failure and chronic ischemic heart failure respond poorly.

23. **B,** Page 1651.

Beta-blockers should be avoided in patients with acute heart failure. Chronic heart failure leads to elevated catecholamine levels, activation of the renin-angiotensin system, and beta-adrenergic receptor downregulation. These neurohormonal mechanisms, which can exacerbate heart failure, are inhibited, not enhanced, by beta-blockers. They are of benefit in selected patients such as those with angina, hypertension, or arrhythmias. Beta-1–specific agents are preferable because of their decreased side effects from beta-2 receptor activation.

24. **C,** Page 1647.

Heart failure occurs frequently in end-stage renal disease. It occurs in up to 10%-20% of patients with ESRD. Half of ESRD patients with heart failure have hypertrophic, hyperkinetic ventricles and a normal ejection fraction, and half will have a dilated cardiomyopathy. Both types of heart failure are difficult to distinguish initially. The ED physician should search for a precipitating cause of heart failure in ESRD. Some ESRD-specific causes include fluid overload from improper dialysis, electrolyte imbalance, toxicity, and uremic pericardial effusion. Treatment options vary; however, standard preload reduction with morphine, nitrates, and furosemide can be effective. Furosemide is an effective vasodilator, even in anuric patients, and should be used.

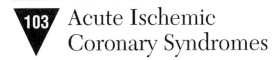

## 103 ▼ Acute Ischemic Coronary Syndromes

*Richard J. Harper*

1. **B,** Page 1656.

Most deaths from AICS happen outside the hospital within 2 hours of the onset of symptoms. About half of all deaths in the United States are attributable to ischemic coronary disease. People younger than 65 account for 45% of AMIs, and more than 160,000 of these people die. Women account for a greater number of cardiovascular deaths than men. While the rate of death from AMI is decreasing, the cost of treating AMIs appears to be increasing.

2. **C,** Page 1657.

The Canadian Cardiovascular Society Classification for angina addresses existing anginal patterns, not changes in pattern. Class I angina does not limit ordinary physical activity. Class II angina slightly limits normal activity. Class III angina is severe, limiting activity to walking one to two blocks or a single flight of stairs. Class IV constitutes an inability to carry on any physical activity without discomfort; angina may occur at rest.

3. **B,** Page 1657.

Rest angina, according to the Agency for Health Care Policy Research, occurs at rest and lasts more than 20 minutes and occurs within 1 week of presentation. New-onset angina is of at least class III severity with onset within the last 2 months. Increasing angina is previously diagnosed angina that is more frequent, longer in duration, or increased by one class (to at least class III severity) within 2 months.

4. **B,** Pages 1658-1659.

Time to initiation of therapy in acute myocardial infarction is the greatest limiting factor in successful treatment. Patient factors are very important in the delay. Self-treatment delays 32% of patients. Delay varies by race, gender, and age. Mortality has been reported to be as low as 1.3% if treatment is initiated within 70 minutes, but as Rosen Figure 103-3 illustrates, total potential benefit drops to below 25% of maximal at 4 hours.

5. **A,** Page 1663.

Anginal pain is more likely to be a dull pressure than a sharp, stabbing pain. Its duration is 2-5 minutes and always less than 20 minutes unless AMI is present. Pain lasting seconds or many hours is less likely to be anginal. Angina is substernal rather than in the lateral chest wall or back. It is reproducible with exertion, not respiration. Associated symptoms are usually present, and palpitation of the chest wall does not exactly reproduce the pain.

6. **A,** Pages 1666-1667.

Atypical symptoms of myocardial infarction are more common in older patients who do not smoke and have no history of angina. After age 85, atypical symptoms are more common than typical symptoms. Approximately half of these infarctions are silent; the remainder have greatly variable presenting symptoms, with dyspnea being the most common. Because of delayed presentation and advancing age in patients with atypical symptoms, their outcomes are less favorable.

7. **A,** Page 1667.

Up to 5% of patients with acute myocardial infarctions, some 40,000 per year, are released from emergency departments inappropriately. The majority of these patients are young males, ages 30-45, without previous hospitalizations for cardiac disease. While their presentations are atypical, about 49% could be discovered by virtue of ECG changes or a history consistent with angina at rest. Missed AMIs account for 20% of emergency department malpractice claims.

8. **B,** Pages 1668-1669.

Agreement on ECG interpretation between emergency medicine residents, staff, and cardiologists is very good. Of particular importance, clinically significant disagreement has been shown to be rare. Unfortunately, the ECG has a sensitivity of only between 25% and 50% in patients eventually diagnosed with acute myocardial infarction. The availability of previous ECGs may assist in preventing existing abnormalities from being identified as new. This reduces over-diagnosis of acute myocardial infarction. About 5% of patients eventually diagnosed with AICS have a normal emergency department ECG. Both short- and long-term outcome are proportional to the degree of abnormality on the initial ECG.

9. **D,** Pages 1674-1675.

An ECG with a prominent R wave in $V_1$, a current of injury in the inferior leads, or a patient with unexplained hypotension with symptoms of acute myocardial infarction should prompt a physician to repeat the ECG with a $V_{4R}$ lead. An elevation of the ST segment in lead $V_{4R}$ (fourth right intercostal space in the midclavicular line) is a specific and sensitive sign of right ventricular infarction.

10. **C,** Page 1679-1688.

This tracing shows a combination of benign early repolarization (BER) and benign variant T wave changes. Elevated ST segments with upper concavity are seen in leads $V_1$ to $V_4$, and a notch J point, the hallmark of BER, is evident in left precordial leads. Slight ST segment depression is present in limb leads. T wave inversions are evident in bipolar limb and left precordial leads. In addition, prominent, asymmetric T waves are seen in right precordial leads. This tracing has some features of BER, acute pericarditis, and acute myocardial ischemia. Absence of pathologic Q waves and T wave inversion in all three bipolar limb leads contradicts the diagnosis of AMI. Absence of PR segment deviation, heart rate of 66 beats per minute and prominent T waves in right precordial leads contradict the diagnosis of acute pericarditis.

11. **D,** Pages 1682-1684.

Electrical alternans (alternately smaller QRS, QRST, or P and QRST in every second or third beat) is uncommon but virtually pathognomonic of pericardial effusion with tamponade. This ECG finding signifies an immediate life threat, and its prompt recognition is imperative. Electrical alternans is most often associated with a malignancy, but it may occur with tuberculosis, rheumatic fever, and other infectious diseases of the pericardium.

12. **B,** Pages 1686-1687.

In this tracing, P waves are absent, and RS complexes are prolonged, blending into oppositely directed ST-T waves to produce sine wave appearance. S deflections and ST segment elevation in right precordial leads resemble the appearance of anteroseptal AMI. This patient's potassium level was 9.2 mEq/L. Hyperkalemia can produce a pseudoinfarction pattern beyond prominent T waves. Elevated ST segments, indistinguishable from those of anterior septal wall injury, may appear in the right precordial leads and lead $aV_R$, with reciprocal ST segment depressions in the left precordial leads and various limb leads. Associated ECG findings often include the absence of P waves, a prolongation of QRS complexes, and Q waves in the leads displaying ST segment elevation. The pathogenesis of hyperkalemic ECG changes has not been resolved. However, the absence of P waves and the presence of prolonged QRS complexes are clearly related to the hyperkalemic depression of cardiac conduction.

13. **C,** Pages 1679-1681.

This tracing demonstrates left bundle branch block (LBBB) with left axis deviation and concordant secondary ST-T wave abnormalities. The QRS complex is prolonged to 0.18 seconds with R deflection in lead 1 and QS deflection in lead $V_1$. Normal sinus rhythm is present, and septal Q waves are absent in leads 1, $V_5$, and $V_6$. This characterizes LBBB. Anterior forces are absent or small in leads $V_1$-$V_4$ because of LBBB. STT waves are concordant and generally opposite to terminal QRS deflection. Note the elevated ST segments blending into upright T waves in leads 3, $aV_F$, and $V_1$-$V_4$. These ST-T changes are consistent with LBBB alone. LBBB can mimic or mask an AMI.

14. **D**, Pages 1679-1681.

The initial 0.04- to 0.06-second QRS forces remain unchanged before and after the onset of right bundle branch block because the normal left-to-right initial activation of the ventricular mass, which is a result of the normal functioning left bundle branch, is intact. This preservation of the initial QRS complex permits the recognition of pathologic Q waves caused by AMI, which is not possible in the presence of LBBB. The characteristic signature of RBBB is that the terminal forces are directed rightward and posterior. The repolarization ST-T abnormalities of AMI are also more easily recognized in the presence of RBBB than LBBB. The mass of the late depolarizing right ventricle is much smaller than that of the late depolarizing left ventricle, thereby allowing primary ST-T wave changes to be more readily seen in RBBB than LBBB. ST elevation in RBBB is considered pathologic and potentially indicative of infarction if it does not follow the rule of direction for secondary ST-T wave changes. In particular, ST elevations in $V_1$ or the inferior leads are not expected as a result of RBBB.

15. **C,** Pages 1687-1688.

Hypothermia produces the Osborne wave, or J wave. The heart rate is usually slow, with a prolonged QT interval. The Osborne wave is broad and upwardly convex and may be mistaken for an injury pattern. It is usually present with core temperatures less than $32°$ C ($89.6°$ F). The diminution of these changes with rewarming is pathognomonic for hypothermia. The Osborne wave may rarely be found in normal individuals and in patients with subarachnoid hemorrhage.

16. **C,** Page 1670.

Pathologic Q waves are negative QRS deflections of 0.04 seconds or more in leads other than $aV_R$ and $V_1$. They commonly develop 24 hours after infarct. When present, they represent transmural myocardial necrosis and are directed away from the area of infarct. Q wave patterns are used to localize the area of infarct. Q waves found in leads $V_1$-$V_4$ localize an infarct to the anterior septal area, whereas Q waves in leads II, III, and $aV_F$ indicate an inferior wall infarct. About 20% to 50% of patients with an acute myocardial infarct exhibit nondiagnostic ST wave changes without pathologic Q waves.

17. **D,** Page 1670.

The ECG shown is representative of an acute inferior wall infarction with concomitant precordial ST segment depression. The ST segment elevation in the inferior leads is representative of an inferior injury pattern, and diagnostic Q waves are not yet present. The 0.04-second R wave in $V_1$ is consistent with a true posterior wall infarction. Depression of the ST segments in the precordial leads $V_1$-$V_4$ in the context of an acute inferior wall infarct is ominous. The precordial lead pattern of injury likely represents left anterior descending coronary artery disease.

18. **B,** Pages 1679-1681.

New right bundle branch block is associated with a higher incidence of complete heart block and a higher mortality than new left bundle branch block. Since both the right and left bundles may be supplied by the LAD, either may be associated with anterior myocardial infarction. Left but not right bundle branch block masks the changes associated with acute myocardial infarction.

19. **D,** Pages 1690-1691.

Digitalis toxicity causes concave ST segment depressions. Pulmonary embolism may produce a Q wave in III, along with an S wave in lead I and an inverted T wave in lead III. It also may produce signs of right ventricular strain with ST elevation in leads $V_1$ and $V_2$. Unlike cerebrovascular accident, pulmonary embolism does not elevate CK-MB.

20. **A,** Pages 1692-1693.

CK-MB has a sensitivity and specificity greater than 90% within 3 hours after ED presentation. The initial sensitivity is low at 34%-62% and increases to 77%-97% at 3 hours. The sensitivity approaches 100% at 10-11 hours after presentation. The specificity is 84%-99% at initial presentation and remains essentially unchanged (83%-99%) at 3 hours. Its negative predictive value is approximately 90% at presentation to the ED and increases to 96%-99% at 3 hours after presentation. The positive predictive value ranges widely from 42%-83% at initial presentation and remains low at 52%-91% at 3 hours after presentation.

21. **A,** Pages 1693-1694.

Myoglobin is an intracellular, oxygen-carrying protein found in all muscle tissue. Its presence in the serum is a sensitive indicator of muscle damage resulting in a negative predictive value of nearly 100%. This protein is smaller than CK. Its serum levels rise within 1-2 hours after onset of infarct and peak at 4-5 hours. Elevated myoglobin lacks specificity for an MI because the myoglobin of skeletal muscle is indistinguishable from that found in myocardial tissue. Due to renal clearance, renal failure elevates myoglobin levels.

22. **C,** Page 1694.

Troponins have initial release kinetics similar to CK-MB, but levels remain elevated much longer, up to 5.5 days. Troponin I is a smaller molecule with a weight of 23,000 daltons compared with 39,000 daltons for troponin T. Cardiac troponins are specific to cardiac muscle and are not elevated in skeletal muscle injury. Troponins may be less specific for myocardial infarction than CK-MB because they can be elevated in unstable angina.

23. **B,** Page 1696.

Few studies have evaluated emergency department exercise testing. Those which have suggest it is safe and effective. The sensitivity for exercise-induced ischemia is approximately 60%-70%. Patients may have either a normal or nondiagnostic ECG. False-positive test results are common in young women, limiting the utility of testing in this group. Fixed lesions of the circumflex may be difficult to identify through exercise testing.

24. **E,** Page 1697.

Current time to treatment of ischemic chest pain ranges from 60 to 90 minutes in most U.S. hospitals. The goal for treatment of the National Heart Attack Alert Program is initiation of therapy within 30 minutes. An ECG should be obtained and interpreted within 10 minutes. Chest Pain Evaluation and Treatment units are an attempt to reduce cost and provide early identification and treatment of acute myocardial infarction and cardiac ischemia. The management of potential cardiac chest pain seems to be an area where protocol-driven care may provide timely and appropriate emergency department treatment.

**25. D,** Page 1698.

The typical process of injury during myocardial ischemia includes initiation of ischemia by plaque rupture. This is followed by platelet aggregation and thrombus formation. Coronary artery vasospasm contributes to damage, and finally reperfusion causes damage through free radicals, calcium release, and the action of neutrophils. Spontaneous thrombolysis occurs during myocardial ischemia and may minimize the degree of damage.

**26. A,** Pages 1699-1700.

The high efficacy of aspirin coupled with its relative safety has led to a search for even more effective antiplatelet agents. All the agents listed are antiplatelet agents with the exception of argatroban, an arginine derivative that is an antithrombotic agent.

**27. E,** Pages 1704-1705.

The ED physician should be well versed in the indications and contraindications for thrombolytic therapy. Absolute contraindications for thrombolytic therapy include gastrointestinal hemorrhage, prolonged or traumatic CPR, recent (2 months) intracranial or intraspinal surgery, intracranial neoplasm, previous cerebrovascular accident known to be hemorrhagic, and pregnancy. There are several relative contraindications, including poorly controlled severe hypertension, recent trauma or surgery, peptic ulcer disease, previous CVA, known bleeding diathesis, hepatic insufficiency, diabetic retinopathy, and prior exposure to streptokinase. Menstruation should be considered a compressible site of bleeding and therefore not an absolute contraindication.

**28. A,** Page 1706.

Cocaine-induced myocardial infarction is treated in a manner similar to standard acute myocardial infarction. The patient should receive thrombolytic therapy if the ECG is appropriate and there are no other contraindications. Nitroglycerin reduces vasospasm and increases blood flow to ischemic tissue. Lidocaine remains the treatment of choice for ischemia-induced dysrhythmias, but sodium bicarbonate, not usually used in acute myocardial infarction, may be administered to decrease QRS prolongation due to cocaine. Beta-blockade, standard treatment in acute myocardial infarction, should be avoided in cocaine-induced infarction because it allows for unopposed alpha effect by cocaine.

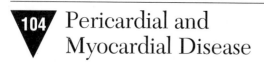

# 104 Pericardial and Myocardial Disease

### *Richard S. Hartoch*

**1. C,** Page 1718.

There are many causes of pericarditis, including trauma, infections (viral, bacterial, fungal, and amebic), radiation, cancer, uremia, collagen vascular disease, drugs, and myocardial infarction. Each of these disorders may also produce a pericardial effusion. Esophageal rupture does not produce pericarditis.

**2. E,** Page 1719.

All of the statements are true regarding chest pain associated with pericarditis. The pain is usually substernal and varies with respiration but it is not necessarily sharp or pleuritic in nature. The pain generally does not radiate to the arms but often radiates to the trapezius muscle ridges, producing isolated shoulder pain. The pain is exacerbated by lying down and relieved by sitting and leaning forward.

**3. D,** Page 1720.

The ECG in pericarditis typically evolves through four stages. In stage I, which occurs in the first hours or days of the disease, the ST segments are elevated in all leads except $AV_R$ and $V_1$, where there is reciprocal depression. The ST segments have an upward concavity, and the J point is indistinct. In addition, there is PR segment depression in 82% of these patients. During stage II, the ST and PR segments transiently return to baseline and produce a normal-appearing ECG. In stage III, there are deep, symmetric, inverted T waves throughout the tracing. These T wave inversions may normalize in stage IV, or they may become permanent. Pericarditis does not produce Q waves.

**4. D,** Page 1722.

Unlike the ECG changes seen in most cases of pericarditis (i.e., viral or idiopathic pericarditis), ST elevations are rare in post-MI pericarditis. Dressler syndrome, which previously was believed to be a late complication of myocardial infarction, probably represents a continuum between early and delayed pericarditis. Like early post-MI pericarditis, pericarditis associated with Dressler syndrome responds to 1 to 3 days of nonsteroidal antiinflammatory therapy.

**5. C,** Page 1721.

Unlike the ECG in acute MI, the ST elevations in acute pericarditis are concave upward rather than convex upward. It is vital to differentiate the two entities because thrombolytic therapy is contraindicated in pericarditis and may lead to acute cardiac tamponade.

**6. D,** Page 1726.

Tachycardia is the earliest sign of cardiac tamponade and occurs as a result of adrenergic stimulation produced by a decrease in cardiac output. As the size of the effusion increases and the stroke volume continues to decrease, there is an increase in the systemic vascular resistance and a narrowing of the pulse pressure. Increased atrial pressures result in jugular venous distention. Pulsus paradoxus and hypotension are both late findings of cardiac tamponade.

**7. D,** Page 1726.

Beck first described his triad of findings in 1935. These findings included hypotension, jugular venous distention, and muffled heart sounds. Tachycardia, although the earliest sign of tamponade, was not described by Beck. Due to the noise in the ED, muffled heart sounds are often difficult to appreciate, and jugular venous distention may be absent in patients who are hypovolemic.

**8. C,** Page 1726.

Electrical alternans, an alternating pattern of high and low voltage on the ECG, is pathognomonic of pericardial tamponade. It is produced by the anteroposterior swinging of the heart within a large pericardial effusion. The amplitude of the voltage alternates between high and low with each beat. Small or early pericardial effusions will not produce sufficient swing of the heart to produce electrical alternans, and pericarditis may not be associated with an effusion.

9. **C,** Page 1726.

The only definitive therapy for cardiac tamponade is drainage of pericardial fluid by means of pericardiocentesis or pericardiotomy. Drainage of only a small amount of fluid will usually result in a dramatic hemodynamic improvement. Although the use of volume expanders or nitroprusside is physiologically sound, in practice these agents have little benefit in cardiac tamponade.

10. **B,** Page 1726.

In constrictive pericarditis, thickened pericardial tissue compresses the myocardium and results in impaired ventricular filling. The signs and symptoms of constrictive pericarditis, which include dyspnea, fatigue, weight gain, jugular venous distention, peripheral edema, and hepatomegaly are indistinguishable from congestive heart failure. The most common cause of constrictive pericarditis is previous viral or idiopathic pericarditis, but any previous cause of pericarditis may produce constrictive pericarditis. Pulsus paradoxus is absent because the constricted pericardium does not transmit intrathoracic pressure variations associated with respiration. Pericardiectomy is the treatment of choice.

11. **A,** Pages 1734-1737.

A normal ECG is seen in only approximately 15% of patients with hypertrophic cardiomyopathy. Evidence of left ventricular hypertrophy (LVH) is usually present. Other abnormalities include left atrial enlargement, Q waves, inverted T waves, or ventricular dysrhythmias. Diastolic dysfunction is the result of a hypertrophied, poorly compliant left ventricle with a prolonged and incomplete phase of relaxation. Chest pain results from the increased oxygen demands of the enlarged left ventricle in association with high left ventricular pressures. High pressures also result in increased pulmonary venous pressures, which ultimately produce dyspnea. Syncope may be due to dysrhythmias or, more commonly, decreased cardiac output as the result of a systolic gradient that is exacerbated by exertion.

12. **E,** Pages 1734-1737.

Sudden death occurs in approximately 1%-2% of all patients with HCM. Dysrhythmias are the most common cause of death. 80% of HCM patients have asymptomatic ventricular dysrhythmias on Holter monitoring. Beta-blockade is the treatment of choice because all major symptoms of HCM, including angina, dyspnea, and syncope, are responsive. Calcium channel blockers are also useful but are contraindicated if conduction blocks are present. Amiodarone is the drug of choice for treatment of ventricular dysrhythmias associated with HCM. 5% of patients with HCM develop subacute endocarditis; therefore patients should receive antibiotic prophylaxis before undergoing invasive procedures.

13. **E,** Page 1738.

Whereas systemic sarcoidosis is most common in blacks, the incidence of myocardial sarcoidosis is equal among whites and blacks. The peak incidence is in the second and third decades of life. Symptoms include dyspnea, palpitations, and chest pain. Sudden death occurs in one half to two thirds of the patients.

 ## 105 Infective Endocarditis and Acquired Valvular Heart Disease

*Brian Holt*

1. **E,** Page 1749.

Many dysrhythmias are associated with prolapse of the mitral valve. Paroxysmal supraventricular tachycardia and premature ventricular contractions are the most common and often cause the palpitations these patients experience. Third-degree heart block is rarely if ever associated with mitral valve prolapse. Cerebral ischemia is thought to be due to embolic events to the cerebral vessels from sterile emboli. These embolic events and rarely ventricular tachycardia can be causes of syncope in patients with mitral valve prolapse.

2. **E,** Pages 1745-1746.

Streptococcus viridans is the most common cause of native valve endocarditis followed by *Streptococcus bovis* and *Enterococcus* sp. Coagulase-negative *Staphylococcus* is the most common cause of prosthetic valve endocarditis, with most infections occurring early in the postoperative period. *Staphylococcus aureus* is the most common cause in IV drug users.

3. **A,** Page 1746.

All of the listed associations are correct with the exception of Janeway lesions, which are non-tender maculopapular lesions of the palms and soles that blanch with pressure.

4. **D,** Page 1746.

The recommendation is to obtain two to four blood cultures when evaluating a patient for suspected endocarditis.

5. **D,** Page 1747.

All are instances in which patients with valvular or congenital heart disease should have prophylaxis except insertion of a Foley catheter without evidence of a urinary tract infection. When a UTI is present, the patient should receive prophylaxis. Mitral valve prolapse without a murmur does not require prophylaxis, in contrast to all other valvular and congenital heart disease.

6. **C,** Page 1748.

Erythema marginatum and subcutaneous nodules represent major diagnostic criteria. They are not pathognomonic for rheumatic fever but are uncommon in other settings. The other major criteria are carditis, polyarteritis, and chorea.

7. **A,** Pages 1748-1751.

Rheumatic heart disease is a common cause of mitral stenosis and chronic regurgitation but not of acute mitral regurgitation. Acute and chronic mitral regurgitation are different disease processes with different etiologies, treatments, and prognoses. Acute mitral regurgitation is usually a result of a ruptured chordae tendineae or papillary muscle or perforation of the valve, and ECG changes are rare. Infectious endocarditis is rare in isolated mitral stenosis but more frequent with associated regurgitation. Chronic regurgitation and mitral stenosis are both associated with left atrial enlargement. Chronic regurgitation is associated with left ventricular hypertrophy.

8. **E,** Pages 1750-1751.

Left ventricular hypertrophy is a usual finding, but atrial enlargement is not typical. Significant obstruction is defined as a valve orifice less than 25% of its original size or a pressure gradient exceeding 50 mm Hg. In patients older than 65 years, stenosis is usually the result of calcified degeneration of the valve cusp.

9. **A,** Page 1751.

Connective tissue diseases may cause either acute or chronic aortic regurgitation. The most common cause of chronic aortic regurgitation is rheumatic heart disease. Chronic regurgitation results in a widened pulse pressure and therefore the finding of a rapidly rising and falling carotid "water-hammer" pulse. Congestive failure is less common than in acute aortic regurgitation because the heart has time to adapt. Acute aortic regurgitation is most commonly caused by endocarditis, aortic dissection, or trauma. In acute aortic regurgitation, the systolic and diastolic pressures are normal to low, pulse pressure is not widened, and the degree of heart failure corresponds to the amount of regurgitation. Medical stabilization involves not pressors but afterload reducers and/or intraaortic balloon pump to improve cardiac function.

10. **A,** Pages 1751-1752.

Chronic low-grade hemolysis occurs in up to 70% of patients with prosthetic valves and may predispose these patients to biliary disease. Severe hemolysis may indicate either primary valve failure or a paravalvular leak.

11. **B,** Pages 1752-1753.

Most patients have ECG changes that may include LVH and Q waves in the inferior, anterior, or lateral leads. Calcium channel blockers and beta-blockers may be useful in the treatment of hypertrophic cardiomyopathy but preload reducers such as diuretics and nitrates, as well as inotropes such as digoxin, should be avoided. The most common symptom is dyspnea, but exertional chest pain and syncope also occur. The Valsalva maneuver will often increase the intensity of the murmur by decreasing left ventricular diastolic volumes.

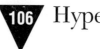

# 106 Hypertension

*Richard S. Hartoch*

1. **B,** Page 1755.

Emergency providers must have a working knowledge of the pathophysiology, natural history, and therapeutic interventions needed for appropriate care of hypertension. Primary responsibilities include recognizing hypertensive emergencies, arranging appropriate long-term follow-up for newly diagnosed cases, and managing the vast array of complications that may arise from long-standing hypertension. Successful management of hypertension requires an established relationship with a primary care provider. Treatment of hypertension on an outpatient basis is usually not the responsibility of the emergency physician.

2. **A,** Page 1756.

The renin-angiotensin system is important in the pathophysiology of hypertension. Renin is an enzyme produced in the kidney that splits angiotensin I from a precursor. Angiotensin I is then acted upon by a converting enzyme (ACE) in the lung to form angiotensin II, a powerful vasoconstrictor that also stimulates the release of aldosterone from the adrenal gland. Angiotensin's effects are dependent on sodium levels. Inhibition of angiotensin markedly decreases blood pressure in patients who are sodium depleted and will have no effect on hypertensive patients with normal total body sodium stores. Patients with high plasma renin levels have a better therapeutic response to beta-blockers and ACE inhibitors than patients with low plasma renin levels, who respond best to calcium channel blockers and diuretics.

3. **C,** Page 1757.

Most cases of hypertension are considered essential. Of the identified causes of hypertension, renal disease is the most prevalent. All types of renal disease have been associated with hypertension including chronic pyelonephritis, polycystic renal disease, glomerulonephritis, and renovascular disease.

4. **C,** Page 1759.

Hypertensive emergencies require reduction of blood pressure within 1 hour. The box on page 1759 of Rosen lists criteria for hypertensive emergencies. Answer C is considered a hypertensive urgency, in which diastolic blood pressure reduction is recommended within 24 hours to reduce risk to the patient. Hypertensive urgency is defined as a diastolic pressure of 115 mm Hg or greater without evidence of end-organ disease. All other answers are examples of hypertensive emergencies.

5. **D,** Page 1763.

Nitroprusside has a direct effect on smooth muscle of both resistance and capacitance vessels. It does not worsen angina. Its effect on venous dilation lowers preload, and cardiac output often improves in patients with congestive heart failure or limited cardiac function. Prolonged use can lead to build-up of the toxic metabolite thiocyanate, especially in the presence of renal failure. Nitroprusside undergoes breakdown in the presence of ultraviolet light and should be wrapped in a protective cover. Administration should be through a free-flowing intravenous catheter, because extravasation can lead to severe skin necrosis. The safety of nitroprusside during pregnancy has not been established (category C).

6. **A,** Page 1762.

A diastolic blood pressure >100 mm Hg during pregnancy is considered a hypertensive emergency. The agent of choice for blood pressure reduction in this case is IV hydralazine, starting with a 5 mg test dose and repeating 10-mg doses every 20 minutes until a diastolic blood pressure <100 mm Hg is obtained. Intravenous, rather than oral, hydralazine is indicated for judicious reduction of blood pressure. Diazoxide in 30-mg boluses is an effective alternative agent in this situation. Nitroprusside is contraindicated because of potential side effects to the fetus.

7. **C,** Page 1762.

Preeclampsia is defined as the onset of hypertension, edema, and proteinuria after 20 weeks of gestation. It occurs most often in young primigravida and older multiparous women of lower socioeconomic class. It usually has a gradual onset, manifesting after 32 weeks of gestation. Preeclampsia may occur up to 7 days after delivery. Emergency providers must be aware of normal blood pressure limits during pregnancy and refer all affected women for early follow-up. Blood pressures <140/90 mm Hg do not require immediate treatment. If the blood pressure is >140/90 mm Hg with signs of preeclampsia, intravenous magnesium sulfate, which acts to reduce central nervous system irritability, is the initial agent of choice. Oral antihypertensive agents are needed but can be delayed until after the patient is admitted.

8. **C,** Pages 1762-1763.

This patient has signs and symptoms most consistent with a proximal aortic dissection involving the carotid artery, which accounts for his syncopal episode and hemiplegia. Aortic dissection is often not obvious. MRI, CT scan, or aortography is needed to confirm the diagnosis. Most cases occur in middle-aged men with a history of hypertension. Twenty-five percent will have aortic insufficiency. Treatment involves judicious lowering of systolic blood pressure to 100-120 mm Hg with nitroprusside and/or trimethaphan as the agents of choice. Surgical intervention is required if the process involves the ascending aorta or if there is leaking from the dissection, compromised cerebral circulation, aortic regurgitation with heart failure, continuing dissection, or failure to control pain and blood pressure. This patient should not be managed with medical therapy alone because of his obvious cerebral compromise. Immediate surgical consultation should be obtained.

9. **E,** Pages 1763-1764.
10. **D,** Pages 1763-1764.
11. **B,** Pages 1763-1764.
12. **C,** Pages 1763-1764.
13. **A,** Pages 1763-1764.

Emergency physicians need to be aware of the potential side effects and complications that may arise from the use of antihypertensive agents.

Labetalol is both an alpha- and beta-blocker that may cause bronchospasm and worsen AV block. It is contraindicated in patients with pheochromocytoma.

Nitroprusside at high doses >800 μg per minute for long periods can accumulate cyanide/thiocyanate byproducts, leading to toxicity.

Diazoxide, a thiazide–like smooth muscle relaxant, should be used with caution in congestive heart failure secondary to marked sodium and water retention. Its use also may lead to hyperglycemia and hyperuricemia.

Trimethaphan affects adrenergic control of all smooth muscle, which explains its effect on the gastrointestinal tract and bladder.

Clonidine causes profound rebound hypertension 16-48 hours after acute withdrawal.

14. **E,** Page 1758.
15. **C,** Page 1758.

Tyramine, an amino acid found in many foods such as beer, wine, cheese, and chocolate, causes release of norepinephrine stores. It is degraded by the monoamine oxidase system. Small amounts of tyramine can cause severe, prolonged hypertension. In the presence of monoamine oxidase inhibitors used to treat depression, tyramine breakdown is blocked, leading to a prolonged hypertensive syndrome. Certain foods rich in tyramine should be avoided during treatment with monoamine oxidase inhibitors. Hypertension due to catecholamine excess is best controlled with phentolamine, a peripheral alpha-blocker. Rosen Box 106-1 lists foods and drugs associated with hypertensive crises in the presence of monoamine oxidase inhibition.

16. **A,** Page 1759.

Malignant hypertension is defined as severe hypertension associated with evidence of end-organ damage. The syndrome may occur at any time in the course of hypertension. The diagnosis can not be made on the basis of blood pressure alone. Patients must display evidence of end-organ damage. The combination of necrosis of arteriolar smooth muscle, leaking plasma, and fibrin deposition is known as fibrinoid necrosis. This is the pathologic change responsible for end-organ damage in hypertension. Retinal changes, such as cotton-wool spots and linear hemorrhages, are commonly seen in patients with malignant hypertension. Blood pressure must be lowered judiciously by 30%-40% of pretreatment levels within 1 hour.

17. **B,** Page 1765.

Evaluation of the patient with hypertension should include a complete history and physical (including funduscopic examination), determination of BUN, creatinine, serum electrolytes, EKG, and urinalysis to identify evidence of end-organ disease. If there is no evidence of end-organ disease, the Joint National Committee on Detection, Evaluation, and Treatment of High Blood Pressure's recommendations for treating hypertensive urgencies include lowering the blood pressure within 24 hours to reduce potential risks to the patient. The most commonly used medications are labetalol and clonidine. Sublingual nifedipine is considered to be a potentially dangerous medication in this setting because of its often profound and unpredictable effect on blood pressure. The use of nitroprusside is reserved for hypertensive emergencies.

18. **E,** Pages 1766-1767.
19. **D,** Pages 1766-1767.
20. **F,** Pages 1766-1767.
21. **C,** Pages 1766-1767.
22. **A,** Pages 1766-1767.
23. **B,** Pages 1766-1767.

Rosen Table 106-2 lists commonly used antihypertensive medications. It is important for the emergency provider to be familiar with these medications, their mechanism of action, and common side effects. Furosemide is a diuretic with actions at the ascending loop of Henle. Clonidine acts centrally to block sympathetic output. Captopril is an angiotensin-converting enzyme inhibitor with actions in the renin-angiotensin system. Prazosin acts at the postsynaptic membrane to block alpha-receptors, leading to lowered blood pressure. Nifedipine is a first-generation calcium channel blocker with actions on arterial smooth muscle. Propranolol is a beta-adrenergic blocker having direct effects on the cardiovascular system.

# 107 Pulmonary Embolism

### *James E. Thompson*

1. **B,** Page 1773.
Pulmonary thromboembolism is a complication of underlying venous thrombosis and may arise from many sources. Autopsy results have shown that 70% of patients with pulmonary emboli have clot demonstrated in the veins of the lower extremities. Other sources include right heart thrombus, upper extremity thrombus, and veins of the lower leg. More than 30% of patients with pulmonary embolism have no clearly demonstrable source of thromboembolism. Estimates of risks of pulmonary emboli from thrombus below the calf remain an area of controversy. The frequency of PE from DVT isolated to the calf appears to be between 33%-46%. The estimated frequency of deep calf vein thrombosis propagating above the knee is 87%.

2. **D,** Page 1775.
Other substances besides thrombus are capable of passing through the systemic venous circulation and lodging in the pulmonary vasculature. These include amniotic fluid, fat, and air. Cases of pulmonary emboli have been reported from sources such as bullets, barium, catheters, tumor, and bile. Non-thrombotic emboli are treated with supportive measures. Anticoagulants and thrombolytic therapy are not indicated in the management of emboli from such sources.

3. **E,** Page 1774.
Amniotic fluid pulmonary emboli are serious complications that can occur with abortion, immediately postpartum, or, most frequently, near the end of the first stage of labor. Management includes supportive measures with evacuation of the uterus. Thrombolytic agents are of no benefit in the treatment of amniotic fluid emboli. Infusion of fresh frozen plasma, platelets, cryoprecipitate, or whole blood may be necessary because DIC is a common complication and accounts for a mortality rate of up to 80%.

4. **C,** Page 1774.
Fat emboli most commonly occur after fractures of the long bones. Fat globules obstructing the end-capillaries throughout the systemic circulation may lead to petechiae, most often noted on the thorax, fundi and conjunctivae.

5. **B,** Page 1774.
The described patient reveals multiorgan involvement of emboli. Fat emboli are capable of passing through the pulmonary circulation and can lodge in any vascular bed. The cerebral circulation is commonly involved, with central nervous system symptoms ranging from headache and confusion to seizures and coma. Petechiae are common and frequently seen on the chest, neck, axillae, and fundi. Respiratory distress is frequently noted. Numerous treatment modalities have been used, including steroids, heparin, emulsifying agents, Dextran, and hypothermia. Of these, the only therapy of potential value has been high-dose steroids. Heparin therapy may have a potential risk of toxic fatty acid production in the lungs and should be avoided.

6. **E,** Page 1774.
Air emboli can originate from multiple sources, the vast majority being iatrogenic. Circulatory collapse and death may result from as little as 5 ml/kg of air, forming an air lock in the right ventricle or in the pulmonary circulation. Sources described include the use of pressurized diving equipment, surgical air powered tools, and vaginal insufflation originally used to treat trichomonal vaginitis. More recently the syndrome has been associated with orogenital sex during pregnancy when air may pass more easily between the fetal membranes and the subplacental sinuses, ultimately leading to circulatory collapse.

7. **E,** Page 1774.
Air embolus is often an iatrogenic event occurring with invasive procedures. A patient with air emboli may have circulatory collapse and a loud churning murmur over the precordium. Echocardiography may reveal air bubbles within the heart. Management involves placement of the patient in the left lateral decubitus position in an attempt to trap the air in the right atrium. Removal may be accomplished with right heart catheterization and aspiration. In full arrest situations, emergency thoracotomy with direct needle aspiration may be successful. Hyperbaric oxygen therapy may be used in stable patients to decrease the size of the air bubble in the pulmonary tree, decreasing the affected areas of pulmonary and cerebral circulation.

8. **B,** Page 1777.
The Urokinase and Urokinase/Streptokinase trials indicate that the presentations of PE are nonspecific. Dyspnea was the most common symptom (84%), followed by pleuritic chest pain (74%), apprehension (59%), cough (53%), and hemoptysis (30%).

9. **E,** Page 1777.
The Urokinase Pulmonary Emboli Trial (UPET) study provides a generally accepted guideline to the signs and symp-

toms of pulmonary emboli as listed in Rosen Tables 107-2 and 107-3. It should be noted that this study suffers from overrepresentation of hospitalized, terminally ill patients, which may differ from ED populations. This study has shown the most common symptom to be dyspnea, occurring in 84% of angiographically proven PE, with pleuritic chest pain being the second most common at 74%. The most common sign was found to be tachypnea >16 per minute in 92% of patients, with rales being the second most common finding present in 58% of patients.

10. **B,** Page 1777.

The classic triad of hemoptysis, pleuritic chest pain, and dyspnea has been reported in only 20% of patients with pulmonary emboli. Of patients who die from PE, only 60% have dyspnea, only 17% have chest pain, and only 3% have hemoptysis. The presentation of pulmonary emboli is quite variable with initial presentations including complaints of abdominal pain, high fever, hiccoughs, new onset atrial fibrillation, DIC, or a host of other varied symptoms and signs.

11. **A,** Page 1779.

Risk factors of thromboembolic disease are based on Virchow's triad of venostasis, hypercoagulable state, and vessel wall inflammation. Although pulmonary emboli most often occur in patients between 50 and 65 years, age has not been found to be an independent risk factor. This age predominance may result from other independent risk factors, such as prolonged immobilization, postoperative period, deep vein thrombosis, CHF, trauma, burns, obesity, previous pulmonary emboli, malignancy, and hypercoagulable states. When a patient with these risk factors presents with symptoms consistent with PE, the diagnosis must be sought aggressively.

12. **E,** Page 1779.

Hypercoagulable states may be responsible for approximately 50% of clinically detected venous thromboembolic events; however, these hypercoagulable states are usually not diagnosed until a patient has had a clinically significant DVT or PE. Common hypercoagulable states include pregnancy, oral estrogen therapy, polycythemia, protein C or S deficiency, antithrombin III deficiency, underlying malignancy, and cigarette smoking.

13. **E,** Page 1779.

Antithrombin III deficiency is a familial disorder that causes thrombotic events. It frequently occurs in the third decade of life. It should be considered in young patients with multiple deep vein thromboses or in patients with recurrent thromboembolic disease. Heparin is ineffective as an anticoagulant in the absence of antithrombin III. Appropriate treatment involves anticoagulation using warfarin.

14. **A,** Page 1794.

Protein C is a naturally occurring anticoagulant, the deficiency of which can lead to thrombosis. Protein C is a vitamin K–dependent protein, like factors II, VII, IX, and X, in which synthesis is inhibited by warfarin therapy. High doses of warfarin given to patients with protein C deficiency may cause a thrombotic state secondary to a critical suppression

of protein C levels that may occur prior to the suppression of other vitamin K–dependent factors. High-dose warfarin therapy should therefore be avoided in patients known to be protein C deficient.

15. **E,** Page 1781.

Pulse oximetry is a useful and rapid method of determining a patient's need for supplemental oxygen; however, there is no role for it in the diagnostic work-up for suspected pulmonary embolism (PE). The alveolar-arterial gradient is a reliable measure of impaired gas exchange. Its use, along with arterial blood gases, may be helpful in the diagnosis of PE. Studies have shown that a high percentage of patients with PE have elevated A-a gradients as well as a decreased $PaO_2$. However, 50% of patients may have a normal ABG or a $PaO_2$ >80 torr. Some experts suggest that the diagnosis of PE may be made with the use of spirometry and calculation of the ratio of dead space to tidal volume (Vd/Vt). A Vd/Vt ratio <40% is regarded as low probability, whereas a ratio >40% is regarded as high probability for PE if the remainder of the spirometry results are normal.

16. **B,** Page 1783.

The most common ECG changes are tachycardia and nonspecific ST and T wave abnormalities. In the presence of PE, the classically described ECG changes are those related to right heart strain. A tall peaked P wave in lead II (P pulmonale), right axis deviation, RBBB, an S1-Q3-T3 pattern, or new-onset atrial fibrillation. Only 20% of patients with PE will have classic ECG findings; another 25% will have ECGs unchanged from baseline.

17. **D,** Page 1783.

Chest radiography is both nonsensitive and nonspecific for pulmonary thromboembolism. Westermark's sign is a dilation of the pulmonary vessel proximal to the emboli with distal blood vessel collapse and if present, is the earliest detectable chest radiograph finding. Another classic radiographic finding suggestive of PE is Hampton's hump, a triangular, pleural-based infiltrate frequently found at the costophrenic junction. A highly specific finding on serial radiographs in a patient with suspected PE is a focal infiltrate that develops within 3 days of onset of symptoms. Up to 30% of patients with PE will have a normal chest radiograph, while 50% will have an elevated hemidiaphragm and 50% eventually develop parenchymal infiltrates mimicking pneumonia.

18. **E,** Page 1785.

The V/Q scan is the single most important diagnostic modality for pulmonary thromboembolism available to the emergency physician. Ventilation scans combined with perfusion scans may reveal an area of mismatch, indicative of pulmonary emboli. Many pathologic processes other than PE can cause perfusion defects on a lung scan. For example, local parenchymal collapse, consolidation, vasoconstriction, COPD, and CHF may cause an asymmetry of perfusion. A V/Q scan with two or more segmental perfusion defects without ventilation defects, however, provides sufficient evidence for the diagnosis of PE.

19. **B,** Page 1788.

The PIOPED study provides guidelines for interpreting V/Q scans. It is based on the results of 877 patients enrolled in a prospective trial with angiographically proven PE who underwent V/Q scanning. Rosen Figure 107-7 defines the PIOPED V/Q classifications. A non-segmental perfusion defect is considered a low-probability scan. All other answers are high-probability classifications. It is important for the emergency physician to be familiar with these classifications and the radiographic findings with which they correspond.

20. **A,** Page 1789.

In a patient with multiple risk factors for PE and symptoms suggestive of the diagnosis, a high-probability V/Q scan reading is convincing enough (95% combined predictive value) that angiography is not needed to confirm the diagnosis of PE. The only other clinical situation in which a V/Q scan result provides an end-point involves a patient with a low clinical suspicion for PE who has a normal V/Q scan. This is sufficient to rule out the diagnosis. All other patients must undergo further work-up.

21. **D,** Page 1787.

Only normal or high-probability V/Q scans in the clinical setting of low or high clinical suspicion respectively may be acceptable end-points for work-up of PE. An intermediate V/Q scan does not change the clinical likelihood of PE. An intermediate V/Q scan has a sensitivity of 41% and a positive predictive value of only 30%. Therefore, if presumed positive, it will be wrong 70% of the time and, if presumed negative, it will miss 41% of PEs.

22. **A,** Page 1787.

The PIOPED study concluded that a V/Q scan, in combination with clinical assessment, will diagnose or exclude only a small number of patients. This study showed that a normal V/Q scan pattern excludes the possibility of embolism with a specificity of 96%. If a normal V/Q scan is presumed to be negative, it will be correct 96% of the time but will miss 2% of cases of PE. 4% of patients with a normal pattern will be found to have PE if angiography is performed. A normal V/Q scan (no perfusion defects) is not a guarantee, but is an acceptable end-point for the work-up of PE when the clinical likelihood is not high.

23. **E,** Page 1790.

In the PIOPED study, 1100 patients underwent pulmonary angiography. There were 60 minor complications (5.4%), 9 major complications (0.8%), and 5 deaths (0.4%) that occurred with angiography. Complications reported in the PIOPED and other studies include anaphylactoid reactions, dysrhythmias, endocardial injury including perforation, and cardiac arrest.

24. **D,** Page 1790.

Pulmonary angiogram is the most invasive, yet most reliable, test for diagnosing PE. It is considered the gold standard test for PE. However, it is not without complications; reported complication rates range from 1% to 5%, and the expected mortality is 1 to 4 per 1000. Complications that may occur include anaphylactoid reactions, dysrhythmias, cardiac arrest, and vessel perforation by the catheter. Complications are more frequent in patients with pulmonary hypertension, allergic histories, ventricular ectopy, left bundle branch block, and serious underlying disease. A false-positive test may result from extraluminal tumors or extrinsic masses compressing vessels that produce angiographic lesions similar to PE. In the presence of anticoagulation, a positive angiogram may be found up to 1 week after initiating therapy. However, lytic therapy may produce complete resolution of the clot within 90 minutes. Therefore, delayed angiography should not be performed when using thrombolytics.

25. **E,** Pages 1793-1799.

Once the diagnosis of PE is proven or presumed correct, several different treatment options are available. The treatment depends on the clinical stability of the patient and the presence of underlying disease states. Treatment options include anticoagulation if the patient is hemodynamically stable; the presence of circulatory collapse is an indication for more aggressive measures including thrombolytic therapy, catheter embolectomy, or open embolectomy.

26. **D,** Page 1793.

Patients with submassive PE may have hemodynamic instability and shock. Simple volume expansion is usually not helpful because although this will raise the systemic blood pressure, such patients are already facing acutely increased right ventricular afterload. Massive volume infusion may therefore exacerbate this situation, leading to worsened right ventricular function. If an inotropic agent is required, there is evidence that isoproterenol may be the preferred cardiotropic agent in these situations. As a pure beta agonist, it is a more effective dilator of pulmonary arterioles and thus leads to decreased right ventricular outflow resistance while also improving myocardial contractility.

27. **A,** Page 1793.

Anticoagulation therapy with heparin remains the traditional treatment for PE. Its aggressive use has been shown to reduce the overall mortality of PE to <10%. It acts to prevent clot progression and reduces the risk of further embolic events, but it is not capable of dissolving an already formed clot. Heparin can safely be used in pregnancy because it does not cross the placenta. In the absence of any contraindication, anticoagulation with heparin should be started as soon as the diagnosis of PE is seriously entertained, before completion of any diagnostic tests. Complication rates of up to 15% have been noted and include an immune-mediated thrombocytopenia, which appears 1-2 weeks after initiation of therapy.

28. **B,** Page 1795.

In the 1990s thrombolytic therapy has replaced surgery in the management of the hemodynamically unstable patient with PE. There are three distinct groups for whom thrombolysis is mandatory: the hemodynamically unstable patient, the group of patients who have exhausted cardiopulmonary reserve, and those in whom multiple recurrences are anticipated. The UPET trial demonstrated a 2-week case fatality rate of 18% in patients with PE and shock versus 73% for patients at the same institutions who were not enrolled in the study. Thrombolytic therapy has a bleeding risk almost twice as high as that for heparin therapy. Thrombolytic agents can rapidly normalize hemodynamic instability because they act to dissolve the clot directly, whereas a non-thrombolysed clot will eventually recanalize, leaving the affected vessels with permanently reduced elastic distensibility. Thrombolytics have been shown to improve the long-term complications as well as reduce the recurrence rate of DVT and PE. The long-term benefit of thrombolytic therapy outweighs the increased risks of bleeding.

29. **E,** Page 1797.
As the use of thrombolytic agents becomes more common, emergency physicians should be aware of the absolute contraindications to their use. These include active internal bleeding, neurosurgery within the past 8 weeks, active external bleeding, recent renal or hepatic biopsy, or ocular surgery within 8 weeks. A recent cerebrovascular accident is a relative contraindication, and thrombolytic therapy may be used in selective cases, although the clinician must bear in mind that the rate of intracranial bleed in all patients given thrombolytics for PE is 0.4%. The benefits of therapy must exceed the risk of intracranial bleed in order to be justified.

30. **D,** Page 1797.
A patient with suspected PE with sudden cardiac arrest may benefit most from emergent bilateral thoracotomy with massage of the pulmonary vessels to dislodge a saddle embolus and restore pulmonary blood flow. This must be performed immediately, because no oxygenated blood will perfuse the brain until pulmonary circulation is restored. Should no saddle embolus be appreciated in the pulmonary vessels, at least open-chest CPR may be performed while other reversible causes of sudden cardiopulmonary arrest are sought.

 **108** Abdominal Aortic Aneurysm

*James E. Thompson*

1. **D,** Page 1806.
Asymptomatic patients with abdominal aortic aneurysms can appropriately be referred to a surgeon for elective repair. AAAs are classified as being intact, leaking, or ruptured. The key to improving the outcome of patients with AAAs is early diagnosis of the condition before a rupture occurs. Whereas the mortality for elective repair has decreased since the early 1960s, the mortality rate for repair of the already ruptured aneurysm remains near 50%.

2. **E,** Pages 1813-1814.
Delay in making the diagnosis of acute rupture of abdominal aortic aneurysm in the ED is a significant predictor of poor outcome. Goals include all of those listed, as well as the appropriate selection of diagnostic imaging studies. Attempts to fully resuscitate patients with ruptured AAA in the ED should be avoided. Hypotensive patients need definitive treatment in the operating room, initially cross-clamping of the aorta and controlling hemorrhage.

3. **A,** Page 1806.
The aorta is composed of three layers of tissue: the intima, media, and adventitia. Compliance in large vessels such as the aorta is provided primarily by the elastic lamina, which is found in the media. A pseudoaneurysm or false aneurysm is a collection of blood that is in communication with the aortic lumen but is not enclosed by intima. The pseudoaneurysm is contained by the adventitial layer or the surrounding soft tissues. The natural course of abdominal aortic aneurysms is to enlarge gradually, at a rate of 0-1.8 cm per year, with a mean expansion rate of 0.5 cm per year. Most AAAs arise below the renal arteries and involve the lower abdominal aorta. Seventy percent involve the iliac arteries, whereas only 2% extend proximally to involve the renal arteries and other branches.

4. **B,** Page 1806.
Aortic aneurysms are frequently confused with aortic dissections. Aneurysms occur almost exclusively in the abdomen, while dissections are predominantly located in the thoracic aorta. Most dissections that involve the abdominal aorta are actually extensions of the dissections of the thoracic aorta. Isolated abdominal aortic dissections, like thoracic aortic dissections, occur in middle age, affect more men than women, and occur more in hypertensive patients. Unlike thoracic aortic dissections, other associated conditions such as medial dysplasia, Marfan's syndrome, congenital cardiovascular lesions, and pregnancy are rarely associated with isolated abdominal aortic dissections.

5. **D,** Page 1806.
The two major proteins responsible for the structural integrity of the aorta are elastin and collagen. Elastin contributes to blood vessel compliance, which helps maintain normal diameter. The current concept of the etiology of AAA is that loss or failure of elastin leads to aneurysm formation. In AAA, elastin concentration is decreased by up to 92%. The role of collagen in the development of AAAs is less clear. Collagen appears to provide the aortic wall with tensile strength, and collagen content in the AAA is usually increased. Most AAAs occur in patients with advanced atherosclerotic disease of the aorta; however, the exact role that atherosclerosis plays in the process of aneurysm formation and rupture is not clear. Most patients with atherosclerosis in other blood vessels have occlusive disease, not aneurysms.

6. **E,** Page 1810.
In patients presenting with the classic triad of pain, hypotension, and a pulsatile mass, the diagnosis of ruptured AAA is easily made. Few patients, however, present in the classic fashion. The sudden onset of pain often leads to the diagnosis of renal colic. Epigastric abdominal pain and tenderness suggest pancreatitis. Presentation with epigastric pain and hypotension may lead to the diagnosis of acute MI. This may be further complicated in an elderly patient with coexistent coronary disease having new ECG changes secondary to the diminished coronary perfusion from the ruptured AAA. Ischemic chest pain and ECG changes consistent with myocardial ischemia do not rule out the presence of a ruptured AAA.

7. **B,** Page 1807.

Abdominal aortic aneurysms occur predominantly in males, with the male-to-female ratio being 7:1. White males are affected substantially more frequently than black males, whose incidence of AAAs is approximately the same as that of white and black females. The incidence of AAAs increases with age, and approximately 80% of patients with AAA are between 61 and 80 years old. Most patients with AAAs are cigarette smokers, and approximately 50% have a past history of hypertension and coronary artery disease. Genetics seem to play a role in the development of AAAs. A sevenfold increase in the likelihood of having an AAA occurs if a close relative has an AAA. In a family with a history of AAAs, the risk of rupture increases if a female member is affected.

8. **C,** Page 1808.

Because the aortic bifurcation lies at the level of the umbilicus, most aneurysms are palpated above the navel. Most patients with AAA have full femoral pulses, and most have only mild abdominal tenderness and guarding. Most intact AAAs are non-tender to palpation and have a gradual onset with a dull, vague quality. Severe pain or tenderness on palpation are ominous signs of imminent or actual rupture. Most patients with AAA are entirely asymptomatic, and their aneurysm is discovered incidentally on physical examination or with a radiographic procedure done for other reasons.

9. **B,** Pages 1810-1813.

The sensitivity of ultrasonography approaches 100% for detection of AAA, and the measurements of AAA size correlate within 3 mm of surgical specimens. Advantages of ultrasound include its emergent use at the bedside and quickness of detection and lack of dye load. Although the sensitivity of both the CT scan and ultrasound is near 100% in detecting AAA, the CT scan is more accurate than ultrasound in determining aortic size, detecting traumas, defining cranial-caudal extent, and demonstrating the involvement of the visceral arteries, inferior vena cava, and suprarenal aorta. Disadvantages of CT are cost, technician availability, longer study time, and complications of IV contrast. Angiography provides a detailed view of the arterial anatomy and demonstrates occlusive lesions. Because only the aortic lumen is seen on angiograph, thrombus can create an image that underestimates the size of the aneurysm. Digital subtraction angiography is an alternative to conventional angiography that requires less time, uses less contrast material, and is less invasive. MRI is an excellent modality for imaging the aorta, because contrast material and ionizing radiation are not needed, and the image produced is equal or superior to a CT image. Limited availability for routine use, increased costs, prolonged scan times, and inability to scan patients with pacemakers, intracranial clips, monitors, and ventilators limit the use of MRI for AAAs. Radiographic signs of AAA are seen on plain film in 66%-75% of cases. The most common positive findings are curvilinear calcification of the aortic wall.

10. **C,** Page 1380.

Hypotension is the single most significant preoperative factor associated with increased mortality, and avoiding or limiting hypotension must be a high priority for the emergency physician in the treatment of ruptured AAA.

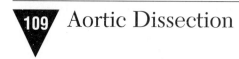

# 109 Aortic Dissection

*James E. Thompson*

1. **E,** Page 1819.

Blunt trauma is usually associated not with aortic dissection but with aortic rupture. This is a separate entity which typically occurs with deceleration injury rather than longstanding media degeneration secondary to hypertension or congenital disorders of elastin. In blunt deceleration trauma, the thoracic aorta may continue to move forward while being anchored in two places, the aortic root and the ligamentum arteriosum. The resultant shearing forces usually produce a tear at the fixation points, typically just distal to the left subclavian artery.

2. **D,** Page 1820.

Dissection is not only the most common, but also the most lethal catastrophe involving the aorta. Aortic dissection occurs two to three times more frequently in males than females, and may have a higher incidence in blacks. Although aortic dissection has been reported in patients as young as 14 months and as old as 100 years, the majority of cases occur in patients between 50 and 70 years of age. Aortic dissection is relatively rare before age 40, except in association with specific predisposing syndromes, such as Marfan syndrome, Ehlers-Danlos syndrome, congenital heart disease, familial incidence, pregnancy, coarctation of the aorta, Turner's syndrome, and trauma. The type of trauma that is usually associated with aortic dissection is iatrogenic, such as cardiac surgery and cardiac catheterization. Blunt trauma to the chest from high-speed deceleration injury usually causes aortic rupture, an entity distinctly different from aortic dissection. The incidence of aortic dissection is nine times higher in patients with a bicuspid valve, compared with a tricuspid aortic valve. Aortic dissection occurs more often in patients with a history of coarctation.

3. **D,** Page 1820.

An aortic dissection is a longitudinal cleavage of the aortic media by a dissecting column of blood. Because the affected aorta is infrequently aneurysmal, the term *aortic dissection* is preferred to *dissecting aortic aneurysm.* The aortic wall is composed of three layers: the intimal, the media, and the adventitia. The media is composed of elastic and smooth muscle tissue and can undergo a process of degeneration characterized by a loss of smooth muscle cells and elastin, accompanied by fibrotic scarring and hyaline-like changes.

4. **D,** Page 1821.

The anatomic classification of aortic dissection is important from both the diagnostic and therapeutic standpoints. The Stanford classification is based on the involvement of the ascending aorta. Type A dissections involve the ascending aorta; type B dissections do not. Dissections that involve the ascending aorta are much more lethal than those limited to the distal aorta and have a different therapeutic approach. Type A dissections are managed surgically, while type B dissections may be managed medically, depending on the presence of complications or uncontrollable hypertension. About two thirds of the patients have type A dissections, and one third have type B. Generally, patients with type B dissections tend to be older, frequently are heavy smokers with chronic lung disease, often have generalized atherosclerosis, and are more often hypertensive than their counterparts with proximal aortic dissection.

5. **E,** Page 1821.

Pain is by far the most common presenting complaint and is present in more than 90% of the cases. It is typically described as tearing, ripping, or knifelike but may be characterized by different patients in many different ways. Typically the pain occurs quite abruptly, with maximum intensity at the onset. In about 20% of the patients, neurologic deficit is the presenting manifestation of aortic dissection. The neurologic presentations are cerebrovascular accidents, spinal cord ischemia, and peripheral nerve ischemia. Pulse deficits and discrepancies in blood pressure between limbs are key diagnostic clues. Pulse deficit, a unilaterally weakened or absent pulse, occurs in almost half of patients with proximal dissections. Patients with type A dissections can present with aortic regurgitation. The usual signs of chronic aortic insufficiency may not be present in this setting. Neurologic findings are common in aortic dissections. The most common abnormality, however, is an altered sensorium. The most common focal neurologic abnormalities are hemiplegia, hemianesthesia, and gaze preference to the affected side. Ischemic paraparesis occurs in only about 4% of dissections and is a result of the interruption of blood flow in the intercostal, lumbar, and anterior spinal arteries.

6. **E,** Page 1821.

Two different classification systems for describing aortic dissection exist. DeBakey classifies aortic dissection into three types: type I dissections involve the ascending aorta, the aortic arch, and the descending aorta; type II dissections are confined in the ascending aorta; and type III dissections are confined in the descending aorta distal to the left subclavian artery. Type III is sometimes subdivided into dissections that stay above the diaphragm (type IIIA) and those that propagate below it (type IIIB). The Stanford classification system is based on involvement of the ascending aorta. Type A dissections involve the ascending aorta whereas type B do not. These classification systems are important from both a diagnostic as well as a therapeutic standpoint.

7. **B,** Page 1824.

All patients with suspected acute aortic dissection should receive careful monitoring of cardiac rhythm, blood pressure, and urine output. The objective of early management is to eliminate the forces favoring progression of the dissection by maintaining systolic blood pressure between 100 and 120 mm Hg. Trimethaphan is effective in the initial treatment of acute aortic dissection and is generally used as a single agent. It is the preferred drug in the patient who has a contraindication to beta-blockers. Labetalol has both alpha- and beta-blockage properties and may be used as a single agent for the management of aortic dissection. Prompt reduction of blood pressure can be accomplished with sodium nitroprusside; however, it increases the heart rate and may also increase the rate of rise of the arterial pulse, which may worsen the dissection. A beta-adrenergic blocker must be used in conjunction with sodium nitroprusside. Propranolol is often utilized to aid in reducing the heart rate to 60-80 beats per minute. A more selective beta blocking agent, such as metoprolol or esmolol, may cause fewer undesirable side effects.

8. **A,** Page 1824.

Type A acute aortic dissections require surgical treatment. The only contraindication to immediate surgical repair of a type A dissection is the simultaneous occurrence of a progressing stroke. Definitive treatment of type B acute aortic dissections is less clear. Generally, these patients tend to be greater surgical risks, and the hospital mortality in patients treated without surgery who have acute type B dissections is 15%-20%, which is comparable to or better than the mortality rate with surgery in most institutions. Uncomplicated distal dissections have in general been treated with blood pressure control, with surgery being reserved for those patients who have persistent pain, uncontrolled hypertension, occlusion of a major arterial trunk, frank aortic leaking or rupture, or development of a localized aneurysm.

9. **B,** Page 1822.

No laboratory test is routinely abnormal in an acute aortic dissection. Serial cardiac enzymes are rarely elevated, unless the dissection has involved the coronary arteries. Routine chest radiography will be abnormal in 80%-90% of cases. The most common abnormality is mediastinal widening, which occurs in 75% of cases. Other radiographic findings include the calcium sign and a double-density appearance of the aorta suggesting a true and false lumen. The use of transthoracic echocardiography has an unacceptably low sensitivity, ranging from 70% to 80%, and is not typically used in imaging patients with suspected dissection. Transesophageal echocardiography, however, has a dramatically improved sensitivity and specificity and can be quickly performed at the ED bedside, but requires sedation and is operator dependent. CT is a reliable modality in a hemodynamically stable patient, and one of its advantages is that it requires no arterial cannulation, unlike aortography. Despite the newer diagnostic modalities available to the emergency physician and the limited role aortography may now play in many emergency departments, it is the modality by which all others are compared and is therefore the gold standard.

# 110 Peripheral Arteriovascular Disease

*Hans Notenboom*

1. **B,** Page 1827.
Atherosclerosis is a disease of large and medium-size muscular arteries. All of the listed vessels are commonly affected except those of the upper extremities.

2. **E,** Page 1827.
Most (85%) arterial emboli originate from the heart, with the left ventricle responsible for 60%-70% and the atria for 5%-10%. Atrial fibrillation is present in 60%-75% of patients with arterial emboli. The bifurcation of the common femoral artery is the most common site for emboli, with the larger aorta and the iliac arteries less frequently involved than the smaller femoral and popliteal arteries.

3. **C,** Page 1842.
In Raynaud's disease, triggers such as cold and emotion result in arterial vasospasm. The arteries are histologically normal, and tissue loss does not occur. Treatment may include reserpine, phenoxybenzamine, or pentoxifylline. Ergots may induce or worsen attacks. Regional sympathectomy provides little lasting benefit in patients with secondary Raynaud's phenomenon.

4. **D,** Pages 1829-1830, 1835.
Rest pain usually involves the foot from the metatarsals distally. It is improved by dangling the legs or standing. The location of claudication correlates well with the level of arterial disease. Calf pain is usually more severe than proximal pain. The majority of those with severe disease causing bilateral claudication will also be impotent.

5. **C,** Page 1830.
Emboli usually have an identifiable source, often the heart. Signs of severe and diffuse vascular disease are less often present in emboli than in thrombosis. The occlusion with emboli is sharply defined, both by symptoms and arteriography.

6. **A,** Page 1836.
Shionoya's criteria for definition of thromboangiitis obliterans include age younger than 50 at onset and a history of smoking. The other choices are common findings in Burger's disease.

7. **C,** Pages 1838-1839.
Popliteal aneurysms are the most common peripheral aneurysm, with up to 60% found bilaterally. The finding of a popliteal aneurysm should result in a search for other aneurysms, including abdominal aortic aneurysms. Incidence of aortic aneurysm is 80% in those with bilateral popliteal aneurysm identified. Aneurysmal dilation causing compression of deep veins can produce deep venous thrombosis. Limb-threatening thromboembolic events, claudication, and atherosclerotic events are associated with popliteal aneurysm.

8. **A,** Pages 1840-1841.
Aneurysmal rupture is inevitable without surgical repair. The other choices are correct, although life-long treatment after successful surgical repair has been advocated by some authors.

9. **D,** Pages 1843.
Temporal arteritis is a disease of older persons, with females twice as commonly affected as males. It classically involves one or more branches of the carotid artery but may involve any artery. The irreversibility of visual loss drives the urgency for steroid treatment. Biopsy should be completed within 48 hours of initiating treatment, or the characteristic giant cells may not be found.

10. **E,** Pages 1844-1845.
About 95% of cases of thoracic outlet syndrome are a result of brachial plexus compression. This most commonly compresses the C8 and T1 nerve roots, mimicking ulnar nerve complaints. Bony abnormalities are associated with arterial compression. Bedside arterial testing is insensitive, but the EAST test is a sensitive means for diagnosing all forms of thoracic outlet syndrome.

11. **C,** Pages 1847-1848.
Arterial injury in intravenous drug abusers is most common in the upper extremities, but pseudoaneurysms form more often in the lower extremities (80%). Distal ischemia is usually associated with a preserved pulse but decreased skin temperature. Ultrasound is not reliable in distinguishing abscess from aneurysm. Angiography is the test of choice. Therapy is usually conservative; surgery is reserved for tissue loss and pseudoaneurysm resection. Anticoagulation has not been demonstrated to be of benefit.

12. **E,** Pages 1848-1849.
The first step in evaluation of a totally occluded central venous catheter is a chest roentgenogram to evaluate placement. A fibrin sheath will cause withdrawal occlusion, but not total occlusion. Subclavian vein thrombosis may be suspected because of catheter malfunction and is not always associated with limb swelling. Hickman-Broviac catheters broken closer than 4 cm from the skin insertion site must be removed.

# 111 Peripheral Venous Disease of the Extremities

*Hans Notenboom*

1. **A,** Page 1873.
Most lower extremity venous thrombi begin around the valve cusps in the deep calf veins or within the soleal plexus. Some thrombi also arise in the iliofemoral veins or as simultaneous multifocal clots.

2. **C,** Pages 1876, 1878.
Although it is widely believed that DVT confined to the veins below the knee is unlikely to cause PE, this is untrue. Calf DVT can cause serious PE without propagating above the knee. At autopsy, 35% of patients with PE have isolated calf DVT. Heparin anticoagulation was introduced into clinical practice in the 1930s, reducing the mortality of PE from 30% to less than 10% by reducing thrombus propagation and thus reducing the size and frequency of recurrent emboli. Post-

phlebitic syndrome develops in 20%-41% of patients with deep calf vein thrombi.

3. **A,** Pages 1873-1876.

Diabetes is not directly related to risk for venous thrombosis. Heparin may induce heparin-associated thrombocytopenia. This can precipitate thrombosis more often in the arterial circulation than in the venous system.

4. **B,** Pages 1865-1867.

Contrast venography is neither perfectly sensitive nor specific in the diagnosis of venous pathology, but it is nonetheless the standard to which all other diagnostic tests are compared. Ultrasound imaging is not as sensitive or specific as contrast venography and will miss venous thromboembolism in as many as 40% of cases, depending on the location. Doppler sensitivity and specificity increases in the hands of an experienced operator. MRI has been shown to reliably detect thrombus in deep veins in the calf, thigh, and pelvis. In addition, MRI can identify other anatomic causes for leg pain and edema when clinical findings incorrectly suggest DVT.

5. **E,** Pages 1872-1876.

Recurrent DVT without apparent cause should result in an evaluation of the clotting system. In this case, a cause is present. The other answers require further evaluation.

6. **E,** Page 1874.

Subclavian and axillary vein thrombosis were rare and reportable entities, but increases in the prevalence of IV drug use, transvenous pacemakers, and long-term central venous catheters have made this a fairly common clinical entity. Up to 40% of patients receiving chemotherapy or hyperalimentation through subclavian catheters have thrombosis. It is also seen in association with Swan-Ganz catheterization and may produce significant morbidity.

7. **B,** Page 1878.

Heparin is the most commonly used drug in the treatment of acute venous thrombosis. It does not dissolve existing clots but interferes with the coagulation cascade to inhibit the action of thrombin and slow or prevent the progression of DVT. Heparin works by activating antithrombin III; thus a deficiency of antithrombin III renders heparin useless as an anticoagulant. aPTT levels must be 1.5 times the control value to have therapeutic heparin effect. Sub-therapeutic heparin levels require the patient to have immediate rebolus.

8. **D,** Pages 1871-1872.

The lifetime incidence of superficial thrombophlebitis in patients with untreated varicose veins has been estimated at 20%-50%. This is not a benign condition; as has been noted, unrecognized DVT is present in up to 45% of patients with what appears to be a solely superficial phlebitis. The risk of DVT has been reported to be three times higher in patients with superficial varicosities. Clinical examination alone cannot distinguish pure superficial vein phlebitis from thrombophlebitis involving the deep system, nor can superficial vein thrombosis be counted on to remain superficial.

# 112 Acute Abdominal Pain

*Craig Lauder and Donnita M. Scott*

1. **A,** Page 1888.

Patients with acute abdominal pain represent 5% of all ED visits. The most common diagnosis made in these patients is nonspecific abdominal pain, representing 34%-53% of all cases. The next most common diagnosis is gastroenteritis (6.9%), followed by pelvic inflammatory disease (6.7%). Ureteral stones account for 4.3% of diagnoses, and appendicitis and acute cholecystitis account for 4.3% and 2.5% respectively.

2. **C,** Page 1888.

Gender and age modify the ED physician's diagnosis for those that present with acute abdominal pain. Men are found to have conditions such as gastritis, appendicitis, and perforated ulcers, whereas women are more likely to be diagnosed with acute cholecystitis, nonspecific abdominal pain, and diverticulitis. Diagnoses among pediatric patients vary by age, although they fall into two main categories: acute appendicitis and nonspecific abdominal pain. In the elderly population, patients are more likely to have acute cholecystitis, malignant disease, and bowel obstruction.

3. **E,** Page 1895.

Amylase is not a specific marker for pancreatitis and can be elevated in many other conditions such as liver disease, bowel infarction, ectopic pregnancy, and diabetic ketoacidosis. If pancreatitis is suspected, a serum lipase study should be added because it has a higher sensitivity and specificity for pancreatitis than amylase.

4. **C,** Page 1890.

Visceral pain is propitiated through nerves in the walls of hollow organs and capsules of solid organs; it tends to be vague and poorly localized. Visceral pain is accompanied by autonomic responses such as nausea, vomiting, and diaphoresis. Somatic pain arises from pain fibers specific to certain dermatomes, and the pain is characterized as sharp and more localized. Referred pain is pain at a distant site from a diseased organ secondary to the embryologic origin of the organ.

5. **A,** Page 1901.

Acute appendicitis (36.9%) is the most common cause of acute abdominal pain that requires an emergent operation, followed closely by intestinal obstruction (35.9%). Perforated ulcer represents 8.2%, while acute cholecystitis and diverticulitis account for 6.2% and 1.5%, respectively.

6. **C,** Page 1894.

Murphy's sign represents right upper quadrant pain upon palpation during inspiration, causing cessation of breathing. This sign is a helpful physical finding in diagnosing acute cholecystitis. Iliopsoas sign and obturator sign are both maneuvers that when elicited indicate an overlying inflammatory disease such as appendicitis or pelvic inflammatory disease. Rovsing's sign is pain elicited in the right lower quadrant while palpating in the left lower quadrant and is significant for appendicitis. Kehr's sign is pain in the shoulder or neck mainly on the left side secondary to irritation of the diaphragm from splenic injury.

7. **E,** Page 1893.

Emergency physicians most often look at the temperature to aid in finding the source of the abdominal pain; however, fever is a nonspecific marker. Yet, processes such as appendicitis with perforation usually have a temperature >38.3° C, and temperatures >38.5° C can signify a bacterial infection. Blood pressure, respiratory rate, and heart rate aid the physician in gauging the severity of the illness.

8. **C,** Page 1888.

95% of the diagnoses of acute abdominal pain in children are nonspecific abdominal pain and acute appendicitis. Children are divided in subgroups (infants, preadolescents, and adolescents), and diagnoses vary based on these subgroups. Yet in all three subgroups, nonspecific abdominal pain predominates. Appendicitis is diagnosed in 32% of cases. However, the prevalence in this age-group is only 0.4%.

9. **D,** Page 1895.

Serum phosphate is consistently elevated in the early development of acute intestinal ischemia.

10. **D,** Page 1897.

The primary imaging study for a patient with right upper quadrant pain is ultrasonography because the hepatic and biliary systems are well visualized. Thus cholelithiasis, cholecystitis, and obstruction can be well delineated using this noninvasive test. CT scan, endoscopy, and laparoscopy are more invasive secondary tests that have a higher complication rate.

11. **E,** Page 1901.

The patient has a distal small bowel obstruction causing her abdominal pain, nausea, and vomiting. The proper management of this patient is to establish IV access, place a nasogastric tube, administer analgesia, and then obtain a surgical consultation. IV fluids are necessary secondary to volume contraction, third spacing of fluids, or GI losses. A nasogastric tube is important to decompress the stomach and prevent vomiting. Giving analgesia does not alter the patient's examination and may actually make the patient more cooperative. If small bowel obstruction is suspected, a surgeon must be involved in the management of the patient.

12. **A,** Page 1896.

The symptoms described are of those of a child with intussusception, and the imaging study that is both diagnostic and therapeutic is barium enema. This test allows visualization of the "telescoping" pattern, and in more than 70% of cases, the barium will reduce the intussusception. CT scan and endoscopy may diagnose the condition but are not therapeutic; MRI and radionuclide scanning have no role if intussusception is suspected.

 **113** Gastrointestinal Bleeding

*John R. Leisey and Thomas A. Sweeney*

1. **D,** Pages 1903-1904.

The most common presentation of UGIB in patients with peptic ulcer disease is melena; however, hematochezia may occur if bleeding is brisk. Gastric or duodenal ulcer bleeding may also present as hematemesis. Bleeding from peptic ulcers is often painless. Persistent pain may indicate another diagnosis or may be the result of perforation. Syncope is less common and would indicate significant acute hypovolemia.

2. **E,** Page 1904.

In patients hospitalized for bleeding varices, the rate of rebleeding ranges from 42% to 70%, and mortality is directly related to the number of blood transfusions required regardless of the severity of the liver disease. Rebleeding occurs in 10%-32% of patients with significant bleeding from peptic ulcer disease. The range of rebleeding following a Mallory-Weiss tear is 9%-13%. The probability of rebleeding with esophagitis is 10%; it is 6% with gastritis.

3. **E,** Page 1906.

Meckel's diverticulum is the most common cause of LGIB in children, with up to 3% of children affected. Although symptoms may occur at any age, bleeding will usually occur in the first 2 years of life. Painless rectal bleeding is the most common presentation. Angiodysplasia is more common in adults than in children. LGIB from an incarcerated hernia or intussusception is usually associated with abdominal pain. Henoch-Schonlein purpura may be associated with LGIB but would include characteristic skin findings.

4. **E,** Page 1908.

Sampling gastric contents to determine whether the hemorrhage is proximal or distal to the ligament of Treitz is an important component of the initial evaluation of GI bleeding. The presence of bile in an otherwise clear gastric aspirate reliably excludes UGIB. However, duodenal hemorrhage may be present despite a clear gastric aspirate. Nasal trauma is the most common cause of a false-positive gastric aspirate result for blood. There is no evidence that gastric tube placement will aggravate bleeding from varices or Mallory-Weiss tears.

5. **B,** Pages 1908-1909.

Endoscopy is the most accurate diagnostic procedure for the evaluation of UGIB. If endoscopy is performed within 12-24 hours of the onset of UGI bleeding, it will identify a lesion in 78%-95% of patients. Aggressive diagnostic evaluation is indicated if UGIB is ongoing or recurrent. Gastric aspirate is not required in this patient because the vomitus can be examined. Angiography is able to detect the location of UGIB in up to two thirds of patients but rarely diagnoses the cause of bleeding. Radionuclide imaging is most useful for localizing the area of hemorrhage in stable patients with LGIB. Radiology is a useful adjunct to diagnose concurrent problems or complications but is unlikely to provide the diagnosis of the cause of gastrointestinal bleeding.

6. **D,** Page 1910.

This patient is showing signs of decompensated hemorrhagic shock. Initial fluid resuscitation should consist of a 20 cc/kg bolus of normal saline or lactated Ringer's solution. Patients with unstable vital signs or shock following the administration of 30-40 cc/kg of crystalloid fluid should be transfused with blood. Whole blood has been reported to be superior to packed red blood cells in hypovolemic, hypotensive patients with acute blood loss. Crossmatched blood is the least likely to cause transfusion reactions but the use of un-crossmatched blood is appropriate in patients with persistent signs of shock after initial fluid resuscitation. Following infusion of 10 cc/kg whole blood, the patient should be evaluated to determine the need for additional blood and crystalloid.

7. **E,** Page 1912.

Emergent surgery is indicated in patients with active GI bleeding who remain hemodynamically unstable following appropriate intravascular volume replacement. Emergency surgery is also recommended when blood replacement exceeds five units within the first 4-6 hours or when two units of blood is required every 4 hours to maintain stable vital signs. Initial presentation in hypovolemic shock is not necessarily an indication for emergent surgery if the patient stabilizes in response to initial volume resuscitation.

8. **E,** Page 1903.

Although the frequency of the common causes of upper gastrointestinal bleeding varies by population, the most common overall cause is peptic ulcer disease.

9. **E,** Page 1908.

Both upper and lower GI bleeds will stop spontaneously in 80% of cases, however, it is impossible to predict which patients will be included in the group that will continue to bleed.

10. **B,** Pages 1904-1905.

The most common cause of significant LGIB in the adult is diverticulosis, which occurs in about half of adults over the age of 60. Significant hemorrhage develops in less than 5%. Three fourths of bleeding diverticulae are found on the right side of the colon. Many patients with bleeding diverticulae will complain of mild cramping abdominal pain and may have either melena or hematochezia. Angiodysplasia is believed by some to be as frequent, or nearly as frequent, a cause of LGIB in the adult. Malignancy accounts for 5% of significant LGIB.

11. **E,** Page 1905.

In the young adult, the most common cause of massive LGIB is ulcerative colitis. Diverticulosis and angiodysplasia are also important structural causes of massive LGIB. Infectious causes, such as *Campylobacter jejuni,* may cause bloody diarrhea that mimics ulcerative colitis.

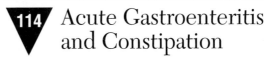

# 114 ▼ Acute Gastroenteritis and Constipation

*David M. Morrison and Thomas A. Seeney*

1. **E,** Page 1918.

Infection is by far the most common cause of acute diarrhea. Viruses cause 50%-70% of all infectious cases, bacteria 15%-20%, parasites 10%-15%, and the remaining 5%-15% are of unknown etiology. Of diarrhea cases seen in the ED, a much higher percentage are caused by bacteria or parasites due to the typically mild nature of viral cases.

2. **D,** Page 1921.

The emergency physician is rarely able to pinpoint the exact cause of a patient's diarrhea in the ED; however, acute diarrhea can be divided into two syndromes. The first category is diarrhea caused by mucosal invasion and resulting inflammation. Invasive diarrhea typically has the following characteristics:

- Incubation period of 1-3 days
- Gradual onset
- Duration of 1-7 days
- Fever
- Significant abdominal pain
- Nausea, vomiting, malaise, myalgia
- Toxic appearance
- Fecal blood, mucus, and leukocytes

The second category is caused by toxins that induce mucosal hypersecretion. Toxigenic diarrhea typically has the following characteristics:

- Incubation period of 2-12 hours
- Sudden onset
- Duration of 10-24 hours
- No fever
- Mild abdominal pain
- No systemic symptoms
- No toxic appearance
- No fecal leukocytes

3. **E,** Page 1922.

Indications for stool culture are (1) historical markers such as immunocompromised patient, travel history, or homosexual history; (2) public health concerns (food handler, daycare worker, health-care worker), nosocomial infection, potential for fecal-oral spread to the public, institutionalized patients; (3) clinical assessment consistent with infectious diarrhea; and (4) stool examination positive for fecal leukocytes.

4. **C,** Page 1923.

Four objectives are present in the management of the patient with diarrhea:

1. Rehydration and prevention of dehydration
2. Symptomatic therapy
3. Prevention of spread of infection
4. Treatment with antibiotics when appropriate

Fluid and electrolyte replacement is the most crucial of these for most patients. In mild dehydration the recommended oral rehydration formula is 1L water with 20 gm glucose, 3.5 gm NaCL, 2.5 gm NaHCO$_3$, and 1.5 gm KCl. Pedialyte and Gatorade are not ideal because of their low electrolyte content and high glucose concentration, but they are superior to tap water. For patients with moderate dehydration, D5/LR or D5/NS are adequate, but patients with severe diarrhea should be given 50 mEq NaHCO and 10-20 mEq KCl in 1L D5/.5NS for adults and D5/0.25 NS for children.

5. **C,** Page 1925.

Empiric antibiotic treatment with ciprofloxacin or norfloxacin is recommended in patients clinically diagnosed with invasive or infectious diarrhea who are significantly ill or appear toxic. The quinolones are effective against all the usual bacterial causes of infectious enteritis: *Campylobacter, E. coli, Salmonella, Shigella, V. parahaemolyticus, Yersinia,* and probably even *Aeromonas* and *Plesiomonas.* Treatment significantly lessens intensity and duration of symptoms and decreases shedding of organisms. Other antibiotics do not have sufficient coverage and have marked resistance. Empiric antibiotics are not recommended in patients whose diarrheal illness falls in the toxigenic category.

6. **B,** Page 1926.

Most patients with acute diarrhea can be managed safely at home. For discharge, patients should be hemodynamically stable, without orthostatic signs and symptoms, and able to tolerate oral fluids. Indications for admission include patients who are unable to compensate for fluid loss and patients who appear toxic or bacteremic. Concomitant medical conditions such as sickle cell anemia, splenectomy, or immunocompromise are not automatic indications for admission but such patients should be more readily admitted because they are predisposed to bacteremia. Infants and the elderly are also more prone to electrolyte abnormalities and their complications; caution must be exercised.

7. **A,** Page 1927.

This boy presents with typical signs and symptoms of *Campylobacter* infection. *Campylobacter* organisms are the most common bacterial cause of diarrhea in patients who seek medical attention, being found in the stools of 5%-14% of patients. Young children have the highest incidence, but all ages are affected and the disease is more common in the summer months. The incubation period is 2 to 5 days. Disease onset is usually rapid and consists of fever, cramping abdominal pain, and diarrhea; flu-like symptoms are generally present, and the clinical picture can mimic appendicitis. The diarrhea often lags 24-48 hours behind onset of symptoms, and stools are loose, bile colored, and become watery and bloody in more than 50% of cases. Diagnosis is made by stool culture. Treatment with antibiotics is generally not indicated, and antimotility agents are not recommended. Should antibiotics be necessary, ciprofloxacin is the agent of choice.

8. **D,** Page 1928.

Humans are infected with *Salmonella* organisms almost solely by the ingestion of contaminated food or drink. It is among the most prevalent communicable bacterial illness and accounts for 10%-15% of all cases of acute food poisoning reported to the Centers for Disease Control and Preven-

tion (CDC). Poultry products are the most common source of *Salmonella,* although unpasteurized milk and domestic pets are another source. Cooking food decreases but does not eliminate the possibility of infection. The typical presenting signs and symptoms are fever, colicky abdominal pain, and loose, watery diarrhea, occasionally with mucus and blood. Most patients have mild abdominal pain; however, some patients can have severe tenderness with rebound. Incubation period is 8-48 hours, and duration of symptoms is 2-5 days. Diagnosis is made by stool culture. Most patients do not require antibiotic therapy; however, for those who do, ciprofloxacin is the agent of choice.

9. **B,** Page 1931.

This boy has typical presentation of hemorrhagic *E. coli* serotype O157:H7. Two serious complication are of concern: hemolytic uremic syndrome (HUS) and thrombotic thrombocytopenic purpura (TTP). *E. coli* is acquired mainly from ingestion of undercooked meat; outbreaks have also occurred from raw milk, contaminated water supply, and person-to-person spread in daycare centers. Typical presentation is watery diarrhea that becomes bloody hours to days later. Patients also note severe abdominal cramps and often vomiting. Diagnosis is made by stool culture. Of the two serious complications, HUS is more common in children, occurring in 20%-25% of cases but also seen in 5%-10% of cases in the elderly, with 50%-80% mortality. TTP is seen in 2%-3% of cases, most often in immunosuppressed patients. Either complication occurs 5 to 20 days after onset of symptoms and can be present long after the diarrhea has resolved. Antibiotics have not been demonstrated to shorten the clinical course and may increase the risk of HUS by eliminating competing bowel flora.

10. **D,** Page 1935.

This patient has typical sign of scombroid fish poisoning; treatment is antihistamines. Scombroid results from ingestion of bacterial toxins found on dark meat fish, most commonly mahi-mahi, tuna, and bluefish. Presenting symptoms resemble histamine intoxication and consist of facial flushing, diarrhea, throbbing headache, palpitations, and abdominal cramps. Dizziness, nausea, vomiting, and urticaria can also occur. Duration of symptoms is usually 6 hours or less, and course is usually benign. Treatment consists of diphenhydramine 50 mg IM or cimetidine 300 mg IV. Rarely IV fluids are necessary. The disease is preventable with proper handling and refrigeration of fish. Since this is not an allergic reaction, patients should not be told that they are allergic to fish.

11. **B,** Page 1937.

The first step of treating *Clostridium difficile* enterocolitis associated with antibiotics is cessation of all antibiotics. *C. difficile* enterocolitis is seen in patients receiving antibiotics, particularly clindamycin, but also ampicillin, cephalosporins, tetracyclines, sulfa products, and erythromycin. Patients treated with constipating agents, especially diphenoxylate hydrochloride or narcotics, are particularly susceptible. Disease is caused by eliminating competing bowel flora, allowing *C. difficile* to proliferate and produce a cytopathic toxin. Patients typically present with fever, crampy abdominal pain, and watery diarrhea that can sometimes be bloody. Onset can occur during the course of antimicrobial therapy or up to 3 weeks later. Diagnosis is made by stool culture. The first step in management is discontinuation of the offending antibiotic. If this does not relieve the diarrhea, the antibiotic therapy should be started with metronidazole or vancomycin.

12. **D,** Page 1940.

This woman presents with typical signs and symptoms of *Giardia lamblia* infection. *Giardia* is the most common cause of water-borne diarrheal outbreaks in the United States, and is also seen commonly in patients with a history of travel to the Soviet Union, Caribbean, and Latin America. It can also be spread by the fecal-oral route. Most patients harboring this parasite are asymptomatic. Most common symptoms on presentation are abdominal distention, colicky pain with audible borborygmi, flatulence, and frequent stools that are pale, loose, explosive, often offensive smelling. Onset is usually sudden following incubation of 1 day to 3 weeks. Examination of the stool will identify the organism in 95% of symptomatic cases, but is less reliable in asymptomatic patients. All patients with *Giardia* infection should be treated, regardless of symptoms, and all household members of an infected patient should be tested and then treated if infected. Treatment is quinacrine hydrochloride 100 mg PO tid for 5 days in adults, 2 mg/kg PO tid in children. Metronidazole is also highly effective at doses of 250 mg PO tid for 5 days in adults, 5 mg/kg PO tid in children.

13. **D,** Page 1942.

This girl has typical signs and symptoms of infestation with *Enterobius vermicularis,* also known as pinworm, perhaps the most prevalent parasite in the United States; 20% to 30% of all children are infected. The human body is the only natural host, and spread is typical by the fecal-oral route. The most common symptom is pruritus ani. This usually occurs at night in relation to nocturnal migration of the gravid female parasite for deposition of eggs onto the perianal area. Migration of the worms into the female genital tract can lead to symptoms of genital infection. The most reliable diagnosis is made by applying a strip of cellophane tape to the perineal area and looking for ova under the microscope. A single test will detect 50% of infections. If done daily for 3 days, the test will detect 95% of cases. All infected individuals and family members should be treated simultaneously with a single dose of mebendazole 100 mg PO or pyrantel pamoate 11 mg/kg. With either drug a second dose should be administered 2 weeks later because young worms may not be susceptible to treatment.

14. **E,** Page 1943.

Compared with patients who are immunocompetent, patients with AIDS have a vastly different profile of pathogens that cause diarrhea, and the ramifications are significantly more serious. A known pathogen can be identified in 80%-85% of patients with AIDS who have diarrhea, and multiple organisms may be present in as many as 20%-25% of patients. All patients with AIDS and diarrhea should have one or more stool samples sent for culture and examination for ova and parasites. Blood cultures should be obtained from all patients, and proctosigmoidoscopy should be considered in patients with clinically severe colitis. Empiric treatment with antibiotics is not indicated. Treatment should be dictated by the causative organisms.

15. **A,** Page 1944.

Patients with chronic persistent diarrhea most often have one of the coccidia, *Cryptosporidium* or *Isospora belli.* CMV and *Mycobacterium avium-intracellulare* also produce a chronic illness, although most patients die within 6 months of diagnosis. *Salmonella* infections are also much more common in the immunocompromised host.

16. **C,** Page 1947.

Travel to areas such as Mexico, Latin America, Africa, the Middle East, or Asia is associated with diarrhea in 30%-50% of travelers. The syndrome is caused by infection acquired by ingestion of fecally contaminated food or water. High-risk items include raw leafy vegetables, undercooked meats or seafood, unpeeled fruits, unpasteurized dairy products, tap water, and ice. Following ingestion, the organism changes the constituency of the bowel flora. *E. coli* is responsible for 40%-50% of all cases; other common organisms include *Shigella, Salmonella,* and *Campylobacter.* Traveler's diarrhea typically begins abruptly and results in loose, watery stools for 1-3 days. Associated symptoms include abdominal cramps, nausea , bloating, urgency, and occasionally vomiting, fever, chills, and headache. Travelers should be advised of high-risk foods and avoid unboiled tap water and ice. Prophylactic treatments include bismuth subsalicylate in patients who tolerate salicylates, and ciprofloxacin in patients with underlying medical conditions or short travels to very–high-risk areas. Treatment of symptomatic patients is achieved with TMP-SMX with loperamide, or ciprofloxacin in patients with high fever or bloody stools or patients refractory to treatment with TMP-SMX.

17. **B,** Page 1949.

Constipation is a common complaint. The most important external factor is diet; an adequate intake of fluids and fiber is essential in preventing constipation. A thorough history and physical examination are crucial, including medication history. The causes of constipation are numerous. In the emergency setting, patients will most often present with acute constipation caused either by drugs or painful perianal lesions. Plain abdominal radiographs are accurate in documenting colonic loading. The treatment of acute constipation is directed toward eradicating the underlying cause and providing adjunctive symptomatic therapy. Adequate fluid and fiber are the keys to prevention. Irritant laxatives should be avoided because long-term usage may decrease bowel motility. Oral mineral oil lubricants may be helpful in patients with painful perianal lesions or elderly patients with chronically hard stools; however, it is contraindicated in patients with swallowing difficulties because aspiration can lead to lipoid pneumonia. Stool softeners have not been shown to be helpful and may be hepatotoxic. Osmotic agents are most often used for colonic preparation for bowel procedures, but they do have a role in treating constipation. Magnesium salts should be avoided in patients with renal conditions and are not indicated for chronic use. Suppositories and enemas are especially helpful in patients who have difficulty expelling soft stool from the rectum.

18. **E,** Page 1951.

Fecal impaction occurs when a large compacted mass of stool cannot be passed by a bowel movement. It is a complication of constipation. Patients at especially high risk are the debilitated elderly. Common symptoms include rectal fullness and discomfort, abdominal pain, tenesmus, anorexia, nausea, fever, and fecal incontinence. Continued passage of some stool does not preclude an impaction, and commonly patients have overflow evacuation of liquid feces around a partially obstructing impaction. Urinary symptoms of frequency, retention, and overflow incontinence are common. Diagnosis is made by palpating the mass on rectal examination, although it may be in the more proximal regions of the colon. Treatment includes manual disimpaction in the ED before discharge, and identification and management of the underlying cause. Mineral oil enemas and whole-gut irrigation may also be used in conjunction with manual disimpaction. Patients whose impactions cannot be removed in the ED should be admitted.

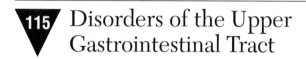

# 115 Disorders of the Upper Gastrointestinal Tract

*Elizabeth A. Moy and James K. Bouzoukis*

1. **E,** Page 1962.

The loss of hydrogen ions in the vomitus results in metabolic alkalosis, and this is maintained by increased reabsorption of bicarbonate in a volume-depleted state. A decrease in extracellular fluid (ECF) and volume contraction activates the renin-angiotensin-aldosterone system, leading to extreme sodium reabsorption by the kidney. This is accomplished by exchanging potassium for the sodium, which leads to hypokalemia. Expansion of the ECF volume enhances renal bicarbonate excretion and corrects the metabolic acidosis.

2. **A,** Page 1966.

Dysphagia from the upper esophagus usually occurs 2 to 4 seconds after the initiation of swallowing. Lower esophageal dysphagia begins 4 to 10 seconds after swallowing and is often described as a sticking sensation. Dysphagia localized to the retrosternal area may be anatomically correct, but localization to the neck may be referred from anywhere in the esophagus.

3. **B,** Page 1966.

This patient describes symptoms of lower esophageal dysphagia. Carcinoma is the most common cause of lower esophageal dysphagia. Dysphagia in a patient over 40 years old should be assumed to be caused by carcinoma until proven otherwise. The dysphagia starts with solids and progresses to liquids. Weight loss is usually prominent. Advanced cases may include hoarseness, Horner's syndrome, or tracheoesophageal fistula.

4. **B,** Page 1969.

Immediate endoscopy should be undertaken for patients with significant distress, children with alkaline button bat-

teries lodged in the esophagus, objects larger than 5 cm long or 2 cm wide (they will not pass the stomach) and with sharp or pointed objects in the esophagus. Oropharyngeal foreign objects can usually be removed with forceps and direct visualization. Smooth upper esophageal objects may be removed using the Foley technique. Glucagon IV, up to 2 mg, may relax the smooth muscle of the esophagus, allowing passage of the object, and is effective in as many as half of patients. It is contraindicated in those with pheochromocytoma and Zollinger-Ellison syndrome. The administration of carbonated beverages results in passage of food boluses in 65% to 80% of patients.

5. **D,** Page 1972.

In cases of esophageal perforation, the early chest x-rays may be normal. Eventually, there may be mediastinal widening, pleural effusions, or mediastinal emphysema. Although barium sulfate is superior in identifying small perforations, it may cause an inflammatory mediastinitis. For this reason, water-soluble agents such as gastrografin should be used. CT scans are not sensitive enough to detect all perforations but will show air-fluid levels or abscesses.

6. **B,** Pages 1970-1971.

Postural exacerbation of reflux symptoms causing esophageal chest pain is seen in most patients and is not commonly seen in chest pain caused by ischemic heart disease. Common precipitants include stooping, bending, assuming a supine position, leaning forward, and straining with bowel movements. The other findings are less specific because they may be due to either esophageal or coronary artery disease.

7. **A,** Page 1967.

Achalasia is a disorder in which there is a marked increase in the resting pressure of the lower esophageal sphincter and absent peristalsis in the esophagus. Dysphagia, odynophagia, and esophageal spasm may be seen early in the course of the disease. Symptoms worsen with rapid eating and stress. A dilated esophagus with air-fluid levels may be seen on chest x-ray.

8. **A,** Page 1973.

Gastric pain is usually visceral and perceived near the midline or the left side of the epigastrium. Lesser sac penetration gastric pain may be referred to the back. The nature of gastric pain is usually cramping, burning or gnawing. Duodenal bulb pain is also visceral, perceived in the epigastrium, often to the right of the midline. Middle and distal duodenal pain is localized to midline low epigastrium. It often radiates straight through to the back, and back pain may predominate.

9. **C,** Page 1978.

Misoprostol is a prostaglandin that inhibits gastric acid secretion and increases secretion of mucus and bicarbonate. It is used to prevent NSAID-induced gastric ulcers in high-risk patients. It is an abortifacient and is contraindicated in women who might become pregnant. Sucralfate binds to epithelial cells and protects from further acid damage. Antacids neutralize acid and should be given after meals and at bedtime. Cimetidine is the oldest of many H2 blockers that inhibit the parietal cells' production of acid. Omeprazole is an $H^+/K^+$ ATPase inhibitor that inhibits the production of hydrogen ions in the apical portion of the parietal cells.

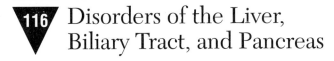

# 116 ▼ Disorders of the Liver, Biliary Tract, and Pancreas

*Brent Passarello and James K. Bouzoukis*

1. **C,** Page 1997.

The differentiation of patients with cholangitis from those affected by cholecystitis is often difficult on clinical grounds alone. Although the classic triad of physical findings first described by Charcot of right upper quadrant pain, fever, and jaundice can be seen in both cholangitis and cholecystitis, an elevated bilirubin is uncommon in cholecystitis. Ultrasonographic evaluation is often required to help distinguish the two entities and in the case of cholangitis will display evidence of dilated common and intrahepatic ducts. Treatment of cholangitis includes hemodynamic stabilization and broad-spectrum antibiotic coverage against gram-positive, gram-negative, and anaerobic organisms. The key to successful treatment is early biliary tract decompression via endoscopic retrograde cholangiopancreatography (ERCP), surgery, or via a percutaneous transhepatic approach.

2. **C,** Pages 1981, 1982.

Approximately 50% of patients with hepatitis C go on to develop chronic hepatitis, and cirrhosis develops in 20% of this group within a decade. The incubation period for the disease is between 30 and 90 days, with a mean of 50 days. Although the disease has been most prominently associated with transfusions, only approximately 10% of patients with this disease report a prior history of having received blood products. Approximately 4%-8% of cases are linked to occupational exposure, 23%-42% are associated with IV drug abuse, and 40%-57% of cases have no identifiable source.

3. **C,** Page 1997.

Sclerosing cholangitis is an idiopathic inflammatory disease affecting the biliary tree. It is characterized by diffuse fibrosis and narrowing of the intrahepatic and extrahepatic bile ducts. It is commonly associated with inflammatory bowel disease, particularly ulcerative colitis.

4. **A,** Pages 1985, 1986, 1988.

Alcoholism is a major medical and social problem in the United States, where an estimated 10 million people are chronic alcoholics. Alcoholic liver disease is ranked as the fourth leading cause of death among men ages 25 to 64 years living in urban areas. The most common variety of alcohol-induced liver disease is steatosis, which generally is reversible with cessation of ethanol use. Jaundice is usually not detectable in patients until their bilirubin levels are at least 2.5 mg/dl. Liver enzyme tests reveal only a moderate elevation, and values in excess of 10 times normal are unusual. Compared with viral hepatitis, a relative predominance of AST over ALT is expected.

5. **A,** Page 1991.

Hepatic abscesses fall into two broad categories, pyogenic and amebic. Pyogenic hepatic abscess is an uncommon entity, present in only 8-16 cases per 100,000 hospital admissions. These abscesses are most commonly associated with biliary tract obstruction or cholangitis, but they may also be related to diverticulitis, pancreatic abscesses, inflammatory bowel disease, omphalitis, appendicitis, or bacteremia of any cause. Clinical presentation is characterized by the subacute onset of high fever, chills, right upper quadrant pain, nausea, and vomiting. Potential laboratory findings include leukocytosis, an elevated alkaline phosphatase, hyperbilirubinemia, and elevated serum aminotransferase levels. Chest x-ray may reveal a right pleural effusion, basilar atelectasis, or an elevated right hemidiaphragm.

6. **D,** Pages 1981-1987.

Hepatitis B is a DNA virus that is transmitted as a consequence of parental exposure or via intimate contact. The highest rates of infection are among IV drug abusers and homosexual men. The typical interval between exposure and onset of clinical illness is between 60 and 90 days, however, serologic markers of infection generally appear within 1-3 weeks. Approximately 10% of adults infected with HBV will become chronic carriers of HBsAg, and will then serve as the major reservoir of infection. The management of health-care workers exposed to blood or other infectious secretions is clearly outlined on Rosen page 1987. In the question scenario, the emergency physician's hepatitis serology revealed HBsAb to be positive. This marker indicates that the earlier immunization has provided protective antibody and therefore no further treatment is necessary with regard to HBV infection.

7. **D,** Page 2002.

Cancer of the pancreas is the fourth most common cause of cancer death in the United States, and this rate is steadily increasing. Tumors are classified as endocrine and non-endocrine, with the latter being far more common. Ductal adenocarcinoma is the most common variety of pancreatic cancer, with a 3-year survival of 2%. Etiologic factors for non-endocrine malignancy include cigarette smoking, diabetes mellitus, and consumption of high-fat, high-protein diets. Pancreatitis does not appear to be an independent risk factor.

8. **A,** Page 1990.

The pathophysiology of SBP remains speculative, but it is probably related to a combination of impaired phagocytic function in the liver and portal systemic hypertension, which can cause bowel mucosal edema and transmural migration of enteric organisms. Additional contributing factors may include impaired opsonic and complement activity in ascitic fluid. The bacteriology of SBP reveals a predominance of gram-negative enteric organisms. *Escherichia coli* is most common, isolated in 47%-55% of cases, followed by *Streptococcus pneumoniae* in 8%-20% of cases.

9. **C,** Pages 1989-1990.

This is a typical case of hepatic encephalopathy. Lactulose or neomycin are the agents of choice. However, neomycin is never given intravenously. It is used orally or rectally to decrease bowel flora. Paracentesis is a diagnostic procedure, and this patient has no indication of bacterial peritonitis. Transfusion or furosemide may both worsen encephalitis by increasing the protein content (transfusion) or decreasing potassium levels (furosemide).

10. **C,** Pages 1999-2000.

Amylase is elevated in the vast majority of cases of pancreatitis, with a reported sensitivity of 95%. The major limitation of this test lies in its relatively poor specificity due to the association of hyperamylasemia with a myriad of diseases and its reported diminished sensitivity in cases of alcohol-related pancreatitis. An alternative to amylase is serum lipase measurement. Lipase is found primarily in the pancreas and proves to be a very reliable test for pancreatitis. It is easily and rapidly measured, has a sensitivity comparable to that of amylase, and is almost 100% specific for pancreatic disease.

11. **D,** Page 2000.

Prognostic signs in patients with acute pancreatitis include those listed in Rosen Table 116-6. The presence of fewer than three signs is associated with a mortality of approximately 1%; mortality is 15% for three or four signs, 40% for five or six signs, and 100% for seven or more positive signs. Serum amylase and lipase have no prognostic value.

12. **B,** Page 1996.

Acalculous cholecystitis occurs in about 5% of cases. It is more common in the elderly and tends to have a more acute, malignant course. Emphysematous cholecystitis is an uncommon variant of cholecystitis, occurring in about 1% of cases. It is characterized by the presence of gas in the gallbladder wall, presumably consequent to the invasion of the mucosa by gas-producing organisms such as *E. coli, Klebsiella,* and *Clostridium perfringens.* It is more common in diabetics, has a male predominance, and is without calculi in 28% of cases. Antibiotic coverage should include penicillin, an aminoglycoside, and clindamycin or metronidazole. Although plain radiographs may reveal calcified stones, gas in the gallbladder, or an upper quadrant sentinel loop, these findings are so uncommon that plain radiographs are not recommended unless there are other diagnostic considerations.

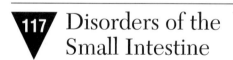

# 117 Disorders of the Small Intestine

*Maria C. Vergara and Steven Kushner*

1. **B,** Page 2006.

The pathophysiology of appendicitis is thought to involve obstruction of the appendiceal lumen followed by the rising intraluminal pressure and subsequent vascular congestion. Gangrenous appendicitis occurs when arterial stasis leads to infarction of the appendix. Perforation will usually occur within 24-36 hours, most commonly resulting in localized peritonitis and abscess formation. Diffuse peritonitis is less common, and small bowel obstruction is a rare complication.

2. **E,** Pages 2006-2009.

Appendicitis is the most common surgical problem requiring emergency intervention in pregnant women, and the highest incidence is in the second and third decades of life (the childbearing years). However, it is no more common in pregnant than in non-pregnant women. The greatest mortality from this disease is seen in the elderly, in whom there is often a delay in diagnosis. More than 50% of all deaths from appendicitis occur in patients who are older than 65 years of age. An appendicolith may be found in the normal, asymptomatic population. Graded compression ultrasound is the most valuable diagnostic test in the assessment of possible appendicitis. A visualized appendix more than 6 mm in diameter is abnormal and consistent with the diagnosis of appendicitis.

3. **E,** Pages 2008-2009.

Patients with definite or probable appendicitis should undergo prompt surgical exploration without diagnostic testing that will delay definitive management. However, when the diagnosis of appendicitis is unclear, ancillary tests, observation, and serial examinations may help confirm or exclude the diagnosis of appendicitis. Although most patients with appendicitis have a WBC count above 10,000/mm³, a normal WBC count does not exclude the diagnosis of appendicitis. Evaluation of erythrocyte sedimentation rate and C-reactive protein have not been shown to improve diagnostic accuracy. Graded compression ultrasound is the most valuable, inexpensive, and safe diagnostic test available to assess possible appendicitis. Mild, sterile pyuria (<20 WBC/HPF) often accompanies appendicitis, and all patients suspected of having appendicitis should have a urinalysis performed.

4. **A,** Pages 2011-2012.

Aggressive treatment of small bowel obstruction has a marked effect on reducing the mortality rate. The development of strangulation increases the mortality rate from 3%-5% to 10%-37%. In the setting of complete small bowel obstruction, the normal secretory and resorptive functions are disrupted. Bowel distention increases the secretory process but decreases the ability of the bowel to absorb fluid and electrolytes. This leads to increased fluid accumulation and worsening bowel distention proximal to the site of obstruction. Peristalsis typically becomes hyperactive at the early stages of the disease process as the bowel attempts to overcome the obstruction. However, with persistent complete obstruction, the bowel becomes atonic and peristalsis ceases. Eventually, there is lymphatic stasis, causing bowel wall edema and third-spacing of fluid. The final stages involve venous and arterial obstruction leading to gastrointestinal bleeding, sepsis, and death.

5. **A,** Pages 2011-2015.

Pain generally precedes vomiting. The lack of rebound tenderness does not exclude possible infarction. High-pitched peristalsis concurrent with colicky pain is a helpful finding in early small bowel obstruction. Although the absence of colonic gas is seen with complete small bowel obstruction, the rate of colonic emptying beyond obstruction varies. Passage of flatus and stool can continue until the large bowel is evacuated.

6. **C,** Page 2011.

Adynamic ileus is the temporary cessation of intestinal peristalsis that is caused by a number of processes, most commonly after laparotomy or abdominal trauma. It can also be associated with intraabdominal, intrathoracic, pelvic, and retroperitoneal infections, as well as metabolic derangements such as hypokalemia. A focal decrease in peristaltic activity may result in gas and fluid collection in an isolated segment of bowel forming a "sentinel loop" on radiography. The "coffee bean sign" suggests the presence of a closed loop obstruction. Adynamic ileus usually resolves after the underlying cause has been treated. Amyloidosis is a condition associated with pseudoobstruction rather than adynamic ileus.

7. **B,** Page 2012.

Typically, the more proximal the small bowel obstruction, the shorter the delay in diagnosis secondary to greater patient discomfort. The patient usually presents with painful abdominal spasms occurring every 3 to 5 minutes and may have several hours of severe colicky pain associated with bilious vomiting. In general, mild abdominal distention occurs with proximal small bowel obstruction, whereas progressively worsening pain and abdominal distention occur with distal small bowel obstruction.

8. **C,** Pages 2013-2014.

Abdominal plain films demonstrate the presence of small bowel obstruction in 50%-60% of cases. However, the cause of the obstruction is rarely demonstrated on conventional films. Strangulated obstruction cannot reliably be distinguished from simple obstruction, and it may be difficult, if not impossible, to distinguish between adynamic ileus and mechanical obstruction on the basis of plain films alone. There are several radiologic aids on plain abdominal films that are helpful in diagnosing small bowel obstruction. These include distended loops of bowel proximal to the site of obstruction, air-fluid levels, and the lack of colonic gas. Subtle findings include the "coffee-bean" sign, a sentinel loop of U-shaped bowel whose lumina are separated by edematous bands of ischemic tissue; and the "pseudotumor" sign, a fluid-filled loop of bowel that resembles a mass. When plain films are equivocal or nonspecific, CT scan may be performed; it is definitively diagnostic in more than 80% of the cases.

9. **C,** Pages 2014-2015.

Initial management of small bowel obstruction consists of aggressive fluid resuscitation, bowel decompression, antibiotics, and a timely surgical consultation. IV hydration should consist of isotonic crystalloid solution though large-bore IV catheters. Enteral decompression should be via a nasogastric tube; it has not been shown that the use of a long intestinal tube is more effective than a nasogastric tube. In the absence of evidence of strangulation, a trial of conservative therapy may be performed. Up to 75% of patients with partial small bowel obstruction and 16%-36% of those with complete small bowel obstruction will have complete resolution of symptoms when treated conservatively.

10. **E,** Page 2016.

The source of SMA emboli is most often either left atrial or ventricular thrombi that fragment during dysrhythmia. Emboli typically lodge four to seven centimeters from the vessel's origin at a point of anatomic narrowing such as the takeoff of a major arterial branch. In the presence of prolonged occlusion, vasospasm develops both proximal and distal to the obstruction. This persists even after the obstruction is relieved and is responsible for continued ischemic damage. The mucosa of the bowel wall is very sensitive to changes in blood flow, and necrotic changes can occur as soon as 10-12 hours after the onset of symptoms. Peristaltic activity increases in response to acute intestinal hypoperfusion, resulting in increased oxygen demand and worsening ischemia. Intestinal infarction secondary to mesenteric venous thrombosis is uncommon even when the portal and superior mesenteric vein junction is occluded, as long as the branches of the peripheral arcades and the vasa recta are patent.

11. **A,** Page 2016.

Sudden occlusion of the superior mesenteric artery is the most common cause of acute mesenteric ischemia. Rheumatic heart disease was once the most common source of systemic emboli, but today most emboli and thromboses arise secondary to atherosclerotic heart disease. Other causes include regional splanchnic vasospasm associated with the use of vasoactive drugs; mesenteric venous thrombosis associated with malignancy, abdominal trauma, and hypercoagulable states; hypovolemia; and sepsis.

12. **E,** Page 2018.

Angiography remains the most useful diagnostic test for suspected occlusive forms of acute mesenteric ischemia. Embolic phenomena cause mesenteric ischemia more often than does thrombosis, but the distinction between the two forms based on clinical or angiographic criteria is no longer clear. One of the benefits of angiography is that it permits the evaluation of the vascular bed distal to obstruction. The study is both diagnostic and therapeutic. Papaverine reduces or eliminates persistent vasospasm and can be infused through the same catheter used to perform angiography.

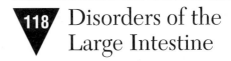

# 118 ▼ Disorders of the Large Intestine

*Tuananh Vu and Steven Kushner*

1. **C,** Page 2026.

This patient's symptoms are consistent with acute diverticulitis. The examination of choice to discover the extent of the diverticulitis is abdominal CT scan. Furthermore, a CT scan may reveal a different diagnosis, such as appendicitis or tuboovarian abscess. The CT scan is also useful when the clinical picture is confusing as is often the case in the elderly. In general, contrast x-ray studies and endoscopy are avoided in acute diverticulitis for fear of inducing a perforation. After resolution of the acute diverticulitis, barium enema examinations are indicated to exclude other colonic pathologic conditions and to look for some of the complications of diverticulitis, such as fistula formation. With careful and appropriate use of the available ancillary studies, unnecessary surgical procedures may be avoided.

2. **C,** Page 2026.

The most common fistula that develops after diverticulitis is colovesical. Patients commonly have symptoms of pneumaturia, fecaluria, or dysuria.

3. **A,** Page 2028.

Figure 118-1 shows the characteristic "bird's beak" seen on barium enema indicative of sigmoid volvulus, and colon cancer is not a risk factor for volvulus. In the United States, sigmoid volvulus occurs in patients with severe psychiatric or neurologic disorders, as well as in the elderly with debilitating disease and inactive lives. There is usually a history of chronic constipation in these groups. Chagas' disease is common in parts of South America, which leads to megacolon and volvulus.

4. **C,** Pages 2027-2032.

The most common causes of large bowel obstruction are carcinoma and diverticulitis. Volvulus and Crohn's disease are less common etiologies. Hernias and adhesions rarely cause colonic obstruction.

5. **B,** Page 2030.

Intussusception is seen in children ages 3 months to 5 years, but the great majority of patients are 5 to 10 months old.

6. **D,** Page 2032.

Toxic megacolon is a manifestation of fulminant colitis seen in ulcerative colitis. The other choices listed are included in the differential diagnosis of ulcerative colitis.

7. **C,** Page 2033.

For acute non-fulminating ulcerative colitis, colonoscopy with biopsies is the most useful diagnostic study. Barium enema of the colon is no longer the diagnostic study of choice in the initial diagnosis of ulcerative colitis, but it may be helpful in chronic cases. Both colonoscopy and barium enema should be avoided when fulminating colitis is suspected because of the risk of perforation. In addition, barium enema may lead to toxic megacolon. Plain film radiographs of the abdomen are not very useful in the diagnosis of non-fulminating ulcerative colitis. However, they can be used to diagnose toxic megacolon, a complication of fulminant colitis.

8. **C,** Page 2032.

Ulcerative colitis always arises first in the rectum and it is confined to the rectum in 10% to 38% of cases.

9. **C,** Pages 2030, 2033-2035.

Marginal thumbprinting is diagnostic of ischemic colitis and is caused by mucosal hemorrhage and pericolic fat inflammation. In Crohn's disease, a barium enema reveals changes consistent with regional enteritis: skip areas of inflammation and non-involvement of the rectum. In uncomplicated intussusception, a barium enema can be both diagnostic and therapeutic. It reveals a characteristic "coiled spring" appearance from a thin layer of barium trapped around the invaginated intestine. If a barium enema is performed in ulcerative colitis, it might reveal a rigid, shortened colon, with loss of haustrations and destruction of the mucosal pattern, the "horse-like" colon.

10. **A,** Pages 2030, 2033-2035.

Ischemic colitis usually presents with acute generalized lower abdominal pain followed by bloody diarrhea or rectal bleeding. Vomiting and fever are rare.

11. **E,** Page 2027.

The patient's clinical picture is diagnostic of large bowel obstruction. The pain out of the proportion to the abdominal examination and the white blood cell count of 25,000 indicate dead bowel. Surgical resection is the definitive treatment; however, the other options listed are appropriate treatments to be performed while waiting for the surgeon.

12. **A,** Pages 2032-2033.

For ulcerative colitis, the drug of choice is IV corticotropin. For patients already receiving steroids, the treatment of choice is either hydrocortisone or methylprednisolone. Cyclosporine is a second-line agent used when IV steroids fail. Cytoxan is not used in the treatment of ulcerative colitis.

---

## ▼119 Disorders of the Anorectum

*Henry E. Wang and Howard Rubinstein*

1. **E,** Page 2037.

The superior and middle hemorrhoidal veins drain into the portal system, and the inferior hemorrhoidal vein drains to the inferior vena cava. Therefore, infectious adenopathy and metastatic spread are different for these areas of drainage.

2. **D,** Page 2037.

The superior, middle, and inferior hemorrhoidal arteries arise from the inferior mesenteric, internal iliac, and pudendal arteries, respectively.

3. **E,** Page 2040.

Portal hypertension does not cause hemorrhoids in adults; the incidence of hemorrhoids in adults with and without portal hypertension is similar. This is not the case with children; children with portal hypertension are prone to hemorrhoidal exacerbations. Pregnant women commonly experience hemorrhoids. Hemorrhoids are not varicose veins; they are normal structures that manifest symptoms when the muscularis submucosa weakens and the anal cushions are displaced distally. Constipation in combination with straining may be a cause of hemorrhoids by producing increased venous backflow.

4. **A,** Page 2041.

Anal fissures result when a hard piece of feces is forced through the anus, resulting in a superficial tear of the anoderm. Anal fissures are most commonly encountered in the 30- to 50-year-old age-group and are the most common anorectal problem in pediatric patients, especially infants.

5. **E,** Page 2042.

99% of anal fissures in men and 90% of anal fissures in women occur along the posterior midline where the skeletal muscle fibers that encircle the anus are weakest. Fissures in women are sometimes found in the anterior midline. Fissures located elsewhere should alert the physician to other diseases such as leukemia, Crohn's disease, HIV, tuberculosis, or syphilis.

6. **B,** Page 2042.

Anorectal abscesses are commonly caused by *Staphylococcus aureus*, *E. coli*, *Streptococcus*, *Proteus*, and *Bacteroides* species.

7. **C**, Page 2043.

Only perianal and ischiorectal abscesses can be safely drained in the ED. Intersphincteric, supralevator, and postanal abscesses occur in deeper structures and are best left to surgical drainage in the operating room. Horseshoe-shaped abscesses may occur in the ischiorectal, intersphincteric, and supralevator spaces. Horseshoe abscesses are frequently large with communications and are best left to surgical drainage in the operating room.

8. **C**, Page 2042.

The WASH regimen consists of warm water, analgesic agents, stool softeners, and high-fiber diet, and may be helpful for hemorrhoids or after drainage of perirectal abscesses.

9. **B**, Pages 2040-2041.

External hemorrhoids originate below the dentate line and receive blood from the inferior hemorrhoidal plexus. Thrombosed external hemorrhoids should be *excised* in the ED within 48 hours of symptom onset; incision and drainage will result in rebleeding and swelling. Internal hemorrhoids occur above the dentate line and derive blood supply from the superior hemorrhoidal plexus. Second- and third-degree internal hemorrhoids can often be reduced non-surgically. Fourth-degree hemorrhoids are permanently prolapsed and require surgery to reduce.

10. **C**, Pages 2046-2047.

Although all of the listed conditions can cause pruritus ani, fecal irritation is the most common cause. It is important to take a careful history to identify possible causes. Prevention of recurrent bouts of pruritus requires impeccable anal hygiene.

11. **D**, Pages 2050-2051.

It is important to promptly remove rectal foreign bodies in order to prevent mucosal lacerations, intestinal obstruction, sepsis, and peritonitis. Hence, it is probably not prudent to wait several days while the patient self-expels the object. Removal of rectal foreign bodies requires creativity and individualized strategy for each patient. After removal of a foreign body, all patients should undergo sigmoidoscopy to look for mucosal tears and perforation.

# 120 Anemia, Polycythemia, and White Blood Cell Disorders

*Michael Baram and Howard Rubinstein*

1. **E**, Page 2054.

Fevers and mental status change are two of the five elements of thrombotic thrombocytopenia (TTP). The others are hemolytic anemia, thrombocytopenia, and renal failure. Oxidants, such as antimalarials, sulfonamides, and nitrofurantoin, can cause individuals with G-6-PD to develop hemolytic anemia. Toxins such as the brown recluse spider and cobra venom can cause hemolysis. The most common cause of transfusion reactions is clerical error.

2. **C**, Page 2061.

Chronic disease causes a hypochromic microcytic anemia

3. **B**, Page 2061.

Iron deficiency causes a hypochromic microcytic anemia

4. **D**, Page 2060.

Vitamin B12 deficiency results in a macrocytic anemia

5. **E**, Page 2060.

Chronic lead poisoning results in a hypochromic microcytic anemia

6. **A**, Page 2064.

Cell fragments can be seen on smear with a positive Combs' test, which indicates immune-mediated cell destruction.

7. **E**, Page 2060.

This patient has a macrocytic anemia with neurologic signs and symptoms. Vitamin B12 is unique in that it is the only megaloblastic anemia to produce neurologic signs and symptoms. Vitamin B12 deficiency is most commonly due to malabsorption.

8. **E**, Page 2071.

Bleeding, bruising, thrombotic episodes, cerebrovascular accidents, myocardial infarction, or deep venous thrombosis are the most common manifestations of primary polycythemia.

9. **C**, Page 2073.

With current treatment, chronic myelogenous leukemia is often followed like a chronic disease. However, progression of the disease that results in blast crisis seen on a peripheral blood smear is an indicator of poor prognosis. Blast crisis is defined as 50,000 blast cells per cm.

10. **A**, Page 2073.

ALL is the most common malignancy of childhood. Treatment has increased mean survival by more than 15 years.

11. **B**, Page 2074.

Any child under 2 years old brought to the ED with a white cell count >15,000 WBC/cc merits a thorough work-up for bacteremia. Although not specific, 15,000 WBC/cc is a fairly sensitive level.

12. **B**, Page 2064.

Haptoglobin binds free hemoglobin on a molecule-for-molecule basis. Its absence implies saturation and degradation after binding with free hemoglobin and is an early finding in hemolysis. LDH is released when the red blood cell is broken down peripherally or in the marrow, thus elevating the serum level. Indirect bilirubin is a reflection of unconjugated bilirubin, and this is increased due to the increased red blood cell hemoglobin breakdown. The reticulocyte count, a reflection of how well the bone marrow can respond by producing more red blood cells, is increased in purely hemolytic states.

13. **B**, Page 2054.

The initial hematocrit value in a patient with emergent anemia may take hours to correctly reflect the degree of blood loss. The most common cause of emergent anemia is blood loss. Hemolytic states are rare causes. Folate, B12, TIBC, and reticulocyte count will be affected after blood transfusions. Vital signs may initially be normal despite significant blood loss; thus emphasizing the importance of serial physical examinations.

14. **E,** Page 2067.

CBC, electrolytes, blood culture, and chest x-ray are all useful as diagnostic adjuncts, but there is no single best test available to detect whether a patient is in sickle cell vaso-occlusive crisis. A complete history and physical examination are thus very important. The physical examination should evaluate every organ system.

# 121 Disorders of Hemostasis

### *Brian K. Lentz and George R. Zlupko*

1. **D,** Pages 2078-2081.

Platelet disorders usually occur as acquired petechiae or mucosal bleeding and are more common in women. While platelet levels below 20,000/mm³ may be associated with spontaneous hemorrhage, the count gives no information about the functional capability of the platelets. The bleeding time is a test of both vascular integrity and platelet function. Two standard incisions 1 mm deep and 1 cm long are made with a template on the volar aspect of the forearm while under 40 mm Hg pressure from a blood pressure cuff. The time is measured from the incision to the moment when the blood oozing from the wound is no longer absorbed by the filter paper. The normal time is 8 minutes and it is independent of the coagulation pathways. With ITP the bleeding source is usually capillary, with resultant cutaneous and mucosal petechiae or ecchymosis. The bleeding is usually mild and occurs immediately after surgery or dental extractions. Deep muscle hematomas and hemarthroses are commonly presenting signs associated with hemophilia A or B. The acute form of ITP is seen most often in children 2-6 years of age. A viral prodrome commonly occurs within 3 weeks of the onset. The platelet count falls, usually to less than 20,000/mm³. The course is self-limited, with a greater than 90% rate of spontaneous remission.

2. **B,** Page 2080.

Fibrinogen is present in sufficient concentration to be measured directly. Because it is the final coagulation substrate, its level reflects the balance between production and consumption.

3. **D,** Page 2081.

Digitoxin, sulfonamides, phenytoin, heparin, and aspirin are drugs commonly implicated in drug-induced thrombocytopenia. The patient has usually ingested the drug within 24 hours. The platelet count may fall below 10,000/mm³ and be complicated by serious bleeding. Laboratory testing may confirm the presence of platelet antibodies, especially in the cases of quinine and quinidine. The count improves slowly over 3-7 days after stopping the drug. A short course of corticosteroid therapy may facilitate recovery.

4. **D,** Page 2086.

Von Willebrand's disease has both a decreased factor VIII:Ag level and a decreased VIII:C activity secondary to underproduction. The patient's platelets are normal in number, mor-

phologic condition, and other functions, but in the absence of circulation factor VII:vWF, their adhering properties are diminished, thus increasing the bleeding time.

5. **B,** Page 2084.

Desmopressin acetate (DDAVP) has been shown to increase levels of factors VIII:C and VIII:Ag in patients with hemophilia A and in some with von Willebrand's disease. Its benefits are primarily noted in patients with mild disease, and it is given intravenously in a 0.3 μg/kg/dose. Recent studies evaluating the anabolic steroid danazol preclude its use as routine therapy for hemophilia.

6. **A,** Page 2086.

In von Willebrand's disease, the patient's platelets are normal in number and morphology, but because of the lack of factor VIII:vWF, their adhesive properties are diminished, causing increased bleeding time. The disease is usually milder than hemophilia A or B. Bleeding sites are usually mucosal, and hemarthroses are rare.

7. **E,** Page 2082.

The mnemonic FAT RN helps to remember the classic pentad of TTP: fever, anemia, thrombocytopenia, renal disease, and fluctuating neurologic symptoms. The platelet count ranges from 10,000/mm³ to 50,000/mm³, with generalized purpura and bleeding. Anemia is almost universal with hemolysis and jaundice. Neurologic symptoms vary widely from altered level of consciousness to stroke to coma. Fever is present in 90% of affected people. Renal disease varies from hematuria and proteinuria to acute renal failure. If untreated, there is an 80% mortality 1-3 months after diagnosis. Initial therapy should consist of prednisone, antiplatelet agents, and—most important—plasma exchange. Platelet transfusion should be avoided because it may cause additional thrombi in the microcirculation.

8. **B,** Pages 2085-2086.

Head trauma is potentially life threatening to hemophiliacs, and central nervous system bleeding is the major cause of death for patients in all age-groups. Studies find a 3%-13% risk of intracranial hemorrhage, yet no patient given replacement therapy within 6 hours had an intracranial bleed. Any patient with an altered level of consciousness or focal neurologic signs should be started immediately on factor VIII therapy and have an emergent CT scan obtained (In emergent therapy, the present level of factor VIII is assumed to be zero). It is recommended that head trauma patients have factor VIII therapy initiated to a 50% activity level and be admitted for 24 hours of observation. While these patients will be treated in joint consultation with their primary physician, hematologist, and/or neurosurgeon, emergent care of the patient should not be delayed and is the responsibility of the emergency medicine specialist.

9. **A,** Page 2086.

In patients with severe disease, replacement therapy with factor VIII in the form of cryoprecipitate is the method of choice. Because the VIII/vWF content of each bag is unavailable, the standard dose is 1 bag or cryoprecipitate per 10 kg of body weight. It has large amounts of VIII:C and a factor influencing VIII:vWF. DDAVP's benefits are primarily noted in patients with mild disease. Platelets are normal in number and morphology in this disease. Ristocetin is an antibiotic used in vitro to demonstrate platelet adhesion and aggregation activity as a function of vWF. Parenteral vitamin K is used to reverse warfarin's effects on vitamin K–dependent coagulation factors such as II, VII, IX, and X, and proteins S and C.

10. **B,** Page 2086.

Hemophilia B is a deficiency of factor IX activity. Its genetic pattern and clinical presentation are indistinguishable from those of hemophilia A, but its incidence is only one fifth that of hemophilia A. Its deficiency is diagnosed by a factor IX assay, usually after the factor VIII:C assay is found to be normal.

11. **D,** Page 2086.

Cryoprecipitate is assumed to have 80-100 units of factor VIII:C per bag. This is in contrast to purified factor VIII:C concentrates that list the units per bottle on the label.

12. **B,** Pages 2086-2087.

DIC is a relatively commonly acquired coagulopathy most often encountered in a critical care setting. Hemostasis is a fine balance between procoagulants and inhibitors, thrombus formation, and lysis; this balance may be disturbed by pathologic processes that result in an out-of-control coagulation and fibrinolytic cascade within the systemic circulation. In this abnormal clotting sequence, platelets and clotting factors are consumed, especially fibrinogen, V, VIII, and XIII. The result is thrombocytopenia, prolonged PT/PTT, and low fibrinogen levels with resultant elevated fibrin degradation or split products. The thrombin time is also prolonged secondary to the low levels of fibrinogen.

# 122 Oncologic Emergencies

*Jason E. Nace and George R. Zlupko*

1. **A,** Pages 2090, 2091.

Although it has been reported that significant tumor burden can predispose to fever, most fevers (55%-70%) occurring in cancer patients have an infectious etiology, especially when the patient has granulocytopenia. Therefore cancer patients with significant fever should be presumed to have an infectious etiology, and antimicrobial therapy should be started immediately after appropriate cultures have been obtained. Patients with two or three low-grade elevations above 38° C orally or a single elevation above 38.3° C and polymorphonuclear leukocytes fewer than 500/mm³ are particularly at risk. Occasionally fever without a source may be due to the underlying disease. In a prospective evaluation of 140 febrile, granulocytopenic patients, it was impossible to differentiate patients with bacteremia-induced fever from those with unexplained fever by their age, sex, underlying malignancy, or the types of therapeutic modalities or invasive diagnostic procedures they had received.

2. **B,** Page 2091.

The gram-negative organisms, especially *Pseudomonas aeruginosa, Klebsiella* species, and *E. coli,* are the most predominant bacterial pathogens, although *P. aeruginosa* had been declining in incidence, most probably because of empiric antibiotic regimens and protocols. In some centers, gram-positive organisms, like *S. aureus* and *S. epidermidis* have become dominant isolates. Once believed to be a contaminant, *S. epidermidis* has arisen as a major pathogen and may be resistant to antistaphylococcal penicillins and cephalosporins. In contrast to patients with AIDS, in patients with solid tumors parasitic infections are not a common source of infection. In addition, the absence of physical findings indicative of infection does not exclude a potentially life-threatening septic event. More than 50% of septic patients will not have any physical findings. Despite this possibility, a meticulous physical examination is required.

3. **E,** Pages 2092, 2093.

Superior vena cava syndrome (SVCS) is the obstruction of the superior vena cava secondary to compression, infiltration, or thrombosis. SVCS occurs in 3% and 8% of patients with cancer of the lung and lymphoma respectively. Between 85% and 95 % of all SVCS cases result from malignancy. The chest radiograph reveals a mass in approximately 10% of patients. Early signs may include periorbital edema, conjunctival suffusion, and facial swelling, which will be most evident in the early morning hours and subside by midmorning. In one study, the most common symptom is shortness of breath (>50%), with swelling of the face, trunk, and upper extremities observed in roughly 40% of patients. Airway obstruction does not occur in the absence of tracheal compression by extrinsic tumor, and there is no evidence that SVCS is a life-threatening event. Venous access may be preferable in the lower extremities.

4. **D,** Page 2093.

Radiation therapy has been emphasized as the primary treatment for SVC compression. Current treatment also uses chemotherapy because of the increased incidence of tumor sensitivity to newer antineoplastic agents. Diuretics have been used with transient symptomatic relief, but they must be used judiciously because overzealous administration can result in hypovolemia and further slowing of blood flow. The prognosis for patients treated for SVCS depends on the tumor type, with better survival with lymphoma than with bronchogenic carcinoma. In a recent series, 10% of patients with lung tumors survived, compared with 45% of lymphoma patients. The overall survival of the entire series is approximately 25% at 1 year and 10% at 30 months after treatment.

**5. D,** Pages 2093-2094.

Acute tumor lysis syndrome most commonly occurs within 1 to 5 days of instituting chemotherapy or radiation therapy of rapidly growing tumors that are extremely sensitive to antineoplastic drugs. It is most commonly seen after chemotherapy of hematologic malignancies. A correlation between a very high blood lactate dehydrogenase and the development of tumor lysis syndrome has been observed. Biochemical hallmarks of this syndrome include hyperuricemia (DNA breakdown), hyperkalemia (cytosol breakdown), and hyperphosphatemia (protein breakdown). Hypocalcemia develops secondary to hyperphosphatemia. The integrity of renal function is a critical factor in determining the degree of metabolic derangements. In patients with preexisting renal insufficiency, the metabolic derangements of tumor lysis are more likely to be severe. Chemotherapy should be delayed, if possible, until metabolic disturbances are corrected.

**6. C,** Page 2095.

Hyperviscosity syndrome (HVS) occurs when excessive elevations in certain paraproteins or marked leukocytosis result in elevated serum viscosity and the development of sludging, decreased perfusion of the microcirculation, and vascular stasis. The most common causes are the dysproteinemias, leukemias, leukemoid reactions, polycythemia vera, and the abnormal hemoglobins in sickle cell disease. IgA has the highest intrinsic viscosity and the greatest tendency to form unstable circulating aggregates. On clinical examination, patients exhibit retinopathy, bleeding from mucosal surfaces, neurologic disturbances, hypotension, respiratory failure, and congestive heart failure. Initial therapy should focus on adequate rehydration and diuresis. An immediate temporizing measure for patients in frank coma and known dysproteinemia is a two-unit phlebotomy and replacement with saline.

**7. D,** Pages 2096-2097.

Hypercalcemia is a common feature in many malignancies and occurs in about 20% of cancer patients. It can occur in the absence of bony metastases and may be a reaction to various substances such as prostaglandins, parathyroid hormone, and steroids. There are also many benign causes. With acute onset, patients may be comatose, with calcium levels of only 12-13 mg/dl. Signs and symptoms include marked CNS effects leading to personality changes, lethargy, and eventual coma. Patients may also develop anorexia, nausea, vomiting, constipation, polyuria, polydipsia, and abdominal pain. ECG shows a shortened QT interval. Half of hypercalcemic cancer patients also have hypokalemia before therapy and should have potassium replacement.

**8. A,** Page 2097.

Emergency treatment of hypercalcemia includes hydration with normal saline and, when urine flow equals 100 ml per hour, furosemide 40-80 mg intravenously to increase excretion of calcium. Mithramycin, calcitonin, and prednisone are all long-term agents. Intravenous phosphates are not recommended because of their serious complications.

**9. B,** Pages 2099-2100.

Pericardial tamponade should be suspected in any patient in the ED with a history of known carcinoma, shortness of breath, and hypotension. The most common cause of neoplastic pericardial tamponade is malignant pericardial effusion, with postirradiation pericarditis, fibrosis, and effusion, or a combination thereof. Only rarely does a tumor or radiation fibrosis cause a neoplastic constrictive pericarditis with resultant tamponade. The most common symptoms include extreme anxiety and apprehension, a precordial oppressive feeling, or actual retrosternal chest pain with varying degrees of dyspnea. True orthopnea and paroxysmal nocturnal dyspnea are uncommon, but when they occur the patient assumes a variety of positions to get relief from the chest pain and dyspnea. Low voltage and the nonspecific findings of pericardial effusion, sinus tachycardia, ST elevation, and nonspecific ST-T wave changes may occur. Electrical alternans with 1:1 total atrial-ventricular complexes has been considered pathognomonic. Radiographic signs of tamponade suggestive of pericardial effusion include an enlarged cardiac silhouette with clear lung fields and normal vascular pattern. The "water-bottle" heart is often present. Echocardiography is the simplest and most sensitive of diagnostic tests and can be done at the bedside. The long-term prognosis, even for those who respond to treatment, is quite poor, with mean survival time of 12-16 months in one study.

**10. D,** Page 2100.

Three distinct herniation syndromes have been described: uncal, central, and tonsillar. In uncal herniation a lateral mass displaces the temporal lobe, which compresses the upper brain stem. A rapid loss of consciousness is seen in conjunction with unilateral pupillary dilation and ipsilateral hemiparesis. Central herniation results from slowly expanding multifocal lesions that cause a downward and lateral shift of the diencephalon and upper pons. It is marked by slowly decreasing level of consciousness, small, reactive pupils, and Cheyne-Stokes respirations. There are no focal neurologic signs. Tonsillar herniation is produced by a large posterior fossa mass that pushes the cerebellar tonsils through the foramen magnum, compressing the medulla and resulting in a rapidly decreasing level of consciousness, occipital headache, vomiting, hiccups, hypertension, meningismus, and abrupt changes in the respiratory pattern. Treatment involves intubation with hyperventilation to produce cerebral vasoconstriction. Mannitol should be given and may be repeated in 4-6 hours. Dexamethasone is generally also recommended. Abscess and metastasis formation are usually managed with antibiotics and antineoplastics, respectively.

**11. E,** Page 2101.

Epidural spinal cord compression from metastatic cancer is common, serious, and potentially treatable. Most cases (68%) occur in the thoracic spine, 15% occur in the cervical spine, and 19% in the lumbosacral spine. Back pain, either local or radicular, is the initial symptom in 95% of these patients. Plain films will show evidence of tumor in the vertebral body in 90% of patients with vertebral metastases. In cases with questionable findings on plain films, tomograms, coned-down views, or a CT scan may reveal bony metastases not otherwise appreciated. Myelography usually demonstrates a complete or near-complete obstruction of contrast dye flow at the level of vertebral body involvement. High-resolution CT scans may prove equal to myelograms, but this has not yet been established. The initial treatment involves corticosteroids (usually dexamethasone, 100 mg IV) followed by radiation. Surgery is indicated only if the diagnosis is in doubt, if a tissue diagnosis is required, if the spine is unstable, or when radiation has already been given to the maximum allowable level.

12. **C,** Pages 2101-2102.

Patients with cancer are susceptible to a variety of CNS infections. Most CNS infections occur in patients with leukemia, lymphoma, or head and neck cancer. Important CNS infections include meningitis, brain abscess, and encephalitis. All cancer patients with fever and an altered mental status require a lumbar puncture. A head CT, however, should precede this, if cerebral metastases are suspected, and thrombocytopenia and coagulopathy should be considered and managed first as well. Absence of WBCs in the CSF does not preclude meningitis, especially in neutropenic patients. Neutropenic patients with either leukemia or lymphoma usually have a gram-negative infection and should be covered with a third-generation cephalosporin or a semisynthetic penicillin. Infections with *Haemophilus influenzae* and *Neisseria meningitidis* are rare, so coverage with ampicillin alone is generally sufficient. Brain abscess is usually seen in patients with leukemia or head and neck tumors and accounts for 30% of CNS infections in cancer patients. Encephalitis is rare in patients with cancer and is most often caused by herpes zoster or *T. gondii,* but its presenting symptomatology is very similar to that of meningitis.

# 123 ▼ Coma

*Lars Blomberg*

1. **A,** Pages 2106-2107.

The ascending reticular activating system (ARAS) and one of the cerebral hemispheres are required for consciousness; the other structures are not. The proximity of the cranial nerves to the RAS makes it unlikely for them to remain intact if the RAS is damaged. When the ARAS is nonfunctional, coma occurs because the cerebral cortex cannot be aroused.

2. **D,** Page 2112.

Pupillary response is generally resistant to toxic or metabolic insult. Local hypoxia, such as that caused by a vascular event, is most likely to cause the described abnormality. Pupillary response is maintained in metabolic coma.

3. **B,** Page 2114.

Cold caloric testing cannot be resisted. A comatose patient whose eyes deviate toward the stimulus and remain there tonically has no cerebral hemisphere function with which to jerk the eyes back to midline (nystagmus directed away from the side of stimulus). The alert patient would show the nystagmus to the left as described. A patient with right medial longitudinal fasciculus (MLF) dysfunction would not toni-cally bring the right eye toward the left from the stimulation because the MLF, which allows the connection between the eyes, is not intact. A patient with right oculomotor nerve dysfunction cannot bring his eye to the left; instead, the unopposed cranial nerve VI will keep his right eye tonically deviated toward the right, while his left eye moves tonically toward the side of stimulus.

4. **C,** Pages 2107-2108, 2114.

Nystagmus in response to caloric testing implies an intact cortex. Active resistance to eye opening and closing is highly suggestive of a conversion reaction. Akinetic mutism is a chronic state that usually results from diffuse frontal lobe disease. Catatonia is a symptom complex characterized by withdrawal, mutism, muscular rigidity, grimacing, and bizarre posturing. Locked-in syndrome results from hemorrhage or infarct of the ventral pons. The patient is incapable of all motor activity that is controlled distal to the pons.

5. **D,** Page 2107.

The description is of stupor. Delirium is a state of disturbed consciousness, motor restlessness, hallucinations, and perhaps delusions. Obtunded patients are awake but not alert, and have associated psychomotor retardation. Coma is defined as a state of unarousable unresponsiveness.

6. **C,** Pages 2107-2109.

In general, supratentorial lesions are a more common cause of coma than subtentorial lesions. Rosen Box 123-2 lists the etiologies of unexplained coma by incidence. Poisoning is the most common cause, accounting for 30% of cases. Supratentorial hemorrhage makes up 15%. Only 3% of comas of undetermined etiology are believed to be secondary to subtentorial hemorrhage, such as those listed.

7. **B,** Pages 2109, 2110.

Rosen Table 123-1 lists the criteria for the Glasgow Coma Scale. The patient's eye and verbal responses both give scores of 1, leaving a motor score of 3. The patient's motor score must be one of decorticate posturing or flexion response.

8. **C,** Page 2111.

The respiratory rate of patients with coma is often abnormal and can yield clues to the underlying etiology. Of the causes listed, only hepatic coma leads to tachypnea through a direct CNS effect.

9. **A,** Page 2113.

Oculocephalic responses are tested by briskly moving the head from side to side. Reflex eye movements are evoked in the opposite direction of the head turning. This response requires the integrity of cranial nerves III and VI as well as an intact medial longitudinal fasciculus. CN II (optic nerve) is involved in the assessment of pupillary response but is not involved in oculocephalic testing.

10. **B,** Pages 2115-2116.

Hypoglycemia accounts for 8.5% of pre-hospital encounters of altered mental status. IV glucose and thiamine (for prevention of Wernicke-Korsakoff syndrome) should be administered to all comatose patients. Complications related to naloxone administration are extremely rare, and thus empiric use poses little risk other than inducing narcotic withdrawal. Many patients in coma have taken a mixed overdose of several medications. Although benzodiazepines may be involved, the increased risk of seizures in a patient with an overdose of an unknown substance precludes the empiric use of flumazenil.

 ## 124 Headache

### *Lars Blomberg*

1. **A,** Pages 2119-2120.

Compression is not recognized as one of the three major groupings of conditions that affect pain-sensitive structures of the head and neck.

2. **C,** Page 2128.

The majority of patients with temporal arteritis have elevated erythrocyte sedimentation rates. None of the other laboratory tests are as useful in confirming the diagnosis.

3. **A,** Page 2129.

Acute narrow-angle glaucoma or angle-closure glaucoma may cause all of the symptoms described; the diagnosis is confirmed by tonometry. The other answers may cause some of the symptoms, including severe, boring pain, but do not include ocular changes.

4. **D,** Page 2124.

Pain is generally less intense than in classic migraine, and it is usually seen in young adults. Extraocular muscle palsies that usually involve the third cranial nerve may be present.

5. **A,** Pages 2123-2124.

Homonymous hemianopsia is seen with classic migraine. Specific visual findings are usually not involved with common migraine. The other answers are present in both classic and common migraine.

6. **C,** Pages 2123-2124.

Cluster headache, also known as histamine headache or migrainous neuralgia, has a male predominance of 4 or 5 to 1. It involves excruciating unilateral pain that rarely lasts longer than 2 hours. Attacks often follow ingestion of alcohol and the use of nitroglycerin- or histamine-containing compounds.

7. **C,** Page 2124.

Cocaine hydrochloride placed in the sphenopalatine fossa can effectively relieve cluster headache 80% of the time. Similar results have been obtained with breathing 100% oxygen. The other choices are therapies for migraine but may also be helpful with cluster headaches.

8. **A,** Page 2128.

Benign intracranial hypertension produces nonspecific headaches, often associated with transient visual loss and pa-

pilledema. Pseudotumor cerebri is most common in young obese females with abnormal menstrual cycles.

9. **B,** Pages 2121, 2123, 2128.

This group of symptoms is consistent with subarachnoid hemorrhage. Diagnosis is definite if retinal hemorrhages and subhyoid hemorrhages are present. Cluster headache is unilateral, excruciating, short-lasting fascial pain with specific triggers. Chronic subdural hematoma may occur with headache, and there are usually changes in personality or mental status. Trigeminal neuralgia is hyperesthesia of the trigeminal sensory fibers, which causes severe, stabbing pain.

10. **A,** Pages 2121, 2123, 2126.

Carbon monoxide poisoning is the leading diagnostic consideration whenever two or more patients present with similar complaints of headache. Symptoms are believed to be due to anoxia. CO levels can easily be obtained in the emergency department and treatment initiated accordingly.

11. **A,** Pages 2124-2126.

Ergotamine preparations are potent vasoconstrictors. They are contraindicated in pregnancy and should be used with caution in any hypertensive patient.

 ## 125 Organic Brain Syndrome

### *Lars Blomberg*

1. **A,** Page 2134.

Electrolyte disturbance, hepatic failure, and hypoxia can all be causes of, or contributing factors to, delirium. However, prescribed and recreational drug use causes the majority of delirium cases.

2. **A,** Page 2135.

Although disorientation often accompanies cognitive impairment such as deficit attention, it is not always present.

3. **C,** Page 2138.

Patients who are immunocompromised for any reason may not exhibit the typical meningeal symptoms of headache, fever, and stiff neck. Laboratory and clinical evaluation of the patient should include the other choices, but they are unlikely to be diagnostic.

4. **B,** Page 2139.

Acute delirium frequently occurs with abnormal vital signs, clouded sensorium, and cognitive defects that can include visual hallucinations. Acutely psychotic people usually have normal vital signs and primarily auditory hallucinations, and they are not tremulous.

5. **C,** Pages 2141-2144.

A rapidly progressive deterioration of cognitive function describes delirium. Acute psychosis can be differentiated from delirium with the help of Rosen Table 125-2 on page 2139. Pseudodementia (depression) usually has a more rapid course.

6. **B,** Pages 2135, 2144-2145.

Asterixis and myoclonus are usually not found in functional syndromes such as dementia. They are associated with the organic syndromes of delirium.

7. **B,** Pages 2140-2141.

Butyrophenones and, in particular, haloperidol have become the drugs of choice for control of agitation in acute delirium. Benzodiazepines have a longer half-life, cause respiratory depression, and create the risk of drug accumulation with repeat dosing. Narcotics can induce dysphoria and exacerbate acute brain failure. Phenothiazines can cause orthostatic hypotension and also lower the seizure threshold.

8. **A,** Pages 2142-2145.

Dementia is defined as a gradually progressive deterioration of cognitive function, and may be caused by more than 50 different disease states. Rosen Table 125-3 on page 2145 lists characteristics that may be helpful in distinguishing cortical from subcortical dementia. Of the symptoms listed, only anomia is consistent with a cortical etiology.

9. **C,** Page 2140.

This patient has a presentation consistent with Wernicke's encephalopathy. Appropriate treatment includes IV glucose and thiamine. Magnesium is a cofactor for thiamine transketolase, and as such hypomagnesemia may result in resistance to thiamine treatment.

10. **B,** Page 2142.

Dementia is not a single disease entity. Although there is a tendency to approach all patients with a chronic dementia with the assumption that treatment will be futile, approximately 20% of dementias are potentially reversible.

11. **B,** Page 2146.

Progressive dementia, ataxia, and urinary incontinence constitute the classic triad of symptoms associated with normal pressure hydrocephalus. A CT scan may be diagnostic in this instance.

## 126 Seizures

*Lars Blomberg*

1. **A,** Pages 2153-2154.

Patients between the ages of 6 months and 5 years have 95% of febrile convulsions. These seizures tend not to occur in series, have no focal features, last less than 15 minutes, appear soon after a sudden rise in temperature, and have a high familial incidence.

2. **D,** Pages 2150-2151.

Simple partial seizures are usually brief, beginning and ending abruptly, and involving little or no alteration of consciousness. With the other choices, there is a more profound alteration of consciousness.

3. **C,** Page 2153.

Causes of pediatric seizures include all of the answers listed. However, hypoxia is the leading cause in the first few days of life. Rosen Box 126-2 lists pediatric seizure causes by age of onset.

4. **A,** Page 2154.

Both hypernatremia and hyponatremia are associated with seizure activity, most commonly at levels of 160 and 120 re-

spectively. Significant hypocalcemia may also precipitate seizure activity and typically is associated with hypomagnesemia. In contrast, hypercalcemia reduces neuronal excitability and rarely produces ictal activity.

5. **C,** Page 2156.

The cause of new-onset seizure in 54% of elderly patients is stroke. Although the other choices are possible etiologies, they occur much less frequently.

6. **C,** Page 2157.

Pseudoseizure patients tend to have an underlying anxiety or hysterical personality disorder. Although post-ictal states have been documented following pseudoseizures, it is much more characteristic for them to be absent.

7. **A,** Pages 2158-2159.

ED evaluation of a first-time seizure should focus on any possible medical, toxicologic, or neurologic cause for the event. Routine screenings such as a CBC, however, have little use in the initial evaluation, with the exception of a blood glucose determination. Other diagnostic tests such as a lumbar puncture or toxicology screen should be ordered if there is a suspicion of meningitis or substance abuse, but these are not essential to the initial work-up.

8. **B,** Page 2159.

Benzodiazepines are the drug class of choice for the initial management of patients in status epilepticus. In comparison studies, no one drug has been shown to be clearly superior; however, lorazepam is generally recommended for alcohol withdrawal seizures because of its longer duration of action. Phenytoin is a second-line abortive treatment in the emergency setting.

9. **A,** Pages 2161-2162.

Numerous side effects are associated with anticonvulsant therapy. Rosen Table 126-2 lists potential adverse effects and drug-to-drug interactions for the more common anticonvulsants.

## 127 Vertigo

*Lars Blomberg*

1. **B,** Page 2170.

The question describes the triad of Ménière's disease. Vestibular neuronitis and vertebrobasilar insufficiency are not generally associated with hearing loss. Acoustic neuroma is not episodic.

2. **C,** Pages 2168-2169.

The Weber test screens for asymmetric sensorineural hearing loss. Audiology, although not a screening test, aids in locating the site of a vertigo-causing lesion. Electronystagmography allows measurements of induced nystagmus.

3. **D,** Pages 2170-2171.

The patient's symptoms describe an occlusion of the posterior inferior cerebellar artery (Wallenberg syndrome). Eaton-Lambert syndrome mimics myasthenia gravis without a decrease in sensation. Multiple sclerosis has a wide range of symptoms reflecting its widespread lesions, and its symptoms are not generally confined to one anatomic location. Subclavian steal syndrome can cause vertebrobasilar insufficiency and vertigo, but it does not cause diminished sensation.

4. **B,** Pages 2165-2167.

Disturbances in the statokinetic system (semicircular canals, utricle, vestibular division of the eighth cranial nerve, and vestibular nuclei) cause true vertigo. Posterior columns are part of the proprioceptive system, along with tendons, muscles, and joints. Eye muscles and the eyes constitute the visual system. The visual system, proprioceptive system, and statokinetic system constitute the equilibrium triad.

5. **A,** Page 2172.

Intravenous diazepam has a sedative effect, acting on the limbic system, the thalamus, and the hypothalamus. The other drugs are less effective and do not act as quickly.

6. **B,** Pages, 2170-2171.

Bilateral internuclear ophthalmoplegia, weak adduction with normal abduction, indicates brain stem pathology and is highly suggestive of MS. Cerebellar hemorrhage is characterized by HA, vertigo , and ataxia. Episodic flares with fluctuating but progressive hearing loss suggest a perilymphatic fistula, while VBI is usually characterized by transient pontine symptoms and focal neurologic abnormalities.

7. **C,** Pages 2169, 2170.

The corneal reflex tests cranial nerves V (afferent) and VII (efferent). A diminished or absent corneal reflex can be an early sign of an acoustic neuroma, most easily diagnosed using an MRI scan.

8. **D,** Page 2170.

The symptoms listed suggest a peripheral cause of vertigo, most likely vestibular neuronitis. Both Ménière's disease and toxic labyrinthitis present with severe vertigo but are associated with hearing loss. BPV is extremely common, and most patents can usually identify a head position that precipitates their vertigo.

 **128** **Weakness**

*Greg Harders*

1. **D,** Pages 2174-2175.

Botulism, myasthenia gravis, Eaton-Lambert syndrome, and the Miller-Fisher variant of Guillain-Barré syndrome are characterized by proximal, bulbar onset. Generally, Guillain-Barré has a rapid, distal onset.

2. **C,** Page 2176.

Signs and symptoms of myasthenia gravis are improved by cold, and an ice pack may relieve partial ptosis in a bedside test. Atropine is of no value in treating the neuromuscular blockage. ELISA and electrocardiographic testing are of benefit in Lyme disease.

3. **B,** Page 2179.

Carcinoma of the lungs is frequently, but not necessarily, associated with Eaton-Lambert syndrome. Tick paralysis is associated with an adherent gravid tick, and tick-borne spirochetes can cause erythema chronicum migrans in Lyme disease.

4. **D,** Page 2180.

The seventh cranial nerve is most often affected in Lyme disease, but the third, fourth, sixth, and eighth are also known to be affected.

5. **B,** Page 2174-2175.

There is symmetric leg weakness with Guillain-Barré syndrome, but distal weakness is more common. CSF protein is >400 mg/L. Fever is distinctly unusual when the patient is seen, although one may be present if there was a viral illness 2 to 4 weeks previously. Deep tendon reflexes are almost always absent in the affected extremities.

6. **C,** Pages 2176-2177.

Edrophonium (Tensilon) is a very–short-acting acetylcholine inhibitor. It will worsen muscle strength in cholinergic crisis but improve it in myasthenic crisis. Cholinergic crisis is secondary to over-treatment, and the patient must be supported until the drug wears off. With cholinergic crisis, muscarinic effects, such as excessive sweating and salivation, may also occur. Dysarthria and dysphagia are symptoms of bulbar muscle weakness, which is common. Initial symptoms are usually ptosis, diplopia, and blurred vision.

7. **D,** Pages 2178-2179.

Constipation may be the first symptom of botulism noted by the parents, followed by weakness. Antitoxin has not been proven useful for infant botulism. Completely or predominantly breast-fed infants have a higher risk of developing infantile botulism because of their lower intestinal pH and different flora as compared with formula-fed babies. The contrast between the infant's alert mental status and normal vital signs on the one hand, and the feeble cry and limited motor activity on the other hand, is characteristic.

8. **C,** Page 2179.

The toxin described is a saxitoxin, and it is also known as paralytic shellfish poisoning. It is heat resistant, produces profound symptoms, and requires supportive care.

9. **C,** Page 2181.

Abnormalities in all the listed electrolytes may cause weakness. Hypokalemia is probably the most common. Generally potassium levels <3 produce symptoms. A less common entity, periodic paralysis, is also associated with hypokalemia and should be considered.

10. **B,** Page 2180.

Tick paralysis does not produce fever, and its presence should alert the emergency physician to seek another etiology. This can be fatal if not recognized

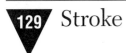 Stroke

*Greg Harders*

1. **D,** Page 2185.
Elevated glucose levels are associated with worse outcomes. Increased lactate is a marker for severe intracellular acidosis. A rapid increase in intracellular calcium occurs with ischemia, which also causes rapid depletion of ATP.

2. **A,** Page 2185.
Occlusions of the middle cerebral artery cause paralysis of the contralateral side of the body, usually worse in the arm and face than the leg. The posterior cerebral artery does not supply the motor strip, and occlusion affects vision and thought processing. Vertebrobasilar artery system occlusions demonstrate bilateral motor deficits.

3. **B,** Page 2187.
Lacunar strokes account for 13%-20% of all strokes. Eighty percent of strokes are ischemic in origin, and 10% are the result of hemorrhage.

4. **A,** Page 2187.
Myocardial infarction can lead to mural thrombus formation in a hypokinetic ventricle and subsequent embolization. Risk factors for hemorrhagic stroke are long-standing hypertension and cerebral artery disease (for intracerebral hemorrhages) and rupture of cerebral aneurysms or bleeding AVMs with subarachnoid hemorrhages. Lacunar strokes are related to hypertension and diabetes. Thrombotic infarcts are secondary to thrombus formation and atherosclerosis.

5. **A,** Pages 2187-2188.
Clinically "silent" prior infarcts may be seen on scans of acute TIA patients. Only 5%-20% of TIA patients experienced a stroke within 1 month. Fifty percent of patients with TIAs in the carotid artery distribution have no angiographically demonstrable arterial disease. Some patients with symptoms consistent with TIAs have well-defined infarcts by angiographic or radiographic evaluation.

6. **A,** Page 2188.
Brain stem infarcts can cause acute loss of consciousness. Cerebral edema occurs 24 to 48 hours after an infarct and can cause coma. A decreased level of consciousness requires bilateral hemispheric involvement.

7. **C,** Page 2189.
Graphesthesia is an easily tested cortical function that distinguishes between subcortical lacunar infarcts and a stroke in the MCA distribution. Babinski's sign indicates only corticospinal tract dysfunction, which would be common to both syndromes. Pronator drift tests subtle motor weakness only. Asymmetric sensation to pain and light touch may be subtle and difficult to detect.

8. **D,** Page 2190.
Hemorrhagic transformation of an ischemic infarction is usually clinically silent. It is most commonly detected radiographically several days after the initial event.

9. **C,** Page 2192.
The majority of arteriovenous malformations that become symptomatic do so after a hemorrhage. Arteriovenous malformations in patients younger than 50 almost always bleed. Arteriovenous malformation hemorrhages are less disruptive to cerebral function than hypertensive bleeds.

10. **B,** Pages 2192-2193.
A grading scale for evaluating subarachnoid hemorrhage has four stages based on the presence of headache, meningeal signs, and focal deficits. The vast majority of subarachnoid hemorrhages occur before the age of 50. Preexisting hypertension may or may not be present and does not affect prognosis. The size of the hemorrhage on CT does not correlate well with the clinical condition.

11. **B,** Page 2193.
The CT scan done immediately will miss 5% to 10% of subarachnoid hemorrhages. Lumbar puncture is the gold standard for acute detection of subarachnoid hemorrhage. MRI scanning currently has an undefined role in the diagnosis of acute hemorrhage. CT scanning is less sensitive as time elapses. This patient should not be discharged on the basis of a CT scan alone.

12. **D,** Page 2193.
The clinical course of cerebellar hemorrhages is notoriously unpredictable; they can lead to sudden coma and death. Surgery also benefits lobar hemorrhages of certain sizes causing deterioration. However, in most cases of intracranial hemorrhage, surgery is not beneficial. Prompt control of hypertension is critical in the management of intracranial hemorrhage.

13. **B,** Page 2195.
A patient with these symptoms whose condition is deteriorating needs to be treated for meningitis immediately. The diagnostic workup can then proceed. CT should precede lumbar puncture if elevated intracranial pressure is a concern. It is incorrect to treat only for comfort and then observe.

14. **D,** Page 2194.
Approximately 3%-4% of strokes occur in patients between the ages of 15 and 45. Younger patients will typically have irreversible causes. In addition to blood dyscrasias, amphetamine (cocaine), and pregnancy, other causes include demyelinating diseases, valvular disease, and hypercoagulable states.

15. **A,** Pages 2186-2191.
Although there are lengthy lists of risk factors for stroke, several are well established and clearly linked to ischemic strokes. Cardiac factors such as atrial fibrillation, valvular disease, and recent myocardial infarction all can provide embolic sources. Hypercoagulable states lead to sludging and thrombosis. Aneurysmal disease and uncontrolled severe hypertension are linked most closely with hemorrhagic stroke.

16. **D,** Page 2189.
A variety of tests exist to assess cerebellar function. Classically finger-to-nose, heel-to-shin, and gait are used as screening examinations. More subtle focal deficits may be ascertained by observing routine ambulation and heel-to-toe walking. Pronator drift is a sign of motor weakness.

## 130 Meningitis, Encephalitis, and Central Nervous System Abscess

*Greg Harders*

1. **C,** Page 2202.
CT scan is the cornerstone of diagnosis of brain abscess. It may be useful in assessing meningitis complications, but in the diagnosis of meningitis, it is not helpful. Focal neurologic deficits and subacute course over 2 weeks are findings present in the majority of patients with brain abscess and a large number of patients who exhibit papilledema, which is rare in meningitis. In brain abscess, nuchal rigidity is present less than 50% of the time.

2. **A,** Page 2203.
With increased sophistication in the analysis of CSF, immediate antibiotic therapy may be initiated in patients with indications for CT scan before lumbar puncture in suspected bacterial meningitis.

3. **D,** Pages 2203-2205.
The normal CSF-to-serum glucose ratio is greater than 0.5 in normoglycemic patients. The normal opening pressure varies from 50 to 200 mm $H_2O$. Normal CSF should have no more than 5 leucocytes/mm$^3$ with no more than 1 PMN. The normal CSF protein is 15-45 mg/dl.

4. **D,** Page 2203.
CSF cell counts of greater than 200 cells/mm$^3$ usually cause clinically detectable changes in CSF clarity.

5. **B,** Page 2205.
A positive India ink preparation is virtually diagnostic, but it occurs in only one third of cases. Pretreatment with antibiotics has little effect on CSF leukocyte counts but may increase the misidentification of gram-positive bacteria as gram-negative.

6. **C,** Pages 2207-2208.
Cefotaxime offers coverage for the likely pathogens *S. pneumoniae, N. meningitides, H. influenzae,* and gram-negative enteric bacilli.

7. **D,** Page 2209.
Rifampin is not recommended for health care workers unless they have had mucosal contact with the patient's secretions, such as in mouth-to-mouth resuscitation.

8. **C,** Page 2202.
The incidence of Waterhouse-Friderichsen syndrome, acute adrenal failure from hemorrhage into the adrenal glands, is dramatically higher in meningococcemia.

9. **C,** Page 2203.
The preferred algorithmic approach is to either perform immediate lumbar puncture followed by initiation of antibiotic or to initiate antibiotics followed by CT and then lumbar puncture.

10. **B,** Pages 2204-2205.
Xanthochromia is an abnormal pigment. It results from the lysis of RBCs and formation of oxyhemoglobin, bilirubin, and methemoglobin. It develops as early as 2 hours and may last up to a month. Its presence is suggestive of a SAH.

## 131 Special Neurologic Problems

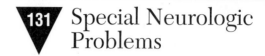

*Greg Harders*

1. **B,** Pages 2213-2214.
The patient has a clinical picture consistent with Guillain-Barré syndrome. Treatment is supportive, but plasmapheresis may help decrease the length of disease.

2. **A,** Pages 2214-2215.
Gaze paralysis suggests a seventh nerve motor nucleus lesion. Depending on the level of the lesion of the peripheral seventh nerve, motor fibers to the stapedius, secretory fibers to the lacrimal gland, and taste fibers to the anterior tongue may all be affected. Patients with Bell's palsy often complain of a vague numbness, but objective sensory findings are rare.

3. **C,** Page 2215.
Bilateral facial weakness may be caused by sarcoidosis, multiple sclerosis, and Guillain-Barré syndrome.

4. **D,** Page 2216.
Intravenous acyclovir is recommended for patients with more than one dermatome involved as well as patients who are immunocompromised. Involvement of the tip of the nose, which is innervated by the nasociliary branch of the ophthalmic division of the maxillary nerve, may indicate potential corneal involvement. The combination of prednisone and acyclovir has not been proven effective in decreasing the incidence of postherpetic neuralgia. Oral treatment with acyclovir of early herpes zoster is just as effective as intravenous acyclovir in decreasing pain and increasing healing.

5. **A,** Pages 2216-2219.
Patients may be able to stand a great deal of pain without withdrawal. Optokinetic nystagmus is a normal finding in sighted or hysterically blind individuals. Bell's phenomenon (upward deviation of the eyes in response to forced voluntary contraction of the eyelids) will be present if a patient has voluntary eye closure that is forcibly opened. Loss of sensation at joint line and vibratory sense only on one side of the skull are not present in organic neurologic disease.

6. **D,** Page 2220.
Optic neuritis is typically unilateral, with loss of vision, preservation of venous pulsations, pain, and photophobia. Papilledema is typically bilateral, with loss of venous pulsations, intact vision, and no pain.

7. **D,** Page 1872.
The patient has pseudotumor cerebri (idiopathic intracranial hypertension), which often responds to therapeutic lumbar puncture. Occasionally, repeated lumbar puncture is needed. Ventriculoperitoneal shunting is rarely needed and only if progressive visual changes are present.

8. **D,** Page 2215.
The scenario represents the classic presentation of the Ramsey-Hunt syndrome. That is, involvement of the peripheral seventh nerve with varicella zoster.

9. **D,** Page 2218.

Findings consistent with psychogenic unconsciousness include upward deviation of the eyes, resistance to eyelid opening, voluntary eyelid contraction, and "nasal tickling." Recommendations are not to establish the diagnosis by inflicting painful stimuli. A slow eyelid closure versus a quick blink suggests a true unconsciousness.

10. **D,** Page 2222.

Syringomyelia is a cavitation in the spinal cord. Involvement of the pain and temperature fibers occurs because they cross centrally as they travel from the ipsilateral to the contralateral side. The proprioceptive and light touch fibers do not cross at this level and are therefore spared.

 ## 132 Urologic Emergencies

### Greg Harders

1. **C,** Page 2234.

The history of a new sexual partner, the gradual onset of symptoms, the discharge from the os, and the sterile pyuria are all consistent with chlamydial urethritis.

2. **C,** Page 2232.

Young adult females with a classic presentation of cystitis do not require urine culture unless immunocompromised. Neonates require culture even if urinalysis is negative.

3. **B,** Page 2241.

A 2-week course of trimethoprim-sulfamethoxazole is a good choice for outpatient management. However, if the patient is seriously ill, he may require admission. The prostate should never be massaged in acute prostatitis, because this may induce bacteremia. If urinary retention is present, suprapubic catheterization is preferred for the same reason. Urine culture usually yields the responsible pathogen in prostatitis.

4. **C,** Pages 2231-2232.

With new onset of fever, the catheter must be changed because of the colonization of the catheter. Patients should also be admitted for IV antibiotics. Bacteriuria is extremely common and, unfortunately, prophylaxis is of unproved benefit beyond 3 days of therapy.

5. **A,** Page 2244.

If manual detorsion is successful, the patient must still undergo exploration. The urologist should be called immediately if torsion is suspected. Valuable time should not be lost while the patient is undergoing nuclear imaging. Prehn's sign is notoriously unreliable.

6. **B,** Page 2238.

Fever alone is not an indication for admission; there should also be other indications before admission is considered for pyelonephritis.

7. **C,** Page 2231.

The risk of pyelonephritis in pregnancy is 20%-40% in those diagnosed with UTI. Asymptomatic bacteriuria is associated with a 10% incidence of prematurity if left untreated, and a full 10-day course of antibiotics is recommended. Ampicillin, cephalexin, and nitrofurantoin are all considered safer in pregnancy than trimethoprim-sulfamethoxazole.

8. **C,** Pages 2229-2232.

In the infant younger than 1 year of age, the preferred method of collection is either catheterization or suprapubic aspiration. It is not appropriate to catheterize an adult or adolescent male. Not all patients require culture in suspected urinary tract infection, and this is especially true in the young healthy female; there is poor clinical correlation between in vitro culture results and patient response to prescribed antibiotics.

9. **D,** Page 2245.

Seizures usually cause urinary incontinence, not urinary retention. Sympathomimetic agents such as decongestants may cause bladder neck hypertonicity. Benign prostatic hypertrophy is the most common contributing factor in elderly men.

10. **D,** Page 2253.

Repetitive films should be avoided, because this does not contribute to localization of the obstruction and is uncomfortable for the patient. If renal insufficiency is present, ultrasound is the procedure of choice.

11. **A,** Pages 2249-2251.

Stone disease is more common in males by a 3-to-1 margin. Recurrence is seen in 37% of patients within 1 year and 50% by 5 years. Most renal stones (90%) are radiopaque. Microhematuria may be present in 20% of patients with documented nephrolithiasis.

12. **B,** Page 2243.

The most common organisms in bacterial orchitis are *Klebsiella*, *E. coli*, and *Pseudomonas*. Mumps is a viral orchitis. Mumps typically causes unilateral (70%) testicular involvement, leading to atrophy. Infertility after mumps orchitis seldom occurs

13. **C,** Pages 2241-2242.

Features of epididymitis include gradual onset of scrotal and/or groin pain. Pain is often localized to the spermatic cord, and swelling of the cord is variable. Fever and toxicity may be seen, and urethral discharge may be present.

 ## 133 Renal Function Evaluation and the Approach to the Patient With Acute Renal Failure

### Greg Harders

1. **E,** Pages 2270-2271.

Renal tubular epithelial cells are present in acute tubular necrosis. The other findings are typical for poststreptococcal glomerulonephritis.

2. **B,** Pages 2271-2272.

Prostatitis is a cause of postrenal obstruction. HSP may cause nephrotic syndrome. Scleroderma may cause intrarenal disease secondary to vasculitis. There are multiple causes of acute tubular necrosis, of which nonketotic hyperosmolar coma is one.

3. **A,** Pages 2272-2273.

Urine dip stick is positive for heme in only 50% of the cases, because myoglobin is rapidly cleared. The BUN-to-creatinine ratio is often less than 10:1 because of increased creatinine released by muscle. However, this is not a very sensitive test for detecting rhabdomyolysis. The potassium may or may not be elevated. CPK is the recommended diagnostic test.

4. **C,** Page 2274.

No consistent beneficial effect has been proven with furosemide.

5. **A,** Pages 2270, 2274.

Irreversible loss of function is gradual; therefore a delay in diagnosis is acceptable if necessary. Ultrasound is extremely sensitive and is a very good test for detecting obstruction. The serum creatinine usually returns to baseline within 1-2 weeks. Full renal recovery is the normal course once the obstruction is relieved.

6. **B,** Page 2276.

A creatinine greater than 10 mg/dl is usually used as the cut-off point for dialysis in acute renal failure.

7. **B,** Page 2262.

Acute tubular necrosis results in granular casts. Nephrotic syndrome may show fatty casts. Prerenal azotemia shows no formed elements or hyaline casts. Red cell casts are typical for glomerulonephritis.

8. **D,** Page 2266.

Hemorrhagic cystitis may not show WBCs on urinalysis; therefore, culture is still needed to rule out an infectious etiology. Coagulation studies and platelet count are rarely helpful in the initial management of hematuria.

9. **C,** Pages 2262-2265.

Hyaline casts are seen after exercise, dehydration, or with glomerular proteinuria. Rifampin classically causes pseudohematuria. A $FE_{Na}$ value of <1 is seen in prerenal azotemia. The presence of even a few red cell casts is significant and represents renal involvement.

10. **C,** Page 2271.

Characteristic features of AIN include fever, rash, eosinophilia, eosinophiluria. It is not uncommon, however, for one of these signs to be absent. Treatment is removal of the inciting agent or infection. Jaundice is not a feature and should suggest further work-up.

11. **D,** Page 2275.

The electrolyte abnormality most responsible for death is hyperkalemia. Because of decreased renal synthesis of 1,25-dihydroxyvitamin D there is associated hypocalcemia. Hyperphosphatemia is seen secondary to decreased urine excretion. Hypermagnesemia is seen in ESRD. Therefore magnesium-containing compounds such as laxatives and antacids should be avoided.

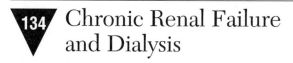

# 134 Chronic Renal Failure and Dialysis

*Greg Harders*

1. **C,** Page 2281.

All of the drugs listed except nitrates have potential renal toxicity and may contribute to worsening renal function in a patient with chronic renal insufficiency.

2. **B,** Page 2280.

The qualitative platelet dysfunction results in increased bleeding time. There may be mild thrombocytopenia; however, this is not usually a significant contributing factor. The prothrombin time is unaffected. The decreased erythropoietin causes the anemia seen in chronic renal disease.

3. **E,** Page 2282.

The peaked T-waves indicate hyperkalemia, which is a common problem in patients with chronic renal failure. In pulmonary edema, volume overload must be avoided; therefore, sodium bicarbonate is contraindicated. Other methods of treating hyperkalemia would include glucose and insulin, inhaled albuterol, furosemide, and calcium gluconate.

4. **B,** Page 2286.

If the patient does not appear seriously ill, close outpatient management is an acceptable alternative to in-hospital treatment. This is especially true because the patient may be loaded with IV antibiotics such as vancomycin, which will maintain adequate therapeutic levels for 5-7 days after a single dose. Vancomycin is not amenable to removal by hemodialysis. *Staphylococcus* is the most common etiology of access site infections. The access site may appear normal although it is the source of the bacteremia with recurrent fevers.

5. **D,** Page 2286.

Simple pressure will usually stop the bleeding. Cryoprecipitate is an option because it has factors that may contribute to improved platelet function. It is important to document the presence of a thrill after the bleeding has stopped; this confirms patency in the hemodialysis access site. Thrombosis of the vessel is a possible complication if compression is too vigorous.

6. **B,** Pages 2287-2288.

Hypermagnesemia, but not low magnesium, may be a cause of hypotension. All of the other conditions may occur with hypotension following dialysis.

7. **D,** Page 2288.

Pericardial tamponade should be considered in any chronic hemodialysis patient who has a cardiac arrest. CPK and ECG are unaffected by dialysis. Hemodialysis patients are more susceptible to ischemic heart disease compared with the normal population. In this group a 50% narrowing is considered significant, as opposed to the 75% that is usually considered significant in the normal population.

8. **B,** Page 2285-2286.

The creatinine is often chronically greater than 10 mg/dl in the dialyzed patient and is not an indicator for emergency dialysis in this population. This is generally considered the level at which dialysis is indicated for those patients with chronic renal failure who have not undergone dialysis. Other indications for emergency dialysis in the chronically dialyzed patient include acidosis, hypermagnesemia, hypertensive encephalopathy, and pulmonary edema.

9. **B,** Page 2289.

This condition, known as eosinophilic peritonitis, is self-limited and thought to be an allergic reaction. No antibiotic therapy is required.

10. **D,** Page 2286.

Immediate vascular surgery consult is required. The success of reopening a graft is dependent on the duration of thrombosis.

11. **B,** Page 2291.

Constipation should be managed with stool bulking agents and stool softeners. Phosphate-containing enemas may exacerbate the risk of hyperphosphatemia. Tap-water enemas are recommended. Magnesium-containing compounds are to be avoided.

# 135 ▾ Pelvic Pain

### *Greg Harders*

1. **D,** Page 2297.

Ruptured follicular cyst, or mittelschmerz, occurs midcycle, and the pain often occurs with exercise. Pain is usually sharp initially; however, it resolves in a few hours up to 2 to 3 days. A ruptured corpus luteum cyst occurs just before menses. Ovarian torsion is usually a sharp pain with intermittent exacerbations, and it is usually associated with a palpable adnexal mass. Appendicitis is always part of the differential diagnosis in the patient with right lower quadrant pain; however, the sudden onset while exercising and the decreasing intensity makes this diagnosis less likely here.

2. **D,** Page 2298.

Older women and pregnant women are at increased risk of perforation after any type of intrauterine procedure.

3. **D,** Page 2300.

Fibroids are usually painless; however, when they are large enough they may cause symptoms because of pressure on nerve roots and other organs. Dysmenorrhea and endometriosis are usually associated with pelvic pain during menses. Ovarian torsion is a sharp pain associated with an adnexal mass on examination.

4. **B,** Page 2200.

A relatively common cause of chronic pelvic pain is endometriosis (up to 50% of adolescents with chronic pelvic pain). A significant complication is the formation and rupture of an endometrioma, which presents like an acute abdomen.

5. **A,** Pages 2295-2297.

Although all of the listed diagnoses are possible, torsion of the ovary is the most likely because of the history of a preceding similar event that spontaneously resolved. A nega-

tive pregnancy test and a positive ultrasound will confirm the diagnosis.

6. **C,** Page 2297.

Patients with a ruptured follicular cyst (i.e., Mittelschmerz) require observation, analgesia, and reassurance. Culdocentesis and ultrasound may be helpful in ruling out other etiologies, but these are not management strategies. Consultation is unnecessary if the diagnosis is known.

# 136 ▾ Vaginal Bleeding Unrelated to Pregnancy

### *Greg Harders*

1. **D,** Page 2306.

Uterine myomas are the most common pelvic tumor, present in 20%-25% of women over age 35. They are often asymptomatic but commonly cause excessive, prolonged menstrual periods (menorrhagia cyclic bleeding) by interfering with endometrial shedding. Malignant degeneration is rare, occurring in less than 1% of cases. Myomas often atrophy after menopause when estrogen stimulation wanes.

2. **A,** Pages 2307-2308.

Anovulatory cycles are the most common cause of dysfunctional uterine bleeding. Because of the failure to ovulate, the endometrium is continuously stimulated by unopposed estrogen. No corpus luteum is formed, and secretion of progesterone is lacking. Endometrial hyperplasia occurs and builds for several months, resulting in amenorrhea. When bleeding finally occurs, it can be episodic and moderate, or profuse. A pregnancy test must be performed because the symptom mimics spontaneous or threatened abortion. Treatment is with progestational agents (or D&C if severe), which stabilize the endometrium and stop the bleeding, followed by increased bleeding when progesterone levels decline.

3. **C,** Page 2304.

Cycle intervals between menstrual periods vary among individual women, and intervals of 18 to 40 days are considered normal. Once established, the interval may vary by up to 5 days. Normal duration of flow is from 3 to 7 days and is rarely constant. Blood loss averages from 25 to 60 ml and, because of fibrinolysis that occurs in the uterus and cervix, menstrual discharge does not clot.

4. **D,** Page 2307.

Ovaries in the postmenopausal age-group should be atrophic. If an ovary is palpated, an ovarian neoplasm must be ruled out. Ovarian tumors cause vaginal bleeding by hormone-induced endometrial hyperplasia. Adenomyosis is a benign hyperplastic growth of the uterus manifested by a firm, tender, enlarged uterus. Exogenous dysfunctional uterine bleeding is secondary to hormone therapy, such as birth control pills. Non-gynecologic causes of bleeding could be quickly eliminated by examination. Any postmenopausal vaginal bleeding is to be considered malignancy until proven otherwise.

5. **B,** Page 2307.

The most common cause of abnormal vaginal bleeding not related to pregnancy is oral contraceptives. Breakthrough bleeding is caused by endometrial hyperplasia, while withdrawal bleeding occurs from noncompliant use. Bleeding is rarely of hemodynamic consequence; however, other contraceptive measures are indicated for the remainder of the cycle.

6. **A,** Pages 2305-2306.

Cervical polyps are common and benign, with little malignant potential. They can cause intermenstrual bleeding, often aggravated by contact during intercourse. Diagnosis is by direct visual inspection during a speculum examination.

7. **A,** Pages 2306-2307.

By definition, a corpus luteum cyst is formed after ovulation in the follicle from which ovulation took place. Generally, without fertilization, it degenerates into the corpus albicans. However, it may persist in the non-pregnant state and produce hormones. Corpus luteum cysts can enlarge up to 12 cm and when rupturing can mimic an ectopic pregnancy.

8. **B,** Page 2309.

Many options are available for treating dysfunctional uterine bleeding. Commonly progesterone or oral contraceptives are used. Multiple NSAIDs have been proven to reduce bleeding (i.e., mefenamic acid). Definitive management is surgery.

9. **B,** Page 2306.
10. **C,** Page 2305.
11. **D,** Page 2307.
12. **A,** Page 2306.

---

 **137** Genital Infections

*Greg Harders*

1. **C,** Pages 2311-2312.

Primary HSV infection causes a more severe clinical syndrome, with both local lesions and systemic symptoms, than recurrent infections, which are often painless. HSV causes typical vesicles and shallow ulcers in vaginal, labial, and pre-labial skin but can also cause a primary cervicitis or urethritis with discharge. Diagnosis can be made by Tzanck slide preparation showing multinucleated giant cells 50% of the time, but tissue culture is the laboratory standard. Treatment with oral acyclovir decreases duration and severity of signs and symptoms.

2. **C,** Page 2312.

Scrapings of the rash of secondary syphilis reveal spirochetes under dark-field examination, and serologic tests are virtually always positive in this stage. The classic painless chancre of primary syphilis heals spontaneously within a week and is absent in secondary syphilis. Condyloma acuminata lesions (venereal warts) are unrelated. Condyloma lata lesions (flat warts) are moist perineal lesions seen in secondary syphilis and are highly infectious.

3. **D,** Pages 2312-2313.

Lymphogranuloma venereum (LGV) is caused by certain strains of *C. trachomatis* and typically manifests as promi-

nent coalescing and sometimes ulcerative inguinal adenopathy in young men, often with systemic symptoms. Treatment with doxycycline is indicated for suspected LGV. Chancroid (caused by *Haemophilus ducreyi*) may result in a painful, unilateral inguinal bubo in 50% of patients. Granuloma inguinale (caused by *Calymmatobacterium granulomatis*) may cause granulomas (pseudo-buboes) in inguinal nodes. Condyloma acuminata is caused by a human papovavirus.

4. **D,** Page 2315.

The protozoan *Trichomonas vaginalis* causes a malodorous, itchy vaginal discharge, usually white but sometimes grayish green and frothy. Trichomoniasis is a sexually transmitted disease, and treatment of the patient and sexual partner is with metronidazole (Flagyl), either a single 2 g dose or 500 mg bid for 7 days. Metronidazole is contraindicated in the first trimester of pregnancy. Erythromycin can be used safely in pregnancy as an alternative to tetracycline for chlamydial infections, and ampicillin can be used as an alternative to metronidazole for bacterial vaginosis. Neither is acceptable therapy for trichomoniasis.

5. **B,** Pages 2317-2318.

Toxic shock syndrome results from the release of an exotoxin by *Staphylococcus aureus*. Vaginal cultures are usually positive for *Staphylococcus*, but blood cultures are negative. Antibiotics have not been shown to alter the course of toxic shock syndrome, but they may prevent recurrences. Vigorous fluid resuscitation is most important. Diagnostic criteria include fever above 38.9° C; systolic blood pressure below 90 mm Hg; erythematous rash with subsequent desquamation; involvement of four organ systems; and lack of other causes.

6. **D,** Pages 2314-2315.

Gonorrheal infection may be asymptomatic in up to 40% of cases. Recommended treatment is with ceftriaxone and doxycycline or azithromycin or erythromycin because of coinfection with *C. trachomatis* in up to 60% of cases. Gram stain of endocervical exudate is not nearly as sensitive as with penile discharge. *C. trachomatis* is the most common sexually transmitted disease.

7. **C,** Pages 2316-2317.

Predisposing factors to pelvic inflammatory disease (PID) include multiple partners, recent menses or abortion, trauma, and presence of intrauterine device. Intermediate and chronic PID often flares up during menstruation.

8. **D,** Page 2315.

*Candida albicans* is the causative agent in this fungal vaginitis. There are many predisposing factors including recent antibiotic use. The discharge consistency is classically described as "cottage cheese." Therapy is fluconazole. Unlike bacterial vaginal discharge, which is typically malodorous, fungal discharge is described as non-odorous.

9. **A,** Page 2312-2313.

Chanchroid, an increasingly common gram-negative-rod infection produces painful chancres. Lymphogranuloma venereum produces a small, often unnoticed, painless lesion. Granuloma inguinale causes a progressively erosive "beefy red" painless lesion. Syphilis, a spirochetal infection, presents typically with a painless lesion, satellite buboes, and rash.

10. **C,** Pages 2311-2312.

Herpes is a DNA virus and is the most common cause of genital ulcers. Lesions have been associated with urinary retention if severe. Transmission risks during delivery range from 3%-5% (in recurrent HSV) to 33%-50% (in primary genital infections). Because of the severity of the consequences of neonatal infection, cesarean section is indicated. Oral rather than IV acyclovir use is indicated for routine use in primary herpes.

 ## 138 Sexual Assault

### Greg Harders

1. **A,** Page 2322.

The presence of motile sperm is an indicator that intercourse took place within the last 12 hours.

2. **D,** Page 2321.

Nongenital traumatic injuries are found in 30%-50% of rape cases. Minor abrasions and contusions account for 80% of these injuries.

3. **A,** Page 2324.

Ovral may be used up to 72 hours after unprotected intercourse with a failure rate of less than 2%.

4. **A,** Page 2322.

Water is used because it does not affect the results of the acid phosphates test and has no affect on sperm mobility.

5. **D,** Page 2321.

Use of the Wood's lamp is widely known to assist in evaluation for semen stains; it may also assist in identifying subtle contusions and rope marks.

6. **A,** Page 2324

Patients require follow-up for at least 1 year after exposure because seroconversion may be delayed. The risk of transmission is thought to be low, although there have been cases of seroconversion after rape. While testing is necessary, the setting and privacy of the ED is not ideal. The efficacy of prophylaxis is unknown and unproved.

7. **B,** Pages 2323-2324.

Prophylactic treatment for gonorrhea and chlamydia is always indicated. It is cheaper, more effective, and psychologically more reassuring to the rape victim than follow-up testing. Hepatitis B prophylaxis is indicated in high-risk incidents such as when the suspect is an IV drug abuser. Syphilis is reported as a result in up to 1% of rapes. Treating prophylactically for gonorrhea and chlamydia is preferred to testing as indicated above. In addition, positive tests may be used to allege sexual promiscuity on the part of the victim.

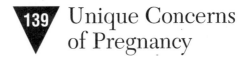 ## 139 Unique Concerns of Pregnancy

### Barbara N. Wynn

1. **D,** Pages 2327-2328.

HCG originates in the trophoblasts and augments corpus luteum production of progesterone. Implantation occurs 6 days after fertilization. Parity refers to the total number of times the patient has given birth regardless of the outcome. Premature labor occurs any time before 30 weeks' gestation.

2. **D,** Pages 2329-2331.

The Centers for Disease Control and Prevention defined anemia in pregnancy as less than 11 gm/dl in the first and third trimesters and less than 10.5 gm/dl in the second trimester. The platelet count decreases as pregnancy progresses. Some believe this is a result of pregnancy-induced platelet consumption. Pregnancy induces a state of peripheral resistance to insulin, and glucosuria can be seen in normal pregnancies. During pregnancy there is a fall in osmolality that is felt to be a result of the resetting of the osmotic thresholds for thirst and vasopressin secretion. The liver structure during pregnancy is unchanged, however, alkaline phosphatase activity is doubled. The increase may be attributed to placental alkaline phosphatase isoenzymes and high levels of circulating estrogens.

3. **E,** Pages 2331-2332.

Braxton-Hicks contractions are painless contractions that occur spontaneously and irregularly early in pregnancy. They are also seen in patients with hematometra and with uterine myomas. They are not reliable in the diagnosis of pregnancy. Chadwick's sign is a pink to blue violet color of the vaginal walls. Hagar's sign is the softening of the lower uterine segment caused by hyperemia. Bleeding before the fortieth day of pregnancy is common and is believed to represent implantation. Fetal heart tones can be auscultated using a Doppler ultrasound usually by 10 weeks, although cardiac activity may be visualized by 8 weeks using ultrasound. Most fetal heart tones can be auscultated by 17 weeks on average and by 19 weeks in nearly all pregnancies in a non-obese patient.

4. **D,** Page 2333.

Normal HCG levels peak at 7-10 weeks of pregnancy with a range of 20-200,000 IU/L. Current pregnancy tests are enzyme-linked immunosorbent assays (ELISA) and have a sensitivity between 25 and 50 IU/L. These tests will not be affected by drugs, with the exception of exogenous HCG used for ovulation induction. Levels of HCG may take as long as 60 days to return to zero after an abortion.

5. **A,** Pages 2332, 2335-2336.

The vital signs of a pregnant patient are essentially the same as for a nonpregnant patient. The only changes seen are in heart rate and blood pressure. Peripheral edema is present in 80% of pregnant women, and a third heart sound and systolic murmurs are common. Diastolic murmurs and systolic murmurs greater than II/VI are not considered normal.

6. **E,** Pages 2337-2338.

Domestic violence is conservatively estimated to occur in 10%-20% of North American spousal relationships. In the pregnant patient, blunt abdominal trauma is the most common type of injury, whereas in the nonpregnant patient the facial area is more commonly involved. Most abused women have no knowledge of the support services available to them, and the fear of offending an abused woman by pursuing direct questions is unfounded. Most abused patients will not volunteer information regarding domestic violence unless specifically asked.

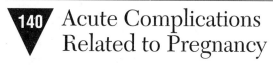

# 140 Acute Complications Related to Pregnancy

*Barbara N. Wynn*

1. **C,** Pages 2344-2345.

Anti-immunoglobulin is indicated if the patient is Rh negative unless the father is known also to be RH negative. Fifty percent or more of women with threatened miscarriage seen in the emergency department ultimately miscarry. Treatment to prevent miscarriage is not useful because most fetuses are nonviable 1 to 2 weeks before actual miscarriage occurs. Therefore patients should be advised that moderate daily activities will not affect the pregnancy. Miscarriages are associated with a significant grieving process and psychologic stress. Because early pregnancy is unannounced and early fetal death is not publicly recognized, it is all the more difficult.

2. **B,** Pages 2345-2347.

Women who have undergone embryo transfer techniques have a much higher risk of heterotopic pregnancy. Fetal heart activity may be seen in either intrauterine or ectopic pregnancies. If culdocentesis is performed and no fluid is obtained, the results should be considered indeterminate because dry taps may be obtained in the presence of peritoneal blood and thus should not rule out the possibility of ectopic pregnancy. The positive predictive value for an intrauterine pregnancy with progesterone level of 25 ng/ml or greater is 99.6%.

3. **E,** Pages 2346-2347.

Ectopic pregnancy occurs simultaneously with intrauterine pregnancy in 1 in 4000 pregnancies. It can be present with very low HCG levels and at times the patient may have no pain and there may be no bleeding or even a missed period. Implantation in the uterine horn is particularly dangerous because the growing embryo can use the myometrial blood supply to grow larger before rupture occurs, usually with severe hemorrhage at 10-14 weeks' gestation. Patients who are bleeding from an ectopic pregnancy may experience endometrial sloughing, which can be mistaken for heavy bleeding or passage of fetal tissue.

4. **E,** Page 2347.

Transabdominal scans have a discriminatory zone of 6500 mIU/ml. Transvaginal scans of gestational sac should be visible by 5 weeks, and fetal heart activity by 7 weeks. A double

ring sign is indicative of an intrauterine pregnancy, and ectopic gestations are rarely visualized on scans.

5. **D,** Pages 2351-2352.

Abruptio placentae is painless approximately one third of the time. Ultrasound is insensitive in the diagnosis of abruptio placentae but is the procedure of choice for diagnosing placenta previa. Most cases of placenta previa identified in the second trimester resolve by the time of delivery as the lower uterine segment elongates.

6. **E,** Pages 2351-2352.

Smoking and maternal hypertension are risks for abruptio placentae. One of the complications of abruptio placentae is DIC, which has a low fibrinogen level. The abdominal examination will show uterine tenderness and irritability. Patients with previous cesarean sections and increased parity are at increased risk for placenta previa, not abruptio placentae.

7. **A,** Page 2353.

The risk for PIH is greatest in women less than 20 years of age, primiparas, and women with twin or molar pregnancies and a family history of PIH. Proteinuria is variable at any given time and may not be detectable in a random urine specimen. This is also a late finding. The LP in the HELLP syndrome stands for low platelet. Eclamptic seizures may be seen postpartum, particularly in the first 48 hours but occasionally as long as 10 days after delivery.

8. **C,** Page 2353.

The most dangerous complication is eclampsia, which is the occurrence of seizure or coma in the setting of signs and symptoms of preeclampsia. The HELLP (hemolysis, elevated liver enzymes, and low platelets) syndrome is a particularly severe form of PIH. Prothrombin time, partial thromboplastin time, and fibrinogen level are all normal.

9. **B,** Pages 2354-2355.

Both intravenous and intramuscular protocols for administration of magnesium sulfate exist. The IV route is preferred because the medication is more easily controlled and the time to therapeutic effect is shorter. Magnesium administration should always be accompanied by clinical observation for loss of reflexes or respiratory depression that occur at toxic levels of magnesium. Magnesium has little direct antihypertensive effect, although by controlling the seizures, the hypertension is usually adequately controlled.

10. **B,** Page 2355.

Hydralazine 5 mg IV should be given and repeated in a dose of 5-10 mg every 20 minutes as needed to keep the diastolic pressure below 110 mm Hg. Nitroprusside and nifedipine have been reported to be safe and effective, although they are much less widely used. Other antihypertensive agents cannot be recommended until concern about uncontrolled lowering of blood pressure and effects on uteroplacental blood flow have been addressed with studies of each in pregnancy.

11. **D,** Page 2356.

Patients with eclampsia should be hypertensive rather than hypotensive. The other processes produce hypotension.

12. **E,** Pages 2357-2358.

The appendix moves out of the right lower quadrant after the third month of gestation and is deep in the right upper quadrant superior to the iliac crest by the last trimester. Proximity to the ureter leads to an increased incidence of sterile pyuria in pregnant patients who have appendicitis. Laxity and displacement of the abdominal wall away from the abdominal viscera especially later in pregnancy result in loss of signs of parietal peritoneal irritation. Leukocytosis is present, although it is rarely high enough to distinguish it from the physiologic leukocytosis of pregnancy.

13. **D,** Pages 2358-2359.

There is an increased incidence of cholecystitis in pregnancy, and because of the potential for other serious diseases, diagnostic studies such as ultrasound should always be performed to verify a clinical diagnosis of cholecystitis. Acute fatty liver of pregnancy is a disorder that may result in fulminate hepatic failure and was until recently almost uniformly fatal. In a normal pregnancy, alkaline phosphatase levels may be double the nonpregnant values.

14. **B,** Page 2360.

The alveolar-arterial oxygen difference may also be abnormally increased, although gradient differences greater than 20 or 25 mm Hg are abnormal. Doppler ultrasonography is useful in the diagnosis of venous thrombosis in the femoral or popliteal veins and provides the least risk. Clinical signs are never good predictors of DVT. Technetium V/Q scans provide negligible radioactive exposure to the fetus, and the diaphragm is symmetrically elevated during late pregnancy.

15. **A,** Pages 2361-2362.

PID is rare in pregnancy and does not occur after the first trimester. The major complication of gonococcal infections in the third trimester is gonococcal ophthalmia of the neonate. Trichomoniasis is rarely aggressive, and only those who have severe symptoms are treated. Treatment with vaginal imidazoles in pregnancy is considered safe, with a cure rate of 85% to 100%.

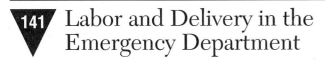

# 141 ▼ Labor and Delivery in the Emergency Department

*Barbara N. Wynn*

1. **D,** Pages 2365-2367.

Bloody show results when the mucous plug is expelled. The bleeding associated with this process is slight, and usually only a few dark red spots are noticed. The significance of a bloody show is that it is a fairly reliable indictor of the onset of stage 1 labor and is not a contraindication to vaginal examination for determination of cervical effacement and dilation. If bleeding continues or is of a large volume, more serious causes should be expected such as placenta previa or placental abruption, which are contraindications for vaginal examination. Emergency department deliveries have a perinatal mortality of 8%-10% compared to 0.04% in patients with good prenatal care and delivery by an obstetrician. In addition, patients who deliver in the emergency department

tend to have more complications such as antepartum hemorrhage, premature rupture of membranes, eclampsia, premature labor, abruptio placentae, precipitous delivery, malpresentation, and umbilical cord prolapse, as well as psychosocial factors such as substance abuse and pregnancy denial. Position is the relationship of the fetal presenting part to the birth canal. Presentation is the anatomic part of the fetus leading through the birth canal.

2. **B,** Pages 2368-2369.

Fetal heart rate tracings have several components that can be accessed: baseline heart rate variability, accelerations, decelerations, and diagnostic patterns. Variability can be beat-to-beat or long term over intervals of a minute or more, but both types of variability are indicators of fetal well-being. Accelerations occur during fetal movement and reflect an alert, mobile fetus. Decelerations in the fetal heart rate are more complicated. There are three types: variable, early, and late, referring to the timing of the deceleration relative to the uterine contraction. Variable and early decelerations are very common and are present on more than 50% of all tracings. Late decelerations are more serious and most often indicate uterine placental insufficiency. A sinusoidal tracing is an ominous finding with a very high associated mortality. Differential diagnosis for this pattern includes erythroblastosis fetalis, placental abruption, fetal hemorrhage, and amnionitis.

3. **E,** Pages 2373-2374.

Preterm labor is defined as uterine contractions with cervical changes before 37 weeks. A viable fetus and a healthy mother are indications for the medical management directed at prolongation of gestation. Exceptions to medical management include the combination of preterm labor and premature rupture of membranes, fetal disorders, and maternal contraindications. Once these criteria are employed, only one fourth of all women with premature labor are candidates for medical management. Magnesium sulfate is the tocolytic of choice for preterm labor in diabetic mothers, those with cardiopulmonary disease, or those with infection. Magnesium sulfate does block shivering, and there is a resultant drop in core temperature that can obscure the diagnosis of intrauterine infection. Cardiopulmonary disease is only a relative contraindication for tocolysis.

4. **B,** Page 2375-2377.

Amniotic fluid pH is 7.1-7.3, and it turns nitrazine paper yellow. A pH above 7.3 turns it blue. Concealed bleeding occurs 20%-30% of the time with abruptio placentae. Breech presentation is the most common malpresentation, occurring in up to 4% of all deliveries. Most premature breech infants deliver spontaneously without difficulty. Shoulder dystocia is the second most common malpresentation and usually develops intrapartum. When shoulder dystocia becomes evident, intrapartum delivery maneuvers can be life-saving. The mnemonic HELPER has been proposed to help keep the appropriate intrapartum steps organized and facilitate a sequential approach. These maneuvers will successfully deliver almost all cases of shoulder dystocia.

5. **A,** Pages 2384-2385.

When a prolapsed cord occurs with a viable infant, cesarean section is the delivery method of choice. If this is unavailable in a timely fashion, however, manual replacement of the cord into the uterus and rapid vaginal delivery may be the only options. Placing the mother in the knee-chest position with the bed in Trendelenburg and digitally elevating the presenting part off the umbilical cord is a maneuver to preserve umbilical circulation. Placement of a Foley catheter and instillation of 500-750 ml saline may help lift the fetus off the cord, particularly in the first stage of labor. Tocolysis with ritodrine will help relieve pressure on the umbilical cord.

6. **A,** Pages 2385-2386.

Postpartum hemorrhage is the most common complication of labor and delivery. Hemorrhage is defined as blood loss in excess of 500 ml. Retained products of conception may cause both immediate and delayed postpartum hemorrhage and thus the timing of the bleeding does not determine this diagnosis. Uterine packing to decrease postpartum hemorrhage was at one time widely used but is no longer common. However, because dilation and curettage and hysterectomy are sometimes not available to the emergency physician, the importance of uterine packing as an option in the emergency department is increased. This approach is only a temporizing measure.

7. **C,** Page 2387.

Uterine rupture is an unpredictable event occurring late in pregnancy or in stage 1 of labor. Uterine inversion is associated with immediate postpartum hemorrhage that can be life-threatening. The highest likelihood for successful repositioning of the inverted uterus is immediately after inversion, and digital pressure should be directed toward the mother's umbilicus along the long axis of the uterus. If the placenta is still adherent, it should not be removed until after repositioning since removal can result in excessive blood loss.

 # 142 Drug Use in Pregnancy

*Bruce W. Nugent*

1. **E,** Page 2392.

Based on currently available human and animal studies plus case reports, the FDA has designated the risk for teratogenicity of the use of various drugs during pregnancy. Class A and B are considered safe for use. Class C and D require the potential for benefit to outweigh the potential for harm. Class X drugs are contraindicated in pregnancy because benefit is clearly outweighed by risk.

2. **D,** Page 2392.

At delivery, mothers who have ingested salicylates are at greater risk of hemorrhage and blood loss. In addition, interference with prostaglandins by salicylates increases the duration of labor and delays its onset. Chronic salicylate use is associated with post-maturity, but there is no increase in the rate of malformations. Salicylates may cause premature closure of the ductus arteriosus.

3. **E,** Page 2393.

Although sulfamethoxazole is a class C drug, it is the best of the choices listed. Sulfonamides are contraindicated near term because of associated neonatal jaundice. Amoxicillin is safe in pregnancy, but the patient is allergic to penicillin. Quinolones should be avoided during pregnancy because of the potential effects on cartilage development. Doxycycline is not a preferred agent for cystitis and is class D. Likewise metronidazole is an inappropriate antibiotic for cystitis and should be avoided during the first trimester of pregnancy.

4. **C,** Page 2394.

All commonly used anticonvulsant agents have been associated with congenital anomalies in as many as 30% of exposed neonates. The physiologic changes of pregnancy result in a lower maternal serum level of most drugs. Fetal hydantoin syndrome occurs in 5%-10% of chronically exposed infants, especially those with low levels of epoxide hydrolase. Anticonvulsants should be continued in pregnancy to avoid the risk of seizures. However, referral to perinatal and neurologic specialists is indicated.

5. **E,** Page 2394.

Neurotubule defects are one of many characteristics in the syndrome of defects associated with the use of valproic acid. Multiple mechanisms have been proposed, but apparently valproic acid inhibits intestinal folic acid absorption. All commonly used anticonvulsants are associated with congenital anomalies, and the combination results in a higher rate of malformation than any individual agent alone.

6. **A,** Page 2395.

Adenosine is the drug of choice in terminating maternal supraventricular tachycardia. Verapamil would be safe to use but is a second-line agent. Labetalol is safe in pregnancy but hemodynamically inappropriate in this case. Both captopril and warfarin are contraindicated in pregnancy.

7. **D,** Page 2397.

The risk of spontaneous abortion increases with dose of alcohol ingested per day, and even two drinks per week has been shown to increase the incidence. The risk of congenital abnormalities also increases in a dose-dependent fashion, and consumption of one ounce of alcohol per day carries an estimated 10% risk for the development of fetal anomalies. Maternal and fetal alcohol concentrations are equivalent, and benzodiazepines are the drug of choice for treatment of withdrawal. Use of one drug during pregnancy is associated with other drug abuse and increases the risk of adverse affects on the fetus.

8. **B,** Page 2398.

Opiates readily diffuse across the placenta, and amniotic fluid is believed to act as a reservoir that prolongs fetal exposure. Opiates have not been associated with an increased risk of structural birth defects; however, there is a greater incidence of low-birth-weight infants in heroin users without prenatal care. More than two thirds of neonates born to opiate-addicted mothers exhibit signs of opiate withdrawal.

9. **B,** Page 2398.

The abstinence syndrome is characterized by signs of CNS hyperactivity, autonomic instability, and gastrointestinal respiratory symptoms. Tachypnea with wheezing is more common than respiratory depression. Methadone-dependent neonates appear to have more frequent and severe symptoms, and clearing of the drug may be delayed for up to 2 weeks after birth because of the higher volume of distribution and slower rate of metabolism of methadone in the neonate. Withdrawal may be treated with methadone or diazepam; however, if seizures occur, methadone is thought to be a better option because they otherwise may be refractory.

10. **A,** Pages 2398-2399.

The toxicity of cocaine is largely caused by its adrenergic effects. Decreased placental blood flow from vasoconstriction results in chronic fetal hypoxemia. Structural defects are presumed to be mediated by the vasoconstrictor effects of cocaine on the developing fetus. Cocaine is an anorexic agent, and malnutrition places the fetus at risk for growth retardation as well.

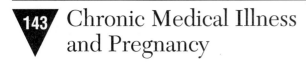

## 143 ▼ Chronic Medical Illness and Pregnancy

*Bruce W. Nugent*

1. **C,** Page 2404.

Physiologic state of hyperventilation is present during pregnancy caused by progesterone stimulation of the medullary respiratory center and decreased functional residual capacity from limited diaphragmatic excursion. Both tidal volume and minute ventilation increase by up to 50% by term. A slight respiratory alkalosis occurs, and the resting $Pco_2$ is decreased by an average of 10 mm Hg.

2. **D,** Pages 2404-2405.

Acute treatment of the pregnant asthmatic patient is largely unchanged from that of the nonpregnant patient. Inhaled beta-agonists are the first-line drugs for an acute exacerbation, and oral or parenteral steroids should be administered if the patient fails to respond to beta-agonists or if the patient is already taking inhaled or oral steroids. Because the fetus is more sensitive to hypoxia than the mother, supplemental oxygen should always be administered.

3. **C,** Page 2406.

The risk of myocardial infarction in a patient with coronary artery disease increases with the duration of gestation and peaks at the time of labor. MI carries a worse prognosis with mortality of 28% overall and 50% during labor. Typical ECG and enzyme changes will occur. Treatment of acute MI during pregnancy is similar to the nonpregnant patient and can include thrombolytic therapy and nitrates. Coronary artery dissection is a rare but often lethal complication in pregnancy. The clinical presentation is similar to MI, but sudden death and cardiogenic shock are more common.

4. **D,** Pages 2406-2407.

The acceleration of pulse seen in normal pregnancy shortens left ventricular diastolic filling time and results in reduced stroke volume. Further increase in heart rate to generate higher cardiac output along with the expanded plasma volume of pregnancy creates a vicious cycle that leads to increased left atrial pressures and signs and symptoms of left ventricular failure. Atrial fibrillation is common and is associated with a maternal mortality of 15% during pregnancy. Treatment is by diuresis, bed rest, and reduction of heart rate. Regurgitant valvular lesions are tolerated well during pregnancy; however, acute aortic insufficiency resulting from acute bacterial endocarditis is an indication for immediate surgical repair.

5. **B,** Page 2407.

The most common complication in pregnancy is anemia, and up to 50% of all pregnancies manifest some type of anemia; without iron supplementation the incidence may reach 90%. Hemoglobin levels less than 11 are associated with increased premature delivery, small for gestational age infants, and hypertrophic placenta, but there is relatively little impact of maternal anemia on perinatal mortality until hemoglobin level of 6.0 gm/ml is reached. Although classically a microcytic hypochromic anemia, these indices are found in only 11% of pregnant patients and are not a reliable screening tool. Megaloblastic anemia is most commonly caused by dietary deficiency of folate and results in an increased incidence of neural tube defects.

6. **A,** Pages 2407-2408.

Many sickle cell anemia patients now live longer than 40 years, and because fertility is usually unaffected are able to bear children. Only 64% of these pregnancies result in a live fetus. Painful crises are more common during pregnancy because vascular stasis in the lower extremities promotes sickling. The Kleihauer-Betke test to distinguish fetal from maternal blood will be falsely positive because of persisting hemoglobin F in the mother.

7. **E,** Page 2408.

Eclampsia generally occurs in the presence of progressive preeclampsia with hypertension, peripheral edema, and proteinuria. Since any immediately post-ictal patient is likely to have hypertension and disorientation and even normal pregnancies may have mild pedal edema, proteinuria may be the only differentiating factor in the initial diagnosis of eclampsia. Noneclamptic patients will revert to normal or low blood pressure after a period of observation.

8. **B,** Pages 2408-2409.

Fewer than 10% of epileptics experience improvement in their seizure disorder during pregnancy. Sub-therapeutic anticonvulsant levels occur due to volume and metabolic reasons as well as from noncompliance to avoid teratogenic effects on the fetus. The risk of status epilepticus to both the mother and the fetus clearly outweighs the potential for adverse teratogenic effects, and standard therapy for status epilepticus is indicated, including phenytoin. Proper positioning to avoid supine hypotensive syndrome and measurement of fetal heart tones should also occur.

9. **A,** Pages 2409, 2410, 2412, 2415.

As pregnancy progresses there is an insulin resistance up to peak demand at 28 weeks. All pregnant women with diabetes are "brittle" and must be followed closely to avoid wide swings in glucose control. Autoimmune diseases such as Grave's disease, multiple sclerosis, rheumatoid arthritis, and myasthenia gravis often may transiently improve during pregnancy because of the relative immunosuppression. After delivery, however, there is a high likelihood of rebound exacerbation of these diseases.

10. **B,** Page 2411.

Hyperemesis and noncompliance or errors in insulin dosage are the most common precipitants of diabetic ketoacidosis in the pregnant patient. Admission is often indicated to correct dehydration and more carefully adjust glucose control. The serum pH may be deceptively normal in the pregnant patient. The initial pH tends to be higher in pregnancy due to physiologic hyperventilation. DKA is rare in patients with gestational diabetes, and insulin and counter-regulatory hormones do not cross the placenta.

11. **E,** Page 2413.

Vertical transmission occurs in 25%-59% of deliveries if the mother is untreated. It is thought to occur in utero, intrapartum through exposure to maternal blood and secretions, and through breast milk. Episiotomy and invasive monitoring should not be routine. Virtually all neonates will have an initially positive HIV antibody test because of transfer of maternal antibodies. Breast-feeding should be avoided because it doubles the risk of fetal infection. AZT therapy of the mother during pregnancy and the neonate decreases the rate of vertical transmission from 25% to 8%. AZT has not been found to cause any specific congenital abnormalities.

12. **B,** Page 2412.

The first priority in treatment of hyperthyroidism is the reversal and stabilization of the end organ and hemodynamic effects of synthetic stimulation. Because the fetal thyroid is extremely sensitive to iodide, its use may result in a large goiter and it should be reserved for only severe cases. $I^{131}$ radionuclide to ablate the maternal thyroid is absolutely contraindicated because it will simultaneously destroy the fetal thyroid gland.

13. **C,** Page 2414.

Screening for syphilis and/or hepatitis B virus infection should be performed on all pregnant patients and repeated at various intervals in high-risk populations. Treatment with benzathine penicillin is highly effective. The occurrence of congenital syphilis is caused largely by inadequate prenatal screening. Link of transmission of hepatitis B virus approaches 90% in untreated cases, and 60%-90% of infected neonates will become carriers into adult life. Routine screening for HBV during pregnancy is cost-effective because treatment with hepatitis B immunoglobulin and hepatitis B vaccine reduces the vertical transmission rate five-fold and in infected neonates the chronic carrier state by 50%.

14. **B,** Page 2409.

The patient is exhibiting signs of autonomic dysreflexia. The response is nonspecific and may be precipitated by disten-

tion of bowel or bladder or any of the other causes listed. However, in certain spinal-cord–injured patients it heralds the onset of labor, which would be most likely in this scenario.

# 144 Acid-Base Disorders

*Jeffrey S. Jones*

1. **E,** Page 2420.

This is an acute process as evidenced by minimal renal compensation. When renal compensation occurs, the plasma $HCO_3$ increases. Initial therapy must be directed toward restoration of ventilation and oxygenation. Induction of $CO_2$ narcosis is unlikely in a patient with acute respiratory acidosis. Blood pressure and cardiac output are usually well-maintained during moderately severe acute respiratory acidosis.

2. **B,** Pages 2424, 2429.

All the others cause metabolic acidosis.

3. **A,** Page 2425.

Metabolic acidosis with a normal anion gap is caused either by an excessive loss of $HCO_3$ (diarrhea) or an inability to excrete H (obstructive uropathy).

4. **E,** Page 2427.

Rapid $NaHCO_3$ replacement may result in paradoxical cerebrospinal and intracellular acidosis. Impaired oxygen delivery, hypokalemia, hypocalcemia, hypernatremia, hyperosmolality, and "overshoot" alkalosis may occur.

5. **D,** Page 2430.

If the electrolyte specimen and the blood gas sample were not obtained at the same time, interventions done to the patient in the interval between blood draws may complicate interpretation of the values.

6. **C,** Page 2424.

Hypoxemia is associated with type A lactic acidosis, the most common type. The others can cause ketoacidosis.

7. **D,** Page 2419.

Serum potassium is directly influenced by serum pH. $K^+$ will rise 0.2-0.6 mEq/L for every decrease in pH of 0.1 units.

8. **E,** Page 2424.

Generalized seizures are a common cause of transient lactic acidosis with a high anion gap. The others can result in a normal anion gap metabolic acidosis.

9. **B,** Page 2429.

There is mineralocorticoid excess and increased $Na^+$ delivery to the distal tubule with $H^+$ and $K^+$ secretion.

10. **A,** Page 2424.

Has a high anion gap.

11. **D,** Page 2428.

This is a primary cause secondary to hypermetabolic state.

12. **C,** Pages 2420, 2422.

This is secondary to acute respiratory center depression.

**145** Electrolyte Disturbances

*Jeffrey S. Jones*

1. **D,** Page 2432.
Water makes up approximately 60% of total body weight.
2. **B,** Page 2432.
Hypotonic saline infusion will lower the ECF osmotic strength, which will then cause a shift of extracellular fluid into the cells until the osmolalities are equalized.
3. **D,** Page 2435.
Relative concentrations are the major determinants of the normal osmotic and electrochemical gradient of all living cells. Ninety-eight percent of the body's $K^+$ is intracellular.
4. **D,** Page 2432.
Mannitol does not penetrate cellular membranes and therefore draws intracellular water into the ECF, resulting in cellular dehydration. All of the other choices readily cross the cell wall and therefore do not cause fluid shifts.
5. **E,** Pages 2433-2434.
Patients with hypovolemic hyponatremia should have volume deficits corrected with isotonic saline (0.9%).
6. **E,** Page 2433.
The hallmark of SIADH is an inappropriately concentrated urine despite the presence of a low serum osmolality and a normal circulating blood volume. Psychogenic polydipsia also causes a euvolemic hyponatremia, but the urine maximally dilutes.
7. **B,** Pages 2433, 2434.
Hyponatremia with dilute urine suggests either an acute water overload or psychogenic polydipsia. Because the patient is not symptomatic, treatment is limited to fluid restriction.
8. **E,** Pages 2434-2435.
The primary goal in the treatment of hypovolemic hypernatremia is to restore volume deficits and to maintain organ perfusion. Treatment should be initiated with an infusion of isotonic saline. Once the patient is hemodynamically stable, the remaining free water deficits can be replaced.
9. **B,** Pages 2434-2435.
Diabetes insipidus (DI) results in the loss of large amounts of dilute urine because of the loss of concentrating ability in the distal nephrons. DI can be central (lack of ADH secretion from the pituitary) or nephrogenic (lack of responsiveness to circulating ADH). Patients are usually able to maintain near-normal serum levels as long as access to water is maintained. Patients will have a low urine specific gravity (<1.005) and low urine osmolality. Those with central DI require the administration of parenteral or intranasal vasopressin.
10. **B,** Pages 2433-2434.
All the others cause hyponatremia. Diarrhea causes it by increased water loss.
11. **B,** Page 2435.
When hypernatremia results from an increase in the total body sodium, diuretic treatment to eliminate the sodium excess should be used in conjunction with water replacement.

12. **C,** Pages 2432-2433.
Hyperlipidemia can cause pseudohyponatremia because the lipids will displace a portion of the plasma water. Therefore there will be less $Na^+$ in a given volume, but the tonicity will be normal. The others result in a reduced sodium concentration relative to plasma water.
13. **C,** Page 2433.
Like hypernatremia, the signs and symptoms of hyponatremia are primarily neurologic. As the serum sodium falls below 120 mEq/L, irritability, disorientation, and confusion are common. Lethargy, apathy, weakness, and seizures may also be seen. Lower levels may be tolerated with chronic hyponatremia.
14. **C,** Page 2434.
When serum sodium is below 120 mEq/L or the patient has CNS manifestations, aggressive treatment with 3% NaCl is indicated. In addition, monitoring of central venous pressure, urine output, and urine electrolytes is important. Acute hyponatremia may be corrected at rates of up to 1-2 mEq/L/hr and chronic hyponatremia should be corrected at a rate not greater than 2.5 mEq/L/hr. Generally, serum sodium should not be corrected to above 120 mEq/L or increased by more than 20 mEq/L in a 24-hour period.
15. **D,** Pages 2433-2435.
Certain antibiotics such as ticarcillin and carbenicillin contain large amounts of sodium chloride. Cushing's disease causes increased sodium absorption. Severe burns, vomiting, and diarrhea all result in increased water loss. SIADH results in euvolemic hyponatremia.
16. **B,** Page 2436.
Antibiotics, such as penicillin or carbenicillin, act as non-reabsorbable anions in the distal tubule and thereby stimulate potassium secretion.
17. **A,** Page 2437.
Addison's disease is a deficiency of mineralocorticoid secretion, which often leads to hyperkalemia. Licorice, a flavoring additive in a number of preparations, including chewing tobacco, contains glycyrrhizic acid. This compound possesses mineralocorticoid properties and historically was used in the treatment of Addison's disease.
18. **A,** Page 2437.
Peaked T waves are seen in hyperkalemia.
19. **A,** Pages 2438-2439.
Acute acidosis, beta-receptor antagonism, alpha-receptor stimulation, digitalis, succinylcholine, exercise, and hyperkalemic periodic paralysis can all cause transcellular shifts. Hypoaldosteronism and $K^+$ sparing diuretics result in hyperkalemia because of impaired renal function. Salt substitute is increased $K^+$ intake. Rhabdomyolysis results in increased $K^+$ because of cellular injury with release of $K^+$ from damaged cells.
20. **C,** Page 2438.
False elevations of potassium may be seen with thrombocytosis, leukocytosis, laboratory error, hemolysis of the blood sample, and abnormal erythrocytes. The others may result in true hyperkalemia.

21. **E,** Page 2439.

Paradoxical aciduria occurs with hypokalemia, not hyperkalemia, because the kidneys will preferentially save $K^+$ and excrete $H^+$, forming more acidic urine.

22. **B,** Page 2439.

This patient warrants aggressive therapy, and the most rapid effect is achieved by the infusion of 10-30 ml of 10% calcium gluconate over 1-5 minutes, which is cardiac protective. It will only last 20-60 minutes, so the other measures need to be instituted. Bicarbonate, glucose and insulin, and beta-2 agonists will all shift potassium into the cells. Kayexalate will remove it from the body.

23. **C,** Pages 2439-2500 and Chapter 148.

Hyperkalemia secondary to mineralocorticoid deficiency is treated with Florinef. If the hyperkalemia were life-threatening, emergency therapy including 10% calcium gluconate should also be administered. Adrenal failure is usually treated with 100 mg of hydrocortisone IV every 6-8 hours.

24. **B,** Page 2440.

A lower albumin level makes fewer sites available for $Ca^{++}$ binding, thus decreasing total $Ca^{++}$ while having no effect on the free ionized fraction.

25. **E,** Pages 2440-2441.

Vitamin D toxicity results in hypercalcemia while insufficiency results in hypocalcemia. Massive blood transfusion (>6 U) results in a citrate load causing hypocalcemia in 94% of patients. In chronic renal failure there is vitamin D deficiency, impaired responsiveness to PTH, and phosphate retention. Secondary hypoparathyroidism can result from hypermagnesemia and neck surgery.

26. **C,** Pages 2442-2444.

The signs and symptoms of hypercalcemia are summarized in the box on Rosen page 2442. The most reliable electrocardiogram change of hypercalcemia is shortening of the QT interval, which is always seen when the $Ca^{++}$ concentration exceeds 13 mg/100 ml. Of the treatment options listed, saline diuresis using furosemide is the most appropriate. Treatment management options are summarized in the box on Rosen page 2444.

27. **B,** Page 2442.

Symptomatic hypocalcemia should be treated with parenteral calcium. Calcium chloride contains 360 mg of elemental calcium in a 10 ml ampule, while calcium gluconate 10% contains 93 mg of elemental calcium. Recommended initial dose is 100-300 mg of either.

28. **A,** Pages 2440, 2443.

Anticonvulsant medications such as phenytoin and primidone are associated with hypocalcemia. All the others can cause hypercalcemia.

29. **D,** Page 2446.

Hypomagnesemia, like hypokalemia and hypercalcemia, will worsen the manifestations of digitalis toxicity. Digitalis-induced dysrhythmias are more likely in the presence of hypomagnesemia.

30. **A,** Pages 2445-2448.

Magnesium absorption occurs mainly in the small intestine and colon. Hypomagnesemia from poor nutrition is rare in the United States. Serum levels of this cation range from 1.8 to 3.0 mg/dl. Hypermagnesemia causes hypotension because it relaxes smooth muscle. Hypermagnesemia and hypomagnesemia cause neuromuscular dysfunction.

31. **C,** Pages 2446-2448.

Loss of deep tendon reflexes will occur as magnesium levels rise above 4 mg/dl. Hypomagnesemia will cause hyperactive deep tendon reflexes, muscular fibrillations, and carpopedal spasms.

32. **A,** Page 2448.

Calcium directly antagonizes the membrane effects of hypermagnesemia and reverses respiratory depression, hypotension, and cardiac dysrhythmias. Dialysis should be considered in patients with coma, respiratory failure, and hemodynamic instability, as well as in those with severe hypermagnesemia associated with renal failure. Hydration with isotonic fluids and furosemide can be used in milder cases. Observation only and stopping the magnesium may be sufficient in some cases.

33. **D,** Page 2449.

Phosphate levels are elevated, not depressed, in hypoparathyroidism.

34. **E,** Page 2449.

Up to 50% of alcoholics are hypophosphatemic. Increased renal excretion and decreased intake are the proposed mechanism.

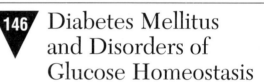

## 146 Diabetes Mellitus and Disorders of Glucose Homeostasis

*Bruce W. Nugent*

1. **D,** Page 2457.

Insulin is the major anabolic hormone and stimulates glucose uptake storage and use in insulin-sensitive tissues. It inhibits hepatic gluconeogenesis and glycogenolysis. Its half-life in the circulation is 3-10 minutes. For incompletely understood reasons, oral glucose evokes more insulin release than does the parenteral form.

2. **D,** Pages 2458-2459.

Non–insulin-dependent diabetes mellitus (NIDDM) has the highest prevalence in Pima Native Americans. The typical patient with NIDDM, or type II diabetes, is likely to be an obese adult or elderly person with varying degrees of pancreatic beta cells dysfunction. All the other answers apply to type I diabetics.

3. **D,** Page 2459.

Insulin-dependent diabetes mellitus (IDDM) is significantly more prevalent in whites than non-whites and has a peak age of onset between 10 and 14 years of age. The patient with IDDM, or type I diabetes, has a virtual absence of pancreatic beta cells, severe insulin deficiency, and predisposition to ketosis. One quarter of diabetics are type I and three fourths are type II.

4. **B,** Pages 2457-2458, 2463-2464.

The catabolic hormone glucagon is the most important of the counter-regulatory hormones and to the anabolic hormone insulin. It is secreted from the pancreatic alpha cells and acts to increase gluconeogenesis and glycogenolysis and increase hepatic ketone production. It is released in response to hypoglycemia, stress, trauma, infections, and starvation and is essential in the pathogenesis of diabetic ketoacidosis where it is elevated to 4 to 5 times normal levels.

5. **C,** Page 2459-2461.

Formal glucose tolerance tests are usually unnecessary to diagnose diabetes. Any random plasma glucose >200 mg/dl or more than one fasting glucose >140 mg/dl establishes the diagnosis. Dipstick methods for testing blood glucose may be inaccurate, especially in the hyperglycemic range or with extremes of hematocrit. Urine ketone dipsticks are a good test for acetoacetate, but they do not measure betahydroxybutyrate. Glycosylated hemoglobin is the most important test in the assessment of degree of diabetic control.

6. **D,** Pages 2461-2462.

Hypoglycemia is the most dangerous acute complication of diabetes and is a life-threatening emergency. Missing meals and increased exercise or insulin are common causes. Symptomatic hypoglycemia in adults occurs at levels of about 50 mg/dl, but symptoms may be blunted in patients with recurrent episodes. Hypoglycemia can be treated with glucagon, 1 mg IM. D50W should not be used in children because it scleroses veins.

7. **A,** Page 2462.

Prolonged hypoglycemia is most likely to occur in patients taking chlorpropamide, especially if renal function is compromised. The duration of action is much greater (60 hours) than for the other oral hypoglycemics. Hypoglycemia induced by any oral hypoglycemic agent should have a minimum observation period of 24 hours and often requires constant infusions of D10.

8. **C,** Page 2466.

In the adult patient who has marked dehydration but without shock, 1 liter of normal saline may be administered in the first hour. Isotonic fluids should be used initially. D5-containing fluids should be postponed until initial fluid therapy has been given and the blood sugar is approximately 250 mg/dl.

9. **E,** Pages 2463-2464; 2460.

DKA occurs in type 1 diabetics. Betahydroxybutyrate predominates over acetoacetate in a ratio of 3:1 to 30:1. An elevated temperature is rarely caused by DKA itself and suggests the presence of sepsis. Acute abdominal pain occurs in half of patients, especially children, and resolves with treatment. Decreased mental status more closely correlates with the degree of hyperosmolarity than with the degree of ketoacidosis.

10. **E,** Page 2465.

The reported serum sodium is often misleading in DKA. The true value of sodium may be approximated by adding 1.3-1.6 mEq/L to the reported value for every 100 mg/dl of glucose over the norm. Acidosis and dehydration contribute to high measured serum potassium despite total body deficits. Correction for acidosis can be made by subtracting 0.6 mEq/L from the laboratory value for every 0.1 decrease in pH.

11. **B,** Pages 2466-2467.

Potassium replacement with potassium chloride is invariably needed in the treatment of DKA, usually early on. Despite theoretical benefits, no clinical benefit from the routine administration of potassium phosphate has been shown. Bicarbonate is indicated only at a pH of 7.0 or below. Isotonic fluids should be used initially. Dextrose-containing fluids should be postponed until initial fluid therapy has been given and the blood sugar is approximately 250 mg/dl. Morbidity of DKA is often iatrogenic, especially hypokalemia, hypoglycemia, alkalosis, and cerebral edema.

12. **E,** Pages 2468-2469.

The patient is developing cerebral edema. Immediate action should be administration of 0.25-1 gm/kg of mannitol at the first sign of a headache or decreased level of consciousness. The patient may require intubation and controlled ventilation, but mannitol is first-line therapy.

13. **A,** Pages 2468-2470.

The prodrome for HHNC is significantly longer than that of DKA. The patient typically manifests more profound electrolyte imbalance and dehydration than those with DKA. A patient with HHNC does not have a ketoacidosis caused by diabetes but may have a lesser degree of metabolic acidosis. The mortality rate is much higher for HHNC as most patients are elderly and have underlying cardiac and renal disease.

14. **A,** Page 2459, 2470.

Diabetes is associated with widespread premature accelerated atherosclerosis. Coronary artery disease is common, and there is an increased incidence of "silent" myocardial infarctions and complicated MIs and congestive heart failure.

15. **A,** Pages 2469-2470.

The patient demonstrates a typical presentation of hyperglycemic hyperosmolar nonketotic coma. Decreased level of consciousness, focal neurologic deficits, and seizures are common. Phenytoin is contraindicated as it is ineffective and may impair endogenous insulin release. Half of the profound fluid deficit can be replaced in the first 8 hours, but CVP monitoring may be necessary. Low-dose insulin is indicated after adequate rehydration is under way. The most commonly associated illnesses are chronic renal insufficiency, gram-negative pneumonia, GI bleeding, and gram-negative sepsis.

16. **E,** Page 2465.

Narcotic overdose may cause coma, but it will not show up with other physical findings and history consistent with DKA.

17. **C,** Page 2470.

Azotemia generally does not begin until 10-15 years after the diagnosis of diabetes and the first appearance of microalbuminuria. Hypertension accelerates renal disease, and angiotensin converting enzyme inhibitors are effective in controlling it and lowering microalbuminuria. Tight glycemic control significantly reduces the risk of microalbuminuria and the progression of nephropathy.

18. **E,** Page 2470.

The severity of diabetic retinopathy is related to the quality of glycemic control. Background or simple retinopathy is characterized by microaneurysms, small vessel obstruction, and hard and soft exudates. Proliferative retinopathy involves new vessel formation, and scarring and complications include vitreal hemorrhage and retinal detachment.

19. **A,** Page 2471.

Autonomic neuropathy is frequent in the gastrointestinal tract manifested by delayed gastric emptying, constipation, or nocturnal diarrhea. Other manifestations include impotence, bladder dysfunction, and orthostatic hypotension.

20. **D,** Page 2471.

Peripheral symmetric neuropathy is a slowly progressive primarily sensory disorder manifesting bilaterally with anesthesia, hyperesthesia, or pain worse at night and more often involving the lower extremities.

21. **B,** Page 2471.

22. **B,** Page 2471.

Mononeuropathy or mononeuropathy multiplex affects both motor and sensory nerves, usually one nerve at a time with a rapid onset and cranial nerves predominant.

23. **E,** Page 2472.

Strict metabolic control is imperative in diabetic pregnancies since perinatal mortality is directly correlated. Hypoglycemia is common because of the tight control. Ketoacidosis is associated with a 50%-90% fetal mortality rate. Pregnancy is associated with progression of retinopathy.

## 147 ▼ Rhabdomyolysis

*Warren F. Lanphear*

1. **C,** Pages 2478-2485.

Rhabdomyolysis is a clinical syndrome caused by injury to skeletal muscle that results in the release of its contents into the circulation. The sarcolemma is the injured skeletal muscle cell membrane. The initial physical examination may be of limited value because muscle weakness, tenderness, and swelling with discoloration of the skin are found only 4%-15% of the time. Creatine phosphokinase (CK) is more sensitive than myoglobin in detecting the presence of rhabdomyolysis in the blood. CK levels of five times normal or greater are diagnostic. The anion gap is characteristically elevated even in patients without acute renal failure.

2. **C,** Pages 2479-2482.

There is a small group of patients who develop idiopathic rhabdomyolysis, sometimes recurrently, but this is not a leading cause of injury to skeletal muscle.

3. **A,** Pages 2482-2485.

Acute renal failure is considered the most lethal complication of rhabdomyolysis. Compartment syndromes may be the cause or a complication of rhabdomyolysis. A great number of patients with acute rhabdomyolysis will demonstrate

laboratory evidence of DIC. Some patients with severe rhabdomyolysis will develop hepatic insufficiency, occasionally requiring liver transplantation. Hyperkalemia is not found universally among rhabdomyolysis patients but rather is a consequence of impaired renal function.

4. **B,** Pages 2484-2485.

The most common cause of acute renal failure associated with rhabdomyolysis is acute intrinsic renal failure (AIRF), formerly known as acute tubular necrosis (ATN). AIRF is defined as a decrease in the GFR caused by a toxic or ischemic event. Increased renal vascular resistance contributes to AIRF. Tubular obstruction, although universally present, is not believed to be the primary event. Hyperkalemia is an effect of diminished renal function.

5. **B,** Page 2486.

The mainstay of therapy is the administration of large volumes of saline very early in the course of the disease. IV sodium bicarbonate to alkalinize the urine prevents crystallization in acid urine. Mannitol and furosemide should be considered if urine output is inadequate despite aggressive fluid therapy. Dialysis may be required if these regimens fail.

6. **D,** Pages 2479-2486.

Hypocalcemia occurs early and is present in up to 63% of cases. Hypercalcemia develops later and is treated if symptomatic. Hypokalemia and hypophosphatemia are reported causes of rhabdomyolysis. Hyperkalemia, hyperphosphatemia, and hyperuricemia are all complications of rhabdomyolysis.

## 148 ▼ Endocrine Disorders

*Jeffrey S. Jones*

1. **B,** Pages 2488-2489.

Thyroid storm will develop in 1%-2% of patients with hyperthyroidism. Most cases are caused by toxic diffuse goiter (Graves' disease) and occur in women in their third and fourth decades. Signs and symptoms reflect adrenergic hyperactivity, but serum catecholamines are not elevated. Thyroid storm is a clinical diagnosis and a medical emergency.

2. **D,** Page 2492.

Blockade of the peripheral adrenergic hyperactivity of thyroid storm is perhaps the most important factor in reducing morbidity and mortality. All the others also need to be given.

3. **B,** Page 2492.

Aspirin should not be used because it displaces thyroid hormone from thyroglobulin and could increase the pool of metabolically active hormone. All the rest may be indicated.

4. **B,** Page 2493.

Precipitating factors other than cold exposure can be identified in fewer than half of patients.

5. **D,** Page 2495.

A high TSH level may be the only laboratory abnormality in hypothyroidism.

6. **A,** Pages 2496-2497.

The single most important factor in survival is prompt IV administration of significant doses of thyroid hormone. All the rest also need to be done after $T_4$ administration.

7. **C,** Pages 2497-2498.

The most common etiology of adrenal insufficiency with which patients come to the ED is suppression of the hypothalamic-pituitary-adrenal axis as a result of long-term glucocorticoid therapy.

8. **C,** Pages 2499-2500.

Two thirds of cases of adrenal failure have associated hypoglycemia. Decreased gluconeogenesis and increased peripheral glucose use are secondary to lipolysis.

9. **A,** Page 2500.

A 48-hour ACTH stimulation test can confirm the diagnosis of adrenal insufficiency and differentiate primary from secondary causes. It is more accurate than the rapid ACTH stimulation tests.

10. **B,** Page 2500.

If the diagnosis of adrenal failure is unconfirmed, dexamethasone is the treatment of choice. It may be administered while an ACTH stimulation test is performed. It is 100 times more potent than cortisol, and this amount of dexamethasone will not falsely elevate serum cortisol determinations. Replacement with hydrocortisone could compound interpretations of serum cortisol determinations.

# 149 Bacterial Infections

*Michael D. Brown*

1. **C,** Pages 2504-2506.

Transmission is by person-to-person contact via nasopharyngeal secretions and is associated with crowded indoor living conditions. Initial signs and symptoms are often indistinguishable from those of URIs. Sore throat, fever, and dysphagia are common. There can be significant swelling of the cervical lymph nodes resulting in a "bull-neck" appearance. Diphtheritic membrane of the throat results from the exotoxin produced by the bacterium. This membrane can lead to airway obstruction. The exotoxin also can affect the cardiovascular and nervous systems. Myocarditis can occur, as can a peripheral neuropathy manifested by muscle weakness. Thirty percent of patients with diphtheria test positive for streptococcal infection. Treatment must include antitoxin with sensitivity skin testing along with intravenous erythromycin or penicillin. To maintain effective immunization, emergency departments should administer diphtheria toxoid along with tetanus toxoid for wound management.

2. **A,** Pages 2505-2506.

Mostly a tropical disease, cutaneous diphtheria has been reported in alcoholics and indigents in temperate climates. These patients generally do not become acutely ill. The infected wounds resemble other chronic skin conditions and are quite contagious. The skin has an ulcer with a grayish membrane. Treatment consists of vigorous cleansing of the lesion and a course of antibiotics. Antitoxin is of questionable value. ECG changes suggestive of myocarditis commonly occur with respiratory tract but not cutaneous diphtheria.

3. **B,** Page 2506.

If the patient has diphtheria, the immunization status needs to be updated and completed, but it does not guide antitoxin usage. Duration, toxicity, and membrane location and appearance are used to determine the dosage of antitoxin. The antitoxin is administered intravenously after conjunctival or intradermal sensitivity skin testing. Actual immunization should also be initiated because clinical injection does not necessarily confer immunity.

4. **D,** Page 2507.

Elevated WBC count with lymphocytosis is common. Fever is absent during the paroxysmal phase unless a secondary infection occurs. The catarrhal phase precedes the paroxysmal coughing and resembles a nonspecific upper respiratory infection. Between episodes of coughing, the patient does not appear acutely ill. After the paroxysm of coughing, a sudden forceful inhalation occurs that produces the "whoop."

5. **E,** Page 2508.

Pertussis vaccine is 80%-90% effective, but protection is absent in many people 12 years after immunization. A great percentage of children vaccinated develop fever, irritability, behavioral changes, and local discomfort at the injection site. The problems associated with the vaccine are more common than those with other childhood vaccinations. Moderately severe reactions are uncommon but include fever of 40° C or greater; persistent, high-pitched crying; and seizures. Severe neurologic complications (prolonged seizures, encephalopathy) occur rarely but have led to a reduction of use of this vaccine in some countries.

6. **E,** Page 2511.

Rabies does not cause trismus, which is the first obvious symptom in the majority of tetanus cases. Both diseases cause brain stem dysfunction, leading to drooling, dysphagia, and respiratory muscle dysfunction. Diphenhydramine is useful for dystonic reactions but will not alleviate symptoms in rabies or tetanus.

7. **D,** Page 2512.

TIG also neutralizes toxin circulating in the bloodstream as well as at the site of toxin production. It does not neutralize toxin in the nervous system and does not treat existing symptoms of tetanus. TIG provides antitoxin (antibodies), which is passive immunity. Active immunity is induced by tetanus toxoid.

8. **E,** Page 2512.

The half-life of TIG is 25 days; therefore repeat injections are not required. Local injection is of no value. Neuromuscular blockers may be used if benzodiazepines do not provide adequate muscle relaxation. A shorter incubation period is associated with a worse prognosis. There is no wound or obvious portal of entry in 10%-30% of cases.

9. **A,** Page 2514.

Infant botulism is caused by the ingestion of spores with in vivo production of toxin. Honey has been implicated as a source of *Clostridium botulinum* spores. Most cases occur in the 1 week to 11 month age-group. Constipation is a common presenting symptom, followed by weak suck, feeble cry, and hypotonia. Fever is usually absent.

10. **C,** Page 2515.

Pupillary response is preserved in myasthenia gravis but not in botulism. Botulism neurotoxin blocks the presynaptic release of acetylcholine throughout the body, whereas myasthenia gravis involves autoimmune destruction of the acetylcholine receptors on the muscle membrane. Both diseases share the findings of ptosis, extraocular palsies, and peripheral weakness.

11. **E,** Page 2516.

Antitoxin is not recommended in infant botulism because of the lack of proven efficacy and risk of anaphylaxis. Adverse reactions to use of the antitoxin occur in 20% of patients because of its derivation from horse serum; hypersensitivity testing is needed. The antitoxin works on circulating toxin but not bound toxin. Antitoxin should be given before wound care with antibiotics to provide prophylaxis against further release of toxin.

12. **D,** Page 2518.

The child needs prompt reevaluation if a blood culture is positive. Amoxicillin may very well be appropriate if the child has improved. Admission is not automatic if the child has improved and amoxicillin is being given properly. Telephone follow-up and waiting for the sensitivity are not sufficient.

13. **A,** Pages 2518, 2519.

Septic shock, adrenal hemorrhages, and DIC characterize OPSI. The risk for this illness does not decrease with time but does decrease significantly after vaccination. Initial symptoms are indistinguishable from other benign viral illnesses.

14. **B,** Page 2521.

Most often, a maculopapular rash is present initially, with the petechial rash appearing within 24 hours. The petechial rash is most common on the trunk and extremities. Vesicles are only occasionally present, and fever and rash are each present 71% of the time.

15. **E,** Page 2521.

Factors predictive of a poor prognosis include absence of meningitis, a total peripheral white blood cell count <500/mm$^3$, and a platelet count <100,000 mm$^3$. Others are seizures on presentation, hypothermia, development of purpura fulminans, presence of shock, low sedimentation rate, hyperpyrexia, and extremes of age.

16. **C,** Page 2523.

The CDC case definition requires 5 days of fever and at least four of the following criteria: bilateral conjunctival injection, rash, cervical lymphadenopathy, mucous membrane changes, and extremity changes. The specific mucous membrane changes are inflamed lips, injected pharynx, or strawberry tongue. They do not include coryza or large tonsils.

The specific extremity changes do not include nail bed hemorrhages, or petechiae. Transverse grooves in the nails may appear 1-2 months after the fever.

17. **B,** Page 2525.

Gamma globulin and aspirin are both used for their antiinflammatory effects, and aspirin is also an antiplatelet agent. Anticoagulation with heparin or warfarin is not routine but may be used in severe coronary disease. Steroids are not indicated.

18. **B,** Pages 2526-2527.

Fever, macular erythroderma, desquamation, and hypotension are required for the diagnosis of toxic shock. In addition, three major organ systems must be involved. Specific tests such as blood cultures and RMSF titers are not required. However, if these tests are obtained, they must be negative.

 **150** Viral Infections

*Warren F. Lanphear*

1. **B,** Page 2532.

When properly prepared, immune globulin cannot transmit hepatitis B or HIV. It is prepared from large pools of human blood plasma. Given IM, it is used for passive immunization against measles and hepatitis A. IV immune globulin is used as replacement for antibody-deficiency disorders.

2. **C,** Pages 2533-2534.

Adults with the acute onset of fever, cough, headache, and myalgias may be treated with 200 mg initially, followed by 100 mg daily for 5-7 days. Amantadine has no effect against influenza B. Prophylaxis with daily amantadine is indicted for high-risk people when the influenza vaccine is contraindicated. High-risk people given the vaccine need amantadine for only 2 weeks while antibody production is induced. Older persons with impaired renal function have a higher incidence of CNS side effects but can take amantadine at a reduced dose of no more than 100 mg daily.

3. **C,** Pages 2538-2539.

Diagnosis of HSV encephalitis can reliably be made only by brain biopsy and subsequent positive culture or direct fluorescent antibody tests. CSF culture is usually negative. Empiric initiation of IV acyclovir is indicated when HSV encephalitis is suspected because of its minimal toxicity and proven efficacy. It may be clinically indistinguishable from other acute CNS infections. HSV encephalitis is not epidemic and does not have a seasonal predilection.

4. **E,** Pages 2539-2540.

Herpes zoster is highly contagious, like chicken pox. It occurs predominantly in older adults. IV acyclovir therapy is used to treat herpes zoster because of the relative resistance of zoster compared with HSV and the difficulty in attaining therapeutic drug levels with oral therapy. Post-herpetic neuralgia often is refractory to treatment.

5. **A,** Pages 2540-2541.

EBV infection is heterophile positive in 90% of cases. Antiviral chemotherapy is not indicated for immunocompetent patients with CMV or EBV infectious mononucleosis. Organ transplant recipients with CMV may get severe, generalized disease, while those with EBV are at risk for lymphoma. Perinatal CMV and EBV both resemble toxoplasmosis. Liver inflammation can be seen in both EBV and CMV infections.

6. **A,** Page 2541.

The illness begins abruptly with the acute onset of fever up to 41° C, lasting 3-5 days. The fine, evanescent rose-colored maculopapular rash appears after fever lysis and lasts 1-2 days. The rash first appears on the chest and then may spread to the face and extremities. The child usually remains active and alert without other symptoms, although febrile convulsions may occur in conjunction with the fever. Treatment is with acetaminophen. It is the most common exanthem in children younger than 2 years old.

7. **A,** Pages 2542-2543.

Fetal infection also has been recognized, and infections during pregnancy have been associated with hydrops fetalis and spontaneous abortion. Erythema infectiosum is a mild, usually non-febrile disease of children between 4 and 10 years of age characterized by a "slapped cheek" rash. There is usually no prodrome, and constitutional symptoms are generally mild in children. Adults commonly have associated arthralgias and arthritis.

8. **C,** Pages 1145-1146, 2545-2546.

Parainfluenza viruses can reinfect individuals within months of primary infection, so prevention of infection is unlikely. Both viruses may result in pneumonia. RSV is the major cause of bronchiolitis, although it may also occur with parainfluenza. RSV accounts for the greatest number of hospitalizations for respiratory infection in infants.

9. **D,** Pages 2546-2547.

The current measles vaccine is a live, attenuated strain given as a first dose at age 15 months. A small percentage of recipients—2% to 5%—fail to convert after a single dose. The new regimen has resulted in a decreased incidence of measles since 1991.

10. **C,** Pages 2549-2550.

The most common clinical manifestation is that of a nonspecific febrile illness. Exanthems resembling rubella are seen with echoviruses and coxsackie A viruses. Vesicular lesions as in hand-foot-mouth syndrome are caused by some coxsackie A and B viruses. Herpangina caused by coxsackie A has a vesicular rash on the cheeks and soft palate with fever, sore throat, and severe pain on swallowing. Overall, inapparent infections greatly outnumber symptomatic cases. Enteroviruses are spread from person to person via the fecal-oral route.

# 151 AIDS and HIV Infection

*Bruce W. Nugent*

1. **A,** Page 2554.

In the United States, homosexual contact remains the most common risk behavior accounting for AIDS; however, its proportion has decreased. New infections due to injection drug use continue unabated, and the proportion of AIDS cases outside urban areas is increasing. There is disproportionate infection among minority populations and socioeconomically disadvantaged groups. The proportion of adult women among those infected is increasing. Heterosexual transmission is the most common mode of transmission worldwide.

2. **B,** Page 2555.

The initial EIA test should be repeated because false positive results may be the majority of positives when low-risk groups are screened (i.e., the specificity is decreased). The patient should be referred for voluntary testing and counseling. Serologic HIV testing in the ED is rarely indicated since confidentiality and proper counseling are difficult. The Western blot is both more specific and sensitive than the ELISA, but it is more expensive and labor intensive. If the Western blot is inconclusive, it should be repeated and, if it remains inconclusive, testing should be repeated in 3-6 months. The use of the EIA test in an area with high seroprevalence decreases the test's sensitivity because of the "window period" between exposures to the virus and detectability of antibodies.

3. **E,** Pages 2555, 2565.

Large volume of blood (such as with a hollow-bore needle) and deep puncture are associated with greater transmission risks. HIV antibodies may take up to 12 or more weeks after exposure to become detected by standard EIA techniques. Maximal benefit is gained when postexposure prophylaxis with antiretrovirals is begun within 1 to 2 hours of exposure. Postexposure prophylaxis is indicated in significant exposures even from asymptomatic HIV-infected patients, who can still transmit HIV. The average risk of transmission is estimated at 0.3%, or about 1 in 300.

4. **B,** Pages 2557-2558.

The patient most likely has *Pneumocystis carinii* pneumonia. Gallium scanning has frequent (up to 50%) false positives. A majority (60%-80%) of patients will respond to treatment. Initial treatment is with high-dose trimethoprim and sulfamethoxazole, but adverse effects are common, as they are with alternative treatments. Steroids (such as prednisone 40 mg PO bid initially) are recommended for patients with a $PaO_2$ <70 mm³, or an A-a gradient of >35.

5. **A,** Page 2558.

AIDS patients with tuberculosis should receive a four-drug regimen determined in conjunction with an infectious disease specialist. Multidrug-resistant tuberculosis is common. Patients with suspected tuberculosis should be isolated. Chest x-ray findings may be indistinguishable from those for a variety of other opportunistic infections. A negative PPD may occur because of anergy. MTB may be the initial finding in HIV patients since less immunosuppression is required to reactivate it. Extrapulmonary disease occurs in more than 75% of cases.

6. **A,** Page 2560.

*Cryptococcus neoformans* may cause CNS disease in up to 10% of patients. Presenting symptoms may be subtle, sometimes even without fever or meningismus. Diagnosis is by positive CFS India ink preparation or cryptococcal antigen. HIV simplex encephalitis is much less common than cryptococcal meningitis. HIV-associated depression and HIV encephalopathy (AIDS dementia complex) are more slowly progressive syndromes. Sinusitis is frequent in the HIV population but would not be expected to cause diminished affect and memory loss. In general, HIV patients with a change in neurologic status should have an emergency department work-up including an LP, usually preceded by either CT or MRI (always if there are focal findings).

7. **B,** Page 2560.

The most common cause of focal encephalitis in AIDS patients is *Toxoplasma gondii.* The diagnosis is usually made by contrast-enhanced cranial CT showing one or more ring-enhancing lesions often with edema. However, the clinical and radiographic findings cannot reliably distinguish toxoplasmosis from a wide variety of other causes. After treatment, improvement can be expected clinically and radiographically, and failure to improve suggests an alternate diagnosis, such as lymphoma. CSF India ink identifies *Cryptococcus neoformans.* The CSF findings of low glucose, high protein, and lymphocytosis suggest tuberculous meningitis, fungal meningitis, *Listeria* meningitis, or parameningeal abscess.

8. **E,** Page 2561.

The development of oral candidiasis is a poor prognostic sign, and these patients are at risk of developing other opportunistic infections. Oral candidiasis is characterized by white plaques that are easy to scrape away from an erythematous base and typically involves the buccal mucosa and the tongue. Most cases can be treated with clotrimazole troches as an outpatient. Nystatin suspension is not recommended because of its inadequate oral pharynx application duration.

9. **E,** Pages 2561-2562.

Salmonella is a particular problem in patients with HIV, often producing recurrent bacteremia and other significant clinical disease. *Campylobacter* infection usually causes a proctocolitis. *Isospora* and *Cryptosporidium* are protozoal infections, which produce a chronic watery diarrhea. Cytomegalovirus is a viral opportunistic infection associated with diarrhea and other gastrointestinal disease (such as hepatobiliary) in HIV patients. Emergency department treatment of diarrhea focuses on supportive care, fluid and electrolyte repletion, and obtaining of appropriate studies.

10. **A,** Page 2562.

Herpes simplex infections respond well to standard therapy and toxic effects are uncommon. Suppressive therapy is often effective. Intravenous acyclovir is indicated for multidermatomal herpes zoster and ophthalmic zoster. Varicella immune globulin is indicated in patients with primary varicella infection and visceral involvement, but not typically for varicella zoster.

## 152 Occupational Health in the Emergency Department: Principles and Practice

*No questions*

## 153 Parasitology

*Warren F. Lanphear*

1. **D,** Pages 2581-2588.

The first three stages (A, B, C) occur but are not thought to be responsible for the clinical systems. The last stage (E) listed does not occur.

2. **B,** Pages 2588-2589.

This illness, also known as African trypanosomiasis, is caused by *Trypanosoma gambiense* and *T. rhodesiense,* which are transmitted by the bite of the *Glossina* (tsetse) fly. The freshwater amebas *Naegleria* and *Acanthamoeba* cause a meningoencephalitis. *Taenia solium* (pork tapeworm) has a larval form that causes CNS cysts. *Plasmodium falciparum* causes cerebral malaria. *T. cruzi* causes acute Chagas' disease.

3. **E,** Page 2589.

Hookworm larvae penetrate the skin, usually through the feet, so wearing shoes largely prevents infection. The ova and larvae are not present in meat or fish, and they are not a water contaminant. Hand-washing would remove soil, but hand-to-mouth transmission is not their route of infection.

4. **D,** Page 2590.

Swimmer's itch spontaneously resolves since it is not tolerated by the human immune system. It does not cause scarring and is not invasive.

5. **B,** Pages 2591-2592.

Chagas' disease, caused by the South American *T. cruzi,* is transmitted by the triatomid bug bite. These bites cause marked local inflammation. Tissue lysis releases large numbers of trypomastigotes, accompanied by fever. Myocarditis with conduction defects (RBBB is the most common) occurs as disease progresses. Ascariasis, leishmaniasis, schistosomiasis, and onchocerciasis do not cause myocarditis.

6. **B,** Pages 2592-2593.

*G. lamblia* is found primarily in duodenal-jejunal mucosa and requires diagnostic procedures directed in that area. Colonoscopy would not examine their preferred location. Stool culture would not be effective for a protozoan. Metronidazole is potentially mutagenic and should not be used in pregnancy, especially without a definite diagnosis. *Giardia* is not toxigenic.

7. **C,** Pages 2582, 2590.

*L. tropica* causes "Old World" leishmaniasis in the Mediterranean area to western India. The other four parasites have a cosmopolitan distribution and are found in the United States.

8. **B,** Pages 2591-2596.

*E. histolytica* causes amebic dysentery characterized by bloody, mucus-filled diarrhea. Giardiasis usually does not cause bloody stools. Pinworms cause pruritus ani, not bloody diarrhea. Whipworm infestation is usually a mild disorder but, when overwhelming, may cause rectal prolapse. Ascariasis causes liver abscesses, small bowel obstruction, and pneumonitis.

9. **A,** Page 2596.

*T. vaginalis* can localize in the prostate gland, sometimes causing prostatitis and reversible sterility. In females, it causes vulvar pruritus, and it has been associated with postpartum endometritis, which produces pelvic pain. Urethritis occurs in both sexes.

10. **B,** Pages 2594-2595.

Hepatosplenomegaly follows egg deposition in the liver. Giardiasis is not an invasive disease. Onchocerciasis causes blindness from corneal damage. Strongyloidiasis does not commonly cause hepatosplenomegaly. Trichuriasis is caused by whipworms and may lead to rectal prolapse.

# 154 Tick-Borne Illnesses

### Michael D. Brown

1. **A,** Pages 2601-2604.

The most commonly affected age-groups are children and young adults, with a peak incidence between May and August. Less than one third recall having been bitten. The etiologic agent is *Borrelia burgdorferi*, which is a spirochete.

2. **A,** Page 2606.

The patient has a history consistent with stage II Lyme disease with neurologic manifestations. CSF examination usually demonstrates lymphocytic pleocytosis and an elevated protein level. There is often a fluctuating meningoencephalitis with superimposed symptoms of cranial neuropathy, peripheral neuropathy, or radiculopathy. Kernig's and Brudzenski's signs are absent, and CT scan is normal. Bell's palsy is bilateral in approximately one third of patients. Spinal root and plexus and peripheral nerves may be involved in the form of thoracic sensory radiculitis, brachial plexitis, mononeuritis, and motor radiculoneuritis in the extremities.

3. **B,** Page 2606.

The incidence of carditis in patients with Lyme disease is estimated at 4%-8%, and neurologic symptoms are seen in approximately 15%. The most common cardiac abnormality is AV block. Left ventricular dysfunction is usually mild and transient. The AV block is usually high grade and is almost always symptomatic; it gradually resolves.

4. **A,** Pages 2609-2611.

Lyme disease should be aggressively treated during pregnancy. Treatment for pregnant and lactating females is amoxicillin. Erythromycin would be used if the patient were allergic to penicillin, but it is probably less effective. Drug of choice for men, nonpregnant and non-lactating women, and children older than 8 years of age is doxycycline.

5. **A,** Page 2610.

All stages of Lyme disease are responsive to antibiotics. The chronic arthritis stage is treated with either a 30-day course of doxycycline or a 14-day course of IV ceftriaxone. Culture is not clinically useful; serologic testing is more practical. The palms and soles are usually spared with secondary skin lesions. The tick nymph is primarily responsible for disease transmission to humans.

6. **E,** Page 2611.

The relapsing fever is usually less severe with each successive relapse. Tetracycline or erythromycin are the antibiotics of choice. Penicillin G is associated with an increased rate of relapses. The spirochetes are easily visible on routine blood smear during a febrile episode. Diseases caused by rickettsiae include RMSF, Q fever, and ehrlichiosis. Spirochetes are responsible for Lyme disease, tularemia and relapsing fever. The Jarisch-Herxheimer reaction may occur within hours of treatment with antibiotics for both Lyme disease and relapsing fever. This reaction is thought to be secondary to the release of pyrogens upon the death of the spirochetes.

7. **D,** Page 2618.

This patient has a history and examination consistent with Rocky Mountain spotted fever (RMSF). Isolation of *R. rickettsii* from blood is expensive, difficult, and time consuming. Thrombocytopenia is nonspecific. Serologic analysis has little value in immediate diagnosis of an acute case. Weil-Felix is the least sensitive and specific test for RMSF. Immunofluorescent identification can be done rapidly when a skin biopsy is obtained from a rash lesion.

8. **A,** Page 2614.

RMSF poses a diagnostic problem because only 3% present with classic triad. Without a history of tick exposure, the differential diagnosis of fever and rash is extensive. Because of increased mortality with delay in antibiotic treatment, this diagnosis must be considered in patients with unexplained febrile illness.

9. **B,** Pages 2619-2620.

Tetracycline and chloramphenicol are both effective agents. Tetracycline should not be used in children younger than 8 years of age, pregnant women, or patients with renal or hepatic dysfunction. The other antibiotics are ineffective.

10. **C,** Page 2625.

Grasping the tick with tweezers or forceps as close as possible to the attachment site and applying slow gentle traction is the best method for removal. Care must be taken not to crush or squeeze the body because expressed fluid may be infectious. Gloves should be worn to prevent transmission of the infectious agent through skin abrasions or mucous membranes.

---

 **155** Tuberculosis

### Michael D. Brown and Gwen L. Hoffman

1. **E,** Pages 2630-2631.

Transmission of MTB rarely occurs outdoors because of the dilution of infectious particles and the exposure to ultraviolet radiation. The disease is transmitted by airborne infectious droplet. The exchanging of contaminated air using filters and ventilation is important in preventing transmission. However, it is not necessary to decontaminate clothing and eating utensils since fomites are not important in the transmission of the disease. Humans are the only known reservoir for MTB. In the United States the main reservoir is the elderly who harbor dormant infection.

2. **D,** Pages 2632-2633.

In most cases primary tuberculosis is subclinical and self-limited in the healthy individual. Conversion to a positive tuberculin (PPD) skin test may be the only means of diagnosing the infection. The most common symptom of pulmonary TB is cough. Hemoptysis may occur, but is usually minor; it is often an indicator of extensive involvement. Generalized malaise, weight loss, and fatigue are common presenting symptoms. A fever usually develops in the afternoon, with defervescence at night causing the classic night sweats. Infants and young children tend to develop large hilar lymph nodes that may compress a bronchus and result in a "brassy" cough. In contrast, fewer elderly people tend to present with respiratory symptoms.

3. **B,** Pages 2634-2635.

Empyema is rare (1%-4%) and is more common late in the course of disease in debilitated patients. Endobronchial spread is the most common complication of cavitary disease. On x-ray it is seen as poorly defined nodules that rapidly coalesce and consolidate (the so-called galloping consumption). Pericarditis results from the close anatomic relationship of the mediastinal lymph nodes to the posterior pericardial sac. Pneumothorax is seen in about 5% of patients. Superinfection may be seen as a "fungus ball" on x-ray secondary to *Aspergillus fumigatus* and can cause massive and fatal hemoptysis.

4. **E,** Pages 2634-2636.

An aspergilloma can be seen in the right upper lung representing superinfection of healed tuberculous cavity. Cavitary tuberculosis with left-sided pneumothorax is found on Rosen page 2634. Ghon focus can be seen on Rosen page 2636.

5. **B,** Page 2635.

Primary tuberculous infiltrate may occur in any lobe but usually involves a single lobe. Enlarged hilar or mediastinal nodes are often present and in fact are the radiologic hallmark of primary TB in children. A normal chest x-ray does not exclude active TB and is more common in patients infected with HIV. The ESR may be elevated; however, it is very nonspecific. The AFB smear is usually the most rapid test available for establishing the diagnosis for active TB and is helpful if positive. However, a negative smear does not rule out active disease. It is suggested that three initial sputum specimens be obtained to increase the yield and also that a positive smear be confirmed by culture. Tuberculin skin testing is important for establishing the presence of MTB infection but is not a good indictor of active clinical disease.

6. **D,** Pages 2635-2636.

Lymphadenopathy is considered the radiologic hallmark of primary TB in children, and massive hilar adenopathy is more common in young children. Primary tuberculous infiltrate can occur in any lobe. When the healed primary focus is visible on chest x-ray as a calcified scar, it is known as a Ghon focus. A moderate-to-large pleural effusion may be an isolated finding on a primary chest x-ray. Cavitary lesions are seen in post-primary tuberculosis.

7. **C,** Pages 2638-2639, 2648.

In the measurement of PPD skin testing the palpable induration, not the erythema, is measured. In patients with no TB risk factors, an induration ≥15 mm is considered positive. There are numerous factors that may decrease the response to PPD testing, including live virus vaccinations such as measles and mumps. The incidence of false-negative results has been reported to be as high as 25% in patients with active TB. Prior BCG vaccination may produce a false-positive response, but this is usually mild and deteriorates with time.

8. **E,** Pages 2640-2642.

A single lumbar puncture yields a positive AFB culture in only 37% of cases. Tuberculous meningitis is most common in young children; miliary TB, on the other hand, is more common in the elderly and in HIV-infected patients. Tuberculous lymphadenitis (scrofula) is the most common form of extrapulmonary TB and is usually located in the cervical nodes. These nodes are usually large, red, painless, and firm and require complete excision rather than incision and drainage. The early changes of Potts' disease may be difficult to detect on plain films and therefore other imaging studies such as CT or MRI may be required in suspected cases.

9. **C,** Page 2643.

Exsanguination rarely occurs, and the major morbidity is due to asphyxiation from aspirated blood. A large tube (8 mm) can accommodate fiberoptic bronchoscopy. Placement into the right mainstem bronchus is not recommended because of the risk of occluding the right upper lobe bronchus. Emergent consultation is needed for bronchoscopy, surgical resection, or angiography with selective embolization. Besides being positioned above the carina, the tube can be placed into the left mainstem bronchus when bleeding is from the right lung. The patient should be positioned with the bleeding lung in a dependent position.

**10. B,** Page 2644.

Supplemental pyridoxine is recommended for pregnant women, patients with a history of seizure disorder, and for those at risk for neuropathy such as diabetic patients and alcoholics. The standard course of therapy is 6 months using a four-drug regimen for the first 2 months followed by 4 months of INH and rifampin. Medical therapy should be initiated in those patients at high risk for TB regardless of the sputum smear results. It is well known that compliance with the recommended therapy is poor, and up to 50% of patients fail to follow the recommendations.

**11. D,** Page 2645.

Patients with acquired resistance can transmit drug-resistant organisms to previously uninfected (never treated) individuals, a process known as primary drug resistance. Although all drug-resistant TB can be traced back to suboptimal treatment, it is the transmission of primary drug resistance from person to person that allows rapid dissemination of drug-resistant strains. In reports from hospital outbreaks of MDRTB, more than 90% of patients have co-infections with HIV, and case fatality rates are as high as 70%-90%.

**12. C,** Pages 2647-2648.

Most TB patients can be managed as outpatients. The ideal situation is to be at home, on antituberculosis therapy, with any contacts receiving preventive treatment. Hospitalization during the first few days may be needed for acutely ill patients or the elderly who may experience adverse reactions. Comorbidity associated with HIV may require hospitalization. Those with active MDRTB have complex treatment regimens and need close monitoring. Patients with social issues such as homelessness may require hospitalization.

# 156 Bone and Joint Infections

*Michael D. Brown*

**1. B,** Page 2652.

After the first year of life, there is no vascular connection between the metaphyseal and epiphyseal areas. The epiphyseal growth plate in children is avascular and inhibits the spread of infection to the epiphysis and joint.

**2. D,** Page 2654.

Puncture wounds of the feet result in osteomyelitis 2% of the time by direct inoculation. The most common pathogen is *Pseudomonas*, which causes osteomyelitis in both children and adults. Cat bites often result in *Pasteurella multocida* osteomyelitis. Fresh-water wounds are often contaminated by *Aeromonas hydrophilia*. Children with hematogenous osteomyelitis may have infection with staphylococci, group B streptococci, *Haemophilus influenzae*, or *Kingella kingae*. *Neisseria gonorrhoeae* accounts for 50% of septic arthritis in sexually active young adults.

**3. A,** Pages 2654, 2665.

In sexually active young adults, *Neisseria gonorrhoeae* accounts for about 50% of septic arthritis. It is more common in women during pregnancy or just after menstruation. An early complaint is polyarthralgia, and in 66% of patients tenosynovitis and dermatitis occur. Gonococcal septic arthritis responds rapidly to antibiotic treatment. The yield is low for Gram stain and culture of the joint fluid, and is negative approximately 50% of the time. However, in 80% of cases, cultures of the genital tract, pharynx, and rectum will be positive.

**4. C,** Pages 2654, 2660.

Puncture wounds to the feet have about a 2% incidence of developing osteomyelitis from direct inoculation. The most common pathogen, *Pseudomonas*, has been cultured from shoes.

**5. B,** Page 2660.

Diabetic foot osteomyelitis is usually polymicrobial, with the most common organisms being staphylococci, streptococci, Enterobacteriaceae, and frequently anaerobes. A typical patient has advanced insulin-dependent diabetes with a history of indolent ulcers and frank cellulitis.

**6. D,** Page 2661.

The most likely pathogen in sickle cell patients with osteomyelitis is *Salmonella* bacteria, followed by other Enterobacteriaceae and then *Staphylococcus* species. Differentiation of bone infection from bone infarction in sickle cell patients can be challenging.

**7. E,** Page 2654.

*Staphylococcus aureus* is the leading cause of osteomyelitis and septic arthritis in all age-groups except neonates. In neonates, group B *Streptococcus* is the leading causative organism in bone and joint infections.

**8. A,** Page 2655.

Bone scanning is more useful than plain radiographs in early diagnosis of osteomyelitis, becoming positive within 48-72 hours after the onset of infection. The technetium methylene diphosphonate is the most commonly employed radionuclides for bone scanning. However, false-positive scans may result from any process that encourages inflammation and new bone formation such as from trauma, surgery, tumors, or soft-tissue infections. Laboratory data are generally not helpful. The WBC count is often not elevated; typical values range from normal to 15,000/mm³. A more sensitive marker for bone infection is the ESR. Plain radiographs have limited usefulness in the early diagnosis of osteomyelitis, and radiographic resolution usually lags behind clinical resolution.

**9. A,** Page 2663.

It is important to avoid any delay in the inoculation of the joint fluid aspirate culture. Blood culture bottles may be used immediately after joint aspiration. Joint fluid culture results are negative in 20%-25% of suspected septic arthritis. This may be due to inadequate sample, poor culture technique, fastidious organisms or misdiagnosis. In most cases of septic arthritis, the joint fluid WBC is >50,000 cells per mm³ and the glucose level is low. The risk of introducing infection during aspiration is small, less than 1 in 10,000 joint injections or aspirations.

10. **A,** Page 2663.

With a septic joint the joint fluid analysis will show a friable mucin clot, cell count 10,000 to greater than 100,000 mostly PMNs, a reduced synovial fluid–to-blood glucose ratio and a positive Gram stain and culture. Most useful are the Gram stain, WBC count and differential, and the ratio of the joint fluid glucose to serum glucose.

11. **B,** Page 2665.

Predominant early complaint is migratory polyarthralgias. Tenosynovitis occurs in two thirds of patients. Synovial fluid often has <50,000 WBCs/mm³. Cultures of joint fluid are negative about 50% of the time while mucosal surface cultures are positive 80% of the time. Polyarticular arthritis is present in about 10% of cases, but usually it is monoarticular.

---

 **157** Soft-Tissue Infections

*Scoff A. Carlson*

1. **B,** Pages 2670, 2672.

Temperature elevation, increased WBC count, and positive blood cultures are all rare findings with regard to cellulitis. The exception is cellulitis caused by *H. influenzae* B. These infections are frequently associated with elevated WBC counts with a left shift and positive blood cultures. Bacteremia is seen in two thirds of these patients. These infections are usually seen in children under the age of 5 and have a primary predilection for the facial region but can occur in the extremities. Although this description is quite classic for cellulitis caused by *H. influenzae* B, the widespread use of the HIB vaccine appears to be markedly decreasing the incidence of infections from this virulent pathogen (see Rosen page 1088).

2. **D,** Page 2671.

Periorbital cellulitis is usually associated with swelling of the eyelid, discoloration of the orbital skin, redness, and warmth. It may be followed on an outpatient basis for the first 24-48 hours of antibiotic therapy. Patients with orbital cellulitis may have proptosis, loss of trigeminal nerve sensation, decreased ocular mobility, ocular pain, tenderness on eye movement, and increased intraocular pressure. Orbital CT scans are extremely useful to diagnose orbital cellulitis or abscesses; sinus and orbital x-ray films tend to be less specific.

3. **B,** Page 2672.

Fever above 38.9° C, erythematous rash, and hypotension are absolute criteria for the diagnosis of TSS. Skin desquamation appears 1-2 weeks after disease onset. Treatment involves drainage/irrigation of infected areas, IV antibiotics, and pressure support with fluids and vasoactive agents. The incidence of TSS has decreased remarkably since high-absorbency tampons were withdrawn from the market.

4. **A,** Page 2672.

The usual age range in staphylococcal scalded skin syndrome is from 6 months to 6 years. Nikolsky's sign—the easy separation of the outer portion of the epidermis from the basilar layer when pressure is exerted on an apparent blister—is present. Tissue and blister fluids are usually sterile. Mucous membranes are rarely involved. The involvement of mucous membranes should alert the physician to an alternate diagnosis of toxic epidermal necrolysis. Although the syndrome is indeed secondary to a staphylococcal exotoxin, systemic antibiotics with a penicillinase-resistant penicillin are indicated.

5. **B,** Pages 2672-2673.

Topical antimicrobial agents other than mupirocin alone or in combination with scrubs or washes are of limited usefulness. They have proven ineffective in treating impetigo in military populations. Moreover, topical antibiotics may alter antibiotic resistance patterns. Poststreptococcal glomerulonephritis is more likely to follow impetigo than streptococcal pharyngitis. In contrast, acute rheumatic fever is not a consequence of impetigo. The lesions of bullous impetigo generally heal faster than those of impetigo contagiosa. First-generation oral cephalosporins are effective in treating impetigo.

6. **B,** Pages 2673-2674.

Most abscesses contain bacteria. However, approximately 5%, especially those associated with parenteral drug abuse, may be sterile. Hidradenitis suppurativa is a disease consisting of chronic suppurative abscesses in the apocrine sweat glands. *Staphylococcus aureus, Streptococcus viridans,* and anaerobes are usually found. Bartholin cysts are usually mixed aerobic and anaerobic infections, as are pilonidal and perirectal abscesses. Pilonidal cysts may yield *S. aureus,* whereas perirectal abscesses often yield *Bacteroides fragilis.*

7. **A,** Page 2675.

A Bartholin cyst is caused by an obstructed Bartholin duct. The organisms found are usually a mixture of aerobic and anaerobic flora from the vagina. *Gonococcus* is cultured less than 10% of the time. Drainage of the abscess should be from the mucosal rather than the cutaneous surface. Marsupialization, not excision, may be appropriate in the ED, since there is a tendency for abscesses to recur after simple incision and drainage. Signs and symptoms are usually localized.

8. **A,** Pages 2676-2677.

Surgical debridement, coupled with broad-spectrum antibiotics, is the mainstay of treatment for necrotizing fasciitis. Although x-rays and MRI are sometimes helpful, the diagnosis is primarily a clinical one. Fasciitis is an infection of the skin, subcutaneous tissue, and fascia. By definition it does not involve muscle, though it can spread there, causing myositis and myonecrosis. Pain varies because of nerve ending destruction. Decreasing pain can indicate worsening involvement; in addition, pain out of proportion to physical findings is common.

# Dental Disorders

*J. Leibovitz*

1. **D,** Pages 2690-2692.
An avulsed tooth should be reimplanted as soon as possible. Avulsed primary teeth should not be reimplanted because they fuse to bone. An avulsed tooth should be rinsed in saline or water and placed in Hank's solution. If this is not available, the tooth can be placed inside the buccal mucosa or under the tongue. If this is not acceptable or if there are concerns about aspiration, then the tooth can be placed in a glass of milk. Ellis II fractures involve the enamel and dentin but spare the pulp. In an adult they are not emergencies because the dentin-to-pulp ratio is large and the possibility of pulp exposure is low. In children or adolescents, an Ellis II fracture is potentially more dangerous because the pulp occupies a greater percentage of the tooth compared to the dentin, which could lead to exposure of the pulp; this requires a root canal procedure. Calcium hydroxide paste should be applied immediately, and a pediatric dentist should be notified. Subluxation of a tooth requires follow-up with a dentist, but as a short-term procedure, an emergency physician can apply a periodontal pack that will reinforce the tooth for up to 48 hours.

2. **A,** Pages 2688-2690.
Leukemic cells can invade the gingivae. The gingival tissue is at risk for infiltration by bacteria, possibly leading to sepsis secondary to the leukemic cells causing edema and bluish-red gingivae. Pyogenic granuloma is a condition found during pregnancy; it results in the overgrowth of fibrous tissue within the gingivae. SLE can cause painful oral ulcers, but this would be a rare presentation in a 2 year old. TTP patients can present with the sudden onset of bleeding from the gingivae.

3. **B,** Page 2689.
Tooth eruption is usually accompanied by dehydration, irritability, and diarrhea. Low-grade fever is common, but any fever above 37.8° C (100° F) should not be attributed to teething. Pain associated with erupting teeth leads to decreased oral intake; this, in combination with diarrhea, can lead to dehydration. Topical analgesics should be used cautiously because of the potential for sterile abscess formation.

4. **B,** Pages 2683-2686.
Ludwig's angina is an infection involving the submaxillary, sublingual, and submental spaces with an elevation of the tongue that may cause airway obstruction. Acute necrotizing ulcerative gingivitis (ANUG) is a periodontal disease that results when bacteria invade healthy gingival tissue. Periapical abscess is confined within the alveolar bone; therefore, incision and drainage is not possible. Periodontal abscess, on the other hand, requires incision and drainage. Penicillin is the antibiotic of choice for most infections of the mouth, with treatment strategies varying from 250-500 mg qid as in cases of periapical abscess, up to 12-15 million units of IV penicillin as in cases of Ludwig's angina.

5. **D,** Pages 2688.
The diagnosis of this condition is acute alveolar osteitis, or dry socket syndrome. No attempt should be made to restart the bleeding, because this is associated with a high incidence of osteomyelitis. This is in contradistinction from bleeding after tooth extraction, which does require removal of the clot so that a new clot may form. Some degree of pain after extraction is normal, usually within the first 24 hours. In patients with acute alveolar osteitis, there is a pain-free period after extraction followed by severe pain and halitosis usually 3-4 days after extraction. The treatment of dry socket includes anesthetic nerve block, medicated dental paste, and antibiotics.

6. **D,** Page 2687.
Acute necrotizing ulcerative gingivitis (ANUG) is a periodontal disease resulting from bacteria invading healthy gingival tissue. Gingivitis results from inflammation to an irritant such as calculus or bacterial plaque. With gingivitis there is a loss of alveolar bone and overgrowth of the gingiva down the roots of the teeth. With ANUG, a gray pseudomembrane covers the tissue and will result in bleeding if removed. ANUG has been associated with emotional stress, fatigue, smoking, and local trauma. It was common in the trenches of World War I and was referred to as trench mouth. At the time it was thought to be contagious, but there has been no evidence proving this. It can be associated with fever, malaise, and regional lymphadenopathy. Treatment consists of systemic antibiotics, warm saline irrigation, local anesthetics, and improving dental hygiene. In addition, immunologic factors play a role in the pathogenesis of the disease.

# Ophthalmologic Disorders

*J. Leibovitz*

1. **C,** Page 2699.
A pinhole should be used to correct vision on a visual acuity examination when either glasses are not available or the person's vision is 20/30 or worse with glasses. Pinhole corrects only for refractive errors (within the lens or cornea), and failure of pinhole to improve vision suggests disease within the retina or optic nerve. An astigmatism, farsightedness, and nearsightedness are all abnormalities within the cornea or lens and should correct with pinhole testing. Macular degeneration is a retinal defect in which the pinhole examination would have no effect.

2. **A,** Pages 2703, 2706-2707.

An orbital hematoma or retrobulbar hemorrhage can occur after blunt trauma. It can result in a significant elevation in intraorbital pressure within the enclosed space, resulting in compression of the optic nerve and central retinal artery. Symptoms include proptosis, visual loss, and increased intraocular pressure. Any compromise in the retinal blood supply is an indication for emergent surgical decompression. Orbital floor fractures are not usually repaired surgically until 7-10 days after the injury when the swelling has resolved. Indications for surgery include continued double vision or obvious cosmetic deformities; otherwise nonsurgical management is appropriate. Traumatic iridocyclitis is a traumatic iritis that results from blunt trauma to the iris or ciliary body. Ciliary spasm causes symptoms of intense eye pain unrelieved by topical anesthetics, photophobia, and cells within the anterior chamber. Treatment is nonsurgical with cycloplegics and steroids. Vitreous hemorrhage occurs from retinal bleeding due to injury of the retina, uveal tract, or surrounding vascular structure. Treatment is nonsurgical; occasionally an ophthalmologist will preform a vitrectomy if persistent nonabsorbing blood is present.

3. **B,** Page 2702.

The duration of action of cyclopentolate is up to 24 hours. Cycloplegia is always accompanied by mydriasis secondary to inhibition of muscarinic receptors. They cause incomplete paralysis of accommodation, and they reach peak onset within 15-20 minutes.

4. **D,** Page 2705.

It is often difficult and not necessary to remove a rust ring at the time of initial evaluation. Removal is easier after it softens within 24 hours. An electric corneal burr is the ideal tool for removal. Failure to remove the rust ring leads to ferrous oxide diffusion throughout the cornea with reduced vision.

5. **D,** Page 2708.

There is no subcutaneous fat in the eyelids themselves; protrusion of orbital fat into the wound indicates penetration of the orbital septum. Ptosis indicates injury to the levator muscle or aponeurosis of the upper lid. Subconjunctival hemorrhage results from rupture of small subconjunctival vessels and by itself is benign. Bell's phenomenon is the normal upward rotation of the globe with reflex blinking.

6. **C,** Pages 2709-2710.

Allergic conjunctivitis is usually characterized by bilateral involvement and symptoms of eye itching in the absence of significant eye pain or loss in visual acuity. A whitish discharge and eye redness are also found, and a seasonal association is common. Eye pain is a common complaint among patients with either viral or bacterial conjunctivitis. Preauricular lymphadenopathy occurs with viral conjunctivitis. Decreased visual acuity is uncommon in all forms of conjunctivitis.

7. **B,** Pages 2713-2714.

Retinal detachments can present with photopsia (flashing lights), floaters, and vision loss. Pain is not associated with retinal detachments. Risk factors include trauma, age older than 45, female gender, nearsightedness, a family history, previous cataract surgery, and a history of floaters. Vision loss is uncommon unless the detachment involves the macula. Usually the detachment involves peripheral aspects of the retina, sparing the macula.

8. **B,** Page 2712.

Homatropine is a cycloplegic agent that dilates the pupil. Pupil dilation increases the obstruction to aqueous humor flow and exacerbates glaucoma. Pilocarpine constricts the pupil, facilitating outflow of aqueous humor and decreasing intraocular pressure. Mannitol is an osmotic agent that lowers intraocular pressure by acting as an osmotic diuretic, drawing fluid from the anterior chamber in to the intravascular space. Oral glycerol can also be used to lower intraocular pressure by a similar mechanism. Acetazolamide is a carbonic anhydrase inhibitor that decreases the rate of aqueous humor formation.

9. **E,** Page 2713.

Central retinal vein occlusion (CRVO) symptoms are similar to those of central retinal artery occlusion (CRAO) in that there is a painless loss of vision. Brief transient blindness is uncommon. A pale retina and optic disc with box car segmentation is seen in CRAO. CRVO has two clinical appearances. In the nonischemic variety there is macular edema with leaky capillary dilation. This condition has less severe symptoms than the ischemic category and it often resolves spontaneously. In the ischemic variety there are dilated veins with retinal hemorrhages and edema leading to more pronounced visual loss. The degree of vision loss depends on the degree of ischemia and ranges from mild to severe. CRAO results from embolic phenomenon, and a search for embolic foci should be included in the work-up. No treatment is necessary acutely for CRVO other than watching for elevation of intraocular pressure consistent with neovascular glaucoma. Eye massage, acetazolamide, timolol, and increasing the $P_{CO_2}$ are all indicated treatments for CRAO.

# 160 Ear, Nose, and Throat Emergencies

*J. Leibovitz*

1. **C,** Page 2724.

Ramsey-Hunt syndrome is a herpes zoster infection of the geniculate ganglion. Findings include facial paralysis, ear pain, swelling and erythema within the external auditory canal, and grouped vesicles. Hyperacusis (painful sensitivity to sound) is not found in this disorder.

2. **D,** Page 2725.

The table on Rosen page 2725 lists the causes of sudden hearing loss. Examples of sensioneuronal hearing loss include vascular, metabolic, medication toxicity, neoplastic, and infectious. Viruses such as mumps, measles, influenza, HSV, varicella zoster, CMV, and EBV can lead to nonconductive hearing loss. A perforated tympanic membrane is the only choice possible for a conductive etiology of hearing loss.

3. **D,** Page 2725.

The patient has findings consistent with a right-sided conductive hearing loss. Otitis media is the only answer that causes a conductive hearing loss. The other choices cause either a unilateral (A and E) or bilateral (B and C) sensory hearing loss.

4. **E,** Page 2721.

Hearing loss is the most common complication from otitis media. Other less common complications include TM perforation, labyrinthitis, cholesteatoma formation, meningitis, and brain abscess. The use of antibiotics has reduced the incidence of all these complications, especially meningitis and brain abscess. Trigeminal nerve involvement does not occur as a complication of otitis media, but facial nerve palsies do occur because of the location of the nerve as it courses through the middle ear.

5. **A,** Page 2727.

Stones of the salivary glands (Sialolithiasis) are most common between the ages of 30 and 50 years and are rare in children. The submandibular gland is involved in 80%-95% of the cases. Viral (mumps) and bacterial causes have been implicated. The disorder presents with severe pain and swelling of the affected gland.

6. **E,** Pages 2725-2727.

Anterior epistaxis is responsible for 90% of nosebleeds. It usually arises from the anterior-inferior nasal septum from vessels known as Kiesslbach's plexus. While posterior epistaxis requires consultation with an otolaryngologist and hospitalization, most anterior bleeds can be managed on an outpatient basis without immediate consultation of a specialist. The most common site of posterior bleeds is the posterior branch of the sphenopalatine artery.

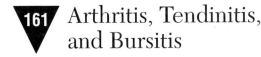

# 161 Arthritis, Tendinitis, and Bursitis

*Patrick Brunett*

1. **C,** Page 2731.

Of the listed arthritides, only pseudogout typically presents as a monarticular arthritis. Other monarticular arthritides are osteoarthritis, septic arthritis, and gout. In addition, trauma and hemarthrosis usually produce monarticular symptoms. Besides those listed, other diseases that produce polyarticular symptoms include rubella, rheumatic fever, Reiter's syndrome, and serum sickness.

2. **D,** Pages 2739-2740.

All of the entities listed are associated with rheumatic fever (RF) except monarticular arthritis. The symptoms of acute RF develop 3-4 weeks after a group A beta-hemolytic streptococcus infection. The arthritis is polyarticular, predominantly involving the knees, ankles, elbows, and wrists. In addition to evidence of a preceding group A streptococcus infection, the revised Jones criteria to diagnose RF state there must be at least two major criteria (carditis, migratory polyarthritis, chorea, erythema marginatum, subcutaneous nodules) or one major (fever, arthralgia, prior history of RF, prolonged PR interval, elevated acute-phase reactants).and two minor criteria

3. **C,** Pages 2733-2734.

The normal synovial fluid glucose is 95% of the serum glucose. Gout, pseudogout, and rheumatoid arthritis, as well as septic arthritis, can produce synovial fluid WBC counts >50,000/mm³. The WBCs in both septic and inflammatory arthritis are predominantly PMNs. Calcium pyrophosphate crystals are rhomboid in shape and positively birefringent, whereas uric acid crystals are long and needle-like and negatively birefringent.

4. **A,** Page 2734.

The presence of crystals in synovial fluid does not rule out septic arthritis. In fact, diagnosis of septic arthritis in a patient with a history of gout or pseudogout is difficult. In these patients, when septic arthritis destroys articular cartilage, crystals may be released into the synovial fluid. In addition, both the crystal arthritides and septic arthritis may produce fever and an elevated synovial WBC count. *Staphylococcus aureus* is the most common cause of septic arthritis, and the knee is the most commonly affected joint. Infants are at risk for *Escherichia coli*, and patients with sickle cell disease are at risk for *Salmonella* arthritis. *Staphylococcus epidermidis*, although frequently thought of as a contaminant, causes infections in prosthetic joints. IV drug abusers are at risk for infections with gram-negative bacteria (*Pseudomonas, Klebsiella, Serratia*) as well as methicillin-resistant *Staphylococcus aureus*.

5. **A,** Pages 2731, 2735.

A uric acid level is not helpful in the diagnosis of gout because it can be normal. Attacks occur most commonly (75%) in the great toe MTP joint, but the tarsal joints, ankle, and knee are also commonly affected. Up to 40% of patients may have polyarticular involvement. Gouty arthritis occurs mostly in middle-aged men and postmenopausal women. Estrogens increase renal excretion of uric acid, while thiazide diuretics decrease excretion.

6. **B,** Pages 2735-2736.

All of the medications listed are used to treat acute attacks of gout except allopurinol. Allopurinol, which decreases uric acid production, and probenecid, which increases excretion, should be used only in the long-term management of gout.

7. **D,** Page 2736.

The knee is the most frequently involved joint, followed by the wrist, ankle, and elbow. Colchicine, although not as effective as in gout, is useful in the treatment of pseudogout. NSAIDs are also useful, and aspiration, with or without steroid injection, can also be used.

8. **C,** Page 2737.

Gonococcal arthritis typically affects young women (4:1 to men) during their menstrual period, last two trimesters of pregnancy, or postpartum. Blood cultures have a very poor yield, while cervical, urethral, pharyngeal, and rectal cultures are positive for *Neisseria gonorrhoeae* in up to 75% of patients. Synovial fluid is positive 50% of the time or less. Symptoms begin with fever, chills, a migratory tenosynovitis, and arthralgias that progress to polyarthritis of the knee, ankle, or wrist. Two thirds of patients have a characteristic hemorrhagic rash that first appears on the distal extremities. Cervicitis and urethritis are rarely symptomatic.

9. **A,** Page 2738.

Lyme disease is caused by the spirochete *Borrelia burgdorferi* and is transmitted by the *Ixodes* tick. The initial illness occurs in the late spring and early summer. Early symptoms include arthralgias, myalgias, headache, fever, fatigue, and lethargy, as well as erythema chronicum migrans (a characteristic skin lesion that develops at the site of the bite and spreads with a bright red border with central clearing). The second stage of the disease begins 4 weeks after the bite and may include neurologic (e.g., Bell's palsy) or cardiac (e.g., fluctuating AV block) abnormalities. Arthritis, which is polyarticular, asymmetric, and most commonly involves the large joints (e.g., knees), is a late manifestation of the disease, occurring up to 6 months after the tick bite.

10. **E,** Page 2739.

All of the statements are true. The arthritis in Reiter's syndrome occurs in genetically susceptible patients after a genitourinary or gastrointestinal tract infection. Arthritis develops 2-6 weeks after an episode of urethritis (due to *Chlamydia trachomatis*) or dysentery (due to *Salmonella, Shigella, Yersinia,* or *Campylobacter*). Tetracycline therapy improves recovery for some patients with chlamydia-induced arthritis but it has no effect on GI-induced arthritis. The arthritis is polyarticular and asymmetric, involving predominantly the knees, ankles, and feet. The ocular component of the disease begins as conjunctivitis and may progress to iritis, uveitis, or corneal ulceration. HLA-B27 is positive in 80% of patients.

11. **B,** Pages 2740-2741.

Joint swelling in rheumatoid arthritis (RA) is polyarticular and symmetric, and usually begins in the hands, wrists, and elbows. Hand swelling involves the MCP and PIP joints but not the DIP joints, which helps distinguish RA from osteoarthritis, reactive arthritis, and psoriatic arthritis. There is a prodrome of fatigue, weakness, and musculoskeletal pain that may last for weeks or months. Synovial fluid analysis is consistent with an inflammatory response, with 4000-50,000 WBCs that consist of 75% PMNs. Rheumatoid factor is positive in approximately 70% of patients.

12. **D,** Pages 2741-2745.

Bursae are sacs lined with synovium that do not communicate with the joint synovium. Olecranon bursitis can be caused by gout, pseudogout, rheumatoid disease, uremia, or infection. *Staphylococcus aureus* is the most frequent cause of both septic olecranon and prepatellar bursitis. Both can usually be treated with oral antibiotics on an outpatient basis. Anserine bursitis occurs mainly in obese older women with large legs, and it usually does not produce swelling or warmth. Steroids should not be injected into any bursa that could potentially be infected, therefore, they should not be used for the olecranon or prepatellar bursae where there is always a moderate risk for infection. Affected joints, especially shoulders, should not be immobilized for more that a few days.

13. **C,** Pages 2741-2744.

Lateral epicondylitis is best treated with a forearm brace and not continued mobilization. The remaining statements are true. DeQuervain's tendonitis, inflammation of the abductor pollicis longus and extensor pollicis brevis, is diagnosed with the Finkelstein's test (the thumb is held in the palm by the fingers, and the wrist is ulnarly deviated).

---

# 162 Systemic Lupus Erythematosus and the Vasculitides

### *Michael D. Shertz*

1. **B,** Page 2748.

SLE has its highest incidence in women of child-bearing age. Specifically, it has an incidence of 1 in 250 African-American women. It has a female preponderance with 53.8 cases per 100,000 women and 40 cases per 100,000 for both sexes. It is an autoimmune condition with many potential complications, including renal failure and steroid-induced disease.

2. **B,** Page 2751.

Drug-induced lupus has been associated with many medications. Hydralazine and procainamide are the most common. However, D-penicillamine, quinidine, and several anticonvulsants (specifically phenytoin) are also of moderate to high risk. Certain antibiotics have rarely been associated with this condition (penicillin, sulfa antibiotics, and tetracycline).

3. **A,** Page 2748.

SLE has many presentations. The American Rheumatism Association Revised Criteria for the Classification of Lupus lists eleven conditions associated with this disease. A patient must have four of these conditions to meet classification. Arthralgias and myalgias almost always occur at some time in the disease. Hand inflammation is common, but it affects the proximal interphalangeal joints and the MCPs. A facial eruption (malar or butterfly rash) is a common first sign. Renal manifestations including nephritis, and neurologic manifestations of seizures, stroke, and peripheral neuropathies are seen. Cardiac manifestations include coronary artery disease, pericarditis, and myopathies.

4. **C,** Page 2750.

Pericarditis is the most common cardiac manifestation of SLE. It has been reported in 30% of patients. Symptoms of fever, tachycardia, chest pain, and transient rubs are seen. Pericardial effusions, however are seen in only 20% of patients. Purulent pericarditis associated with *Staphylococcus aureus* and tuberculosis have occurred in patients taking steroids. Pericarditis in SLE is usually self-limited. Libman-Sacks vegetations on the mitral valve are noninfectious and related to autoimmune deposition. SLE patients with hypertension and hypercholesterolemia are at markedly increased risk of coronary artery disease. Myocarditis is clinically apparent in only 10% of patients; however it is present in 40% at autopsy.

5. **B,** Page 2750.

The diagnosis of SLE is often confirmed by antinuclear antibody testing, although it may be positive in the elderly, with medications like hydralazine and procainamide, and in many other disease states. Antibodies to double-stranded DNA and anti-Smith antibodies are most specific for SLE. The ESR can be 50-100 mm/hr despite minimal disease activity and so is a very poor gauge of disease progression or activity. Patients with SLE may have false-positive RPR and VDRL results.

6. **B,** Page 2751.

Drug-induced lupus is most frequently associated with hydralazine and procainamide. Less than 1% of patients taking those medications will fully manifest this disease. However, more than 50% will have a positive ANA titer. The condition is usually reversible with discontinuation of the drug. Arthralgias are the most common manifestation of drug-induced lupus.

7. **A,** Page 2755.

Hypersensitivity vasculitis is a clinical syndrome characterized by small vessel vasculitis. It is mediated by immune complexes and is associated with penicillin and sulfa antibiotics. The skin of the dependent lower extremities is most involved, demonstrating "palpable purpura." The skin lesions begin abruptly after 1-2 days on the medication. Fever, malaise, and weight loss are common systemic manifestations. A mild leukocytosis and a mildly elevated ESR are nonspecific laboratory findings. Many cases of this condition cannot be attributed to any clear etiology.

8. **B,** Page 2756.

Henoch-Schonlein purpura affects the arterioles and capillaries with peak incidence between ages 4 and 11. It often follows a viral upper respiratory infection. A rash of palpable purpura and arthralgias are classic. GI symptoms including abdominal pain, nausea, vomiting, and bloody diarrhea can occur in 70% of patients. Renal involvement occurs in half of cases, with hematuria and red cell casts. It rarely progresses to renal failure; however, long-term renal involvement occurs in 25% of patients. Because of this, patients with renal involvement should be admitted for IV steroid therapy.

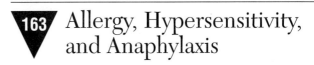

## 163 ▼ Allergy, Hypersensitivity, and Anaphylaxis

*Hans Notenboom*

1. **D,** Pages 2772-2773.

A 24- to 48-hour hospital admission is appropriate for any patient who has experienced a severe form of anaphylaxis, even if he or she has responded quickly and completely to initial therapy. Although clinical deterioration after a severe anaphylactic reaction with complete resolution is uncommon, a small but significant proportion of patients will redevelop symptoms 24 to 48 hours after the initial attack. This may be due to the high-molecular-weight neutrophil chemotactic factor-mediated late-phase reaction of the biphasic allergic response, which peaks in 4-12 hours and lasts up to 48 hours. Also, one should be careful with patients on therapeutic doses of beta-blocking medications, as they may be susceptible to a similar clinical rebound once effects of initial therapeutic interventions wear off.

2. **A,** Pages 2770-2771.

Epinephrine, which is both an alpha- and a beta-adrenergic agonist, is the first drug of choice for anaphylaxis. The severity of presentation of a patient with anaphylaxis determines the route and subsequent dosage given. Mild anaphylaxis (urticaria, rhinitis, conjunctivitis, and mild bronchospasm) allows for an SC injection of 0.01 ml/kg of 1:1000 solution to a maximum of 0.5 ml. This is the same dosage that is used in moderate anaphylaxis (angioedema, generalized urticaria, early laryngeal edema, and hypotension with blood pressure >80 mm Hg), but the route here is IM. In each case, these doses can be repeated every 5-20 minutes for three doses as needed. In severe anaphylaxis (laryngeal edema, respiratory failure, and shock) a dose of 0.1 ml/kg of 1:10,000 solution to a maximum of 5 ml IV over 3-5 minutes can be administered. In adults, 1.0 ml of 1:10,000 solution should be given initially over 3-5 minutes IV, and this dose can be repeated every 3-5 minutes as needed to a maximum of 5 ml every 15-30 minutes. In children, an infusion rate of 0.1 ml/kg/min is advised, increasing to a maximum of 1.5/ml/kg/min.

3. **E,** Pages 2767-2768.

Hereditary angioedema is an autosomal dominant condition due to C1 esterase inhibitor deficiency or functional deficiency. Its cardinal signs and symptoms include edema of the airway, face, or extremities and abdominal pain associated with nausea, vomiting, and diarrhea. Epinephrine may be administered with caution; however, life-threatening attacks have responded effectively only to fresh frozen plasma transfusion that contains C1 inhibitor.

4. **C,** Pages 2762, 2766.

Aspirin and other nonsteroidal antiinflammatory drugs inhibit cyclooxygenase and the subsequent production of prostaglandin, thromboxane, and prostacyclin. This results in a shift in the lipoxygenase pathway with a subsequent increase in production of LTC4, LTD4, and LTE4 . Blockage of leukotrienes with experimental antagonists has indicated that they are primarily implicated in the prolonged airway and secondary cardiovascular response of anaphylaxis. Though onset is slow, on a molar basis leukotrienes possess up to 6000 times the bronchoconstricting potential of histamine. Most aspirin-sensitive patients can tolerate sodium salicylate or acetaminophen as an aspirin substitute.

5. **E,** Pages 2759, 2764.

The first anaphylactic-induced fatality caused by penicillin was in 1949. Since then it has remained the leading cause of fatal anaphylaxis. Studies have shown 1 fatality per 7.5 million injections. This usually amounts to 100-500 deaths per year in the United States. Only six deaths have ever been recorded from oral penicillin. Hymenoptera stings are responsible for about 40-100 deaths per year in the United States. Food-related reactions are fewer still. NSAIDs are one of the most common agents responsible for anaphylactoid-induced fatalities. These reactions present in a similar clinical fashion to true anaphylaxis but are triggered by mechanisms independent of IgE antibodies.

 # 164 Dermatologic Disorders

*Michael D. Shertz*

1. **D,** Page 2779.

Tinea versicolor is a superficial fungal infection of the skin producing lesions that can be a variety of colors from pink to white. The lesions frequently come to medical attention because they do not tan. A subtle scale can often be noted. The organism is *Pityrosporum ovale.* Diagnosis can be confirmed by KOH preparation, which shows short hyphae and spores (the so-called chopped spaghetti and meatballs appearance). The other listed options are fungal infections of other body surface areas.

2. **B,** Page 2779.

Cutaneous candidiasis favors moist and macerated areas of the body and is a superficial infection; fever from this condition would not be expected in an otherwise healthy child. Children frequently develop it in association with diaper dermatitis. Satellite lesions of papules or pustules are very reassuring of the diagnosis. The lesions are prone to secondary bacterial infection. KOH preparation would show the typical budding yeasts or pseudohyphae. Contact dermatitis as well as tinea cruris are in the differential diagnosis. Treatment is with any of the topical antifungal agents.

3. **C,** Page 2780.

Pityriasis rosea is a mild skin eruption found mostly in children and young adults. It is preceded by a "herald patch" in half of cases. The eruption is usually asymptomatic other than mild itching, and oral lesions are very rare. There is no treatment for this condition since it will resolve in 8-12 weeks on its own. The differential diagnosis should include tinea corporis, drug eruption, and secondary syphilis.

4. **D,** Page 2781.

Fever and migratory arthralgias commonly accompany skin lesions. Hospitalization is recommended with septic arthritis, meningitis, and endocarditis. The lesions are usually culture negative; however, Gram stain may reveal organisms. The disseminated form occurs in only 1%-2% of patients with gonorrhea, although females are affected primarily.

5. **A,** Page 2781.

Impetigo is a slowly evolving pustular eruption usually on the face of a preschool child. Malnutrition and poor hygiene are associated with the condition. It is usually due to *Staphylococcus aureus* with group A streptococcal infection a distant second. Topical and systemic therapy are equally effective treatments, though if there is significant skin involvement topical therapy is less convenient. Regional lymphadenopathy is very common. Poststreptococcal glomerulonephritis is a recognized complication of streptococcal impetigo.

6. **D,** Page 2783.

Drugs may cause any type of dermatosis. The most common drug eruption is urticaria followed by a red morbilliform rash. Skin lesions may appear after the drug has been discontinued. Most drug eruptions occur within 1 week; penicillin-related eruption can occur after a longer period.

7. **B,** Page 2786.

Toxic shock syndrome was popularized in the 1980s secondary to tampon use. It is associated with osteomyelitis, fasciitis, peritonsillar abscess, and septic abortion. The diagnostic criteria include fever to at least 38.9° C, hypotension, skin rash, and involvement of at least three organ systems. Supportive care and high-dose penicillin are the cornerstones of therapy. Corticosteroids reduce the severity and duration of treatment if initiated within 3 days. The condition is toxin mediated.

8. **D,** Page 2787.

Lobster, strawberries, fish, eggs, and nuts all release histamine through a nonimmunologic mechanism. The other sources of urticaria, such as pollen inhalation, viral illness, and insect stings, are all related to an immunologic mechanism.

9. **B,** Page 2788.

This is consistent with Rocky Mountain spotted fever, which is a tick-borne disease. It occurs in the southeastern United States as well as South and Central America. Chloramphenicol therapy should be initiated on suspicion of this disease (tetracycline after secondary teeth are in). The involvement of the palms and soles is typical. Measles produces a rash that is maculopapular and starts on the face and trunk, spreading to the extremities. Roseola occurs in infants, and the rash appears after the fever subsides. A sandpaper-like rash is typical of scarlet fever.

10. **C,** Page 2789.

The incidence of scarlet fever has declined in recent years; onset is abrupt with fever, chills, exudative pharyngitis, and a sandpaper-like rash. The rash can desquamate as symptoms resolve. Treatment is aimed at preventing late complications like acute glomerulonephritis and rheumatic fever. Erythema infectiosum is characterized by mild symptoms and a "slapped cheek" rash.

11. **C,** Page 2792.

The nits often attach to the base of the hair shafts, appearing as white dots. Occasionally the adult forms, which appear as blue or black grains, can be found. Any sexual contacts should be treated; household contacts should be examined, and if uninfected no treatment is necessary. Scabies involves the interdigital web spaces and is a mite infestation.

12. **B,** Page 2795.

Multiple skin lesions are associated with internal malignancy. Erythema nodosum is an inflammatory reaction of the dermis-adipose interface characterized by painful nodules. The condition is self-limiting other than local pain. The cause of pemphigus vulgaris is unknown; however, it is thought to be secondary to an immunologic mechanism. Scarlet fever is characterized by a sandpaper-like rash with fever and streptococcal pharyngitis.

13. **A,** Page 2797.

Acyclovir is not routinely recommended for oral herpes, herpes zoster, or varicella infections unless the patient is immunocompromised. Acyclovir reduces the duration of viral shedding and accelerates healing. It does not prevent recurrent episodes.

14. **A,** Page 2795.

Based on the patient's complaint, a sexually transmitted disease seems likely. Primary syphilis is characterized by a painless, smooth-based penile ulcer, whereas the secondary stage is manifested by rash. Painless lymphadenopathy can also occur. Diagnosis is confirmed by VDRL, RPR, or FTA-ABS testing. Dark-field microscopy is the only way to visualize the organism. The Jarisch-Herxheimer reaction occurs 12 hours after treatment of syphilis and is manifested by fever and rash; it is self-limiting. Patients are frequently not told about this reaction and seek treatment in the ED when this occurs. Genital herpes simplex is usually associated with penile vesicles on an erythematous base. However, as those vesicles resolve, they frequently become unroofed and appear as small ulcers. Herpes is associated with generalized lymphadenopathy and flu-like symptoms.

15. **B,** Page 2794.

The Venereal Disease Research Laboratory test (VDRL) is the most commonly used diagnostic test for syphilis. In primary syphilis the test is frequently negative early in disease. In secondary syphilis the test is invariably positive with titers above 1.16. The test can have false-positive results after infections with malaria, mycoplasma, and mononucleosis. The VDRL test usually returns to nonreactive in 6-12 months after treatment of primary disease and 1 to 10 years after secondary disease.

16. **D,** Page 2789.

This is a typical picture of rubella, particularly the involvement of the postauricular nodes. It is important to recognize rubella in order to avoid maternal exposure that can result in severe birth defects. Roseola is a benign disease caused by human herpes 6. It is manifested by high fever for several days. A discrete pink or rose-colored rash occurs in macules on the trunk and then moves to the extremities when the fever defervesces. Rocky Mountain spotted fever is manifested by the abrupt onset of fever, headaches, chills, and malaise; rash develops on the second to fourth day with blanching erythematous macules around the wrists and ankles. They may become petechial. Measles is a febrile illness with rash that starts on the face and spreads to the trunk on the third to fifth day of illness. Koplik's spots—bright red spots with bluish centers opposite the molars—occur early in the course of the measles.

17. **A,** Page 2795.

Most cases of erythema nodosum are idiopathic. Thorough history and physical examination are necessary, and most recommend a chest radiograph and/or a PPD. In an otherwise asymptomatic patient, no further work-up is needed. The association with malignancy is known but not understood. Multiple causes are seen, including drug induced; oral contraceptives are the most common drug etiology.

18. **C,** Page 2791.

Erythema multiforme is an acute but usually self-limiting disease characterized by target-shaped lesions on the soles and palms. Three colors or zones of the lesion is a classic finding. The mild form of this condition will resolve spontaneously in 2-3 weeks. Stevens-Johnson syndrome is a severe, potentially life-threatening form of this condition. It is characterized by bullous lesion and mucus membrane involvement. Patients frequently appear seriously ill.

---

 **165** ## General Approach to the Psychiatric Patient in the Emergency Department

*Michael D. Shertz*

1. **B,** Page 2808.

Ten percent of ED visits are psychiatric emergencies. In addition, most patients are self-referred and are more likely to come to the ED in the evening. The most common symptoms in order of frequency are agitation or anxiety, suicidal or assaultive threats, and psychosis. Some studies have estimated that 4%-20% of psychiatric ED patients are intoxicated.

2. **D,** Page 2811.

See Rosen Table 165-2. It is recommended that CBC, serum electrolytes, blood alcohol, blood glucose, and calcium be checked in most ED psychiatric patients. Studies have shown that up to 20% of these patients are intoxicated during their evaluation in the ED, so a blood alcohol level is recommended. A liver panel might be warranted in substance abusers. In the elderly, a broader approach may be needed including chest x-ray, urinalysis, and BUN/creatinine. A CT scan is not needed in psychiatric patients without altered mental status, neurologic defects, or a history of head trauma.

3. **A,** Page 2809.

Acute psychosis is a description of behavior, without any reference to etiology. The most common cause of anxiety in the ED population is drug withdrawal. Family members are frequently able to provide indispensable information about the psychiatric emergency department patient. Symptoms of depression, delusions, or hallucinations can represent psychiatric or medical illness.

4. **B,** Page 2811.

Auditory hallucinations are common in psychiatric illness; visual, tactile, or olfactory hallucinations are usually indicative of medical illness. Abnormal vital signs, confusion, disorientation, asymmetric neurologic findings, and incontinence should always be considered indications of medical illness.

5. **E,** Page 2812.

See Rosen Box 165-2 for risk factors for suicide: male gender; white race; older; single, divorced, or widowed; childless; socially isolated; any history of depression, substance abuse, or family history of same.

6. **C,** Page 2814.

Antipsychotic medications will improve an organic psychosis just as effectively as a "functional" psychosis, so care must be taken to avoid delaying the organic diagnosis once the psychosis is controlled. Four-point restraints are the safest way to restrain a patient; their intent is unmistakable, they have minimal side effects, and they can be removed immediately. Neuroleptic medications are often used in the ED to control agitated patients. Although effective for this purpose, they have numerous side effects that must be considered before their use. The use of a seclusion or "quiet" room is often helpful; it diminishes external stimuli and provides a safe place to hold psychiatric patients away from other patients who might be frightened by their behavior.

# 166 Thought Disorders

*James Bryan*

1. **A,** Pages 2818-2820.

Patients often present with an apparent acute psychosis that is secondary to an organic (medical) rather than a functional (psychiatric) etiology. Factors that suggest an organic etiology include disorientation, age at onset greater than 35-40 years old, visual hallucinations, lethargy and altered level of consciousness, and abnormal vital signs. Of these factors, orientation to time, place, and person is the most sensitive test for differentiating organic from functional disease; medical patients tend to be disoriented, whereas psychiatric patients remain oriented. Other factors that indicate a psychosis due to an organic etiology include tremor, ataxia, aphasia, occasional periods of perception or lucidity, sudden onset of symptoms, emotional lability, social immodesty, or an abnor-

mal physical examination. Patients with a functional psychosis tend to be awake and alert, oriented, socially modest, and exhibit a flat affect. Patients with schizophrenia have auditory hallucinations that are characteristically pejorative and threatening.

2. **A,** Page 2820.

Because of their potent anticholinergic, antihistaminic, and anti-beta-adrenergic effects, the earlier, less potent antipsychotic drugs thioridazine (Mellaril) and chlorpromazine (Thorazine), produce more sedation, cardiovascular toxicity, and orthostatic hypotension. The newer antipsychotic drugs, such as haloperidol (Haldol) and fluphenazine (Prolixin), have relatively few of these adverse effects and, consequently, are better for elderly patients. The more potent antipsychotics, however, produce more extrapyramidal symptoms such as dystonia and akathisia.

3. **D,** Page 2820.

Haloperidol is the most widely used drug for rapid tranquilization in the United States, but many prefer droperidol. Both drugs are used in the same dosage. Droperidol has a faster onset of action and a shorter duration of action than haloperidol, and it causes slightly more sedation. For these reasons it is ideal for sedating uncooperative patients for diagnostic procedures. Droperidol does not, however, possess any antipsychotic activity, so it is not useful in the treatment of schizophrenia.

4. **C,** Pages 2817-2819.

Patients are usually brought to the ED secondary to a crisis or because their bizarre behavior has attracted someone's attention. The symptoms of schizophrenia include delusions, hallucinations, disorganized speech or actions, and negative symptoms. The delusions tend to be persecutory, religious, or somatic in nature, commonly involving a sense of loss of control of one's mind or body. Hallucinations are usually auditory and pejorative or threatening. Speech exhibits looseness of associations and poverty of content, and the patient may perseverate, use nonsense words, or be totally incoherent (word salad). Patients tend to be disorganized and disheveled, and wander about talking to themselves. Negative symptoms include a flattened affect, poverty of speech with empty replies (alogia), and an inability to persist with goal-directed activities (avolition). Most schizophrenics are socially withdrawn and require a sheltered environment to function (choice C). Scenario A is consistent with mania (see chapter 167), in which the patient exhibits a decreased need for sleep, is involved in activities that have a high potential for negative consequences (e.g., buying sprees), and has an inflated self-esteem or grandiosity. During the active phase of the illness, schizophrenia, schizophreniform disorder, and brief reactive psychosis (choice B), appear very similar and are differentiated by their duration and ultimate prognosis. A brief reactive psychosis has a sudden onset and is usually seen postpartum or secondary to any major stress, such as the loss of a loved one. Symptoms last from several days to a month. Sudden onset, disorientation, visual hallucinations, confusion, and emotional lability are all consistent with an organic rather than functional etiology (choices D and E).

5. **C,** Page 2821.

Akathisia, a state of motor restlessness in which the patient feels the need to move constantly, is a common extrapyramidal side effect of high-potency neuroleptics. Patients usually pace about the room and have a sense of inner tension. Akathisia is frequently misdiagnosed as decompensating psychosis, resulting in an increase in the neuroleptic dose and, therefore, an increase in side effects. Akathisias should be treated with benzodiazepines or beta-blocker, and, if possible, reduced doses of the neuroleptic agent.

6. **C,** Page 2821.

Dystonia is the most common adverse effect of the neuroleptic medications. Dystonic reactions are characterized by involuntary contractions of the neck, face, and back muscles. The patient may exhibit involuntary protrusion of the tongue (buccolingual crisis), deviation of the head to one side (torticollis), upward deviation of the eyes (oculogyric crisis), and, occasionally, laryngospasm. Because the symptoms tend to fluctuate, decreasing with voluntary movement and increasing with stress, physicians often misdiagnose dystonia as hysterical in nature. Motor restlessness is characteristic of akathisia and not dystonic reactions.

7. **D,** Pages 2821-2822.

There are multiple side effects to the neuroleptic medications. Tardive dyskinesia (TD) is a side effect of chronic (several years) neuroleptic medication use. TD is characterized by involuntary movements, especially of the face and tongue, and occurs on average in 20% of patients receiving chronic treatment. The facial movements are usually described as grimacing, writhing, or choreoathetoid in nature. Once TD has developed, there is no effective treatment, although decreasing the dose of the neuroleptic may help some patients. TD differs from dystonia in that dystonia tends to occur early in treatment, and the muscle spasms tend to be sustained. Akinesia is characterized by immobility, withdrawal, and lack of motivation. Neuroleptic malignant syndrome is a life-threatening complication of neuroleptic drug use and occurs in 0.5%-1.0% of patients. Onset is usually within the first few weeks of treatment, after an increase in dose, or after high doses are given in the ED. Patients present with high fever, muscle rigidity, altered level of consciousness, autonomic instability, and elevated serum creatine kinase levels. Treatment consists of cooling, rehydration, supportive measures, and discontinuation of the neuroleptic. Dantrolene, a skeletal muscle relaxant, can be used in severe cases.

# ▼ 167 Affective Disorders

*James Bryan*

1. **E,** Page 2824.

Insomnia is often a symptom of depression, but it is not implicated as a cause of depression. Some individuals are genetically predisposed to major depression, and first-degree relatives and twin siblings of patients with depression are three times more likely to suffer from depression than the general population. Altered levels of neurotransmitters provide a biochemical basis for depression, and current treatment involves the use of drugs that increase neurotransmitter levels. Psychologic factors, including hypercritical or abusive parents, growing up in an emotionally unresponsive environment, and the absence of positive role models in childhood have all been linked to depression.

2. **D,** Pages 2824, 2826.

Patients with major depression often present with a triad of signs and symptoms consisting of a dysphoric mood (loss of interest or ability to experience pleasure in normal daily activities), distorted perceptions of themselves (diminished self-worth or unjustifiable feelings of guilt), and vegetative symptoms (insomnia or hypersomnia, poor appetite with weight loss, loss of energy, diminished ability to think or concentrate). In extreme cases, called psychotic depression, the patient's perceptions become so distorted as to cause delusions or hallucinations. Poor impulse control is characteristic of a personality disorder, not major depression. These patients may have depressive symptoms, but they often fluctuate with environmental changes. In addition, these patients are often manipulative or have a sense of entitlement, as well as a history of unstable relationships.

3. **B,** Page 2826.

Patients with depression often present to the ED with other complaints or for other reasons. Depression should be suspected in any patient who presents after a suicide attempt or with suicidal ideation. Patients may also present with multiple somatic complaints. In addition, depression should be considered in any MVA in which there is a single occupant, especially if it involves striking a stationary object or running off the road.

4. **B,** Pages 2827-2828.

Approximately 65%-70% of patients with severe depression will respond initially to selective serotonin reuptake inhibitors (SSRIs) or tricyclic antidepressants (TCAs). While fluoxetine (Prozac) represents a good initial SSRI, there is little reason to start a patient on medications in the ED. The initial response to antidepressants is not seen for 10-14 days, and a peak response does not occur for 6 weeks. Therefore, there is little advantage in starting medications acutely, and there is always a risk of prescribing medications in potentially suicidal patients. In addition, patient compliance and follow-up is often very poor. In acute overdoses, SSRIs are relatively safe. Severe, life-threatening arrhythmias and neurologic sequelae are seen with TCA overdoses. Patients for whom SSRIs fail can be switched to a monoamine oxidase inhibitor (MAOI), but they should never be given concomitantly. An interaction between SSRIs and MAOIs may precipitate a serious serotonin syndrome, characterized by mental confusion, myoclonus, diaphoresis, and shivering. Death secondary to hyperthermia and cardiovascular collapse has occurred. Waiting at least 2-5 weeks after discontinuation of the SSRI is recommended before initiating treatment with the MAOI.

5. **D,** Page 2828.

While phenytoin is not used in the treatment of depression, carbamazepine and valproic acid have both been used in patients with severe depression that is refractory to other treatment modalities. In patients who do not respond to SSRIs or TCAs, MAOIs and electroconvulsive therapy may be utilized. Bupropion and trazodone are also used but may be limited by their side effects. Bupropion can induce seizures in overdoses or in patients with a history of seizures. Trazodone can cause sedation, priapism, and orthostatic hypotension.

6. **B,** Page 2829.

During manic episodes, patients exhibit a decreased need for sleep. They have an increase in goal-directed activities, but they are easily distracted. Patients are usually energetic, cheerful, and sociable, but they may become irritable and argumentative, especially if their wishes are not met. They exhibit poor judgment and become involved in risky endeavors such as reckless driving, promiscuity, and spending sprees. A major depressive episode immediately precedes or follows a manic episode in more than 50% of cases.

7. **E,** Pages 2830-2831.

All of the medications listed may be used in either the acute or long-term management of mania. Lithium carbonate is the drug of choice, but in an acute manic episode, a benzodiazepine (e.g., clonazepam) or a neuroleptic (e.g., haloperidol) may be used if the patient is agitated or psychotic. In addition, lithium takes 5-6 days to become therapeutic and up to 2 weeks to reach a maximal effect, so haloperidol is often added during the early treatment phase. Valproate and carbamazepine are also used to treat mania.

 ## 168 Anxiety Disorders

*James Bryan*

1. **D,** Pages 2833, 2837.

Patients with a simple phobia have symptoms when exposed to the specific thing they fear. Simple phobia is a subset of phobia—an irrational fear of things that would be considered a normal fear in children (e.g., spiders, snakes, dark rooms). Phobias are considered disorders if the phobia interferes with the person's daily life. Agoraphobia is anxiety in places or situations where escape might be difficult (e.g., theaters, elevators). Panic disorders are characterized by recurrent unexpected panic attacks (intense apprehension, fearfulness, or terror often associated with feelings of impending doom). Posttraumatic stress disorder is an anxiety disorder associated with memories or situations that remind the patient of a previous terrible or traumatic event.

2. **A,** Page 2833.

The symptoms described are those of a generalized anxiety disorder. Anxiety is an unpleasurable state that is painful and persistently stressful. The patient has had excessive anxiety and worry for longer than 6 months.

3. **E,** Pages 2833, 2837.

The fear of public speaking is classified as a social phobia, which is the fear of social or performance situations. This fear often leads to avoidance behavior and an inability to function in social situations or at work. Treatment, as for simple phobias, is best accomplished with behavioral psychotherapy, in which patients are taught to gradually overcome the fearful situation by repeatedly increasing their exposure to the situation.

4. **B,** Pages 2834-2836.

Many organic conditions occur with symptoms similar to anxiety disorders, including coronary artery disease, mitral valve prolapse, hypoparathyroidism, hyperthyroidism, asthma, airway obstruction, hypoxemia, cardiac arrhythmias, pulmonary embolus, and pheochromocytoma. In addition, many drugs, including amphetamines, cocaine, caffeine, and nicotine, may stimulate anxiety attacks. Only after ruling out an organic etiology may a diagnosis of anxiety disorder be considered.

5. **A,** Page 2838.

Benzodiazepines are the drugs of choice for treating acute exogenous anxiety disorders that are likely to be time limited. No more than 1 week of treatment should be prescribed because those patients that do not improve within 1 week are not likely to respond to further benzodiazepine therapy.

## 169 Approach to the Difficult Patient in the Emergency Department

*Michael D. Shertz*

1. **A,** Page 2842.
Countertransference is a term created by Freud to describe the negative reactions that patients can arouse in physicians. This was recognized for its potential impact on the patient-physician interaction. Transference is the reaction the physician causes in the patient. Negative reactions can be triggered by the patient's appearance (unwashed and disheveled), attitude (arrogant or angry), interactive style (whining, manipulative, or demanding) or complaint (self-destructive or drug seeking). Unfortunately, all of the factors come into play when practitioners interact with patients.

2. **A,** Page 2842.
Patient satisfaction is highly correlated with the patients' sense that the physician listened to them and their concerns. However, physicians continue to focus on their own medical agendas, even if such an agenda is unrelated to the patient's concerns. A refusal, intentional or not, to address the patient's concerns is a recipe for an unhappy patient. Studies show that physicians spend approximately 1 minute of a 20-minute encounter educating patients about their illness or diagnosis. This is even more true in emergency medicine when diagnosis is following so closely with disposition. Ultimately, people don't sue people they like. Patients will be more tolerant of a less-than-optimal outcome if they felt that they were treated well.

3. **C,** Page 2843.
Malingering is the intentional production of false or grossly exaggerated physical or psychiatric symptoms, motivated by external incentives that are unrelated to the illness. Narcotics are the most common objective of the malingerer in the ED. Malingering represents manipulative behavior and is coded in the *DSM-IV* as a problem rather than a mental illness. Since emergency physicians should be giving the vast majority of their patients the benefit of the doubt regarding their illness, malingering should rarely if ever be diagnosed in the ED.

4. **C,** Page 2843.
Somatization is the involuntary production of symptoms without the patient's conscious awareness. Unlike the malingerer, the somatic patient is not motivated by any conscious desire for secondary gain.

5. **C,** Page 2844; see Rosen Box 169-1.
Borderline personality disorder is a pattern of instability of interpersonal relationships, self-image, and affect. It is usually marked by impulsive behavior beginning early in adulthood and by fear of abandonment, either real or imagined. Patients' interpersonal relationships fluctuate between extremes of idealization and devaluation. They have an unstable self-image, are recurrently suicidal, have chronic feelings of emptiness, and experience difficulty controlling anger.

6. **C,** Page 2844; see Rosen Box 169-1.
Antisocial personality disorder is a pattern of behavior marked by disregard and violation of the rights of others since around the age of 15. It is also characterized by impulsiveness, irritability, aggressiveness, frequent physical fights, recklessness, and lack of remorse for having hurt or mistreated others.

7. **E,** Page 2845; see Rosen Box 169-2.
General strategies for dealing with the difficult ED patient include being supportive; building rapport with the patient increases the likelihood that everyone will leave the interaction satisfied. Unfortunately, building rapport with manipulative patients is time consuming and requires an attempt to understand the patient's motivation for coming to the ED. This may simply be a desire for a second opinion or confirmation that the primary physician is treating their problem appropriately. Other strategies include structuring the interview and setting limits on what behavior is and is not acceptable. For loud, aggressive, profane patients, pointing out that there are sick children in the room next to theirs (whether there are or not) and that their behavior is frightening those children is sometimes a helpful strategy. Often, it is necessary to simply tell the patient that apparently there will be no agreement on a solution to the problem. This will be better received if the physician has taken the time to build rapport with the patient. Useful books are available on nonverbal communication and body posturing that are directed at how to build rapport.

8. **D,** Page 2849.
Dependent patients see physicians as inexhaustible sources of compassion and understanding. They frequently start with reasonable requests that escalate to greater demands for analgesia or affection. Patients with certain personality disorders (borderline, histrionic, and somatoform) often behave in this way. Dependent patients are best dealt with early in their help-rejection cycle. Establishing with them the limits of the ED and the necessity of follow-up, if needed, is of paramount importance. Overall, the key to dealing with all difficult patients is an understanding that they do not make good decisions. Therefore it is unreasonable for the physician to take their obscenities or demands personally; if these patients could make reasonable decisions, then they would not be engaging in self-destructive behavior.

# 170 Somatoform Disorders, Factitious Disorders, and Malingering

*Hans Notenboom*

1. **A**, Page 2853.

Patients with somatoform disorders are most likely between the ages of 20 and 60. They are most often women, people with less than 12 years' education, widowed or divorced individuals, and those with low self-esteem. These people are prone to be self-conscious, vulnerable to stress, anxious, hostile, and depressed.

2. **A**, Page 2855.

Also known as hysterical neurosis, conversion type, the rarely encountered conversion disorder is characterized by the sudden onset and dramatic presentation of a single symptom, typically simulating some nonpainful neurologic disorder for which there is no pathophysiologic or anatomic explanation. The symptoms, although generally conforming to the patient's own idiosyncratic ideas about illness, are not under the voluntary control of the patient.

3. **B**, Page 2856.

A distinguishing feature of this disorder is that the patient's symptoms actually do exist and often may be confirmed by physical examination but are exaggerated and misinterpreted in the mind of the patient. The other answers correspond with hypochondriasis

4. **D**, Page 2856.

Good premorbid health represents a better prognosis in conversion disorder than does poor premorbid health. The other answers are all good indicators of positive prognosis.

5. **C**, Page 2856.

This condition is similar to other somatoform disorders in that stressful events are translated into somatic symptoms. In this instance the primary, and often exclusive, symptom is distressful pain that has the following characteristics: not intentionally feigned, persistent in nature, limits daily function, involves one ore more organ systems, and cannot be pathophysiologically explained.

6. **B**, Page 2861.

Malingerers are usually reluctant to accept expensive, possibly painful, or dangerous tests or surgery. Otherwise, the other possible answers are all situations that are indicative of possible malingering. Management in the ED begins with an explanation that the symptoms and examination are not consistent with any serious disease. Primary care follow-up should be offered if there is no resolution of symptoms. Malingerers may become threatening when they are denied treatment or are overtly confronted.

# 171 Suicide

*Norm Kalbfleish*

1. **E**, Pages 2863-2866.

Recent studies have shown that panic disorder is the psychiatric diagnosis with the highest rate of suicide—greater than depression and bipolar disorder. Alcoholism is associated with suicide, but if the patient is without a concurrent psychiatric diagnosis, the rate is less than for panic disorder. Both the chronic low back pain patient and the patient with amputations have a slightly higher rate of suicide than the general population.

2. **C**, Pages 2863-2866.

Intoxication in the presence of suicidal ideation significantly increases the risk of suicide. These patients should never be released from the ED without psychiatric evaluation. Many personality disorders are associated with an increased risk of both suicide attempts and completed suicides. The ability of a patient to sign a no-harm contract has been clearly associated with a reduction of suicide. This contract should be between a mental health professional and the patient. Finally, the depressed patient is not more likely to attempt suicide because the subject of suicidal ideation has been addressed.

3. **D**, Pages 2865-2866.

Those at greatest risk for completed suicide are male patients who are recently divorced or separated and are without children. If a patient has a mother, father, or sibling who committed suicide, even in the distant past, that patient has a significantly increased risk of suicide.

4. **A**, Pages 2866-2869.

There is no perfect instrument to assess the lethality of a suicidal ideation. The SAD PERSONS mnemonic, however, has proven valuable to emergency physicians who take under consideration each of the issues represented by the mnemonic. Emergency physicians have considerable liability exposure if they have not taken measures to prevent the potential suicidal patient from elopement before completing the assessment. Finally, intoxicated patients who profess suicidal ideation should be observed until the intoxicant has been metabolized. Only at that time may the emergency physician optimally evaluate the patient for continued suicidal ideation.

## 172 The Violent Patient

*Norm Kalbfleisch*

1. **A,** Pages 2871-2872.
A history of psychiatric illness in violent patients suggests a functional cause of the violence. However, the physician should do a thorough history and physical examination to determine if there is an organic etiology of the behavior. Elderly patients with no history of violence who have threatening behavior probably have an organic etiology for their behavior. The converse, patients under the age of 40 with their first episode of threatening behavior, is more likely to have functional cause if intoxicants are excluded. The intoxicated patient who manifests threatening behavior is thought by definition to have an organic condition.

2. **A,** Pages 2871-2872.
There are few reliable predictors of ED violence; neither ethnicity nor education was associated with violence in one recent study. If the emergency physician experiences fear in exposure to a potentially violent patient, that visceral response should key the provider that indeed this circumstance may be dangerous and a safe distance should be established. A particularly dangerous patient is one who does not verbalize or emote, yet remains uncooperative and brooding. Assessments of these types of patients tend to underestimate the potential for violence and give few clues for impending escalation. Finally, the potentially violent patient may be safely given parenteral medications under limited conditions such as when the patient becomes cooperative and subdued in the presence of a show of force.

3. **C,** Pages 2873-2879.
The ideal room for evaluation of the violent or agitated patient has a safe exit for both the patient and personnel. A long, narrow room is not ideal because either the patient is between the staff member and the door, or the staff member is in the way of the patient if he or she tries to escape. If the person must be physically restrained, a minimum of five people is necessary: one to secure each extremity and one to direct the restraint. The patient is capable of biting personnel if the head is not secured. Obtaining informed consent from the violent patient is problematic; however, the patient should be told what is necessary for him or her to comply.

4. **A,** Pages 2874-2878.
Patients who are violent and intoxicated pose a very significant risk to themselves and health care providers. Although no position is absolutely safe when a patient must be physically restrained, the prone position is thought to afford better protection from aspiration in the likely event of vomiting. Even properly applied restraints may cause compromise of the distal extremity. Physical restraint alone may not be adequate to protect the patient and staff because gurneys have been overturned by restrained patients. Any restrained patient, particularly the intoxicated patient, should have one-to-one monitoring. Close, intermittent monitoring is inadequate. Finally, the emergency physician should be cautious about the release of a patient from physical restraint.

5. **D,** Pages 2874-2878.
When a violent patient is in the ED, it is important that the emergency physician develop a strategy to ensure safety of other patients and ED staff. A violent adult patient with a gun is extremely dangerous and represents an immediate threat to hospital personnel and patients. Under these conditions, a show of force is inappropriate and dangerous; police must be involved without delay. If the patient does not have a weapon, a show of force is very helpful with the appropriate number of personnel. Chemical restraint is sometimes necessary. The ideal agent should be relatively short acting with a fast onset of action and should be given parenterally (IV or IM).

6. **D,** Pages 2872-2876.
All the responses may eventually be required in evaluation and treatment of patients, but often an agitated patient may be brought under control by taking a firm but non-threatening stance. The patient should be encouraged to express her feelings by using such statements as, "What is the matter?" or "You seem upset." However, frankly psychotic or delirious patients typically do not respond appropriately to verbalization; therefore the emergency physician must be prepared to utilize physical or chemical restraint if appropriate.

 ## 173 Substance Abuse

*Patrick Brunett*

1. **C,** Page 2880.
The identification of toxidromes is important in diagnosing unknown ingestions. Adrenergic and cholinergic syndromes are especially significant. Sympathetic overload is suggested by the presence of cool, pale, diaphoretic skin; mydriasis; and hyperactive bowel sounds. Anticholinergic agents cause red, dry, hot skin; dry mouth; and absent bowel sounds.

2. **B,** Page 2880.
"Cotton fever" refers to an acute syndrome of fever, tachycardia, and tachypnea occurring 10-20 minutes after injection, due to pyrogenic drug impurities filtered and trapped in the lungs. The other entities (sacroiliitis, wound botulism, tetanus, and pulmonary abscess) are delayed complications of intravenous injection. Other non-synovial joints (intervertebral disk, sternoclavicular joint) may also become infected by repeated bouts of bacteremia.

3. **A,** Page 2883.
Chronic hydrocarbon abuse leads to permanent neurologic abnormalities including cognitive deficits, cerebellar ataxia, and cranial and peripheral nerve dysfunction. Acute manifestations include wheezing, GI distress, cardiac dysrhythmia, pulmonary edema, hypokalemia, and altered mental status.

4. **C,** Page 2884.

Nitrites oxidize hemoglobin to methemoglobin, which is incapable of binding oxygen. Manifestations include central cyanosis, "chocolate brown" blood, and inaccurate pulse oximeter readings. Methylene blue IV is the treatment of choice for methemoglobin levels >30%. Hypotension, tachycardia, and syncope are generally self-limited and not life threatening. Hemolytic anemia occurs primarily in patients with glucose-6-phosphate dehydrogenase deficiency.

5. **B,** Pages 2886-2887.

Both benzodiazepines and butyrophenones (haloperidol or droperidol) have been proven effective in controlling violent behavior in patients with phencyclidine (PCP) toxicity. Trying to reason with, or "talk down" a combative patient on PCP may be futile and may unnecessarily endanger emergency department personnel. Mild to moderate hypertension may not require specific therapy. In severe hypertension, phentolamine or nitroprusside are therapies of choice. Rhabdomyolysis with elevated creatine kinase is quite common in these patients.

6. **D,** Pages 2888-2889.

LSD, psilocybin, and mescaline produce clinically indistinguishable intoxications. Vomiting is more common with psilocybin and mescaline, especially during the first hour after ingestion. If vomiting occurs 6 or more hours after ingestion, hepatotoxic mushrooms should be considered. All three agents are central nervous system stimulants and produce mydriasis, restlessness, and visual hallucinations.

7. **A,** Pages 2888-2889.

Supportive care and verbal reassurance are usually sufficient in the management of hallucinogen intoxication. Benzodiazepines or neuroleptics are effective if sedation is desired. Detoxification with activated charcoal is indicated in large-quantity mushroom or mescaline ingestions. Standard urine toxicologic screens will not detect most hallucinogens.

8. **E,** Pages 2896-2897.

The seeds of the jimson weed plant are highest in the active ingredients atropine and scopolamine. Anticholinergic effects include pupillary dilation, dry mouth, and urinary retention. Butyrophenones are effective sedative agents without the risk of respiratory compromise posed by benzodiazepines. Physostigmine reverses anticholinergic symptoms in minutes but should be reserved for severe anticholinergic poisoning.

9. **C,** Pages 2880; 2889-2891.

Early deaths from amphetamine toxicity result from cardiac dysrhythmias, seizures, and CNS depression. Late mortality is due to rhabdomyolysis, renal failure, DIC, acidosis, and cardiovascular collapse. Uncontrolled agitation and seizures may lead to rhabdomyolysis and hyperthermia and should be managed aggressively. Beta blockers should be avoided in the treatment of amphetamine-induced hypertension, as this may result in unopposed alpha-adrenergic effects. Hallucinogenic amphetamines stimulate dopaminergic and serotonergic systems. Serotonin syndrome, characterized by hypertension, hyperthermia, and hypertonicity, may be triggered by concomitant use of amphetamines with MAO inhibitors or serotonin reuptake inhibitors such as fluoxetine.

10. **E,** Pages 2890, 2894.

The differential diagnosis of amphetamine and cocaine intoxication is broad and includes the entities mentioned, as well as sepsis, serotonin syndrome, and neuroleptic malignant syndrome. It is important to differentiate generalized sympathetic overdrive without apparent cause from increased sympathetic tone secondary to other causes such as sepsis or drug withdrawal.

11. **C,** Pages 2893-2894.

Obstetric complications of cocaine use include vaginal bleeding, abruptio placentae, preterm labor, and precipitous delivery. Cocaine-induced myocardial ischemia may occur in otherwise healthy young persons. Wheezing, hemoptysis, pneumonitis, pneumomediastinum, and pneumothorax occur principally in patients who smoke crack cocaine. While headache is a common complaint in cocaine users, any patient with persistent altered mental status, complex seizures, neurologic deficits, or severe headache should undergo brain CT to rule out intracranial hemorrhage.

12. **E,** Page 2892.

Cocaine blocks reuptake of norepinephrine, dopamine, and serotonin. Direct sympathetic stimulation of the heart results from adrenergic excess. Platelet aggregation, coronary vasoconstriction, and early coronary atherosclerosis have been described. Cocaine does block sodium channels with resultant myocardial depression, but this effect is overshadowed by its sympathetic stimulant effects.

13. **C,** Page 2895.

Benzodiazepines are the principal agents used to treat cocaine toxicity. Phentolamine and nitroprusside have been shown effective for treatment of severe or refractory hypertension. Although labetalol, an agent with combined alpha and beta adrenergic blockade, provides a theoretical advantage, results of human and animal studies have been inconclusive. Animal studies with calcium channel blockers have also been equivocal. The use of thrombolytics in cocaine-induced chest pain is controversial. Many patients initially meeting ECG criteria for thrombolytics go on to have negative serial cardiac enzyme evaluations. Aspirin, nitroglycerin, and phentolamine are all indicated for cocaine-induced chest pain.

14. **E,** Page 2895.

Phenytoin is not effective in treating cocaine-induced seizures. Benzodiazepines and barbiturates are indicated in status epilepticus and in complex, multiple, or focal seizures. Single, generalized seizures are usually self-limited and require only supportive care.

# 174 Stress, Wellness, and the Impaired Physician

*James E. Thompson*

1. **E,** Page 2902.

A great number of stressors have been cited in the literature as contributing to stress in the practice of emergency medicine. These multiple stressors relate to four aspects of emergency practice:

- Patients in the emergency department often may be difficult and violent and may arouse countertransference amongst practitioners
- Emergency physicians must practice in a diverse environment with respect to rotating shifts, chaotic surroundings, and undifferentiated patients
- The impact of managed care and uncompensated care has put great strain on the emergency physician to practice with limited resources
- Emergency physicians are constantly making difficult decisions, often about critically ill patients, based on ambiguous or incomplete information

2. **A,** Page 2903.

Burnout is a term that was introduced in 1975 to describe feelings of job dissatisfaction caused by work-related stress. Burnout is of special relevance to physicians because it may undermine the relationship between the caregiver and patient that is essential to quality medical care. Furthermore, studies have suggested that physicians experiencing burnout are likely to experience decreased productivity, less job satisfaction, high job turnover, low self-esteem, physical symptoms, family and marital discord, and affective changes including anxiety, hostility, and depression.

3. **C,** Page 2903.

Although the extent of impairment among emergency physicians is unknown, studies have shown that emergency physicians make up 2.8% of California physicians but 6.5% of all physicians identified as chemically impaired. The identification of the impaired physician is often difficult. Long before workplace deficits become apparent, there often is a pattern of family difficulties, extramarital affairs, and divorce. Once impairment in a physician is identified, intervention has an excellent prognosis for recovery when long-term monitoring occurs.

4. **E,** Page 2904.

Qualities that characterize successful physicians (perfectionism, drive to succeed, willingness to work long hours) may dispose them to neglect their own personal and physical needs. Finding a balanced lifestyle allows integration of professional goals and responsibilities with the need for self-care and development. Strategies include promoting wellness in the ED with strategies to address the impact of shift work and violent patients, the cultivation of close family and social relationships, the development and maintenance of physical fitness, and relaxation methods.

5. **C,** Page 2904.

Having strategies for managing difficult patients is a key to maintaining control in the ED. It is important to not block out one's reaction to a difficult patient; rather one's own emotional response to a patient must be acknowledged and the reaction shared with other members of the team. Having clearly set limits for the patient's behavior can aid in maintaining control of the interaction and of the caregiver's own emotional response. Setting limits can aid in not allowing countertransference to interfere with the delivery of quality care. Allowing adequate physical space between the practitioner and the patient, recognizing signs of impending violence, acting promptly should such behavior arise, and allowing the patients to verbally vent their anger can aid in diffusing potentially dangerous situations in the ED.

6. **B,** Page 2905.

Strategies published in the literature for coping with shift work include the following:

- Work an isolated night shift to cause minimal circadian disruption
- Eight-hour shifts are preferable to twelve-hour shifts
- Do not attempt to maintain your day schedule while working night shifts
- Group together the same shifts as much of the time as possible.

Other strategies include scheduling shifts in a clockwise direction; using compromise strategies for sleep such as anchor sleep, split sleep periods, and napping; using bright lights for 2 hours after arising as an adjunct in adjusting to new shifts, and exercising regularly.

7. **C,** Page 2906.

Multiple methods of relaxation exist to aid in coping with stress. It has been demonstrated that physical correlates of stress, such as increased heart and respiratory rates, oxygen consumption, and serum lactate, can be normalized by a variety of relaxation techniques. Studies have shown that regular use of techniques such as Zen, yoga, and progressive relaxation can allow individuals to gain considerable control over the relaxation process.

## 175 Domestic Violence

*J. Leibovitz*

1. **E,** Page 2911.

The lifetime prevalence of battering in the adult female is more than 50% among ED patients. The incidence of current abuse is 12%. The incidence of spousal abuse as a cause of ED visits is estimated to be between 22% and 35%.

2. **A,** Pages 2910-2911.

Abused women are more likely to have low-birth-weight children, miscarriages, premature labor, stillbirths, and injuries to the fetus. Among children of battered women, 34% of boys and 20% of girls show clinically significant behavior problems. During pregnancy the risk of abuse persists. Some pregnant women report a decrease in abuse, whereas 21%-29% report an increase in abuse, and 13% report abuse for the first time. Nearly 40% of homicides are committed by either relatives of the victims, a spouse, or an intimate acquaintance. Two to four million women become victims of domestic violence per year.

3. **E,** Pages 2912-2913.

Victims of domestic violence often develop some somatic complaints such as chest pain, dizziness, or generalized weakness. There can also be profound anxiety and depression, which may lead to suicide, alcoholism, and drug addiction. Chronic pelvic or abdominal pain is a common presenting feature among battered women. African-American women who attempt suicide display a higher rate of domestic violence—approaching 50%—compared to other races.

4. **E,** Page 2912.

According to a survey in emergency departments in California of both nurse managers and physician directors, drugs, alcohol, denial, fear of repercussions, and failure to volunteer information were among the greatest barriers believed to be involved in establishing the diagnosis of domestic violence. Patients who sustain injuries from domestic violence often are reluctant to reveal the real cause of their injuries.

5. **E,** Page 2914.

Accessing safety is extremely important with domestic violence. Although an escalating pattern of violence, possession of a firearm, increased drug and alcohol use, presence of violent behavior outside the home, and stalking behavior show an increased risk for mortality, the greatest risk for potentially lethal domestic violence is when an attempt is made to leave the relationship. Up to 75% of domestic assaults are reported to law enforcement agencies during separation periods.

6. **E,** Page 2916.

The physical abuse ranking scale can be used to determine the risk of extreme danger. Any behavior ranked higher than five or six is considered to be very significant for potential injury.

1. Throwing things, punching the wall
2. Pushing, shoving, grabbing, and throwing things at the victim
3. Slapping with an open hand
4. Kicking or biting
5. Hitting with a closed fist
6. Attempting strangulation
7. Beating the victim up
8. Threatening with a weapon
9. Assaulting with a weapon

7. **B,** Page 2910.

Medication abuse includes the inappropriate use of medication, withholding medication, or overmedication. It may be used as in this case to render the victim more passive and, in general, make life easier for the abuser (caretaker). Physical abuse involves some display of physical force. Financial or economic abuse results when the victim is cut off financially so that the abuser controls all the finances. Psychologic abuse involves either verbal or emotional abuse.

## 176 Ethnicity, Culture, and the Delivery of Health Care Services: Enhancing System Outcomes in a Multicultural Environment

*No questions*

## 177 Differential Diagnosis

*Evelyn Kim*

1. **E,** Page 1145.

The clinical scenario describes the classic presentation of bronchiolitis, a lower respiratory tract infection causing inflammation and obstruction of the small airways. The major etiologic agent is respiratory syncytial virus; the second most common cause is parainfluenza virus. *Haemophilus influenzae* type B is the cause of epiglottitis, an upper airway obstructive disease. Bacteria are almost never responsible for bronchiolitis. Household allergens are often the precipitants of an asthma exacerbation, one of the differential diagnoses in this scenario. Asthma can often be ruled out by a previous history of recurrent wheezing or familial atopy. The infectious prodrome may exclude the diagnosis of foreign body aspiration, although if the physician is unsure, a normal expiratory chest radiograph is helpful.

2. **E,** Pages 1145-1146.

Forty to fifty percent of infants hospitalized with bronchiolitis will develop recurrent wheezing. It is unclear whether bronchiolitis creates abnormalities that predispose a child to develop recurrent wheezing or if underlying abnormalities make a child more susceptible to develop bronchiolitis. The mortality rate for bronchiolitis is less than 1%, and bacterial superinfection is also very rare.

3. **D,** Pages 2107-2108, 2188.

Coma is a result of an abnormality of the reticular activating system or diffuse impairment of the cerebral cortex. Diffuse impairment can occur with intoxication, inflammation, seizures, postictal states, and increased intracranial pressure. Ischemic cerebral infarction, on the other hand, usually presents with a focal deficit. Complete loss of consciousness would be unusual in the absence of brain stem involvement.

4. **B,** Pages 362-363, 610, 1463.

The fat embolism syndrome usually occurs from 12 to 36 hours after a long-bone fracture. Early signs include respiratory distress, restlessness, confusion, and petechial rash. Other clues to the diagnosis include fever, tachycardia, jaundice, and renal involvement. In any trauma patient with a significant mechanism for injury, it is important to evaluate for coexistent life-threatening injuries that could cause an acute deterioration in cardiac and hemodynamic stability. What might seem a minor fall in a younger patient can cause significant injury in a geriatric patient with decreased bone density and less pliable tissues. Nonetheless, as in any trauma patient, continued hemorrhage that creates hemodynamic instability is usually located in the chest, abdomen, or retroperitoneum. Furthermore, elderly patients typically have less physiologic reserve and less ability to compensate for the stress of trauma. Shock, hypoxia, and the stress of acute injury can cause myocardial depression and precipitate a myocardial infarction. As an alternative, syncope or dysrhythmia from an evolving myocardial infarction can be the inciting event of a trauma.

5. **D,** Pages 2168-2172.

Internuclear ophthalmoplegia results from pathology of the medial longitudinal fasciculus, in which each eye fails to adduct with lateral gaze. Like vertigo, it is a common presenting symptom of multiple sclerosis. Ménière's disease is characterized by the triad of hearing loss, vertigo, and tinnitus. Acoustic neuroma often presents as unilateral hearing loss of several months' duration that progresses to involve both the vestibular and auditory functions of cranial nerve VIII. Labyrinthitis usually displays both vestibular and cochlear symptoms, with sudden onset of vertigo, nystagmus, hearing loss, and tinnitus. Vertebrobasilar insufficiency causes episodes of brain stem ischemia, typically manifested as vertigo, dysarthria, ataxia, face numbness, hemiparesis, and diplopia.

6. **E,** Pages 2357-2358.

The physiologic and anatomic changes associated with pregnancy make evaluation of abdominal pain particularly challenging. During the last trimester, the appendix is displaced to the right upper quadrant. This proximity to the ureter and kidney may create a sterile pyuria in pregnant patients with appendicitis. Bacteruria, however, is seen only with urinary tract infection or pyelonephritis. If, after urinalysis, the diagnosis is still unclear, an abdominal ultrasound may be per-

formed to detect appendicitis or gallbladder disease. With proper technique, ultrasound can detect an inflamed appendix up to 90% of the time. Additional tests, such as CBC and ESR, are less useful diagnostic tools in light of the physiologic increase in levels associated with pregnancy. Quantitative hCG levels are not useful in the diagnosis of abdominal or pelvic pain beyond the first 6 weeks of gestation. Upper genital tract infection and pelvic inflammatory disease as causes of abdominal pain are very rare in pregnancy and are virtually never seen beyond the first trimester.

7. **E,** Pages 1266-1267.

Major alcohol withdrawal can occur from 24 hours to 5 days after cessation of drinking. It encompasses the symptoms of autonomic hyperactivity (tachycardia, hypertension, nausea, anorexia, coarse tremor) and mental status disturbances such as confusion, disorientation, and visual hallucinations.

8. **B,** Pages 1431-1433.

Cocaine is a sympathomimetic agent, and acute intoxication or overdose will produce the findings of a sympathomimetic toxidrome. This includes paranoia, tachycardia, hypertension, hyperpyrexia, mydriasis, tremors, and hyperreflexia. Life-threatening sequelae of sympathomimetic overdose include dysrhythmias, acute myocardial infarction, vasomotor collapse, seizures, and cerebrovascular accident.

9. **A,** Pages 1292-1293.

Isopropyl alcohol intoxication is manifested primarily by gastrointestinal and central nervous system symptoms. Both isopropyl alcohol and acetone, its major metabolite, are CNS depressants and can cause headache, dizziness, poor coordination, and confusion. Isopropyl alcohol is also a gastrointestinal irritant, causing symptoms of abdominal pain, nausea, and vomiting.

10. **D,** Page 1389.

The opioid abstinence syndrome follows a typical course that spans from 12 to 72 hours after last use. From 12 to 24 hours, the patient may develop yawning, lacrimation, rhinorrhea, mydriasis, gooseflesh, and twitching. These symptoms typically reach maximum intensity at 48-72 hours and are further accompanied by disheveled appearance, fever, and hypertension. The opioid abstinence syndrome, unlike that of barbiturates and alcohol, is not associated with mortality in the absence of underlying disease.

11. **F,** Pages 1302-1303.

Over-the-counter nighttime sleep aids typically contain H1-receptor blocking agents, such as diphenhydramine, pyrilamine, and cyclizine, which exhibit anticholinergic toxicity in the overdose setting. This toxidrome presents with delirium, tachycardia, dry and flushed skin, dilated pupils, urinary retention, and hypoactive bowel sounds.

12. **G,** Pages 1355-1357.

PCP intoxication can cause a wide variety of signs and symptoms, making it difficult to recognize in the acute setting. More common findings include behavioral changes ranging from bizarre and violent to mute and staring, hypertension, and tachycardia. Nystagmus, either vertical, horizontal, or rotatory, is a relatively consistent finding and an important diagnostic clue.

13. **C,** Pages 1396-1397.
Promethazine is a phenothiazine neuroleptic that is commonly used for its antiemetic properties. The syndrome of intoxication results from various dopamine, muscarinic, histamine, and alpha-adrenergic receptor inhibitions. Signs and symptoms include agitation, hallucinations, CNS depression, and extrapyramidal effects. Acute dystonia (muscle spasms, tremors, oculogyric crisis), motor restlessness, parkinsonism, and tardive dyskinesia are all examples of extrapyramidal effects.